NUCLEAR MEDICINE CASES

The McGraw-Hill Radiology Series
Series Editor: Robert J. Ward, MD

This innovative series offers indispensable workstation reference material for the practicing radiologist. Within this series is a full range of practical, clinically relevant works divided into three categories:

- **Patterns:** Organized by modality, these books provide a pattern-based approach to constructing practical differential diagnoses.
- **Variants:** Structured by modality as well as anatomy, these graphic volumes aid the radiologist in reducing false positive rates.
- **Cases:** Classic case presentations with an emphasis on differential diagnoses and clinical context.

NUCLEAR MEDICINE CASES

Joseph Rajendran, MD, DMRT, FASNC
Associate Professor of Radiology and Radiation
Oncology (Adjunct)
Division of Nuclear Medicine/Department of Radiology
University of Washington &
Diagnostic Imaging Service, VA Puget Sound Health
Care System
Seattle, Washington

Vivek Manchanda, MD
Senior Fellow, Oncologic and Cardiac PET/CT
Department of Radiology
University of Washington
University of Washington Medical Center
Seattle, Washington

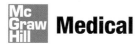
Medical

New York   Chicago   San Francisco   Lisbon   London   Madrid   Mexico City
Milan   New Delhi   San Juan   Seoul   Singapore   Sydney   Toronto

Nuclear Medicine Cases

1 2 3 4 5 6 7 8 9 0   CTP/CTP   14 13 12 11 10

ISBN 978-0-07-147604-1
MHID 0-07-147604-0

Notice

Medicine is an ever-changing science. As new research and clinical experience broaden our knowledge, changes in treatment and drug therapy are required. The authors and the publisher of this work have checked with sources believed to be reliable in their efforts to provide information that is complete and generally in accord with the standards accepted at the time of publication. However, in view of the possibility of human error or changes in medical sciences, neither the authors nor the publisher nor any other party who has been involved in the preparation or publication of this work warrants that the information contained herein is in every respect accurate or complete, and they disclaim all responsibility for any errors or omissions or for the results obtained from use of the information contained in this work. Readers are encouraged to confirm the information contained herein with other sources. For example and in particular, readers are advised to check the product information sheet included in the package of each drug they plan to administer to be certain that changes have not been made in the recommended dose or in the contraindications for administration. This recommendation is of particular importance in connection with new or infrequently used drugs.

This book was set in TradeGothic Light by Glyph International.
The editors were Michael Weitz and Christie Naglieri.
Project Management was provided by Smita Rajan and Somya Rustagi, Glyph International.
The production supervisor was Catherine Saggese.
The index was prepared by Robert Swanson.
China Translation & Printing Services, Ltd., was the printer and binder.

This book is printed on acid-free paper.

Library of Congress Cataloging-in-Publication Data

Nuclear medicine cases / editors, Joseph Rajendran, Vivek Manchanda.
       p. ; cm. — (McGraw-Hill radiology series)
  ISBN-13: 978-0-07-147604-1 (softcover : alk. paper)
  ISBN-10: 0-07-147604-0 (softcover : alk. paper)
  1. Radioisotope scanning—Case studies.   2. Nuclear medicine—Case studies.   3. Diagnosis, Differential—Case studies.   I. Rajendran, Joseph.   II. Manchanda, Vivek.   III. Series: McGraw-Hill radiology series.
  [DNLM: 1. Nuclear medicine--Case Reports. 2. Diagnosis, Differential—Case Reports.   WN 203 N9635 2011]
RC78.7.R4N753 2011
616.07'575—dc22

2010000391

McGraw-Hill books are available at special quantity discounts to use as premiums and sales promotions, or for use in corporate training programs. To contact a representative please e-mail us at bulksales@mcgraw-hill.com.

*To my wife Shakunthala, for her sacrifices and inspiration;
to our children Grace and Vinod, for their support; and to my late
parents, Grace and Edward Sokkiah, who introduced me to the
importance of education.*

Joseph Rajendran

*To my parents, Raj and Dr. HR Manchanda;
Rashna, Rajeev, and Josh.*

Vivek Manchanda

CONTENTS

Each Case Highlights Findings, Differential Diagnoses, and Comments

Icons are used to create a grading system

The innovative grading system indicates the degree to which the images are representative of a case's typical appearance. The scale ranges from "typical" (five circles) to "rare" (one circle). Similarly, the differential diagnoses images are graded "common" (five squares) to "unusual" (one square). The aim is to provide the reader with a sense of appropriateness regarding the practical use of differential diagnoses.

IMAGE KEY

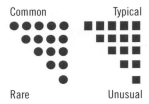

Common — Typical — Rare — Unusual

CONTRIBUTORS

Sidharth Damani, MD
Fellow, Vascular and Interventional Radiology
Department of Radiology
University of Washington
Seattle, Washington

Naoya Hattori, MD, PhD
Assistant Professor
Department of Molecular Imaging
Hokkaido University
Hokkaido, Japan

Christopher J. Hurt, MD
Radiologist
Virtual Radiologic Professionals LLC
Eden Prairie, Minnesota

Bhasker R. Koppula, MD
Department of Radiology
University of Washington Medical Center
University of Washington
Seattle, Washington

Vivek Manchanda, MD
Senior Fellow, Oncologic and Cardiac PET/CT
Department of Radiology
University of Washington
Seattle, Washington

Helen R. Nadel, MD, FRCPC
Department of Radiology
British Columbia Children's Hospital
Vancouver, British Columbia

Marguerite T. Parisi, MD, MS Ed
Associate Professor of Radiology and Adjunct Associate
Professor of Pediatrics
University of Washington School of Medicine
Attending Radiologist and Division Chief, Ultrasound
    and PET/CT
Seattle Children's Hospital
Seattle, Washington

Shawn E. Parnell, MD
Assistant Professor, Pediatric Radiology
Department of Radiology
University of Washington and Seattle Children's Hospital
Seattle, Washington

Grace S. Phillips, MD
Assistant Professor, Pediatric Radiology
Department of Radiology
University of Washington and Seattle Children's Hospital
Seattle, Washington

Joseph Rajendran, MD, DMRT, FASNC
Associate Professor of Radiology and Radiation
Oncology (Adjunct)
Division of Nuclear Medicine/Department of Radiology
University of Washington &
Diagnostic Imaging Service, VA Puget Sound Health
Care System
Seattle, Washington

Nghia Jack Vo, MD
Assistant Professor, Pediatric Radiology and Vascular and
    Interventional Radiology
Department of Radiology
University of Washington and Seattle Children's Hospital
Seattle, Washington

FOREWORD

The best teachers I have had throughout my medical career were the individuals who were not only dedicated educators, but also committed to clinical excellence. They understand the context of the information they are conveying and the points that require special emphasis. They recognize that teaching is a scalable way to have a clinical impact on the largest number of people. And most importantly, they do not rest until they have done the very best that can be done.

Joseph Rajendran is exactly this type of individual. I have had the privilege of working with him for eight years. His unique commitment and talent were clear to me early in my tenure at the University of Washington. Based on his excellence, I asked him to be the Vice Chair and Director of Diagnostic Imaging Service at our Veteran's Administration Hospital. Predictably, he is doing a marvelous job. Did I mention that he is also a well-funded NIH researcher? For those keeping track, that makes him a quadruple threat.

Joseph's collaborators are Meg Parisi and Vivek Manchanda. Meg, similar to Joseph, has a lifelong commitment to excellence in education. She is a local expert and national leader in pediatric nuclear medicine. She has done a wonderful job editing the pediatric section of the book. Vivek is early in his career but we expect him to be a future star given his trajectory. His being earlier in his career ensures that the book is particularly responsive to the readers that are in training. He brings a background in nuclear medicine and radiology.

The passion, commitment, and the knowledge that define these individuals are manifest in this book. They have written this book using a case based format. In so doing, they have been able to cover the field of nuclear medicine with breadth and depth. They have sought out content expertise amongst the individuals that have submitted cases.

They have implemented a compelling approach to the case-based format. Each case takes the reader through the clinical context, including presenting symptoms and patient demographics. Subsequently, the imaging findings are presented followed by an appropriately broad but useful differential diagnoses. This is then followed by a comprehensive discussion of the disease diagnosis that is relevant and complete. The clinical history, the imaging findings and the case summaries are wonderfully written. The important information is emphasized in an engaging format. The images are presented with clarity and are annotated in a way that is facilitating to those early in their career and not distracting to those with more experience. Lastly, and this is my favorite aspect, the authors share pearls that will enable the reader to attain expert status.

In summary, you will love this book. It is thoughtfully constructed and reader focused. You will see manifest the inspiration and commitment of the two editors. Enjoy, learn and ultimately have an impact.

Norman J. Beauchamp
Professor of Radiology and Chair
Department of Radiology
Professor of Neurological Surgery and
Industrial Engineering
University of Washington

SERIES EDITOR'S FOREWORD

It is with great pleasure that I introduce our Nuclear Medicine Cases volume. Joseph Rajendran and Vivek Manchanda are remarkably talented authors who have labored to bring an outstanding breadth and depth of case material that encompasses Nuclear Medicine imaging's most essential entities. Extensive pathology awaits the reader interested in delving deeper into the common and not-so-common entities encountered in every day nuclear imaging practice.

The text is organized systematcially for easy navigation and accessibility. Each case explores common presentations of the entity followed by typical imaging findings, differential diagnoses, a comments section, and useful pearls. The images are strategically formatted with the "index image" (the entity's most representative example) on the left and additional images on the right. A useful and practical differential diagnosis section follows.

The innovative grading system indicates the degree to which the images are representative of a case's typical appearance. The scale ranges from "typical" (five circles) to "rare" (one circle). Similarly, the differential diagnosis images are graded "common" (five squares) to "unusual" (one square). The aim is to provide a reader with a sense of appropriateness regarding the practical use of differential diagnoses.

Our ultimate aim for the series is to create a practical resource for radiologists at the workstation to reference on a regular basis. Please look forward to future Case editions as well as the corresponding Patterns and Variants volumes.

Congratulations to Drs. Rajendran, Manchanda, and their contributors. They have done an exemplary job in creating a practical and comprehensive work.

Robert J. Ward, MD, CCD
Series Executive Editor

Chief, Division of Musculoskeletal Radiology
Department of Radiology
Tufts Medical Center
Residency Associate Program Director
Director, Medical Student Education
Assistant Professor of Radiology and Orthopaedics
Tufts University School of Medicine
Boston, Massachusetts

Consultant
Sullivan's Island Imaging, LLC
Sullivan's Island, South Carolina

PREFACE

Nuclear medicine has taken great strides in recent years, particularly in the field of molecular imaging. Developments in technology and advances in the field of multimodality imaging have made PET/CT imaging the standard of care. It is our opinion that the field of molecular imaging will only expand in the years to come. When we embarked on this project, we decided to highlight a collection of general nuclear medicine and PET/CT cases to provide the readers with the latest information in those areas. The cases are grouped according to organ systems, with a separate section for pediatric cases.

In spite of advances in molecular imaging, the bulk of clinical nuclear medicine practice still comprises of general nuclear medicine cases that form the foundation for the practice. In keeping with this, we have highlighted a number of general nuclear medicine cases that are of the "bread and butter" variety to present the characteristics of these everyday cases. Every case has a comments section that briefly describes the important clinico-pathological features of the case in question as well as possible findings on images. In addition to presentation, findings, and differential diagnoses, we have provided "pearls" of salient points related to the case that would benefit the readers in their daily practice. Our aim is not to cover the entire range of cases or for this book to serve as a reference textbook, but rather to present summary information that focuses on unique presentations of interesting and routine cases—a quick read with individual clinical problems covering a wide range of clinical topics of interest to practicing imaging physicians who can use this book as a guide in their practice.

It is our sincere hope that you will find this book interesting and useful in your daily nuclear medicine practice.

Joseph Rajendran
Vivek Manchanda

ACKNOWLEDGMENTS

This nuclear medicine casebook would not have been possible without the inspiration from all the teachers and trainees in the Department of Radiology at University of Washington. We thank our many colleagues who contributed towards cases and images. Their enthusiasm and interest are reflected in the variety of interesting cases. We are especially thankful to Dr Norman Beauchamp, Chairman of Radiology at University of Washington, for his encouragement to embark on this task, and his continued support, leadership, and vision provided to us during the process. Our thanks are due to Dr Hubert Vesselle, Director of Nuclear Medicine, for his support and for establishing the pool of nuclear medicine cases. Special thanks to Anthony Choi, who helped with case index preparation,

image transfer, and communication with publishers; and Dr. Marguerite Parisi for taking the lead and editing the section on pediatric nuclear medicine cases. We thank all assigned members of of publishers of this book, McGraw-Hill Companies, for their efficient handling of the process from start to finish, as well as to members of Glyph International (India) for their great project and editorial management. Last but not the least, we are deeply indebted to our families who have given us consistently strong support and encouragement during the entire process.

Joseph Rajendran
Vivek Manchanda

Chapter 1

ENDOCRINE

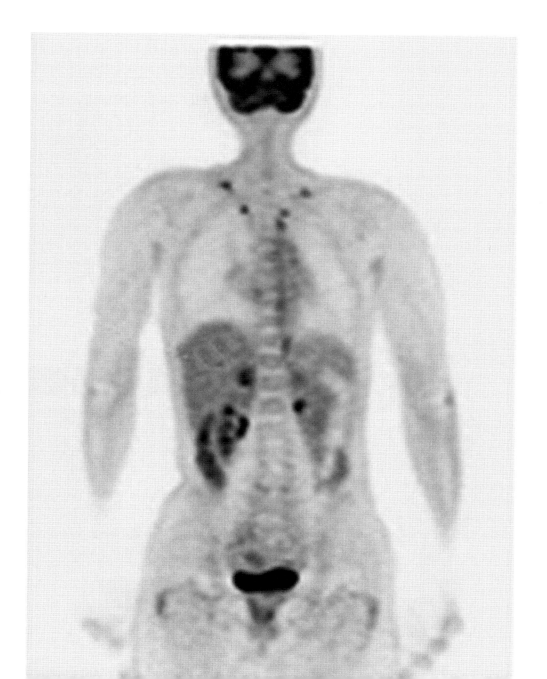

Vivek Manchanda, MD

PRESENTATION

Man in the fifth decade of life, status post parotidectomy for parotid cancer with right adrenal mass and headaches.

FINDINGS

Focal hypermetabolic right adrenal mass with 45 HU (Hounsfield unit) density on noncontrast CT.

DIFFERENTIAL DIAGNOSES

- *Metastasis.*
- *Lymphoma.*
- *Adenoma.*
- *Unilateral hyperplasia.*
- *Adrenocortical cancer* (fluorodeoxyglucose [FDG] avid).
- *Myelolipoma* (may show FDG activity in hematopoietic and adenomatous component).
- *Abscess* (circumferential FDG).
- *Hemorrhage* (cases of false-positive FDG activity reported).

The level of activity is greater than that of liver, so adrenal adenoma or adrenal hyperplasia are unlikely. Increased metanephrine levels indicated pheochromocytoma that was surgically proven.

COMMENTS

Pheochromocytomas are tumors of chromaffin cells which usually arise in the adrenal gland. Paragangliomas are rare (extra-adrenal) neuroendocrine tumors, derived from neural crest and chromaffin cells. Pheochromocytomas are frequently functioning in contrast to parasympathetic chain paragangliomas.

Multiple tumors can be seen with hereditary disorders, such as multiple endocrine neoplasia (MEN) II and III, neuroectodermal syndromes (eg, tuberous sclerosis, von Hippel-Lindau disease, Sturge-Weber syndrome, and neurofibromatosis), or Carney syndrome.

The diagnosis is established by the detection of elevated urine/plasma catecholamines and treatment involves surgery. Malignancy is established by metastasis to lymph nodes, liver, lungs, and bone.

Adrenal pheochromocytomas vary in size. MR typically shows hyperintense T2 signal. CT shows homogeneous/

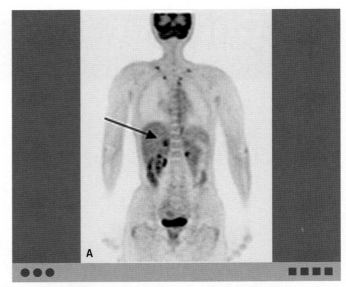

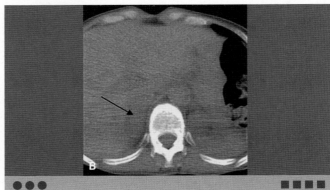

A. and **B. Pheochromocytoma:** Right adrenal hypermetabolic mass, (arrow) with b/l neck and paraspinal brown fat, 45 HU density on noncontrast CT. Increased serum metanephrine levels.

PEARLS

- Between MIBG and FDG, almost all pheochromocytomas are identified.
- FDG-PET is a useful adjunct to MIBG scintigraphy, most useful when MIBG scan is negative.
- FDG activity corresponding to hematopoietic and adenomatous components of myelolipoma have been reported.
- ^{18}F-DOPA has shown excellent sensitivity and specificity in detecting pheochromocytomas, which show dopamine synthesis by means of DOPA decarboxylation.

heterogeneous hypervascular lesion with/without calcifications. Tumor manipulation by imaging or biopsy may precipitate hypertensive crisis.

FDG activity greater than liver usually excludes adenoma and cysts. Most pheochromocytomas are FDG avid. Malignant pheochromocytomas are less MIBG and more FDG avid. FDG-PET is especially useful in detecting pheochromocytomas that fail to concentrate MIBG.

Low density (< 10 HU) on CT or relative loss of signal on out-of-phase (compared with in-phase) images on MRI and rapid washout of contrast on CT are most consistent with adenomas.

Paragangliomas (about 10%) include organ of Zuckerkandl (located at the origin of the inferior mesenteric artery), bladder wall, retroperitoneum, paracardiac region, and carotid and glomus jugulare bodies.

MIBG is superior to In-111 pentetreotide for localizing pheochromocytoma. Carbon 11 (C-11) metahydroxyephedrine (norepinephrine analogue) shows excellent localization of pheochromocytoma, but may be affected by agents that inhibit uptake of MIBG.

ADDITIONAL IMAGES (C-F)

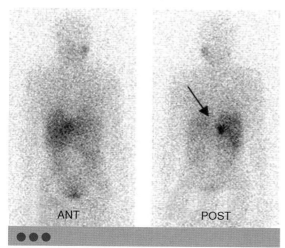

ANT   POST

C. Same patient (as in Figures A and B), MIBG scan (anterior and posterior) with hypermetabolic adrenal mass; pheochromocytoma.

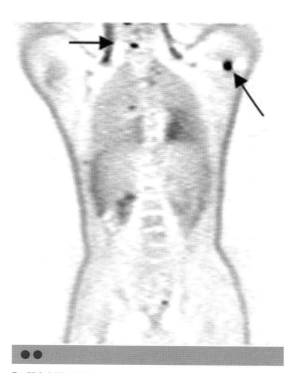

D. FDG-PET, NAC image: Malignant pheochromocytoma with multiple metastases, including left proximal humerus.

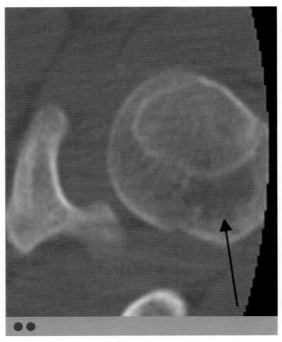

E. Corresponding axial noncontrast CT; lytic left proximal humeral lesion.

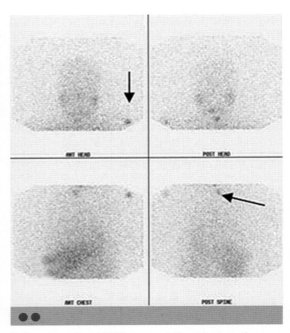

F. Corresponding MIBG; lesser defined lesions than FDG-PET.

DIFFERENTIAL DIAGNOSIS IMAGES (G-I)

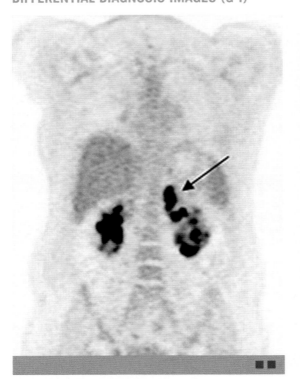

G. Adrenal involvement in lymphoma (*arrow*) along with bilateral kidney involvement.

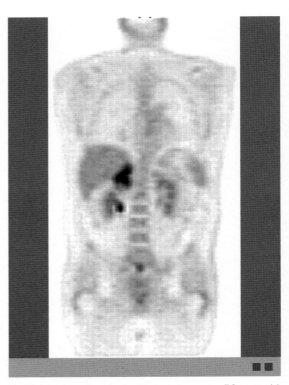

H. Right adrenal metastasis, rectal cancer, 50-year-old male.

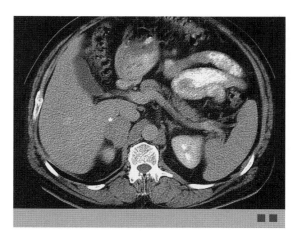

I. Right adrenal metastasis, CT, 50-year-old male with rectal cancer (*small white star*).

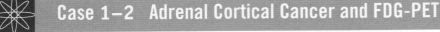

Vivek Manchanda, MD

PRESENTATION

A preteen girl with history of left abdominal mass and fullness.

FINDINGS

Large heterogeneous fluorodeoxyglucose (FDG)-avid (and metaiodobenzylguanidine [MIBG] negative) retroperitoneal mass that extends into inferior vena cava (IVC). Bone marrow stimulation with granulocyte colony-stimulating factor (G-CSF).

DIFFERENTIAL DIAGNOSES

- *Neuroblastoma*: It is less likely; given age, vascular invasion; no MIBG activity (most neuroblastomas are MIBG avid).

- *Adrenal metastasis*: Less likely; no evidence of FDG-avid primary tumor.

- *Sarcoma/rhabdoid tumor.*

- *Malignant pheochromocytoma.*

COMMENTS

Adrenocortical cancer (ACC) is the most likely diagnosis given increased size, FDG uptake and heterogeneous enhancement on CT, and extension of the tumor into renal vein or IVC.

ACC is a rare childhood cancer that can present with hormonal disturbances. The second peak occurs in adults (40-50 years age).

It usually presents as a large abdominal mass with symptoms of pain and fullness. An adrenal tumor larger than 5 or 6 cm is usually malignant. Association of ACC with hemihypertrophy and Beckwith-Wiedenmann and Li-Fraumeni cancer syndromes has been described.

CT features include central necrosis/hemorrhage, heterogeneous enhancement, invasion into adjacent structures, and venous extension into renal vein or IVC.

MR shows a large mass with lower signal intensity than that of liver on T1 and higher signal (often heterogeneous) on T2. No signal loss on out-of-phase imaging is found as it does not contain significant intracellular lipid.

FDG-positron emission tomography (FDG-PET) shows heterogeneously increased FDG uptake (greater than that in liver) in a large mass. This corresponds to the wide range of histological differentiation within the tumor.

Dissemination at the time of diagnosis portends poor prognosis and FDG-PET can aid in such analysis, even though current use of FDG-PET at initial diagnosis of ACC is limited. Commonest sites of distant metastasis of ACC include liver, lungs, lymph nodes, and peritoneum. The

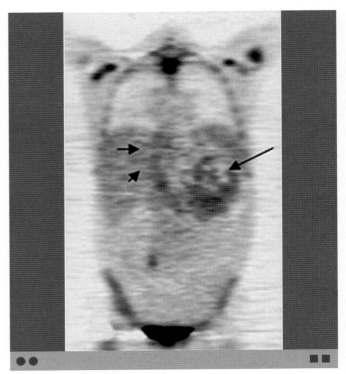

A. Heterogeneous FDG-avid left retroperitoneal mass (ACC, long arrow), invading IVC (*short arrows*). G-CSF-stimulated bone marrow, PET.

intensity of FDG activity in the primary tumor has been shown to correlate with survival in ACC. FDG-PET is very reliable in detecting local recurrent disease, even when anatomic imaging is inconclusive.

ACC is typically non-MIBG avid.

NP-59 (I-131 [iodine-131] norcholesterol) scan visualizes functional adrenal cortex. Nonvisualization of both adrenals (contralateral adrenal shuts down as excessive cortisol shuts down adrenocorticotropic hormone [ACTH]) in patients with Cushing syndrome indicates ACC.

PEARLS

- **Primary ACCs are rare and occur as large masses in children which can present earlier with hormonal disturbances.**

- **Heterogeneously increased FDG uptake in a large adrenal mass is the hallmark. They are typically not MIBG avid, which is primarily adrenal medullary imaging agent.**

- **Increased level of FDG activity in primary ACC has been associated with poorer prognosis.**

ADDITIONAL IMAGES (B–E)

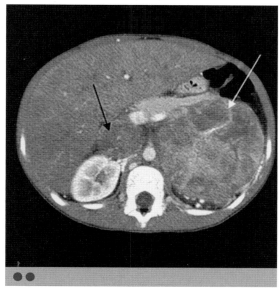

B. Left ACC (white arrow), IVC invasion (black arrow), CT.

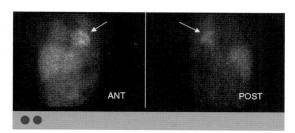

C. MIBG-negative mass. White arrow, normal MIBG in heart.

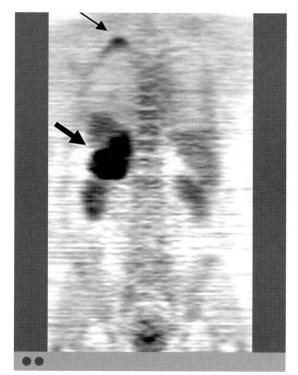

D. Another patient, recurrent ACC (*thick arrow*) with right upper back muscle metastasis (*thin arrow*).

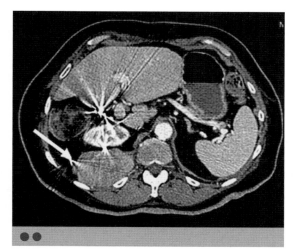

E. Recurrent ACC, corresponding CT.

DIFFERENTIAL DIAGNOSIS IMAGES (F-G)

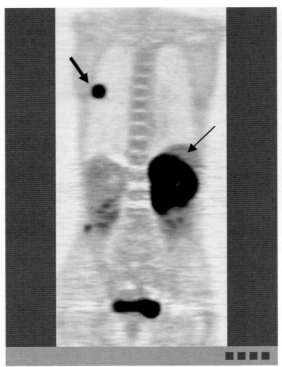

F. Right primary lung cancer (*thick arrow*) with adrenal metastasis (*thin arrow*), coronal PET.

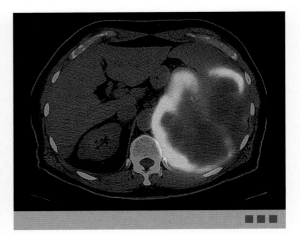

G. Left adrenal poorly differentiated sarcoma, fused PET/CT.

Vivek Manchanda, MD

PRESENTATION

Man in the fifth decade of life with lung cancer, right adrenal nodule.

FINDINGS

Focally hypermetabolic right adrenal nodule. On noncontrast CT, the density is 40 HU (Hounsfield unit).

DIFFERENTIAL DIAGNOSES (UNILATERAL ADRENAL MASS)

- *Pheochromocytoma.*
- *Lipid-poor adenoma.*
- *Unilateral hyperplasia.*
- *Hematoma.*
- *Lymphoma.*
- *Granulomatous disease.*
- *Myelolipoma.*
- *Ganglioneuroma.*
- *Hemangioma.*

Given diffuse increased level of FDG activity (more than that of the liver); adenoma (lipid rich or poor), hematoma,

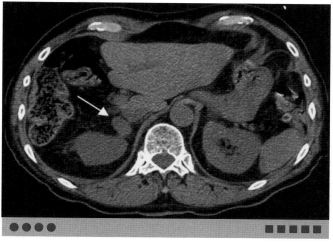

B. Corresponding CT.

ganglioneuroma, hemangioma, and hyperplasia are unlikely. Pheochromocytoma can be excluded with normal metanephrine levels.

COMMENTS

The adrenal glands are a common site of metastatic disease; ranked after lungs, liver, and bone.

The commonest primary cancers that metastasize to adrenals include lung, breast, melanoma, kidney, thyroid, and colon cancers.

Because of increased intracellular fat, adrenal nodules with densities less than 10 HU on unenhanced CT scans are typically benign, whereas lesions with densities greater than 10 HU are considered indeterminate. Contrast medium washout studies can help in the differentiation of adrenal metastases from lipid-poor adenomas (>60%

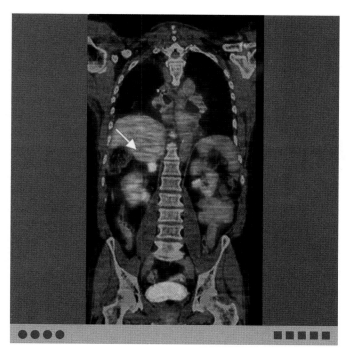

A. Right adrenal metastasis.

PEARLS

- Adrenal adenoma typically has none to low FDG activity (less than that of liver).

- An adrenal lesion's combined FDG activity on PET and density on noncontrast CT has high specificity for adrenal adenoma versus metastasis.

- PET/CT can help detect collision tumors (existence of histologically distinct tumors) in adrenals.

- Asymmetric suprarenal brown fat FDG activity is typically posterior to the kidneys (best seen on sagittal views).

absolute washout). MRI with in- and out-phase sequences can also aid in the characterization of indeterminate adrenal masses. Adrenal metastases are usually T1 hypointense and T2 hyperintense.

On PET, a lesion that shows less FDG uptake than liver, or shows uptake that is significantly higher than that of liver can be interpreted with high confidence as benign or malignant, respectively, unless the patient has pheochromocytoma, which can be excluded by biochemical markers. If adrenal mass shows FDG uptake equal to or slightly higher than that of liver, an additional imaging study may be performed for

further characterization, especially when it is the only area suspicious for metastasis.

Most pheochromocytomas (either benign or malignant) are metabolically active and accumulate FDG, although the uptake is found in greater percentage of malignant than benign lesions. Well-differentiated metastasis, metastasis from neuroendocrine tumors, necrotic metastasis, and early metastasis may have an uptake equal to or slightly more than that of liver.

Unilateral brown fat uptake can be confused with an adrenal lesion.

ADDITIONAL IMAGES (C-D)

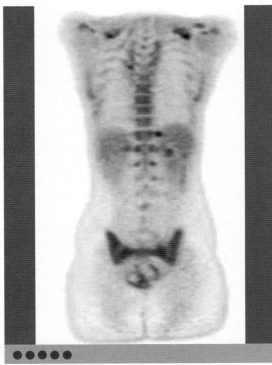

C. Asymmetric brown fat uptake in left paraspinal region, coronal PET.

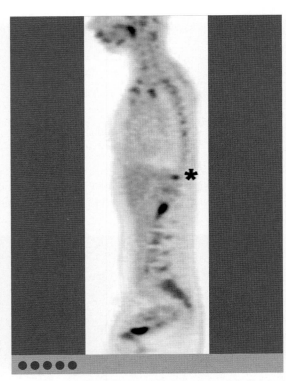

D. Asymmetric focal brown fat, posterior to left kidney (*black star*), sagittal PET.

DIFFERENTIAL DIAGNOSIS IMAGES (E-L)

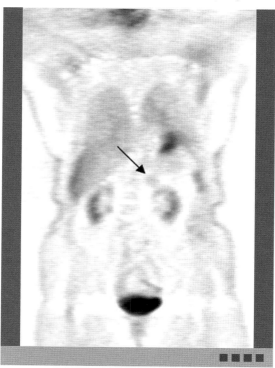

E. Left adrenal adenoma (*arrow*), FDG uptake less than liver, coronal PET.

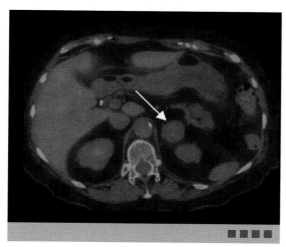

F. Left adrenal adenoma (*arrow*), FDG uptake less than liver, fused PET/CT.

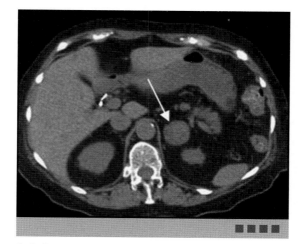

G. Left adrenal adenoma (*arrow*), noncontrast CT.

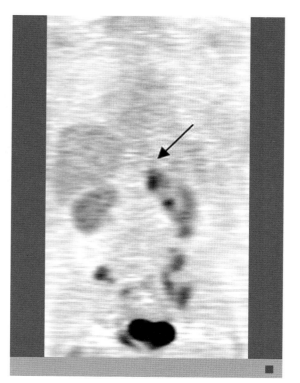

H. Left adrenal plasmacytoma (*arrow*) in a patient with multiple other organ involvement (not shown) coronal PET.

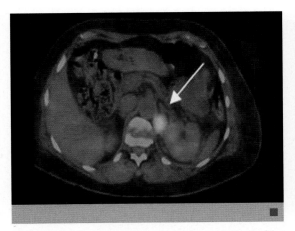

I. Left adrenal plasmacytoma (*arrow*) in a patient with multiple other organ involvement (not shown), fused PET/CT.

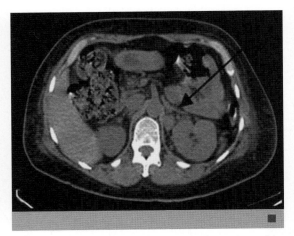

J. Left adrenal plasmacytoma (*arrow*) in a patient with multiple other organ involvement (not shown), noncontrast CT.

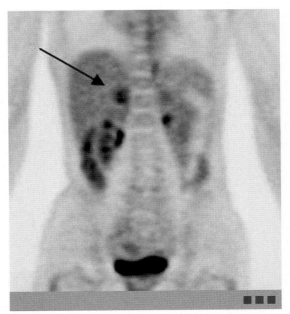

K. Right adrenal pheochromocytoma (arrow), coronal PET.

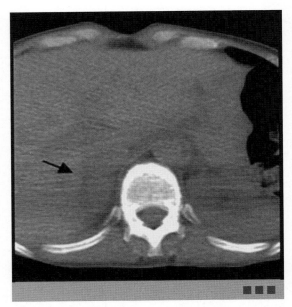

L. Right adrenal pheochromocytoma (*arrow*), noncontrast CT.

Joseph Rajendran, MD

PRESENTATION

A 50-year-old male with diarrhea, right lower quadrant (RLQ) pain, and flushing.

FINDINGS

Following the IV injection of 5 mCi of indium 111 (In-111)-labeled octreotide, whole-body planar images and single photon emission computed tomography (SPECT) images of the abdomen were obtained at 4 and 24 hours. SPECT images help with the localization and enable correlation with other cross-sectional images.

COMMENTS

Carcinoids, with an estimated 1.5 clinical cases per 100,000 population, are the most common neuroendocrine tumors. They are derived from primitive enterochromaffin stem cells in the gut, although they can arise from other organs such as the lungs, mediastinum, and pancreas. Small bowel carcinoid is commonly seen in the sixth or seventh decade, with approximately 6% presenting with carcinoid syndrome. Urinary 5-HIAA (hydroxyindoleacetic acid) levels

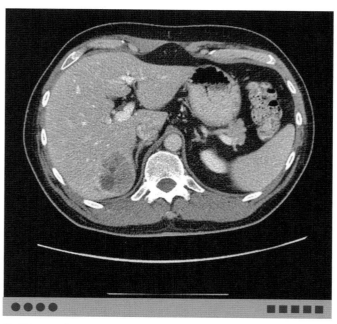

B. CT scan shows the abnormal focus in the right lobe of the liver and the focus in the right lower abdomen.

are usually increased and help aid in the diagnostic evaluation. Octreoscan is an In-111-labeled pentetreotide taken up in somatostatin-expressing tissues and is 80% to 100% sensitive. Imaging is done at 4 and 24 hours with an option to add imaging at 48 hours. The sensitivity of this test is reduced when patients receive systemic octreotide for the control of symptoms. Ideally, patients should stop octreotide treatment prior to getting the scan. However, in patients with severe symptoms it might not be possible, but Octreoscan would provide valuable information if the patient is symptomatic in spite of treatment. Patients with metastatic carcinoid have a survival rate of 36% at 5 years.

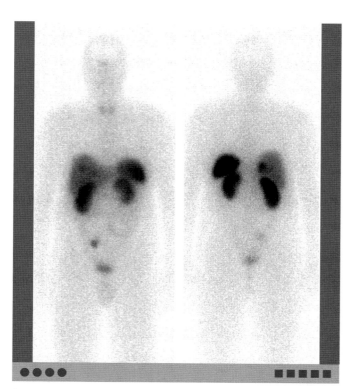

A. In-111 Octreoscan whole-body images (4 and 24 hours) show a focus of increased uptake in the right lobe of the liver and another focus in the RLQ of the abdomen. There is normal physiologic uptake seen in the liver, spleen, and kidneys.

PEARLS

- Urinary 5-HIAA levels are usually increased and aid in the assessment of carcinoid tumors.

- Octreotide is rapidly taken up in the kidneys and has low hepatobiliary clearance.

- Smaller foci (<1 cm) are difficult to diagnose.

- Octreotide therapy to be discontinued to improve sensitivity.

ADDITIONAL IMAGE

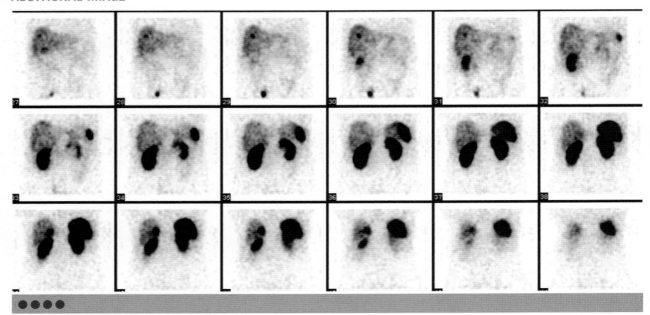

C. Coronal projections of In-111 Octreotide SPECT images at 24 hours show the focus of abnormal radiotracer activity in the right lobe of the liver.

Joseph Rajendran, MD

PRESENTATION

A 36-year-old female with 3 months of syncopal episodes, many associated with hypotension, palpitations, and pallor. Elevated serum norepinephrine and urine metanephrines.

FINDINGS

Following the IV injection of 500 µCi of Iodine 131 (I-131) MIBG, whole-body planar images were obtained at 24 and 72 hours.

DIFFERENTIAL DIAGNOSIS

Adrenal pheochromocytoma: Clinical presentation is identical to current case, but the location of the primary tumor is in the adrenal gland, confirmed by the location on imaging.

COMMENTS

Pheochromocytoma arises from neural crest cells in the adrenal medulla, sympathetic ganglia, organs of Zuckerkandl, and aortic and carotid chemoreceptors. Extramedullary tumors can also be present. Patients typically present with hypertension, headaches, tremors, palpitations, weight loss, and hyperglycemia. Biochemically, there are elevated urine and plasma cate-cholamines, elevated urine vanillylmandelic acid (VMA), and metanephrine. Structurally, MIBG resembles norepinephrine and guanethidine (a neurosecretory granule-depleting agent). MIBG localizes to storage granules in the adrenergic tissue

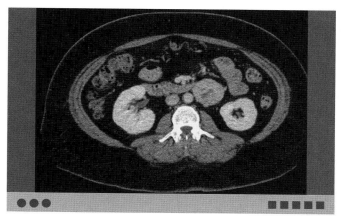

B. CT scan of the abdomen showing a mass anterior to the left kidney not located in the typical location of the adrenal gland.

of neural crest origin, with uptake proportional to the number of neurosecretory granules. When I-131 is used, a dose of 500 µCi is administered intravenously followed by whole-body images at 24 and 72 hours after administration. Certain sympathetic or sympathomimetic drugs need to be withheld prior to starting the test; these drugs include combined alpha- and beta-blockers, guanethedine, antipsychotics, and nasal decongestants such as phenylephrine as these tend to block the uptake of MIBG. In patients with suspected pheochromocytoma, the radiotracer is administered slowly so as not to precipitate a hypertensive crisis. Blood pressure (BP) is measured prior to and after the injection. Thyroid uptake is blocked with Lugol solution or saturated solution of potassium iodide (SSKI) starting the day prior to the test. Iodine-labeled MIBG shows normal uptake in the salivary glands, liver, and bowels, as well as the heart. The latter uptake is as a result of sympathetic innervation of the heart. Iodine-labeled MIBG imaging has a sensitivity of 80% to 90% and a specificity of 95% to 99%.

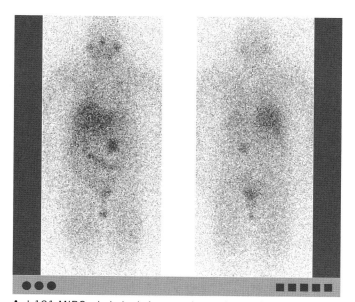

A. I-131 MIBG whole body images show a focus of increased uptake in the left abdomen corresponding to the CT abnormality on Figure B. There is normal physiologic uptake seen in the salivary glands, liver and bowels.

PEARLS

- Drugs that have the potential to interfere with the uptake need to be stopped for a suitable time to increase the sensitivity of this test.

- Smaller foci (<1 cm) are difficult to diagnose especially when I-131-labeled MIBG is used.

- Bowel preparation might be necessary during the test to reduce false-positive results.

- Care should be taken to avoid a rare incident of hypertensive crisis by injecting the drug slowly and taking precautions. Patients need to be observed and their BP be checked prior to and after the injection of the radiotracer.

Joseph Rajendran, MD

PRESENTATION

A 38-year-old female noticed hair loss in 2004. Symptoms of tremors, anxiety, and palpitations started in 2005.

FINDINGS

The Tc-99m pertechnetate thyroid scan shows uniformly enlarged thyroid gland (size 50 g) with homogeneous uptake in both lobes and the uptake is significantly greater than that of major salivary glands. Gland was smooth on palpation. Iodine 131 (I-131) thyroid uptake at 4 hours was 63% and at 24 hours was 88%.

DIFFERENTIAL DIAGNOSES

- *Subacute thyroiditis*: In spite of the thyrotoxic symptoms and low thyrotropin-stimulating hormone (TSH), there is low radioactive iodine uptake and "poor quality" images.

- *Multinodular goiter*: Patchy uptake in irregularly enlarged gland that can have normal or even low uptake levels.

- *Autonomously functioning thyroid nodule*: Focal increased uptake in a dominant nodule with suppressed uptake in the rest of the gland. Radioiodine uptake can be low to normal.

COMMENTS

Graves disease affects 1.4 cases per 1000 persons and the diagnosis is largely based on laboratory results, including an elevated free T3/T4 level and suppressed thyrotropin level prompted by clinical symptoms and signs. The gland is usually diffusely enlarged on physical examination. Normal uptake at 4 and 24 hours can be seen in patients with hyperthyroidism and can be caused by dietary factors such as over-the-counter (OTC) multivitamins and food supplements that contain large amounts of iodine. Often, antithyroid drugs are administered before I-131 treatment to deplete the gland of stored hormone and to normalize serum T3 and T4 levels before therapy. This also reduces the possibility of radiation-induced exacerbation of thyrotoxicosis. The antithyroid drug is discontinued 2 days before therapy. This is particularly done in patients with severe thyrotoxicosis with high T3 or T4 and very high uptake. Beta-blockers, the mainstay of treatment, can be continued throughout. Hypothyroidism occurs after I-131 therapy in 10% to 20% of patients and increases over time, requiring a close clinical and biochemical follow-up. Incidence of hypothyroidism is more frequently related to the amount of administered radioactivity while, on the other hand, a higher radioactivity will result in a greater likelihood of control of the condition with one dose.

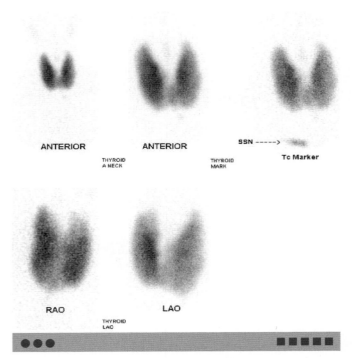

ANTERIOR THYROID A NECK ANTERIOR THYROID MARK SSN -----> Tc Marker

RAO LAO THYROID LAO

A. Uniformly enlarged thyroid gland with diffusely increased uptake (88% at 24 hours) and the presence of a pyramidal lobe are characteristics of Graves disease.

PEARLS

- **Graves disease is under a spectrum of autoimmune disorder.**

- **Higher than normal iodine uptake differentiates it from thyroiditis.**

- **Presence of pyramidal lobe is most commonly seen with Graves disease and is as a result of stimulated thyroid tissue in the thyroglossal tract.**

- **All three treatment methods—antithyroid drugs, surgery, and radiation therapy with I-131—are equally effective in controlling hyperthyroidism. In the United States, I-131 therapy is the most commonly used method for adult patients.**

- **The amount of radioactive I-131 used to treat Graves disease is generally lower than that is required for treating multinodular goiter or autonomously functioning toxic nodule.**

- **In general, it might take around 12 weeks to see the full effect of the radioiodine treatment.**

DIFFERENTIAL DIAGNOSIS IMAGE

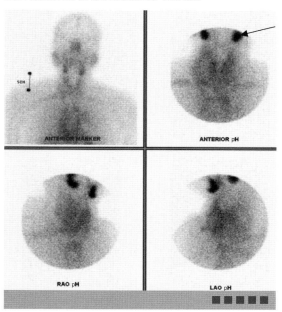

B. Thyroiditis: Paucity of uptake in the thyroid gland with a 24-hour uptake of only 4%. Typically the low uptake levels preclude images to be obtained. Arrow points to normal uptake in the salivary gland.

Vivek Manchanda, MD

PRESENTATION

Right neck mass in a 3-year-old patient with elevated vanillylmandelic acid levels.

FINDINGS

Intense focal hypermetabolic right neck mass on FDG-PET scan.

DIFFERENTIAL DIAGNOSES

- *Infection/abscess*
- *Paraganglioma*
- *Metastasis*
- *Lymphoma*
- *Castleman disease*
- *Granulomatous disease*
- *Infected branchial cyst*
- *Sarcoma: Rhabdomyosarcoma*

COMMENTS

Neuroblastoma is one of the commonest extracranial solid malignant tumors in children, arising from neural cells of sympathoadrenal system.

Local disease assessment can be made with the MR and CT. MIBG (norepinephrine analogue) is used to assess the extent of the disease. Some neuroblastomas may show In-111 pentetreotide accumulation (caused by somatostatin receptors).

Most neuroblastomas accumulate FDG, prechemotherapy, or preradiation therapy. FDG uptake is not dependent on type 1 catecholamine uptake. Neuroblastomas that do not concentrate MIBG (about 30%) may show FDG uptake.

Bone scan is used to detect skeletal (cortical) involvement for staging but cannot distinguish active disease from reparative uptake.

An advantage of FDG-PET is imaging on the same day of radiotracer injection (as compared to 1-2 days postinjection for MIBG).

Mild diffuse FDG uptake can be seen in normal bone marrow, but focally and asymmetrically increased FDG activity indicates metastasis. Pitfalls resulting from physiologic FDG uptake early on in G-CSF therapy include heterogeneous tracer uptake-simulating disease.

The current primary role of FDG-PET is in evaluation of known or suspected MIBG-negative neuroblastoma. In high-risk neuroblastoma, FDG-PET was found superior or equal to

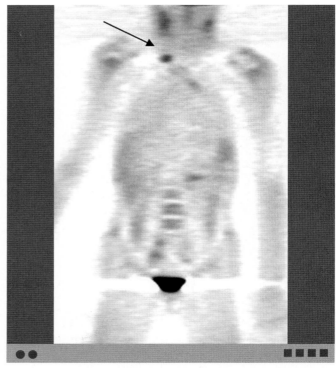

A. Focally increased FDG activity (*arrow*), biopsy-proven poorly differentiated neuroblastoma, coronal PET.

MIBG in determining extraskeletal and soft tissue metastasis, detecting smaller lesions, determining the extent of disease, and localizing disease sites. Detection of cranial vault lesions was found to be difficult owing to physiologic brain uptake.

Some of the other tracers that have been described to evaluate neuroblastomas are 11C-hydroxyl ephedrine and 11C-HED, an epinephrine analogue, and 11C-epinephrine PET.

PEARLS

- **Most neuroblastomas are FDG-avid. The uptake is not dependent on type 1 catecholamine uptake. MIBG remains mainstay for staging neuroblastoma.**

- **Up to 30% of neuroblastomas that are not MIBG avid may be FDG-avid.**

- **FDG may be superior to MIBG for locating neuroblastomas in certain tissues or when a tumor becomes dedifferentiated or loses the noradrenergic transporter system.**

- **Multiple imaging modalities may be required for staging and restaging of neuroblastoma.**

ADDITIONAL IMAGES (B-C)

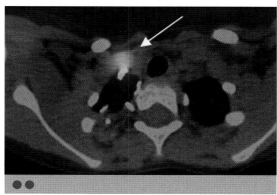

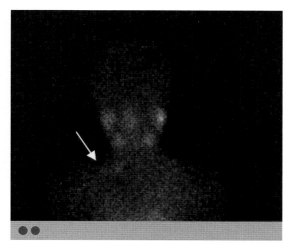

B. Focally increased FDG activity (*arrow*), biopsy-proven poorly differentiated neuroblastoma, fused axial PET/CT. Surgical clips from prior surgery.

C. Focal, only mild MIBG right neck uptake (*arrow*), biopsy-proven poorly differentiated neuroblastoma.

DIFFERENTIAL DIAGNOSIS IMAGES (D-F)

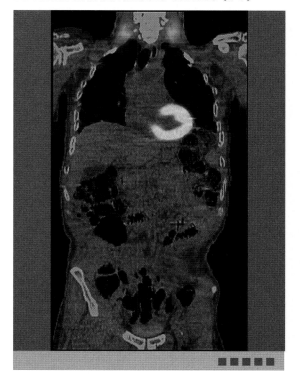

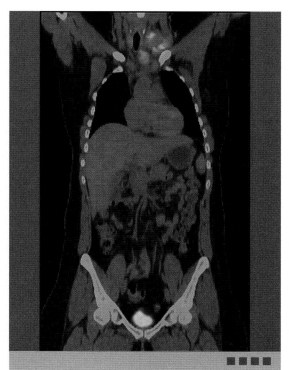

D. Bilateral neck physiologic muscle FDG uptake, coronal fused PET/CT.

E. Left neck Hodgkin lymphoma, 30-year-old female.

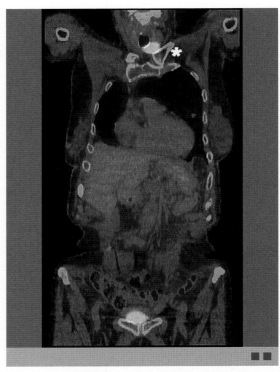

F. Left Hürthle cell (thyroid) cancer (*white star*), 87-year-old-female, coronal fused PET/CT.

Joseph Rajendran, MD

PRESENTATION

Young woman status post-kidney transplant with symptoms of hyperparathyroidism. Evaluation requested for parathyroid adenoma. Past history of radioiodine ablation for hyperthyroidism.

FINDINGS

Tc-99m sestamibi planar images of the neck at 1 and 2 hours postinjection show an absent uptake of the radiotracer in the thyroid gland on all images with a focus of uptake, persisting in the region of the left lower pole that showed increased prominence on later images. Patient also underwent SPECT imaging with limited CT at 1 hour for localization.

DIFFERENTIAL DIAGNOSES

- *Thyroid adenoma*: Unlikely in this case as there is no functioning thyroid gland/tissue as a result of prior Iodine 131 (I-131) therapy.

- *Post-thyroidectomy*: History usually establishes the cause for lack of thyroid uptake.

COMMENTS

Initial images (10-15 minutes) show prominent thyroid uptake although a focal uptake can be seen in a parathyroid adenoma even on this early images. While normal parathyroid generally has a washout similar to that of thyroid gland, abnormal parathyroid tissue has a slower washout—the principle behind these studies and making the contrast. Primary hyperparathyroidism can still occur after treatment with I-131 for hyperthyroidism because radiation dose from I-131 therapy usually spares the parathyroid gland. Clinical presentation is similar to those with functioning thyroid gland. While SPECT imaging provides additional localization information, most cases are diagnosed on planar images. Addition of SPECT and or limited CT (usually at 1 hour) helps to identify the location of the adenoma and will help the surgical procedure. Adenomas can be intra- or retrothyroidal and the confirmation helps with planning the surgical approach. Occasionally, the adenomas can be ectopic. The sensitivity for the detection is 90% to 95% for larger adenomas but is lower for smaller adenomas. Parathyroid hyperplasia

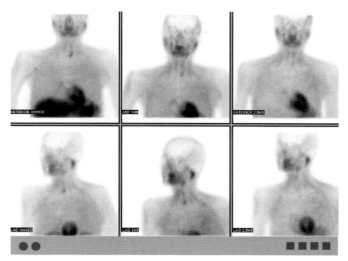

A. Images of the neck at 1 and 2 hours in anterior and oblique projections show the focus of persistent uptake in the region of left lower pole. Note absent uptake in the thyroid gland.

with a sensitivity of about 50% is the usual cause for false-positive results. The main advantage of scintigraphy is not only the identification but also localization of the adenoma to guide the surgeon. Use of handheld radiation probe at the time of surgery provides additional guidance to the surgeon. All or any one of the four parathyroid glands can be involved and presurgical imaging helps the surgeon by localizing the adenoma and will help reduce the duration of anesthesia in high-risk patients.

PEARLS

- **Radioactive iodine therapy for benign thyroid disorders does not affect the function in the parathyroid gland.**

- **Past history will help identify the cause of lack of visualization of thyroid gland.**

- **SPECT images help to localize the position of the gland that will provide additional guidance to the surgeon.**

- **Parathyroid scintigraphy can be performed using a[201] subtraction scintigraphy or Tc-99m sestamibi or Tc-99m tetrofosmin.**

DIFFERENTIAL DIAGNOSIS IMAGES (B-D)

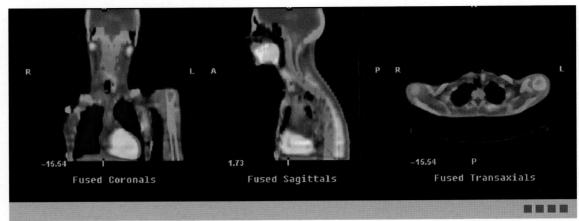

R   L   A   P   R   L

−15.54   1.73   −15.54   P

Fused Coronals   Fused Sagittals   Fused Transaxials

B. Fused images of Tc-99m MIBI and CT shows a focus of increased and retained uptake in the left lobe of the thyroid gland corresponding to thyroid adenoma.

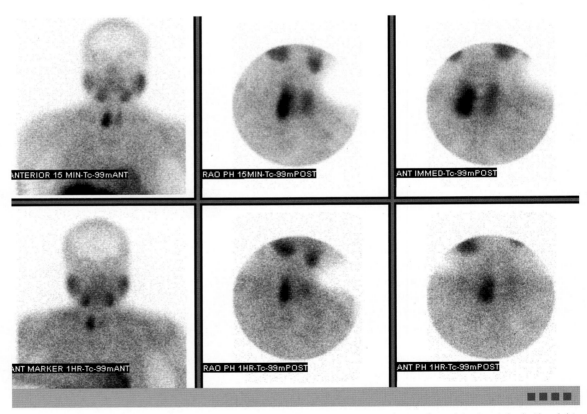

ANTERIOR 15 MIN-Tc-99mANT   RAO PH 15MIN-Tc-99mPOST   ANT IMMED-Tc-99mPOST

ANT MARKER 1HR-Tc-99mANT   RAO PH 1HR-Tc-99mPOST   ANT PH 1HR-Tc-99mPOST

C. Planar Tc-99m sestamibi parathyroid anterior and posterior images show a focus of persistent uptake in the right lower pole consistent with parathyroid adenoma. Note normal uptake in the thyroid gland.

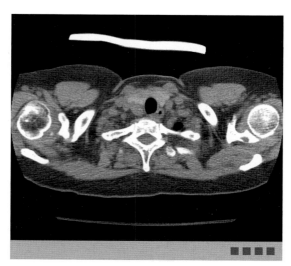

D. Axial slice of CT scan of the neck shows a parathyroid nodule behind the right lower pole of thyroid gland corresponding to the focal uptake on Tc-99m sestamibi scan.

Case 1–9 Autonomous Functioning Thyroid Nodule Diagnosed after I-131 Therapy for Graves Disease

Joseph Rajendran, MD

PRESENTATION

Six months after treatment with 10 mCi of Iodine 131 (I-131) for Graves disease, patient continued to have symptoms of hyperthyroidism.

FINDINGS

The Tc-99m pertechnetate thyroid scan shows a focal hot nodule in the left lobe corresponding to the palpable nodule. Radiotracer uptake is significantly decreased in rest of the gland. I-131 thyroid uptake at 24 hours was only 15%.

DIFFERENTIAL DIAGNOSIS

• *Graves disease with a multinodular pattern*: There is heterogeneous uptake in an enlarged and nodular thyroid gland. Dominant nodule may be felt.

COMMENTS

Most thyroid nodules are not true neoplasms but are caused as a result of hyperplasia and involution in the thyroid tissue. Patients present with no symptoms or severe symptoms of hyperthyroidism. Majority of the patients have a palpable nodule that can be easily confirmed with ultrasonography (USG). Patients with autonomous functioning thyroid nodule (AFTN), unlike those with Graves disease, can show normal ranges of thyroid uptake in a normal-sized gland that shows focal increased uptake in the nodule amidst low uptake in rest of the gland, secondary to suppression of TSH caused by hypersecretion of thyroid hormones by the AFTN. It may also be as a result of previous I-131 therapy as seen in this patient. Patients with symptomatic and biochemical hyperthyroidism need to be treated to lessen systemic complications even with normal 24-hour thyroid uptake. Patients need to be and can be treated with higher amounts of radioactive iodine 131 (RAI-131) without the immediate likelihood of hypothyroidism, because almost all of the administered activity will be localized in the hyperfunctioning toxic nodule, relatively sparing the normal thyroid tissue. It is likely that the glandular tissue in this focal area was autonomous to begin with and was resistant to and spared by the first I-131 therapy ablating the normal-functioning thyroid tissue, resulting in the development of AFTN subsequently. Alcohol ablation of the AFTN has been done with some success, but the majority of these patients respond well to RAI therapy.

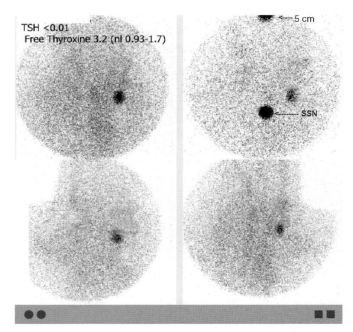

TSH <0.01
Free Thyroxine 3.2 (nl 0.93-1.7)

←5 cm

←SSN

A. Tc-99m pertechnetate thyroid images show no significant uptake in the thyroid gland but a focus of increased uptake in the left lower neck. Thyroid uptake of 24 hours was 15%.

PEARLS

- Theoretical advantage for using RAI-131 for treating AFTN is that almost all of the administered activity can localize in the functioning hot nodule, relatively sparing the suppressed parts of the gland. However, in this patient since the thyroid gland was already treated with I-131, this will not be a benefit.

- In the typical patient with AFTN, higher amounts of radioactive iodine can be used with minimal likelihood of hypothyroidism.

- Surgery, although highly successful, is rarely used in patients with AFTN.

- Unlike in a cold nodule, the incidence of malignancy is very low in AFTN, hence additional evaluation measures are generally not needed at the time of diagnosis.

DIFFERENTIAL DIAGNOSIS IMAGE

Free Thyroxine 5.3 (nl 0.93 - 1.7)

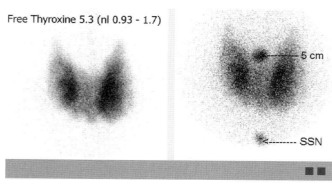

5 cm

SSN

B. Diffusely mildly enlarged thyroid gland with mildly patchy uptake in a normal thyroid gland.

Joseph Rajendran, MD

PRESENTATION

A 48-year-old with recurrent metastatic thymoma which invaded the pleura and pericardium status post surgery, chemotherapy, and radiation therapy. Evaluation for octreotide avidity.

FINDINGS

Following the IV injection of 5 mCi of In-111 octreotide, whole-body planar images and SPECT images of the abdomen were obtained at 4 and 24 hours. SPECT images help with the localization and enable correlation with other cross-sectional images.

DIFFERENTIAL DIAGNOSES

• *Thymic hyperplasia*: Seen in younger patients and can be secondary to chemotherapy. The whole thymus is enlarged and might show increased uptake following chemotherapy.

• *Metastases to thymus:* If octreotide avid, it usually presents as focally increased uptake with evidence of systemic cancer.

COMMENTS

The thymus is a lymphoid organ located in the anterior mediastinum, mainly connected with the development and maturation of cell-mediated immunity. Histologically, the organ is composed mainly of epithelial cells and lymphocytes. Under normal conditions, thymus shows involution after puberty. Thymomas, the most common anterior mediastinal tumors, are composed mainly of epithelial cells; however, there might not be clear histological distinction between benign and malignant thymomas which are usually encapsulated but local spread and invasion is possible. Thymomas are associated with myasthenia gravis (50% of thymoma patients), red cell aplasia, and hypogammaglobulinemia. Patients present with local symptoms (in one-third of patients), incidentally picked up on imaging (in one-third of patients), and myasthenia gravis (in one-third of patients). Following therapy, the 5-year survival rate in patients with noninvasive thymomas is 70% to 85% and decreases at 50% to 67% for invasive thymomas with the worst trend for stage IV (23%).

In-111 pentreotide (octreotide) binds to the somatostatin receptor subtype 2.

Octreotide is a somatostatin analog that binds to tissues with expression of somatostatin receptors—neuroendocrine tumors. Octreotide concentrates in most thymomas, particularly those associated with autoimmune disease in a greater proportion than in normal thymic tissue, but not in benign

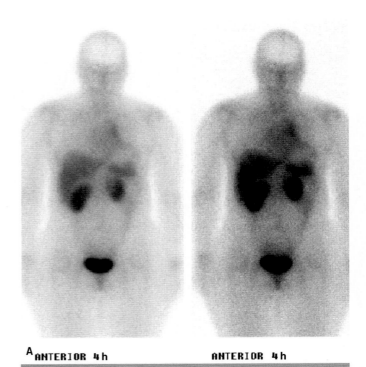

A ANTERIOR 4 h   ANTERIOR 4 h

A. In-111 octreoscan whole-body images (4 hours) show linear uptake in the left paramediastinal and hilar regions that increases in intensity over time. There is normal physiologic uptake seen in the thyroid gland, liver, spleen, and kidneys.

lymphofollicular hyperplasia, a fact that is useful to differentiate the two conditions. Metastases to thymus can occur as a result of direct extension from the lungs or from extrathoracic sites, such as the kidneys, testis, colon, and rectum, as well as ovary, prostate, breasts, bladder, and stomach. Octreoscan can be used to select candidates for targeted therapy as well as in following-up response to therapy.

PEARLS

- **Octreotide is rapidly taken up in the kidneys and has low hepatobiliary clearance.**

- **Smaller foci (<1 cm) are difficult to diagnose.**

- **Octreotide therapy is to be discontinued prior to test to improve the sensitivity.**

- **Higher levels of In-111 octreotide uptake predict good response to octreotide therapy, while lack of uptake shows dedifferentiated tumor which may not respond well to therapy.**

Vivek Manchanda, MD

PRESENTATION

Status post left thyroidectomy and Iodine 131 (I-131) therapy for thyroid cancer with rising thyroglobulin levels.

FINDINGS

FDG-avid left upper anterior chest wall soft tissue mass, I-131 negative. I-131-avid right thyroid lobe.

DIFFERENTIAL DIAGNOSES

- *Metastasis.*
- *Sarcoma.*
- *Lymphoma.*
- *Melanoma.*
- *Plasmacytoma.*

In a patient with prior subtotal thyroidectomy and rising TG levels, FDG-avid (even if I-131 nonavid) recurrent thyroid cancer is the most likely explanation, proven by biopsy.

COMMENTS

Well-differentiated thyroid cancer ranks among the cancers with good prognoses, contributed by effective surgical resection of the primary, slow growth, and I-131 ablation.

Papillary thyroid cancer usually spreads to cervical nodes locally and less commonly to distant sites, such as bone and lungs. Follicular thyroid cancer usually spares cervical nodes and involves bone and lungs about 20% of the time.

The typical indication for FDG-PET/CT is a negative I-131 scan in a patient with rising thyroglobulin levels. It has been advocated with high-risk disease and Hürthle cell cancers. Anaplastic thyroid cancer, thyroid lymphoma, and medullary thyroid cancers tend to be very FDG-avid.

Per studies, TSH stimulation by either withdrawal of hormone or recombinant TSH (rTSH) injections improves sensitivity to detect metastasis.

Well-differentiated thyroid cancer metastasis is typically more I-131 avid. Poorly differentiated thyroid cancers are less iodine and more FDG-avid. Some thyroid cancer metastases may have both poorly differentiated and well-differentiated components.

Studies have suggested that prognosis of I-131-negative (and FDG-positive) metastasis is worse than that of I-131-positive (and FDG-negative) metastasis. Usually, a trial of I-131 therapy is used to get rid of the remaining

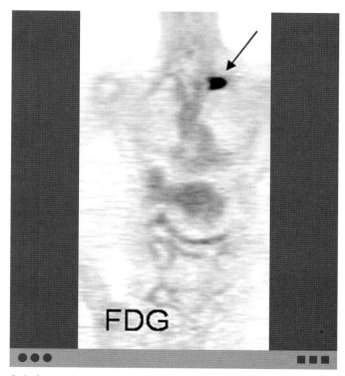

A. Left anterior chest wall hypermetabolic mass, coronal FDG-PET.

differentiated component of the disease. Lithium or retinoic acid can boost the response to I-131 therapy, but the results have been variable. Surgery/radiation are often the mainstay treatment of FDG-avid metastasis.

I-124 PET may be used in future in combination with FDG-PET for management and follow-up of thyroid cancers.

PEARLS

- Increasing post–TSH-stimulated thyroglobulin levels and negative I-131 scan is an indication to obtain FDG-PET/CT

- Some studies have suggested that FDG-negative scan in a patient with increasing thyroglobulin (Tg) levels is a good prognostic indicator.

- Nonbreath-hold CT acquired with PET may miss metastases which are non–FDG-avid because of their small size.

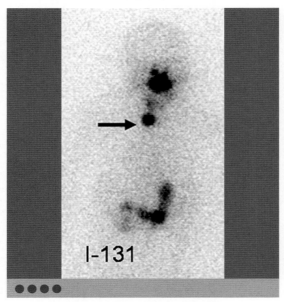

B. I-131 post therapy scan with right neck uptake from remnant thyroid. No uptake in left chest wall mass.

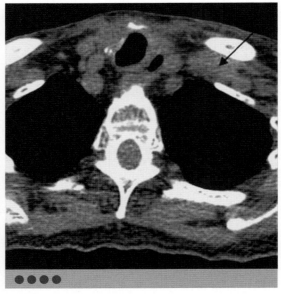

C. Noncontrast CT with left neck mass.

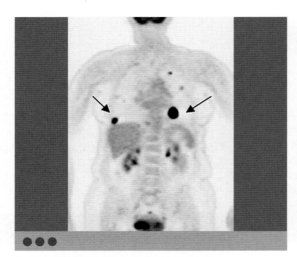

D. Thyroid cancer metastasis in bilateral lungs in a different patient, coronal FDG-PET.

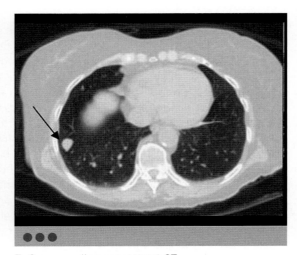

E. Corresponding noncontrast CT.

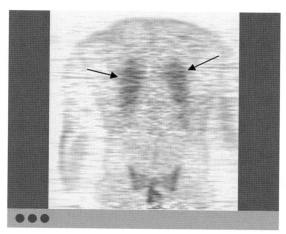

F. Miliary metastasis from thyroid cancer, coronal FDG-PET (filtered back reconstruction).

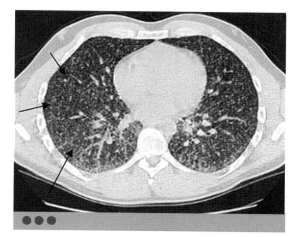

G. Corresponding noncontrast CT with innumerable tiny nodules.

DIFFERENTIAL DIAGNOSIS IMAGES (I-J)

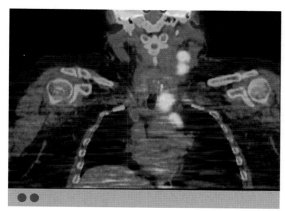

H. Recurrent anaplastic thyroid cancer with nodal metastasis, fused coronal FDG-PET.

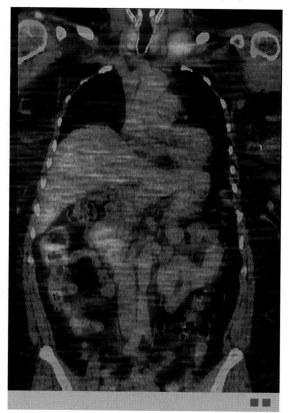

I. Left supraclavicular plasmacytoma; fused coronal PET/CT.

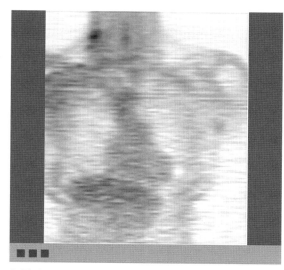

J. Right neck melanoma metastasis; coronal PET.

Vivek Manchanda, MD

PRESENTATION

Left thyroid nodule in a patient with breast cancer.

FINDING

Hypermetabolic left thyroid nodule, corresponding to 1.0-cm thyroid nodule seen on the CT scan.

DIFFERENTIAL DIAGNOSES

- *Metastasis*: Thyroid metastases are very rare. A primary thyroid cancer is more likely.
- *Functioning thyroid adenoma.*
- *Lymphoma.*
- *Focal thyroiditis.*

COMMENTS

Incidental thyroid nodules are seen by the radiologist commonly. The clinically detected thyroid nodules are most often benign. The incidentally detected thyroid nodules on cross-sectional and FDG-PET imaging are a distinct group.

On a CT scan; thyroid calcification, larger size, and younger male patients confer high risk for carcinoma.

Hypermetabolic focal thyroid uptake on an FDG-PET scan has a high likelihood (close to 50% or more) of being a primary thyroid cancer.

Metastasis to the thyroid gland is extremely rare. The commonest cancer to metastasize to thyroid is the renal cancer. Therefore, any focal FDG uptake on a PET scan warrants a biopsy and USG correlation.

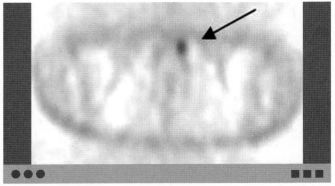

B. Axial FDG-PET with left thyroid hypermetabolic nodule.

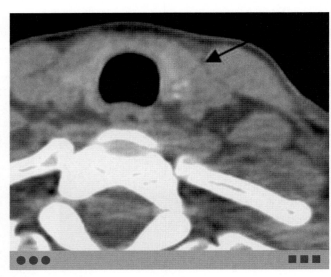

C. Corresponding noncontrast CT, left thyroid nodule with punctate calcifications, papillary thyroid cancer.

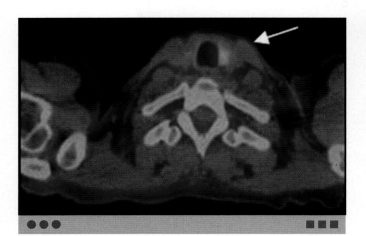

A. Incidental left thyroid primary papillary thyroid cancer.

PEARLS

- Incidental focal thyroid uptake must be investigated with fine-needle aspiration biopsy (FNAB), preferably with USG to exclude incidental primary thyroid cancer.

- Functioning thyroid adenoma (more likely) and metastasis (rare) are included in the differential diagnosis of a hypermetabolic thyroid nodule.

- Diffuse thyroid uptake can be seen as a normal variant or in thyroiditis.

- Non–FDG-avid thyroid nodules which are larger than 1 cm have been reported in literature to be unlikely to be malignant, but more studies are needed.

FDG-PET can play an important role in the management of patients with inconclusive cytologic diagnosis of a thyroid nodule. Fluorine 18 (^{18}F) FDG-PET has been suggested to reduce the number of futile hemithyroidectomies in some studies.

On the other hand, the issue of non–FDG-avid thyroid nodules that are more than 1 cm large on CT has not been adequately addressed. In the author's limited experience, the large (>1 cm) FDG-negative nodules that were biopsied turned out to be benign.

Diffuse FDG uptake in a normal-sized thyroid gland is nonspecific and unlikely to be related to malignancy. This is most commonly seen as a normal variant or in underlying inflammatory conditions, such as Hashimoto thyroiditis.

Thyroid lymphoma (very FDG-avid) is a rare non-Hodgkin lymphoma (NHL), which can present as a solitary nodule, multiple nodules, or homogeneously enlarged and hypoattenuating thyroid gland.

ADDITIONAL IMAGES (D-F)

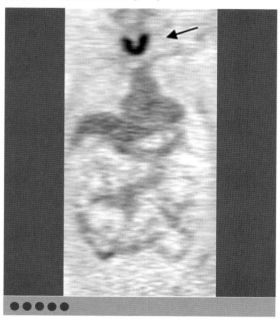

D. Diffuse thyroid uptake, normal variant or thyroiditis (Hashimoto thyroiditis in this instance).

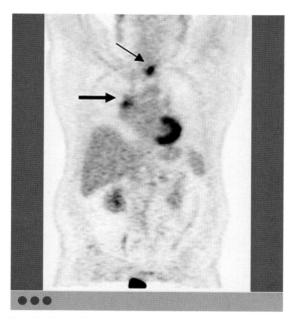

E. Left thyroid Hürthle cell cancer in a patient with right lung primary cancer.

DIFFERENTIAL DIAGNOSIS IMAGES (G-J)

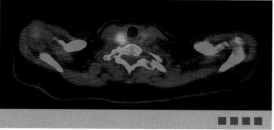

G. Right thyroid lymphocytic thyroiditis, fused PET/CT.

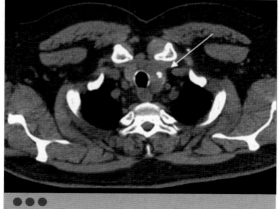

F. Corresponding CT.

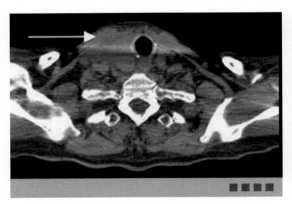

H. Right thyroid B-cell lymphoma in a patient with head and neck primary. Rapidly enlarging right thyroid gland on noncontrast CT.

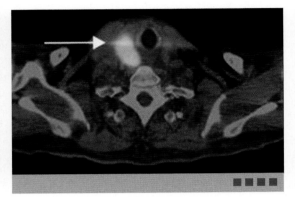

I. Fused PET/CT, right thyroid lymphoma.

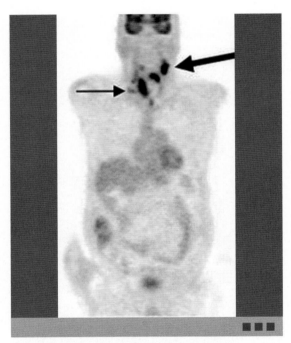

J. Left neck nodal metastasis (thick arrow) from right thyroid primary (thin arrow), coronal FDG/PET.

Joseph Rajendran, MD

PRESENTATION

A 45-year-old female noticed painful swelling in the neck and had symptoms of hyperthyroidism, including tremors and tachycardia.

FINDINGS

The Tc-99m pertechnetate thyroid scan shows poor uptake in the thyroid gland, likely normal sized. The uptake is significantly lower than that of major salivary glands. Gland was smooth on palpation. Iodine 131 (I-131) thyroid uptake at 24 hours was only 4%.

DIFFERENTIAL DIAGNOSES

- *Multinodular goiter*: Patchy uptake in irregularly enlarged gland can have normal or low uptake levels.

- Resolving thyrotoxicosis.

- *Lithium and amiodarone toxicity:* Patient's medical history would clinch the diagnosis

COMMENTS

Hashimoto thyroiditis (also known as autoimmune or chronic lymphocytic thyroiditis) is the most common type of thyroiditis. The thyroid gland is always enlarged in the early stages and might be associated with pain. Damaged thyroid glandular cells enlarge to compensate for the inefficiency in converting iodine into thyroid hormone. The radioactive iodine uptake varies, depending on the stage of the process. By the time these patients are referred for imaging, the uptake is generally very low, indicating an advanced or resolving phase of the process. With progression of disease, the TSH increases as a result of pituitary rebound, but the T4 level continues to fall and the patient eventually becomes hypothyroid. Thyroid uptake can be performed with isotopes of iodine either I-123 or I-131; the advantage of the former is that imaging also can be performed with the same dose. When I-131 is used, thyroid images are performed with Tc-99m pertechnetate; the advantage being the cost. Low radioactive iodine uptake helps differentiate the early stages of this condition from hyperthyroidism. As the condition resolves, the uptake improves but it can stay low for a longer period. When interpreting the

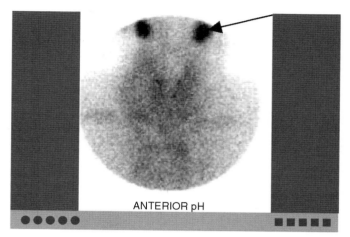

ANTERIOR pH

A. Paucity of uptake in the thyroid glad with a 24-hour uptake of only 4%. Lower uptake in the thyroid gland versus the salivary glands is diagnostic of thyroiditis (anterior). Typically, the low uptake levels preclude images to be obtained.

results, one needs to be aware of other causes for low uptake (eg, iodine intake and overload, thyroid medication that can suppress the uptake). When the uptake is very low, it is typically not possible to perform the thyroid scan, but the uptake values provide very useful clinical information.

PEARLS

- **Patients with thyroiditis and symptoms of hyperthyroidism and suppressed TSH levels can be differentiated from thyrotoxicosis by the presence of low-iodine uptake values.**

- **Iodine load with intake and concurrent thyroid medications should be ruled out as causes for low thyroid uptake.**

- **If I-131 is used to perform uptake, the smallest possible dose is to be used to keep the thyroid radiation exposure to a minimum.**

- **Repeat uptake measurements, although rarely necessary, can be performed if needed but only after the elapse of sufficient time after the test.**

DIFFERENTIAL DIAGNOSIS IMAGE

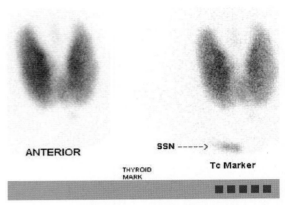

ANTERIOR

THYROID MARK

SSN ----->

Tc Marker

B. Uniformly enlarged thyroid gland with diffusely increased uptake (88% at 24 hours) and the presence of a pyramidal lobe are characteristics of Graves disease.

Chapter 2

MUSCULOSKELETAL

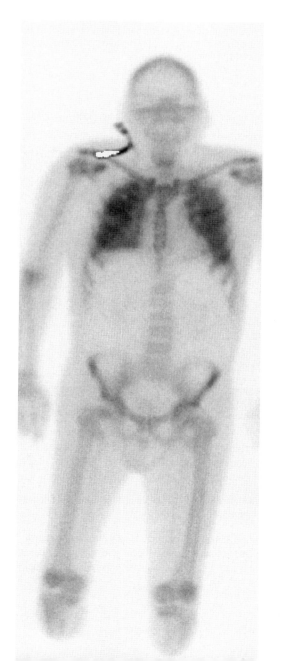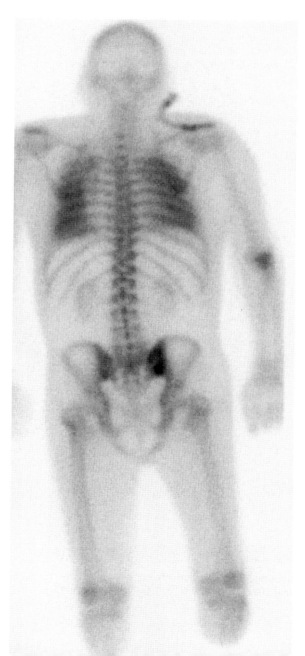

Joseph Rajendran, MD

PRESENTATION

A 56-year-old male with significant weight loss and right upper quadrant (RUQ) and back pain.

FINDINGS

Diffusely increased uptake seen in the right upper abdomen corresponding to the 11 × 9 × 10-cm mass in the liver (segments V/VI) seen on the CT scan.

DIFFERENTIAL DIAGNOSES

- *Prior technetium 99m (Tc-99m) nuclear medicine studies*: Most typically seen after liver spleen scan, but a careful history would help identify the cause.

- *Radionuclide ventriculography (MUGA)*: Presence of radiotracer activity in the blood pool—cardiac and major blood vessels.

- *Hematoma*: Calcified hematoma takes up Tc-99m methylene diphosphonate (MDP) in soft tissues. The history usually establishes the cause.

COMMENTS

Soft tissue uptake on bone scanning can be seen due to either active uptake in a tissue or exaggerated physiologic uptake in tissues that normally show activity. The most commonly seen

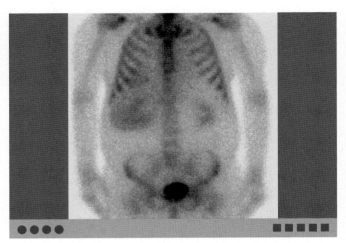

B. Tc-99m MDP anterior abdominal image shows mild diffusely increased uptake in the right upper quadrant corresponding to the metastases in the liver.

abnormal soft tissue uptake of the radiotracer MDP is in the urinary tract. However, abnormal activity can be seen in tissues/organs that normally do not show tracer activity or uptake. A number of conditions can cause this problem: (1) as a result of faulty preparation of Tc-99m MDP, (2) faulty injection, and (3) uptake in soft tissue as a result of processes that have increased blood flow or calcification such as tumors, or metastatic or heterotropic calcification, or hematoma. Soft tissue uptake can also be seen when uptake in hepatic metastases depends on the tumor type and is commonly seen in metastatic disease from colon cancer (adenocarcinoma) as well as primary hepatocellular carcinoma. Other conditions that show uptake in soft tissue on delayed images include sarcomas, meningiomas, and primary breast cancer.

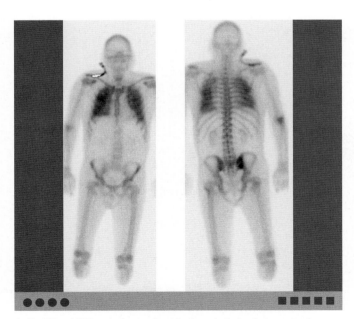

A. Tc-99m MDP anterior and posterior whole body images show diffuse uptake in both lungs consistent with metastatic calcification.

PEARLS

- While bone scan is primarily done for the evaluation of the skeletal system, attention should be given to nonskeletal uptake of the radiotracer as it can direct to the presence of coexisting conditions.

- Pattern and location of the abnormal uptake will help in identifying the pathology.

- Recent history of nuclear medicine imaging with Tc-99m-based tracers will help in explaining the visualization of "abnormal" nonskeletal radiotracer uptake.

DIFFERENTIAL DIAGNOSIS IMAGES (C-G)

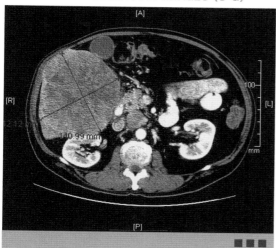

C. CT scan shows enlarged liver, which is widely replaced by metastatic cancer.

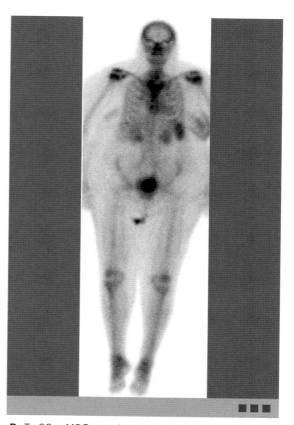

D. Tc-99m MDP anterior whole-body bone scan shows uptake in the breasts (breast cancer), liver, spleen, and cardiac blood pool (previous Tc-99m-labeled RBC for MUGA).

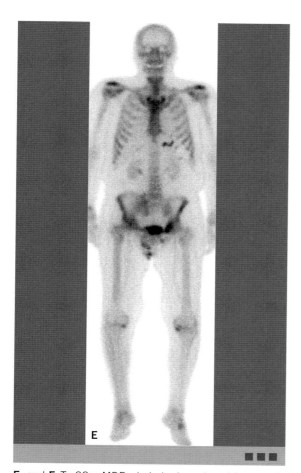

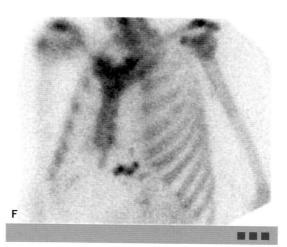

E. and **F.** Tc-99m MDP whole-body and spot images show a curvilinear focus of increased tracer uptake in the soft tissues of the abdominal wall located in the left upper quadrant.

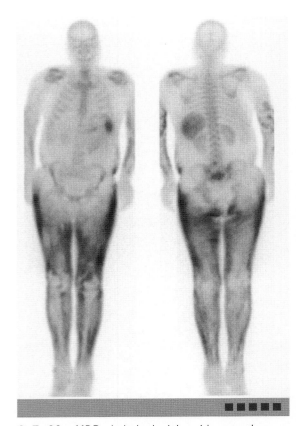

G. Tc-99m MDP whole-body delayed images show diffusely increased uptake in the superficial tissues of bilateral lower extremities in a patient with cirrhosis of the liver and bilateral lower limb edema. Note prominent uptake in the spleen.

Joseph Rajendran, MD

PRESENTATION

Postmenopausal woman with node positive-breast cancer. Long-standing renal failure.

FINDINGS

Bone scan shows diffuse abnormal uptake mainly in the right lung.

DIFFERENTIAL DIAGNOSES

- *Prior Tc-99m nuclear medicine studies*: Macroaggregated albumin (MAA) perfusion lung scan but will show bilateral uptake, and history determines the diagnosis.

- *Metastatic disease*: Rarely can be unilateral from thyroid and osteosarcoma.

- *Metastatic pulmonary calcification*: Usually bilateral involvement.

- *Infection (eg, TB)*: Clinical signs and symptoms point to the diagnosis.

- *Silicosis*: Usually bilateral and there is history of chronic exposure to the causative agent.

COMMENTS

Soft tissue uptake on bone scanning can be seen due to either active uptake in a tissue or exaggerated physiologic uptake in tissues that normally show activity. The most commonly seen abnormal soft tissue uptake of the radiotracer

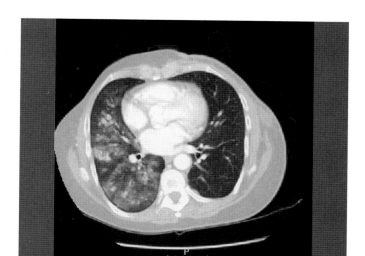

B. CT scan shows diffuse calcification in the right lung.

MDP is in the urinary tract. However, abnormal activity can be seen in tissues/organs that normally do not show tracer activity or uptake. A number of conditions can cause this problem: (1) as a result of faulty preparation of Tc-99m MDP, (2) faulty injection, and (3) uptake in soft tissue as a result of processes that have increased blood flow or calcification such as tumors, or metastatic or heterotropic calcification. Soft tissue uptake can also be seen when uptake in hepatic metastases depends on the tumor type and is commonly seen in metastatic disease from colon cancer (adenocarcinoma) as well as primary hepatocellular carcinoma. Other conditions that show uptake in soft tissue on delayed images include sarcomas, meningiomas, and primary breast cancer.

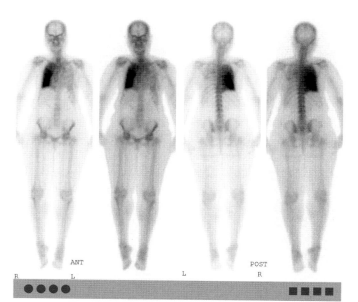

A. Whole-body Tc-99m MDP scan shows diffuse, intensely increased uptake in the right lung (posterior) and probable mild increase in the left lung (anterior).

PEARLS

- While bone scan is primarily done for the evaluation of the skeletal system, attention should be given to nonskeletal uptake of the radiotracer as it can direct to the presence of coexisting conditions.

- Pattern and location of the abnormal uptake will help in identifying the pathology.

- Recent history of nuclear medicine imaging with Tc-99m-based tracers will help in explaining the visualization of "abnormal" nonskeletal radiotracer uptake.

- Metastatic calcification in disease conditions with elevated calcium-phosphate production and deposition of calcium within the soft tissues.

- Can occur anywhere, but predilection is for acidic tissues like lungs, kidneys, stomach.

Vivek Manchanda, MD

PRESENTATION

A woman in early seventies has left distal tibial pain for 4 months. No previous cancer history.

FINDINGS

Mildly hypermetabolic (maximum standardized value [SUV] of 1.8) lesion in distal tibia on FDG PET corresponding to expansile lucent lesion with chondroid mineralization on plain radiograph.

DIFFERENTIAL DIAGNOSES

- *Enchondroma*
- *Bone Infarct*
- *Chondroblastic osteosarcoma*
- *Metastasis*
- *Sessile osteochondroma*

A painful bony lesion with chondroid matrix is highly concerning for chondrosarcoma, even if it is mildly hypermetabolic.

COMMENTS

Chondrosarcomas are primary malignant tumors of cartilaginous origin with chondroid matrix. Many benign etiologies such as enchondroma, osteochondroma, and periosteal chondroma may turn malignant.

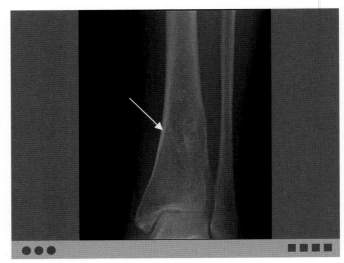

B. Corresponding X-ray showing expansile distal tibial metaphyseal lesion with chondroid calcification.

Fluorodeoxyglucose (FDG) uptake has been used to grade chondrosarcomas. Lower SUVs for grade 1, moderately increased for grade 2, and around 7.10 (+/−2.6) for grade 3 have been described. Some studies have suggested significant differences between patients with and without disease progression, with higher SUVs in patients developing recurrent or metastatic disease compared with lower SUVs in patients without relapse. The combination of SUV and histopathologic tumor grade can improve prediction of outcome, allowing identification of patients at high risk for local relapse or metastatic disease.

However, FDG-PET and receptor-imaging radiopharmaceuticals have low sensitivity in differentiating low-grade chondrosarcomas from benign enchondromas. Low cellularity, mitochondrial specialization, and the presence

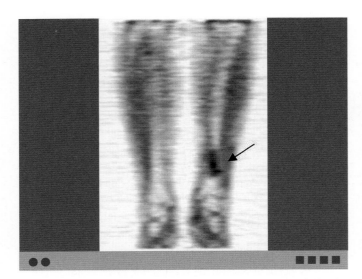

A. Low-grade chondrosarcoma left distal tibia (maximum SUV of 1.8, coronal FDG-PET).

PEARLS

- **FDG-PET scan can be used to differentiate low-grade from high-grade osteochondromas. It is not useful in differentiating enchondromas from low-grade chondrosarcomas, which may show similar FDG activity.**

- **Dedifferentiated chondrosarcomas may not show mineralized matrix and are extremely FDG avid.**

- **Chondrosarcomas can be differentiated from enchondromas by pain, greater endosteal scalloping, osteolysis, and periosteal reaction on the CT.**

of an efflux membrane pump may contribute to poor imaging. A negative FDG-PET scan in a low grade chondrosarcoma should be interpreted carefully.

Features favoring chondrosarcoma over enchondroma in a lesion with chondroid calcifications include location in the axial skeleton and flat bones, pain related to the lesion, deep endosteal scalloping (greater than two-thirds of cortical thickness), cortical destruction (osteolysis around the lesion or in vicinity) and soft tissue mass, periosteal reaction, and tumor size greater than 4 cm.

FDG-PET is a powerful diagnostic tool for detecting high- and intermediate-grade local recurrence. The dedifferentiated chondrosarcomas may not show chondroid matrix and are very FDG avid.

ADDITIONAL IMAGES (C-G)

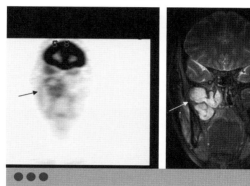

C. Recurrent right maxillary high-grade chondrosarcoma, coronal FDG-PET (attenuation corrected), and coronal T2-W MR images, postcontrast.

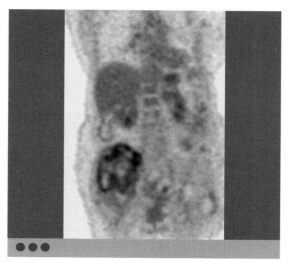

D. Chondrosarcoma of right hip, coronal FDG-PET.

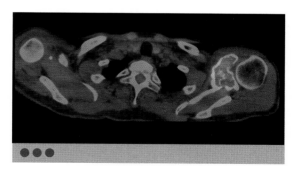

E. Left scapular chondrosarcoma, max SUV of 4.0 (grade 2 out of 3 on path), axial-fused PET/CT.

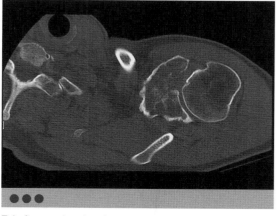

F. Left scapular chondrosarcoma, corresponding axial CT.

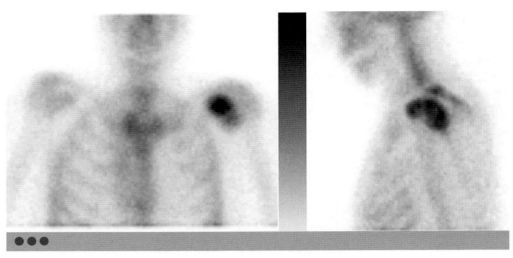

G. Left scapular chondrosarcoma, Tc MDP bone scan.

DIFFERENTIAL DIAGNOSIS IMAGES (H-P)

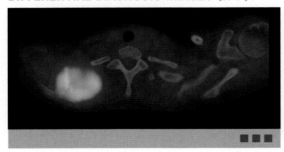

H. Right scapular Ewing sarcoma, 16-year-old female. Axial fused PET/CT.

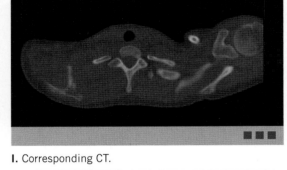

I. Corresponding CT.

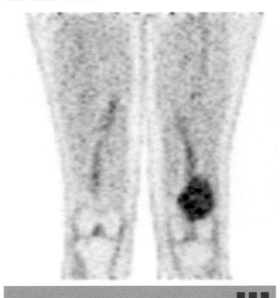

J. Parosteal osteosarcoma, PET, 35-year-old female.

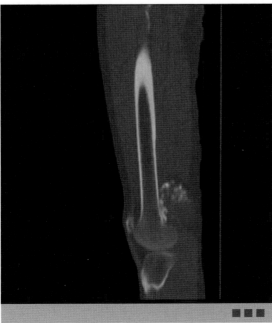

K. Corresponding sagittal CT.

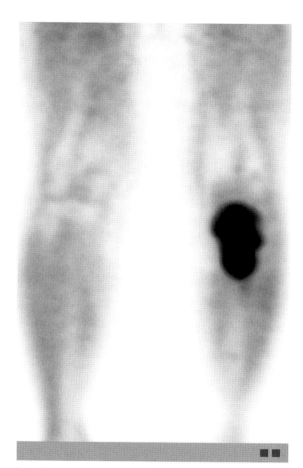

L. Left lower extremity metastasis from colon cancer, 50-year-old male. Coronal FDG-PET.

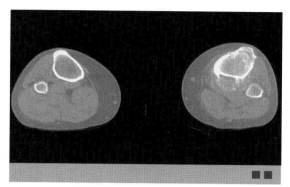

M. Corresponding CT.

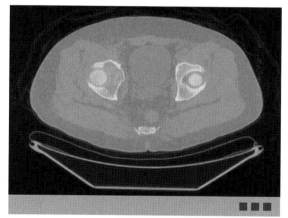

O. Corresponding axial CT, right acetabulum chondroblastoma.

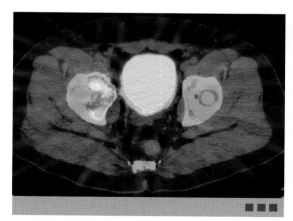

N. Fused axial PET/CT, right acetabulum chondroblastoma.

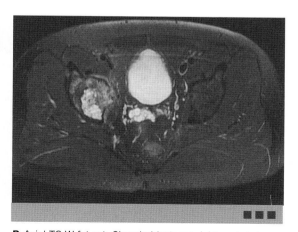

P. Axial T2 W fat sat. Chondroblastoma right acetabulum.

Joseph Rajendran, MD

PRESENTATION

A 72-year-old male post-CVA (cerebrovascular accident), complains of pain and swelling of the distal right upper extremity.

FINDINGS

Tc-99m MDP bone scan images show increased blood pool activity in the distal upper extremity. Delayed images show increased uptake in all the small joints of the right hand.

DIFFERENTIAL DIAGNOSES

• *Chronic degenerative disease*: Blood flow in the three-phase bone scan is usually not increased and delayed

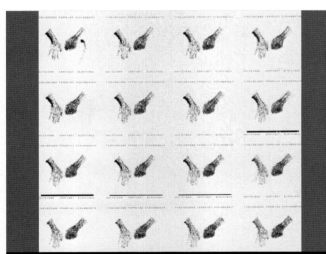

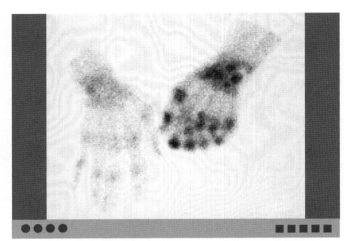

B. Delayed Tc-99m MDP bone scan images of the right upper extremity show uptake in several small joints of the right hand in a periarticular pattern, characteristic of CRPS.

images show bilateral increased articular uptake involving joints randomly. In the distal upper extremity, the first metacarpophalangeal (MCP) joint is the most commonly affected joint.

• *Diffuse inflammatory arthritis (rheumatoid)*: Typically, the blood flow is not as pronounced as that of complex regional pain syndrome (CRPS) except in the very early and acute phases. The classic presentation shows bilateral joint involvement and is typically symmetric. Major joints are also affected by this disease process.

COMMENTS

CRPS, previously referred to as reflex sympathetic dystrophy (RSD), is a neurologic disorder affecting central and peripheral

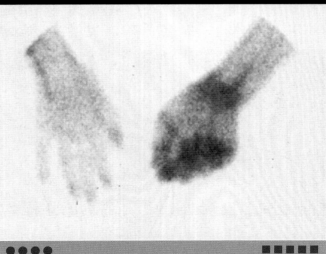

A. Blood flow (*top*) and blood pool (*bottom*) Tc-99m MDP bone scan images show increased blood flow to the distal upper extremity with increased blood pool activity in the same area.

PEARLS

• **Bone scan is very sensitive and shows findings much earlier than other tests and is helpful in the follow-up of patients with CRPS.**

• **Early disease is characterized by increased blood flow, which becomes normal or decreased as the disease progresses.**

• **The classic pattern of increased blood flow, blood pool activity, and increased periarticular uptake is seen in 50% of patients but has the highest specificity and diagnostic accuracy.**

• **Variants of this typical pattern with normal or decreased uptake can be seen in children and some adults.**

nervous systems. It is a chronic pain disorder characterized by intense pain, out of proportion to the severity of the injury or immobilization, which gets worse rather than better over time. In the United States, the incidence of CRPS is approximately 1% to 15% after peripheral nerve injury and 10% to 30% after fractures and contusions. The upper limbs are more frequently affected than the lower. The patient often presents with pain, edema, stiffness, muscle wasting, and discoloration of the affected region. Scintigraphic findings vary, depending on the stage of the disease. Early disease is characterized by increased blood flow, which becomes normal or decreased as the disease progresses. The classic pattern, seen less than 50% of the time but providing the highest diagnostic accuracy, is a unilateral increase in blood flow and blood pool activity with increased periarticular uptake on delayed images. Bone scanning has a sensitivity and specificity of approximately 95%. The degree of these findings decreases with time and eventually shows reduced bone uptake as a result of late vasospasticity. More than 95% of cases show the periarticular uptake on delayed images, although specificity is low if this is seen in the absence of increased blood flow. False positives can be a result of infection or arthritis. Children often have normal or decreased uptake and some adult variants have also been found with cold or decreased uptake.

DIFFERENTIAL DIAGNOSIS IMAGES (C-D)

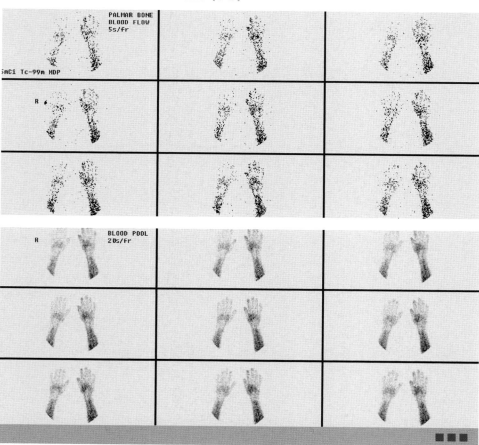

C. Tc 99m MDP blood flow images to the distal upper extremities show reduced blood flow on the right side.

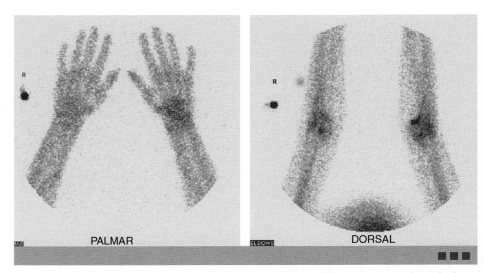

D. Delayed Tc-99m MDP bone scan images of the upper extremities show reduced uptake in the joints of the right hand.

Vivek Manchanda, MD

PRESENTATION

A woman in midthirties with abdominal wall mass and papillary thyroid cancer.

FINDINGS

Moderate to intensely hypermetabolic, well defined mass in the left rectus abdominis muscle.

DIFFERENTIAL DIAGNOSES

- *Metastases*: Leiomyosarcoma, melanoma, thyroid cancer
- *Primary malignancy*: Leiomyosarcoma, fibrosarcoma, spindle cell sarcoma, liposarcoma, lymphoma, fibrous histiocytoma
- *Benign*: Neurofibroma, leiomyoma
- Abscess
- Hematoma

Abscesses, hematomas, and poorly differentiated sarcomas are typically centrally hypometabolic. Neurofibromas are typically only mildly hypermetabolic.

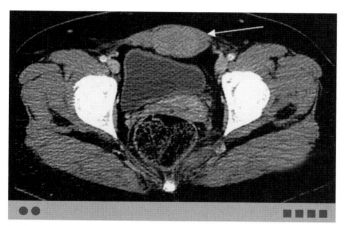

B. Corresponding contrast enhanced axial CT.

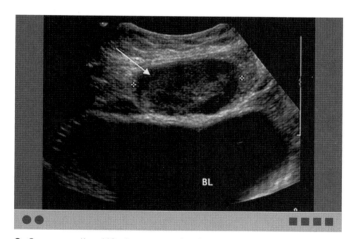

C. Corresponding US shows complex heterogeneous, mixed echogenicity mass.

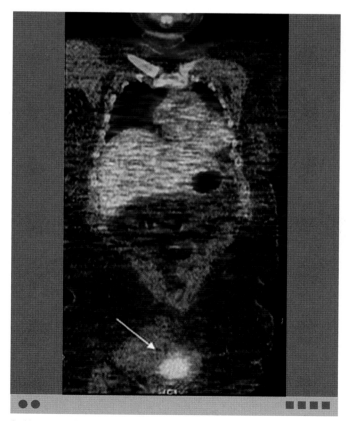

A. Hypermetabolic inferior left rectus abdominis muscle mass (*white arrow*), coronal fused PET/CT.

PEARLS

- Desmoid tumors are locally aggressive, benign fibrous neoplasms that arise from musculoaponeurotic tissues.

- Classic presentation in adults is solid tumor in rectus abdominis muscle in women with previous history of abdominal delivery.

- FDG activity correlates with level of cellularity. It is difficult to differentiate desmoid tumor from fibrosarcoma by PET alone.

- Papillary thyroid cancers are unlikely to metastasize via bloodstream.

COMMENTS

A well-defined, moderate to intensely hypermetabolic mass in the rectus abdominis muscle in a female with prior history of cesarian delivery is very suggestive of desmoid tumor, as the index case turned out to be. Papillary thyroid cancer is unlikely to metastasize via bloodstream.

Desmoid tumors are solid tumors that are locally aggressive and well-differentiated benign fibrous neoplasms that arise from musculoaponeurotic tissues.

Mesentery, rectus abdominis aponeurosis, and internal or external oblique muscles are usual locations. Trauma, surgery, estrogen, Gardner syndrome, and familial polyposis coli are usual associations. The peak incidence is between 25 and 40 years of age (M:F, 1:3). Rare pediatric cases have been reported.

The tumors are composed of abundant collagen surrounding poorly circumscribed bundles of spindle cells. A fibrosarcoma on the other hand has greater mitotic activity and increased nuclear-to-cytoplasm ratio with less collagen. It is difficult to differentiate desmoid tumors from low-grade sarcomas.

Level of FDG uptake correlates with proportion of cellularity, hyalinized collagen, and fibrous composition. The MR features also depend on the features of the lesions. Whereas, initial stage tumors have low signals on T1- and heterogeneously high signals on T2-weighted images (T1- and T2-WI), the later stage tumors have low signals on both T1- and T2-WI owing to increased fibrous composition. Most lesions show marked enhancement after gadolinium infusion. CT features include ill- to well-defined mass with usually higher attenuation than muscle and variable enhancement. On ultrasound, desmoid tumors are well-defined lesions with varying echogenicity.

The desmoid tumor recurrence rate varies from 30% to 70%.

ADDITIONAL IMAGES (D-E)

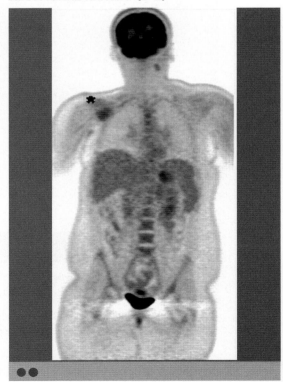

D. Right shoulder desmoid, coronal PET, 16-year-old female (*small black star*).

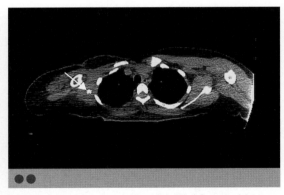

E. Right shoulder desmoid, axial CT, 16-year-old female (*small white star*).

DIFFERENTIAL DIAGNOSIS IMAGES (F-M)

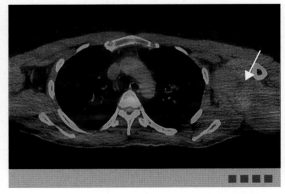

F. Left shoulder myxoid liposarcoma, fused PET/CT, 38-year-old male (*arrow*).

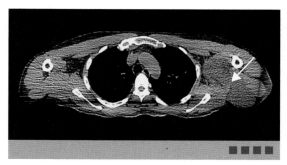

G. Corresponding noncontrast CT (*arrow*).

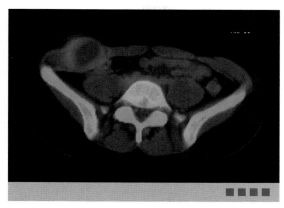

H. Right abdominal wall poorly differentiated spindle cell sarcoma with central necrosis, axial fused PET/CT.

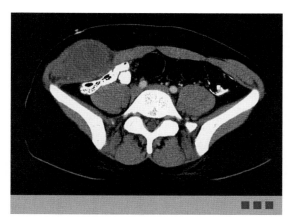

I. Right abdominal wall spindle cell sarcoma with central necrosis, axial contrast CT.

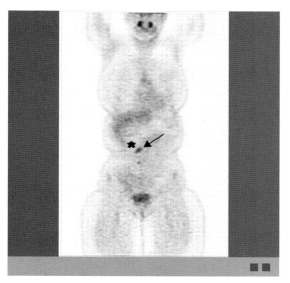

J. Abdominal wall metastatic leiomyosarcoma, PET (*small black star*).

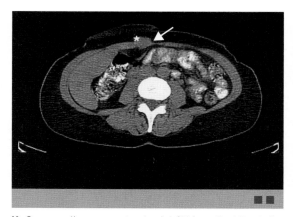

K. Corresonding noncontrast axial CT (*small white star*).

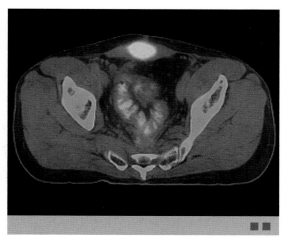

L. Abdominal wall metastatic colon cancer (known peritoneal seeding), fused axial PET/CT.

49

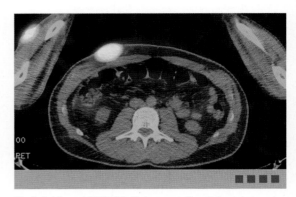

M. Axial fused PET CT. Cutaneous T cell lymphoma, subcutaneous abdominal wall and right arm.

Vivek Manchanda, MD

PRESENTATION

Patient A: Teenager, post therapy FDG-PET scan for Hodgkin lymphoma. G-CSF given 1 week prior to examination.
Patient B: Adult with Neulasta® administered the same day.

FINDINGS

Patient A: Diffuse, homogeneously increased FDG activity in the entire skeleton.
Patient B: Diffuse, heterogeneously mildly increased FDG activity in the entire skeleton.

DIFFERENTIAL DIAGNOSES

- *Leukemia, lymphoma*
- *Metastases*
- *Anemia, thrombocytopenia, leukocytosis* (mild increased FDG)

Uptake associated with diffuse metastases, marrow stimulation from drugs, and lymphomas is higher than that from anemia, thrombocytopenia, and leukocytosis. Smoking has also been attributed with mildly increased diffuse marrow FDG activity.

COMMENTS

Mild diffusely increased FDG uptake in the bone marrow can be seen in patients with marrow hyperplasia as a result of anemia, thrombocytopenia, and leukocytosis. It is commonly seen in patients who are undergoing chemotherapy, as a consequence of supportive therapy with cytokines. Bone marrow stimulants, such as G-CSF (filgrastim), Neulasta, and GM-CSF, and erythropoietin (EPO) can cause diffusely increased FDG uptake in bone marrow (and in the spleen) on PET. If there is concern for marrow metastases or in patients with cancers such as breast or lymphoma or multiple myeloma or melanoma, which can have marrow-based metastases, pharmacologic agents should be stopped for at least 2 to 3 weeks before getting the study.

Diffuse bone marrow uptake of FDG also has been reported in patients with leukemia and lymphoma. Patients with diffuse bone marrow metastases can also present with diffuse FDG uptake in the skeleton. Knowledge of patient's history, including laboratory work and medication history is important to make that distinction.

On contrary, radiation causes marrow to become fatty with fewer residual capillaries, resulting in photopenia on bone scintigraphy and FDG-PET scan.

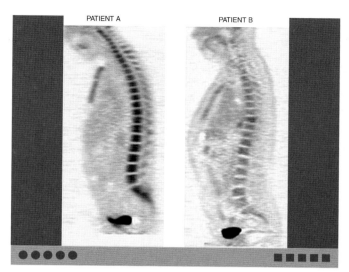

A. Patient A: Diffusely increased FDG uptake in the spine, injected with G-CSF, 1 week before examination. Sagittal FDG-PET.
Patient B: Heterogeneous FDG uptake, injected with Neulasta the same day, sagittal FDG-PET.

In patients who have had both radiation and pharmacologic bone marrow stimulation, a mixed photopenic/diffusely increased FDG uptake may be seen.

Heterogeneously increased FDG activity is concerning for malignancy. Early G-CSF/Neulasta response can appear heterogeneous.

A single intense marrow-based hypermetabolic focus, without corresponding CT finding, may require correlation with MR or biopsy, if it were to change the management of the patient.

PEARLS

- **Diffuse FDG uptake in the skeleton can be seen in marrow stimulation from drugs, leukemia, lymphoma, diffuse metastases (usually intense) and anemia, thrombocytopenia, leukocytosis, and smoking (usually mild).**
- **Radiation therapy usually causes photopenia.**
- **Proper history is very important to distinguish between the patterns of uptake.**
- **Heterogeneous uptake is usually due to metastases, recent marrow stimulation, and radiation combined with marrow stimulation.**

ADDITIONAL IMAGE

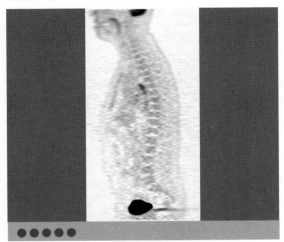

B. Patient B, imaged again without Neulasta. Resolution of heterogeneous mildly increased FDG activity, sagittal FDG-PET.

DIFFERENTIAL DIAGNOSIS IMAGES (C-E)

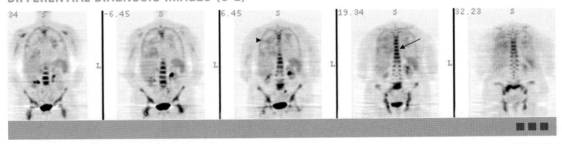

C. Homogeneously increased FDG uptake in diffuse, large B-cell lymphoma involving marrow, coronal FDG-PET.

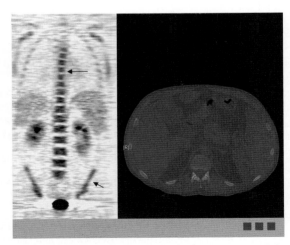

D. Increased FDG activity in marrow disease in Hodgkin's lymphoma, coronal FDG-PET, and corresponding axial noncontrast CT with no obvious abnormality.

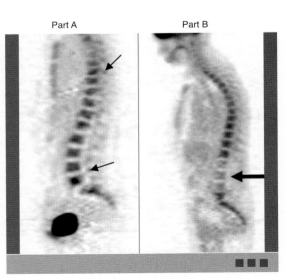

E. Part A: Relatively homogeneous FDG uptake in metastases from breast cancer, sagittal FDG-PET.
Part B: G-CSF-induced increased marrow activity in thoracic spine and photopenia in L2-L4 (*arrow*), from radiation therapy.

Joseph Rajendran, MD

PRESENTATION

A 28-year-old man with acute onset of nontraumatic right ankle edema 3 months prior which gradually progressed to pain, particularly with physical activity.

FINDINGS

Diffuse uptake involving the metaphysis and epiphysis of the long bones and involvement of the calvarium and mandible. Axial skeleton is spared.

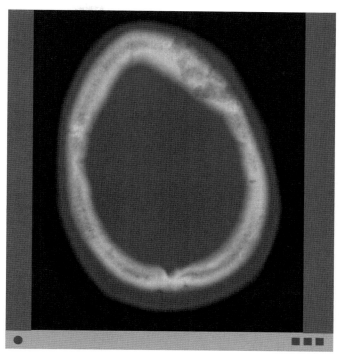

B. CT scan of the skull shows the characteristic radiographic pattern.

DIFFERENTIAL DIAGNOSES

- *Superscan*: Typically involves the entire skeleton and has very minimal to absent renal uptake.

- *Marrow expansion*: Typically involves the long bones, mostly involving areas such as proximal long bones. Axial skeleton rarely shows focal uptake. This process lacks the characteristic appearance of bone expansion.

COMMENTS

Erdheim-Chester disease is a rare form of non-Langerhans cell histiocytosis showing the following pathologic features: irregular thickening of trabeculae in cortical and cancellous bone, marrow fibrosis, and lipid granulomatosis. Pathologic

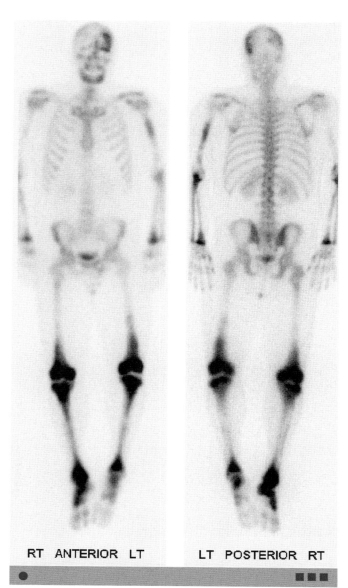

RT ANTERIOR LT   LT POSTERIOR RT

A. Whole-body Tc-99m MDP anterior and posterior scans shows diffuse, intensely increased, abnormal uptake in bilateral forearm bones, distal femora, and proximal and distal tibia and moderately increased uptake in the left frontotemporal region.

PEARLS

- *Triad of presentation*: Diabetes insipidus, exophthalmos, and bone pain

- Generalized diffuse skeletal uptake, involving several long bones, skull, and pelvis

features are similar to Hand-Schüller-Christian and Farber diseases—two types of Langerhans cell histiocytosis. Clinical presentation is highly variable and is mainly due to the extraosseous manifestations. Cardiopulmonary symptoms include dyspnea, ground glass opacities in the lungs, and interlobular septal and pleural thickening. Retroperitoneal: infiltration of fat by histiocytes and associated fibrosis—can cause ureteral obstruction, periaortic fibrosis; neurologic: central diabetes insipidus (most common) secondary to pituitary involvement, cerebellar involvement resulting in ataxia; orbital: large retrobulbar and orbital masses. Variable extraosseous involvement can cause mild or fatal course; however, the classic triad of presentation—diabetes insipidus, bilateral exophthalmos, and bone pain—is seen in many patients.

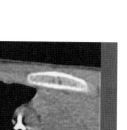

Vivek Manchanda, MD

PRESENTATION

Teenager with painful right rib mass.

FINDINGS

Moderate to intensely hypermetabolic expansile right rib lesion with cortical disruption and soft tissue mass.

DIFFERENTIAL DIAGNOSES

- *Primary bone malignancy:* Ewing's sarcoma, Osteosarcoma

- *Primary lung sarcoma invading bone*

- *Eosinophilic granuloma* (EG) with periosteal reaction

- *Metastases*

- *Multiple myeloma* (MM) (older age group)

- *Lymphoma*

- *Hemangioma*

- *Infection*

Ewing sarcoma (as in the index case) is typically a hypermetabolic chest wall mass with associated bony destruction. FD is usually ground glass expansile lesion and is not

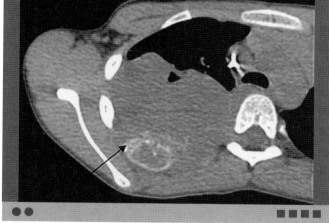

B. Corresponding axial noncontrast CT.

very FDG avid. Primary rib osteosarcomas (hypermetabolic) and rib hemangiomas (usually hypometabolic) are rare. EG, MM, metastases, and lymphoma are usually FDG avid.

COMMENTS

Ewing sarcoma is a small round cell tumor which arises from the undifferentiated mesenchymal cells of bone marrow or primitive neuroectodermal cells. The age group is 5 to 15 years and typical sites include pelvis, scapula, vertebral column, ribs, and clavicle. The commonest site in long bones is femur, followed by humerus, tibia, and bones of the forearm. Ewing sarcoma arises mostly from diaphysis in contrast to commonly metaphyseal origin of osteosarcoma.

It does not have a favorable prognosis among the primary musculoskeletal tumors. Chemotherapy, irradiation, and surgery have increased current long-term survival rates to greater than 50%. In addition, the preferred method of tumor resection has changed; limb salvage has nearly replaced amputation of the affected limb.

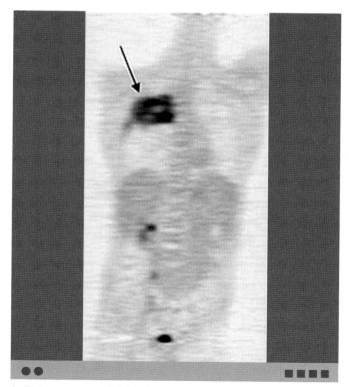

A. Ewing sarcoma of right chest wall, coronal FDG-PET (*arrow*).

PEARLS

- **In evaluation of post-therapy Ewing sarcoma, SUVs lower than 2.5 were associated with a favorable histological response and a 4-year progression-free survival.**

- **A breath-hold CT should be obtained with PET/CT to detect small pulmonary metastases.**

- **PET/CT is more sensitive than bone scan in detecting marrow metastases from Ewing sarcoma.**

Ewing sarcoma has a strong predilection to metastasize, most commonly to the lungs and bone. Bone marrow is another site of metastases, but lymph node metastases is rare.

Most extraskeletal Ewing sarcomas occur during 10 to 30 years of age, with a peak incidence at 20 years. The commonest sites include chest wall, paravertebral muscles, extremities, buttocks, and retroperitoneal space. They can grow and spread like skeletal Ewing sarcoma.

FDG-PET has been successfully used in assessing the therapeutic response prior to surgery. Another potential role is in assessing patients with suspected or known pulmonary metastases.

A breath-hold CT should be included in the protocol for PET/CT for sarcomas to detect small pulmonary nodules.

Patients with lower post-chemotherapy metabolic activity have been shown to have better prognosis with more likelihood of a 4-year progression-free survival.

ADDITIONAL IMAGES (C-G)

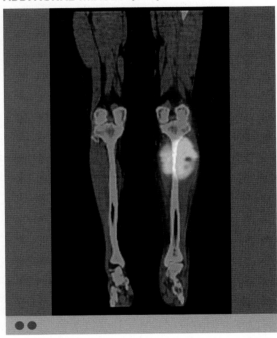

C. Intensely hypermetabolic left proximal tibial Ewing sarcoma, 23-year-old female.

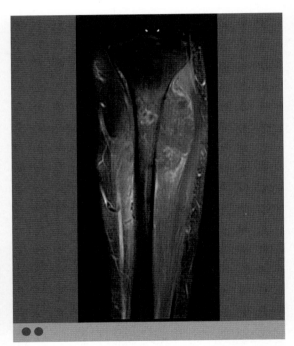

D. Tibial Ewing sarcoma with soft tissue mass, coronal T1W fat sat post contrast, 23-year-old female.

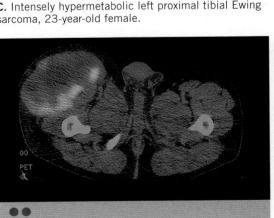

E. Extraskeletal Ewing sarcoma of right hip, axial fused PET/CT in 32-year-old.

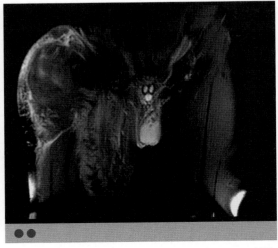

F. Extraskeletal Ewing sarcoma of right hip, coronal T1 fat sat post contrast in 32-year-old male.

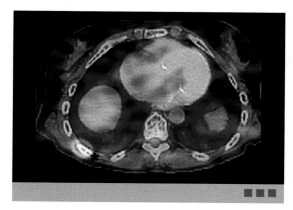

G. Moderately hypermetabolic left ninth rib Ewing sarcoma pre- and post-therapy.

DIFFERENTIAL DIAGNOSIS IMAGES (H-L)

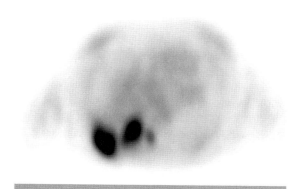

H. Intensely hypermetabolic right chest wall osteosarcoma, axial FDG-PET, 25-year-old female.

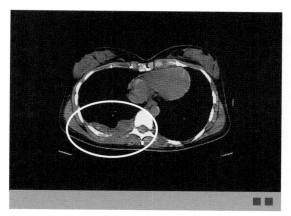

I. Corresponding noncontrast axial CT.

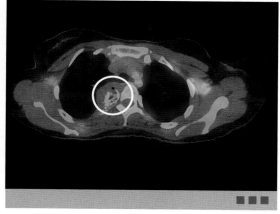

J. Hypometabolic right primary posterior rib hemangioma (*circle*), fused axial PET/CT, and bilateral brown fat uptake.

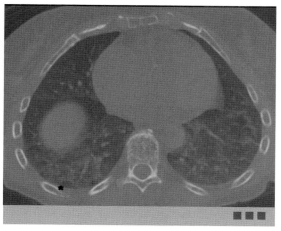

K. Multiple myeloma: Hypermetabolic right eighth rib (*small black star*), 57-year-old-female.

L. Corresponding noncontrast axial CT.

Joseph Rajendran, MD

PRESENTATION

A 28-year-old male status post-crush injury 3 months prior with decreased range of motion in the left hip. Status post-right leg amputation.

FINDINGS

- *Blood flow*: Faint linear uptake adjacent to left femoral shaft

- *Delayed*: Increased radiotracer uptake adjacent to the left femoral shaft

DIFFERENTIAL DIAGNOSES

- *Soft tissue or bone tumors*: Will have characteristic appearances specific to the tumor type on plain films and other cross-sectional imaging.

- *Radioactive contamination*: Foley catheter/urinary contamination can be easily identified by the location of the "uptake" and its disappearance after changing clothes or washing.

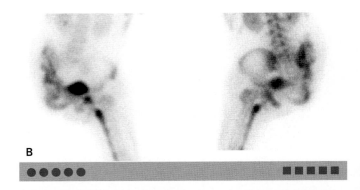

B

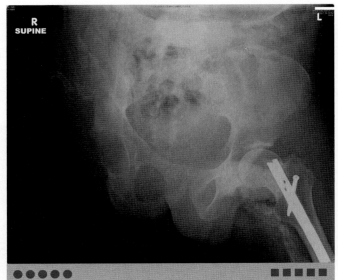

C. Plain radiographs show the presence of HO in the region of left hip joint.

COMMENTS

Heterotopic ossification (HO) is the development and growth of bone tissue in extraskeletal tissues. Contrary to the original

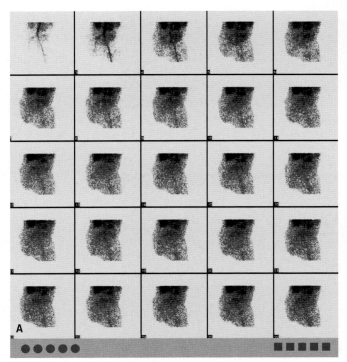

A

A. and **B.** Tc-99m MDP three-phase bone scan shows mildly increased blood flow to the left acetabular region. Delayed images show a linear area of uptake in the same region.

PEARLS

- Serial follow-up bone scanning can be performed to assess the progress of the process. Three-phase bone scan helps establish the maturity of the process.

- Delayed imaging by itself can help establish the maturity of the lesion. Uptake that is equal to that of normal skeleton indicates a matured process.

- Correlation with plain radiograph or CT scan helps plan surgical resection.

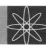

nomenclature (myositis ossificans) that is largely replaced, HO can develop in any soft tissue other than muscles. Under certain stimuli, the osteogenic stem cells in soft tissues that are normally dormant start proliferating and laying down the bone matrix, ultimately resulting in the formation of new bone in varying stages of maturity. HO is typically common in patients after spinal cord injury although other trauma and surgery (hip replacement) are also causative. Clinical symptoms can mimic infection and, depending on the stage of evolution, present with fever, increased erythrocyte sedimentation rate (ESR), and redness and swelling. Following trauma, solitary lesions can undergo spontaneous regression. Biopsy can be falsely positive for sarcoma because of

disorganized cells. In general, biopsy should be avoided as it can further stimulate new bone formation. Level of uptake of MDP is dependent on the stage of heterotopic bone formation—maximal in early stages with equal uptake to that of normal skeleton in late stages. In early stages, perfusion is increased and is normal as the heterotopic tissue matures. Management is usually conservative with surgical resection limited to patients with severely restricted joint mobility and function or those with severe symptoms. Surgery is most successful (without HO recurrence) when HO is mature, and three-phase bone scan is useful to establish maturity—normal blood flow indicating maturity. Uptake on delayed images helps decide the timing of surgery to avoid recurrence.

DIFFERENTIAL DIAGNOSIS IMAGES (D-E)

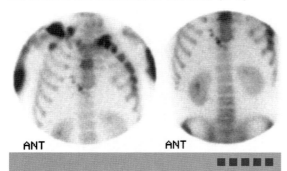

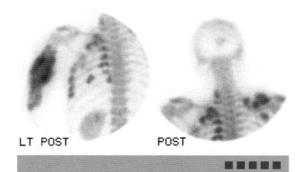

D. Tc-99m MDP bone scan (anterior chest and abdomen) in a patient after motor vehicle accident shows increased uptake in the soft tissues of both arms (HO) and multiple foci of uptake in the ribs and clavicle (fractures).

E. Tc-99m MDP bone scan (posterior chest, head, and neck) in the same patient after motor vehicle accident shows increased uptake in the soft tissues of left arm (HO) and multiple foci of uptake in the ribs and clavicle (fractures).

Naoya Hattori MD, PhD

PRESENTATION

A 49-year-old male patient complains significant bone and joint pain. With bilateral primary non–small-cell lung cancer treated with chemoradiotherapy.

FINDINGS

The Tc-99m MDP bone scan shows multiple non-nodular uptake along the cortex of the long bones in both upper and lower extremities. The symmetrical increase in bone activity and the typical "double stripe sign" can be observed.

DIFFERENTIAL DIAGNOSES

- *Normal bone scan*: Usually seen in younger patients with good bone uptake.

- *Shin splints*: Typically seen in younger patients who are physically active and the findings are mostly located in the posterior aspect of the legs, involving the tibia commonly. Usually seen unilaterally, and accompanied by pain. Plain radiographs do not show any typical findings until in very late stages and when there is focal disease involvement.

- *Periostitis due to stress injury*: Non-nodular periosteal accumulation of Tc-99m MDP.

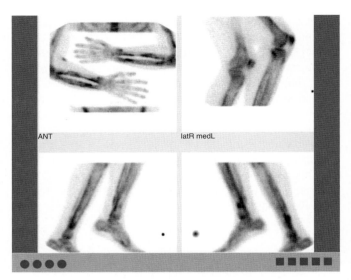

B. Symmetrical uptake in bilateral upper (anterior) and lower extremities.

COMMENTS

Hypertrophic pulmonary osteoarthropathy (HPO) occurs as a nonmetastatic manifestation of lung cancer and can be seen in up to 10% of such patients. It consists of two components: clubbing of the fingers and toes and periostitis of the long bones. Patients may have pain and swelling about the wrists and less commonly the ankles and knees. The pain typically is generalized and mild but can become severe in late stages of the disease. Plain film findings in HPO reveal a thick, lamellar periosteal new bone formation. Bone scan may show patchy or linearly increased activity along the periosteum of long bones.

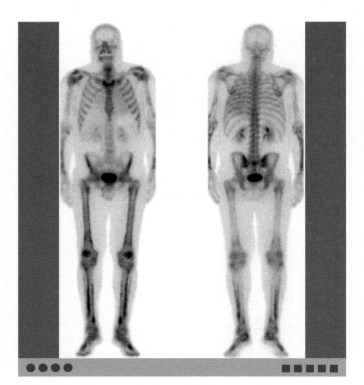

A. Whole-body images showing multiple non-nodular uptake along the cortex of the long bones.

PEARLS

- **Hypertrophic osteoarthropathy is considered to be a paraneoplastic syndrome.**

- **Bilateral uptake or that involving both upper and lower extremities are associated with the risk of neoplasm.**

- **Periosteal involvement of long bones is seen as linearly increased uptake in the cortex of long bones and in a parallel pattern of increased uptake, resulting in the "railroad sign."**

- **Increased uptake can also be seen in the terminal phalanges as a result of increased bone turnover due to clubbing.**

- **There can be associated focal distribution of radiotracer uptake in a pattern typical for the primary cancer in question.**

HPO tends to resolve following tumor resection or chemoradiation. HPO can also be seen in metastatic lung cancer, bronchiectasis, cystic fibrosis, mesothelioma, pneumoconiosis, cyanotic heart disease, and inflammatory bowel disease. Hypertrophic osteoarthropathy can be primary or secondary, both presenting with clinical symptoms of bone and joint pain. Secondary HPO has been described in association with chronic pulmonary disease, neoplasm, hepatopathy, and inflammatory bowel disease. The pathogenesis of the disease is not yet wholly understood, but is considered to be a manifestation of a paraneoplastic syndrome due to high frequency of accompanying neoplastic disease. Scintigraphic findings can be found at the distal ends of metacarpals, metatarsals, and long bones of the extremities. The pattern and intensity of Tc-99m MDP uptake are not necessarily correlated with etiology; however, bilateral upper and lower extremity uptakes are associated with the risk of neoplasm. Lung cancer is a common malignant etiology for HPO.

ADDITIONAL IMAGE

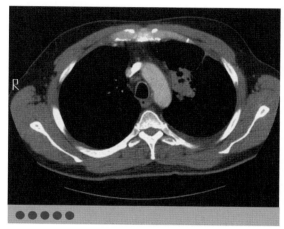

C. Chest CT showing non–small-cell lung cancer in left upper lobe.

DIFFERENTIAL DIAGNOSIS IMAGES (D-E)

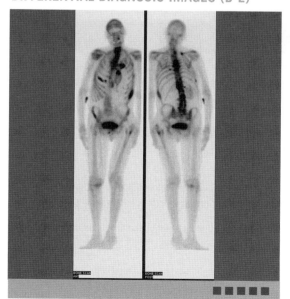

D. Multiple bone metastases: Patient with transitional cell carcinoma of the urinary bladder with widespread metastases in the vertebrae, and ribs. Note lack of periosteal uptake in the extremities. Uptake in the proximal left femur related to left hip prosthesis.

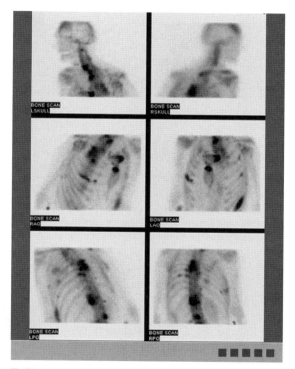

E. Planar spot images showing multiple metastatic disease in the vertebrae, sternum and ribs.

Vivek Manchanda, MD

PRESENTATION

A 21-year-old male with scrotal mass.

FINDINGS

Diffuse mildly increased FDG activity in the right scrotal mass which extends into perineum.

DIFFERENTIAL DIAGNOSES

• Lipoma

• Liposarcoma

Findings favor well differentiated liposarcoma over lipoma given increased FDG activity over background fat FDG activity. Surgery proved same.

COMMENTS

Liposarcoma, a malignancy of fat cells, is one of the commonest soft tissue sarcomas, more commonly seen in men than women. The tumors are of five types: well-differentiated, myxoid, round cell, dedifferentiated, and pleomorphic. Reciprocal gene translocations have been found with round cell and myxoid liposarcoma variants.

Most of the liposarcomas arise de novo. It is rare to develop a liposarcoma from a preexisting lipoma.

The well-differentiated cancer is difficult to differentiate from lipoma, both by FDG-PET and by MR/CT. Irregularly thickened or nodular septae on MR with increased FDG activity (in comparison to normal fat) and heterogeneity on CT is more suggestive of liposarcoma than lipoma. Both well-differentiated and myxoid liposarcomas are low grade and accordingly have lower FDG activity. The commonest finding in the well-differentiated cancer is the presence of fat.

Well-differentiated liposarcomas usually occur in deep soft tissues of both the limbs and the retroperitoneum. They may achieve very large sizes in retroperitoneum before the diagnosis. Myxoid and/or round cell liposarcomas and pleomorphic liposarcomas have a striking predilection for the limbs, and dedifferentiated liposarcomas occur predominantly in the retroperitoneum. Dedifferentiated and pleomorphic liposarcomas are the most aggressive and have the highest FDG activity among the liposarcomas.

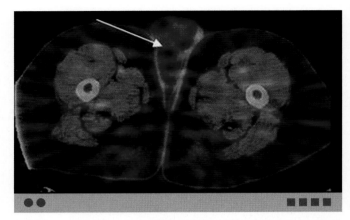

A. Diffuse, mildly increased FDG activity in the right scrotal mass (when compared to subcutaneous fat), which extends into perineum.

In children, liposarcomas account for less than 5% of all soft tissue sarcomas.

Some studies have shown that pretherapy tumor FDG activity is a more important parameter for risk assessment in liposarcoma than tumor grade or subtype. Higher FDG activity resulted in a significantly reduced disease-free survival and identified patients at high risk for developing early local recurrences or metastatic disease.

Spindle cell sarcoma is considered a variant of well-differentiated liposarcoma with abundant spindle cells which can recur locally and dedifferentiate and metastasize.

PEARLS

• **Well-differentiated liposarcomas can be differentiated from lipomas by increased FDG activity than normal fat, by irregular and nodular septae on the MR, and by heterogeneity on CT scans.**

• **Pleomorphic and dedifferentiated liposarcomas are the most aggressive liposarcomas and accordingly have higher SUVs.**

• **In some studies, level of pretherapy FDG activity was the most important parameter for risk assessment.**

• **Myxoid and well-differentiated liposarcomas have predilection for extremities.**

ADDITIONAL IMAGES (B-F)

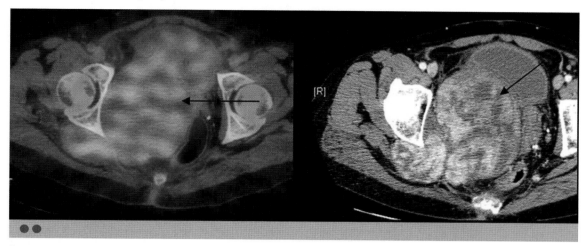

B. Round cell liposarcoma of pelvis.

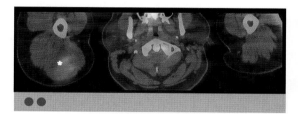

C. Myxoid liposarcoma in right shoulder (*white star*).

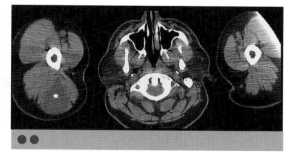

D. Noncontrast CT, myxoid liposarcoma in right shoulder.

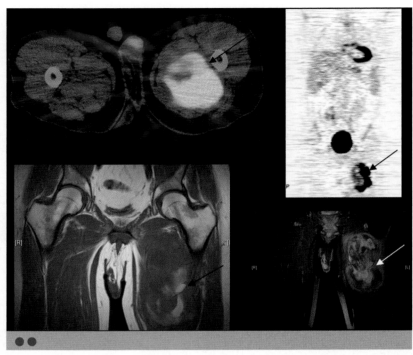

E. Spindle cell sarcoma in left thigh fused axial PET/CT, coronal FDG-PET, coronal T1W, and coronal T1W post contrast images.

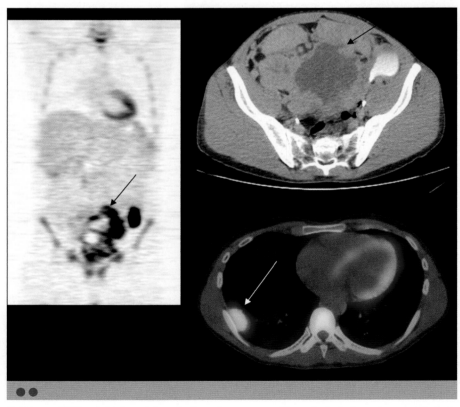

F. Intense FDG uptake in pelvic spindle cell sarcoma with central photopenic necrosis and right lung metastasis. Coronal FDG PET, axial CT, and fused PET CT.

DIFFERENTIAL DIAGNOSIS IMAGES (G-H)

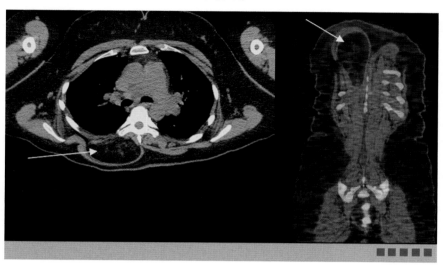

G. Axial noncontrast CT and coronal fused FDG-PET, classic lipoma (*arrows*).

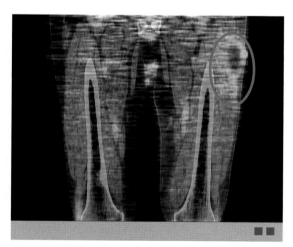

H. Soft tissue malignant fibrous histiocytoma (MFH), left thigh, 77-year-old male, coronal fused FDG-PET (*circle*).

Joseph Rajendran, MD

PRESENTATION

A 21-year-old female with neck pain for 1 year.

FINDINGS

- Radiographs: Sclerotic right C7 pedicle/lamina.

- Technetium 99m methylene diphosphonate (Tc-99m MDP) bone scan: It shows a solitary focal increased uptake in the right posterior elements of the C7 vertebra.

- CT: Lytic lesion with thin sclerotic margins, right anterior portion of C7 lamina. Nidus with small calcifications and no evidence of cortical disruption or soft tissue mass.

DIFFERENTIAL DIAGNOSES

- *Infection/osteomyelitis*: Patients typically present with pain, fever, and leukocytosis.

- *Eosinophilic granulomas*: Characteristic lytic pattern is seen on plain radiographs.

- *Osteosarcoma*: More cortical/periosteal and soft tissue changes noted.

COMMENTS

Osteoblastoma is an uncommon benign tumor of the bone (1% of all bone tumors) and has a lot of similarities to

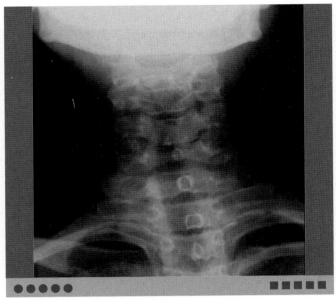

B. Radiographs: Sclerotic right C7 pedicle/lamina.

osteoid osteoma. It is commonly seen in the spine (55% posterior elements alone, 45% posterior elements and vertebral body) and typically in young patients (90% in second and third decades). There is male M>F 2:1. It can present similar to osteoid osteoma, or with paresthesias, paraparesis, paraplegia Tx with excision (recurrence 10%-15%). Well-circumscribed radiolucent lesion contains a thin shell of peripheral new bone that separates it from the surrounding soft tissue. It is larger than 2 cm in diameter and without a large reactive zone of bone around it, unlike osteoid osteoma. Bone scan shows focus of increased uptake and is nonspecific. Biopsy confirms the diagnosis. Osteoblastomas in the spine typically involve the posterior elements. A well-circumscribed lesion with expansion in this location, there is a greater likelihood for it to be osteoblastoma. Treatment is primarily with excision and has a recurrence of 10% to 15%.

PEARLS

- Osteoblastoma is benign tumor of the bone with many similarities to osteoid osteoma.

- Bone scan is not specific but is helpful to clinch the diagnosis when used in conjunction with other imaging methods.

- Biopsy confirms the diagnosis.

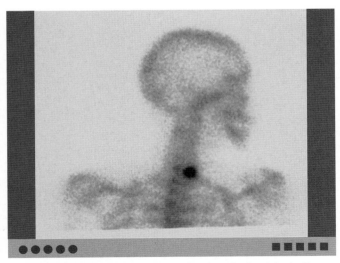

A. Tc-99m MDP bone scan: Solitary focal marked uptake in the right posterior elements at C7.

DIFFERENTIAL DIAGNOSIS IMAGES (C-E)

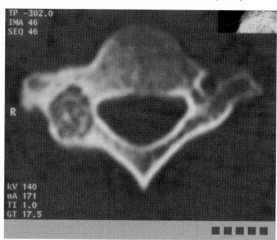

C. CT: Lytic lesion with thin sclerotic margins, right anterior portion of C7 lamina. Nidus with small calcifications and no evidence of cortical disruption or soft tissue mass.

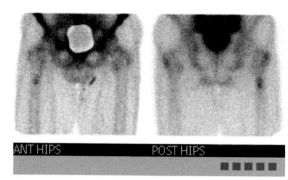

D. Tc-99m MDP bone scan (anterior and posterior hips) shows a focus of increased tracer uptake in the proximal right femur.

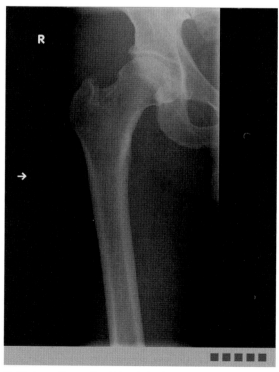

E. Plain radiograph of the right femur shows the location of osteoid osteoma in the proximal femur (*white arrow*).

Joseph Rajendran, MD

PRESENTATION

A 26-year-old female patient presented via outpatient care facility with leg pain. Plain X-ray showed mildly suspicious changes for neoplasm.

FINDINGS

Tc-99m MDP whole-body images show an area of abnormally increased radiotracer uptake in the distal right femur involving both the condyles. There is diffuse mildly increased uptake in the proximal right tibia as a result of hyperemia. Rest of the bones show uptake within normal limits.

DIFFERENTIAL DIAGNOSES

• *Trauma*: In some cases, trauma can precede the development of osteosarcoma and is not an etiology. History and radiological appearance will confirm the diagnosis.

• *Infection*: Typically associated with fever, pain and leukocytosis, and clinical tenderness at location. There typically is lack of soft tissue uptake.

COMMENTS

Osteosarcoma most commonly occurs in the extremities of long bones near metaphyseal growth plates. Femur is the most commonly involved bone—more than 40%. Its incidence increases with the age and reaches its peak in adolescence. While lungs are the most common sites for metastases, other bones of the skeleton can be involved with metastases as well. The role of bone scan is in detecting skeletal metastases rather than in assessing tumor margins or the degree of soft tissue involvement as bone scan does not have the resolution to accurately determine the margins of the tumor and the degree of soft tissue invasion. MRI and CT are superior. Bone scan retains its utility because patients survive longer and hence develop bony metastases more frequently. Besides, it has ability to scan the whole body. The differential diagnosis for nonspecific findings such as this would include infection, that is, osteomyelitis and fracture. In an elderly patient, Paget disease would be a strong possibility. If increased activity were seen on both sides of the joint, inflammatory arthritides could also be considered. Presence of calcified metastases in the lungs can show intense uptake in the lung lesions.

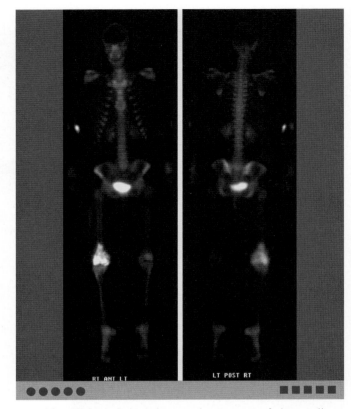

A. Tc-99m MDP whole-body images show an area of abnormally increased radiotracer uptake in the distal right femur involving both the condyles (anterior). There is diffuse mildly increased uptake in the proximal right tibia as a result of hyperemia (posterior). Rest of the bones show uptake within normal limits without evidence of metastases. There is a large focus of bone expansion with new bone formation in the soft tissues matching the mass seen on MRI. The findings are typical for osteogenic sarcoma.

PEARLS

• **Bone scanning helps identify the presence of skeletal metastases more than delineating the margins of the primary tumor. MRI is superior for the latter purpose.**

• **Calcified lung metastases show intense uptake of Tc-99m MDP.**

• **Soft tissue edema may be seen in the limb distal to the primary lesion.**

• **Blood flow as well as delayed images show increased flow and uptake in the affected limb secondary to increased blood flow associated with the osteosarcoma tumor that is typically hypervascular.**

ADDITIONAL IMAGES (B-C)

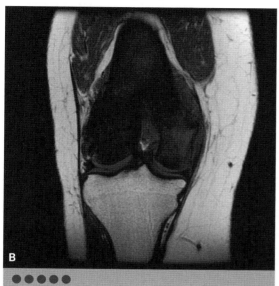

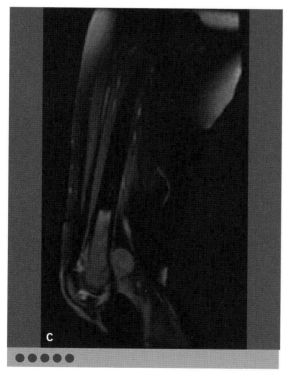

DIFFERENTIAL DIAGNOSIS IMAGES (D-F)

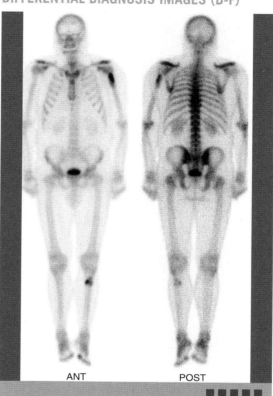

ANT   POST

D. In another case with osteosarcoma, anterior and posterior. Tc-99m MDP whole-body images show a linear area of abnormally increased radiotracer uptake in the proximal left humerus and proximal left tibia.

B. and **C.** There is an infiltrative mass involving the distal femur with an exophytic component extending into the posterior soft tissues. The marrow margin is indistinct and there is infiltration and destruction of the cortex.

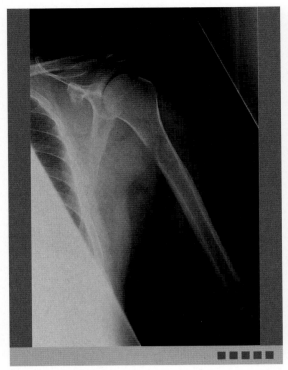

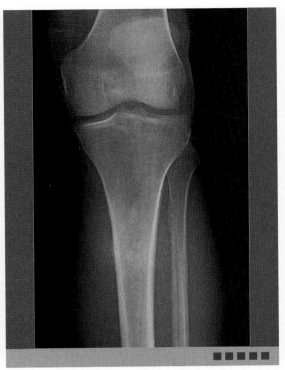

E. Plain radiograph of the left shoulder shows the linear radiolucent area in the proximal humerus corresponding to the bone scan abnormality on Figure D.

F. Plain radiograph of the left knee shows the area of abnormality in the proximal left tibia corresponding to the bone scan finding on Figure D.

Vivek Manchanda, MD

PRESENTATION

Teenager with prior history of left femoral osteosarcoma.

FINDINGS

Multiple hypermetabolic pulmonary lesions, with corresponding CT showing pulmonary nodules.

DIFFERENTIAL DIAGNOSES

- *Metastases such as from osteosarcoma*
- *Infection such as fungal*
- *Lymphoma*

Hypermetabolic pulmonary nodules in a patient with a history of osteosarcoma are most consistent with pulmonary metastases.

COMMENTS

Osteosarcoma is a primary bone malignancy, with two age peaks. Majority of the cases occur in the late teens and the second peak is in the elderly.

Metaphysis of long appendicular bones (distal femur, proximal tibia, and proximal humerus) is involved in younger patients as compared to axial and previously radiated bones in older (7-15 years postradiation) or Paget's disease or fibrous dysplasia. Osteosarcomas are seen in association with retinoblastomas, Li-Fraumeni syndrome, Rothmund-Thomson syndrome, and Bloom syndrome.

Current treatment recommendations for osteosarcoma include neoadjuvant chemotherapy and surgical resection (limb salvage), followed by postoperative chemotherapy.

Osteosarcoma subtypes include conventional osteoblastic osteosarcoma (majority), chondroblastic, fibroblastic, telangiectatic, small cell, and giant cell. The response to chemotherapy is best with fibroblastic subtypes and poorest with the chondroblastic subtypes.

Nonmetastatic disease presentation has good prognosis. Most relapses occur within the first 5 years. The average survival after a recurrence is less than 1 year. Among those who do achieve a second remission, majority develop a second relapse within 1 year.

In a poor responder, often identified by FDG PET, attempts for therapeutic intensification are accomplished by changing chemotherapy agents.

FDG-PET can give valuable information regarding optimal biopsy site and response.

FDG-PET has a good sensitivity in detecting lung and bony metastases. NAC PET images and CT are best to identify lung metastases.

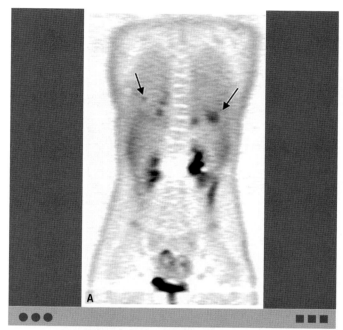

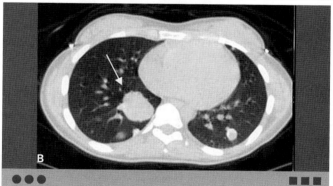

A. and **B.** Pulmonary metastases from osteosarcoma, NAC FDG-PET image and CT, 16-year-old female.

PEARLS

- Pulmonary metastasis is the commonest form of distant spread in sarcomas and osteosarcoma (in 80% of patients), and bone involvement is the second most common (15%).

- A breath-hold chest CT is recommended with PET/CT to detect small pulmonary metastases.

- Some studies have compared both MR and FDG-PET for metastases in bone and have found them complementary.

- PET can play an important role in guiding biopsy.

Prognostic indicators for osteosarcoma include metastatic disease, size and location, response to neoadjuvant chemotherapy, and surgical remission. Per studies, higher level of FDG activity in primary osteosarcoma and post-chemotherapy has been associated with poorer prognosis.

DIFFERENTIAL DIAGNOSIS IMAGES (C-F)

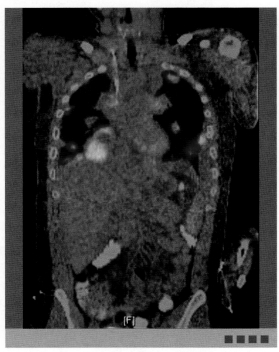

C. Metastases from peripheral neuroectodermal tumor to the lungs, 17-year-old male.

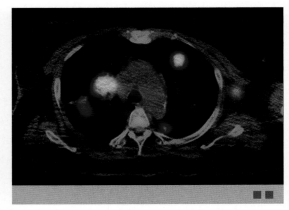

D. Pulmonary and left axillary involvement in non-Hodgkin lymphoma, 17-year-old female.

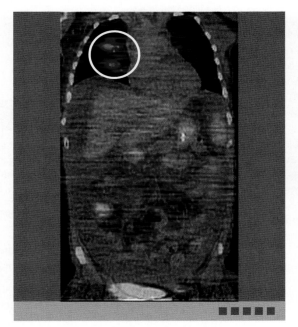

E. Pulmonary infection in a 47-year-old male fused PET/CT, note ascites.

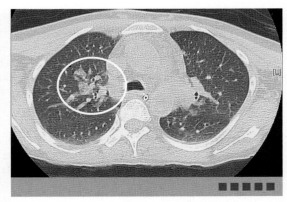

F. Chest CT with right upper lobe pneumonia (*circle*) that resolved in 2 weeks, 47 year old male.

Joseph Rajendran, MD

PRESENTATION

An 82-year-old with invasive urothelial carcinoma of the bladder.

FINDINGS

There is intensely increased uptake in the right hemipelvis involving all the bony components.

DIFFERENTIAL DIAGNOSES

- *Bony sclerosis* without osseous enlargement, including blastic metastases, myelofibrosis, renal osteodystrophy, FD, fluorosis, mastocytosis, and tuberous sclerosis.

- *Calvarial hyperostosis*: Hyperostosis frontalis interna, FD, and metastatic disease.

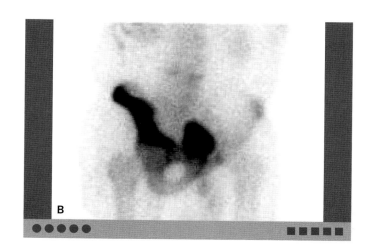

- *Metastatic disease* from prostate cancer has similar appearance, but radiographic or CT appearance and serum tumor markers help differentiate the condition.

- *SAPHO syndrome*: Synovitis, acne, pustulosis, hyperostosis, and osteomyelitis. Hyperostosis is multifocal and the associated findings confirm the diagnosis.

COMMENTS

Paget disease of the bone, also known as osteitis deformans, is a metabolic disorder characterized by abnormal osseous remodeling. A chronic disease of unknown etiology affecting the older population, it results in enlarged, coarsened bones. In the United States, it affects 3% to 4% of the general population older than 40 years and occurs more commonly in the northern United States than in the South. Paget disease may be monostotic but is more commonly polyostotic. The following bones are the most frequently affected: pelvis, femur, tibia, humerus, lumbar and thoracic spine, and calvaria. Patients are often asymptomatic but pain is the

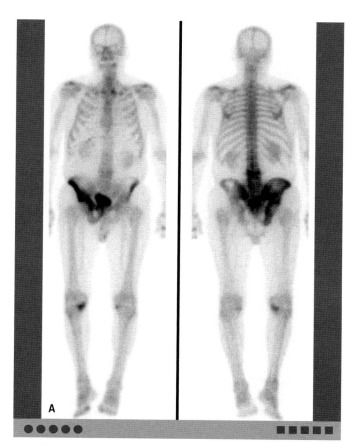

A. and **B.** Whole-body and spot Tc-99m MDP scan images show diffuse intensely increased uptake in the right hemipelvis and L4 vertebra involving the entire bone.

PEARLS

- Imaging and particularly bone scan can be less obvious in very early stages.

- Bone scan is helpful in detecting the polyostotic presentations.

- Bone scanning can not differentiate Paget disease from metastatic disease.

most common symptom. Depending on the site of involvement, headaches and hearing loss can also occur. The most common complications are insufficiency and pathologic fractures. Rare complications of pagetic bone include the development of osteosarcoma. The disease is diagnosed using one or more of the following techniques: X-rays, elevated alkaline phosphatase test, and bone scans. Radiographic findings are often diagnostic in patients with Paget disease. A bone scan is useful in evaluating the extent of the disease. The scintigraphic appearance is striking, with intensely increased tracer localization involving the entire bone.

DIFFERENTIAL DIAGNOSIS IMAGES (C-E)

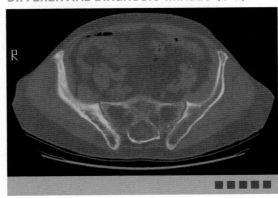

C. CT scan of the pelvis shows expansion and sclerosis of the right hemipelvis, characteristic of Paget disease.

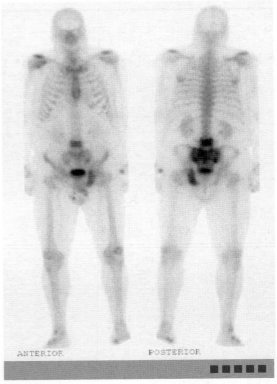

D. Whole-body Tc-99m MDP scan images show diffuse intensely increased uptake in multiple bones-sacrum, L4 vertebra, and left ischium, characteristic of Paget disease.

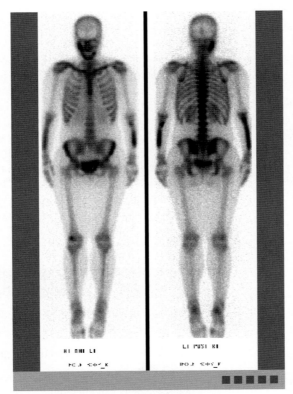

E. Whole-body and spot Tc-99m MDP scan images show diffuse intensely increased uptake in multiple bones in the forearms and right mandible in a patient with SAPHO syndrome.

Joseph Rajendran, MD

PRESENTATION

A 67-year-old smoker with a history of recently diagnosed renal cell cancer or carcinoma (RCC) presenting with diffuse pain in the left hip for several months duration.

FINDINGS

Tc-99m MDP, 3 hours delayed whole-body and spot images show a photopenic area in the left acetabulum with a rim of increased activity at the periphery. There are additional areas of increased uptake in the thoracic vertebrae and adjacent ribs consistent with metastases.

DIFFERENTIAL DIAGNOSIS

• *Solitary plasmacytoma*: Appearances are similar to this but history and clinical, imaging, and pathologic findings will help differentiate.

COMMENTS

RCC accounts for about 3% of adult malignancies and is the most common renal cancer in 90% to 95% of cases. It is frequently diagnosed in late stages, showing metastatic disease at presentation. RCC arises from the proximal renal tubular epithelium. Renal cancer occurs in both sporadic and hereditary forms. von Hippel-Lindau (vHL) syndrome is one of the most common hereditary forms of RCC and is associated with mutations in the vHL protein, causing over-expression of vascular endothelial growth factor (VEGF). This results in multiple angiomatosis. Skeletal metastases from RCC are typically osteolytic in sharp contrast to prostate cancer metastases. Hence the sensitivity for detecting a small metastases from RCC in the bone can be significantly lower. However, larger lesions are clearly seen as photopenic areas with minimal reactive bone activity in the adjacent normal bone.

A. and **B.** Tc-99m MDP whole-body images show a large area of photopenia in the left acetabulum with a thin rim of mildly increased radiotracer uptake. This corresponds to the subtle abnormality seen at the left acetabulum on plain radiograph of the pelvis. There are also other foci of increased uptake—right ninth and left seventh ribs posteriorly, right mid-femur, left scapula (glenoid region), and seventh and eighth thoracic vertebrae.

PEARLS

• Primary presentation can be due to skeletal metastases.

• Careful inspection of the skeleton is needed to detect the presence of photopenic areas (due to purely osteolytic lesions).

• Other tumors associated with purely osteolytic metastases include thyroid, melanoma, lung, and breast cancers.

• It is important to look for photopenic foci in weight-bearing bones that are at greater risk for fracture. Correlative radiographs should always be performed to confirm the structural integrity of the bone.

• Frequently, foci of predominantly increased radiotracer uptake can be seen and are due to the reactive bone process as a result of osteolytic metastases.

• When patients present with metastases as the presenting symptom and photopenic metastases are found on bone scan, it is important to inspect the kidney morphology to detect defects in the kidney structure that might point to the presence of the primary tumor. Renal primary should be the first differential diagnosis in such cases.

ADDITIONAL IMAGE

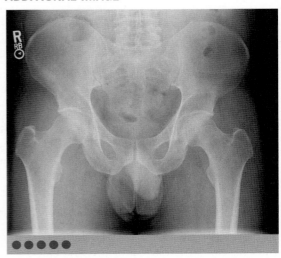

C. Plain radiograph of the pelvis shows an osteolytic area in the left superior acetabulum corresponding to the photopenic area on bone scan.

Joseph Rajendran, MD

PRESENTATION

A 35-year-old male complaining of diffuse muscular pain in both thighs and anterior abdominal wall after strenuous exercise.

FINDINGS

On delayed whole-body Tc-99m MDP images, diffusely increased soft tissue uptake is seen in bilateral thighs and abdomen. Note the uptake shows geographic pattern of the various muscle groups in the thighs and anterior abdomen. Kidneys can show diffusely increased uptake as a result of the process.

DIFFERENTIAL DIAGNOSES

* *Electrical burns*: Usually at the point of contact; history will help with the diagnosis.

* *Myalgias from other etiologies*: Usually generalized and confirmed by the history. Rare complication of statins is rhabdomyolysis; however, imaging is typically not required to diagnose these conditions.

COMMENTS

Rhabdomyolysis is the rapid breakdown of skeletal muscle fibers due to physical or chemical trauma. This results in the release of potentially toxic cellular components, mainly creatine phosphokinase (CPK), into the bloodstream, leading to acute renal failure. In the United States, rhabdomyolysis accounts for 8% to 15 % of the cases of acute renal failure.

Although some patients may present with the classic clinical triad of myalgias, generalized weakness, and dark urine, findings often considerably vary and the clinician needs to pay close attention to the history. Rhabdomyolysis has multiple etiologies, ranging from crush injuries to drug abuse, and is multifactorial. It can be a rare complication of statin therapy when patients present with polymyalgia involving many muscle groups and not related to strenuous exercise. Rhabdomyolysis appears to be a relatively common sequela of strenuous exercise in up to 40% of the time. Tc-99m MDP bone scan is a useful diagnostic test in clinically suspected rhabdomyolysis and can also localize and quantify the muscular involvement. When combined with phosphate, calcium buildup in damaged tissue provides a site for radionuclide deposition. The localization of skeletal tracers in damaged skeletal muscle is similar to that in cardiac muscle and hence the time course of scintigraphic abnormality appears similar to that for acute myocardial infarction. The greatest uptake in the muscles is seen in 24 to 48 hours post-injury and these changes typically resolve within 1 week after the insult.

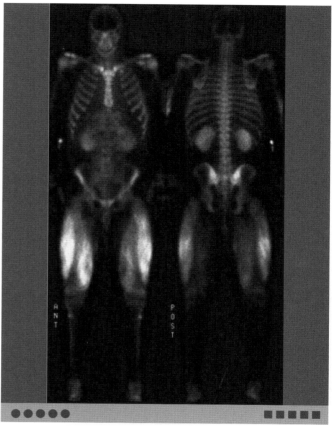

A. Whole-body Tc-99m MDP images (anterior and posterior) show normal uptake in the bones. There is diffusely increased uptake in several muscle groups in both the thighs and anterior abdomen, involving the quadriceps and rectus abdominis. Kidneys show prominent but normal uptake.

PEARLS

* Geographic localization of radiotracer uptake is diagnostic of the etiology.

* Maximum radiotracer uptake is seen in 24 to 48 hours and shows resolution within 1 week.

* Bone scanning is rarely used in the primary diagnosis of rhabdomyolysis as history and other findings are usually able to clinch the diagnosis. But it can be used in situations that are difficult to establish the diagnosis.

* Diffuse renal parenchymal uptake may be seen as part of this disease process.

DIFFERENTIAL DIAGNOSIS IMAGE

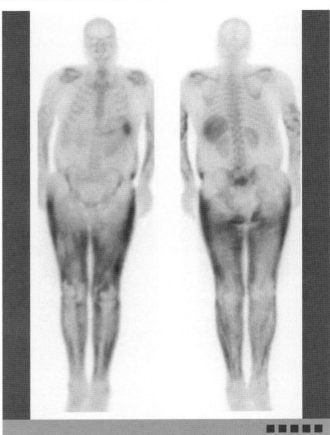

B. Tc-99m MDP whole-body delayed images show diffusely increased uptake in the superficial tissues of bilateral lower extremities in a patient with cirrhosis of the liver and bilateral lower limb edema. Note prominent uptake in the spleen. Note uptake in the subcutaneous tissues is not as geographic as in image A.

Case 2-18 Septic Arthritis

Naoya Hattori, MD

PRESENTATION

A 59-year-old male found to have a low-grade fever, neutrophilic leukocytosis (white blood cell [WBC] count 17 × 10^9) cells per liter, elevated ESR (106 mm), and hyperuricemia (8.9 mg/dL).

FINDINGS

The Tc-99m MDP bone scan shows increased blood flow and tracer uptake in the left ankle region.

DIFFERENTIAL DIAGNOSES

- *Osteomyelitis*: Osteomyelitis presents with either an increased or a decreased uptake which may extend beyond the limits of a joint capsule.

- *Brodie abscess*: Localized and low-grade infection in the bones, typically positive only on the delayed images.

COMMENTS

Septic arthritis can be due to direct invasion of joint space by various microorganisms but majority of the times caused by bacterial infection. Early recognition of septic arthritis is very important to institute treatment that will avoid significant

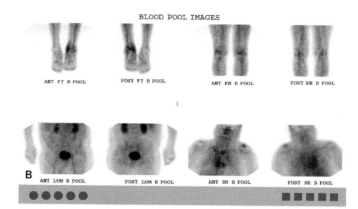

BLOOD POOL IMAGES

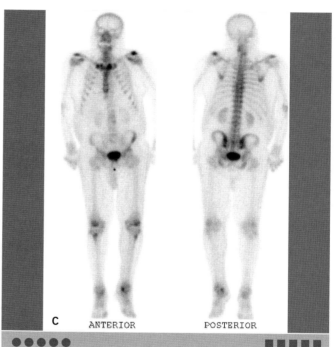

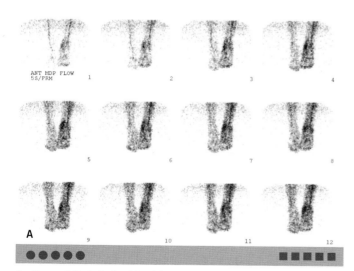

A., B., and **C.** Anterior blood flow images of Tc-99m MDP shows increased blood flow to the left lower extremity. Blood pool images of that region show increased blood pool activity (medial greater than lateral) and in the region of the left acromioclavicular joint. Delayed images show mild, diffusely increased uptake in the left ankle and both knee joints. There are focal areas of increased uptake in the medial left ankle, left acromioclavicular joint, both knee joints, and left sternoclavicular joint. (*Images courtesy of Naoya Hattori, MD, PhD.*)

morbidity. Prosthetic joint infections are becoming a common clinical presentation. Tc-99m MDP bone scan, particularly three-phase, is a highly sensitive tool (sensitivity > 90%) in the diagnosis of bone and joint infection. Scintigraphy is

PEARLS

- Scintigraphy is particularly useful in diagnosing infection in hip, pelvis, shoulder, spine, and foot.

- Diagnosis of septic arthritis is made when an increased or decreased uptake extend a short distance on either side of the joint line, but limited to and uniformly within the joint capsule.

particularly useful in diagnosing infection in hip, pelvis, shoulder, spine, and foot, although diagnosis of osteomyelitis of the long bone is relatively easy and does not require scintigraphic assessment. The infection can be seen as either an increased uptake (hot scan) or a decreased uptake (cold scan). The reported positive predictive value was 86% (82% for a hot scan and 100% for a cold scan) and the negative predictive value was 63%. False-positive scans were sometimes due to contiguous soft tissue infection or may be caused by secondary hyperemia. Diagnosis of septic arthritis is made when an increased or decreased uptake extend a short distance on either side of the joint line, but limited to and uniformly within the joint capsule. If the distribution of uptake within the joint capsule is not uniform or if extension beyond the joint capsule is extensive or asymmetrical, the case is diagnosed as osteomyelitis rather than septic arthritis.

DIFFERENTIAL DIAGNOSIS IMAGES (D-F)

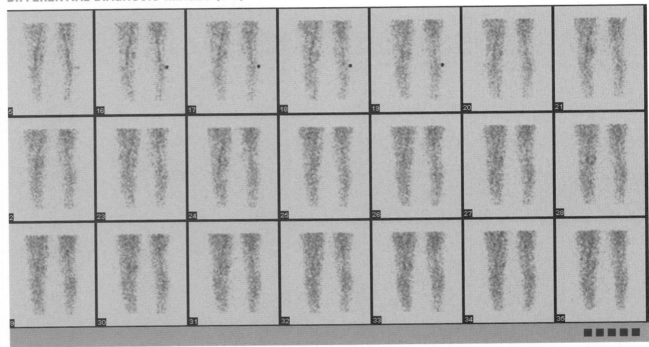

D. Anterior Tc-99m MDP shows symmetric blood flow to both knee regions. (*Image courtesy of Naoya Hattori, MD, PhD.*)

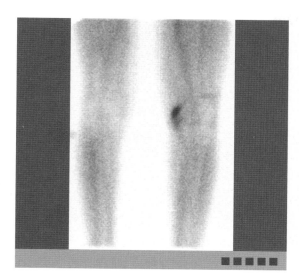

E. Anterior blood pool image shows moderately increased focus of radiotracer uptake in medial left knee. (*Image courtesy of Naoya Hattori, MD, PhD.*)

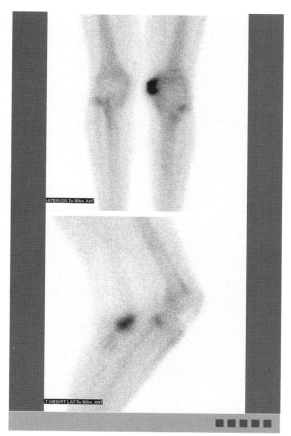

F. Delayed Tc-99m MDP images (anterior and medial) show an intense focus of increased uptake in the medial left knee.

Joseph Rajendran, MD

PRESENTATION

A 25-year-old male marathon runner complaining of pain in the thigh for 3 weeks.

FINDINGS

Three-phase Tc-99m MDP bone scan shows increased blood flow in the region of mid-thigh and is confirmed on blood pool images. Delayed images show a fusiform and focal increase in uptake in the femur corresponding to the painful focus.

DIFFERENTIAL DIAGNOSES

- *Direct trauma*: Typically there is history of direct trauma to the bone and may be associated with other fractures and soft tissue injuries.

- *Hypertrophic pulmonary osteoarthropathy (HPO)*: Typically associated with a systemic pathology such as lung cancer and shows diffuse periosteal uptake in the appendicular skeleton and has the characteristic "tram track" sign.

COMMENTS

Stress fractures are overuse injuries of the bone caused by repetitive subthreshold loading that, over time, exceeds the bone's intrinsic ability to repair itself. In the United States, the incidence of stress fractures is 5% to 30% among athletes and military recruits. Most patients present with activity-related pain corresponding to the location of the fracture. The fractures may be associated with shin splints which typically precede the onset of a stress fracture. Imaging studies are useful in confirming the clinical diagnosis. Conventional radiographic findings may be unremarkable early in the disease course but may show findings of cortical lucency that signify a nonhealing stress fracture. A three-phase bone scan is usually very sensitive when conventional radiology findings are nondiagnostic in the presence of strong clinical suspicion. The bone scan is diagnostic if focal isotope uptake is seen in the area of interest in the third phase of the scan. Scintigraphy is very sensitive and, if there is no focal uptake, the likelihood of a stress fracture is highly unlikely. Drawbacks of scintigraphy include a relative lack of specificity and anatomic resolution.

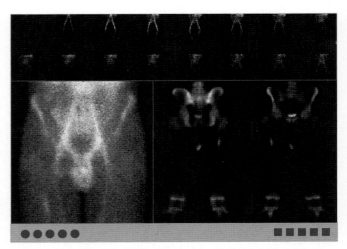

A. Three-phase Tc-99m MDP bone scan shows increased blood flow in the region of mid-thigh and is confirmed on blood pool images. Delayed images show a fusiform and focal increase in uptake in the femur corresponding to painful focus.

Nevertheless, the temporal pattern of uptake on the scan may be useful in distinguishing the etiology of the patient's symptoms and the stage of healing of the fracture. Diffuse, mild periosteal uptake can be seen in patients with shin splints, but a focal and fusiform increase in uptake is diagnostic of stress fracture.

PEARLS

- Bone scanning is very sensitive in diagnosing stress fracture and can be positive even in asymptomatic patients and well before plain radiographs.

- Lack of specificity needs to be taken into account at the time of interpretation as many other conditions can mimic stress fracture.

- Three-phase bone scan is helpful to determine the age of the fracture but is not a necessary technique to diagnose the presence of stress fracture.

- Intensity of uptake usually parallels the degree of symptoms the patient complains of following strenuous exercise.

DIFFERENTIAL DIAGNOSIS IMAGES (B-C)

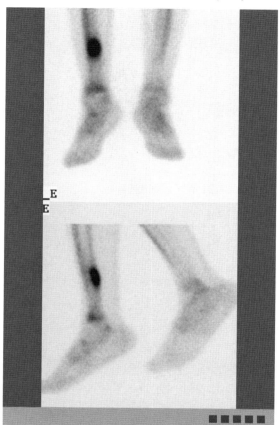

B. Tc-99m MDP bone scan of the distal lower extremities shows a fusiform focus of intensely increased uptake in the lower right tibia.

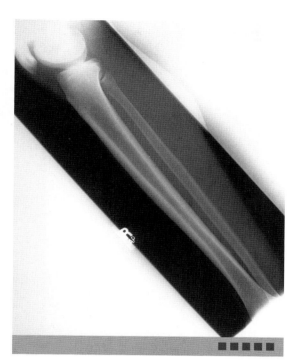

C. Plain radiograph of the right leg shows minimal changes in the bone.

Case 2–20 Super Scan

Joseph Rajendran, MD

PRESENTATION

A 65-year-old male with known prostate cancer and generalized pain.

FINDINGS

Anterior and posterior images of Tc-99m MDP whole body scan show diffusely increased uptake in the entire skeleton with absent uptake in the kidneys.

DIFFERENTIAL DIAGNOSIS

• *Myelofibrosis*: Also can show diffusely increased uptake in the skeleton as a result of diffusely increased marrow activity due to the pathologic process

COMMENTS

Prostate cancer results in osteoblastic metastases that typically involve predominantly the axial skeleton although appendicular skeleton is involved in late stages. These metastases are discernable as discrete foci of tracer uptake in the early stages of the disease process, but, with advancing disease, these disease foci coalesce to involve diffuse areas. With widespread involvement of the bones, tracer uptake is proportionate to blood flow and active bone turnover. Lack of normal uptake in the kidneys is due to higher metastatic tumor burden, resulting in more avid uptake in the skeleton. This causes reduced availability of blood to the kidneys with the resultant decreased excretion via kidneys. Patients with diffuse skeletal involvement are prone to develop bone marrow-related complications such as thrombocytopenia.

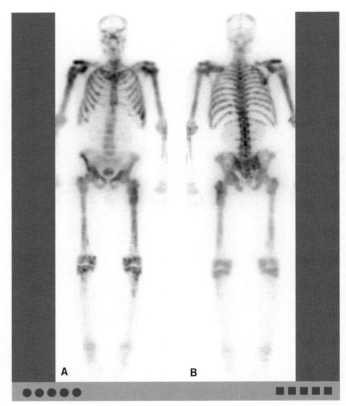

A. and **B.** Whole-body, Tc-99m MDP bone scan shows diffusely increased uptake without obvious focal abnormality and very minimal uptake in the kidneys. This is characteristic of a "super scan."

PEARLS

● Bone scan images have greater contrast and appear to be normal uptake in the skeleton. Lack of focal areas of uptake can be deceiving.

● Even though progression of the metastatic disease can be easily seen on follow-up scans, patients occasionally present initially with diffuse involvement and a "super scan."

● Absence of normal uptake in the kidneys (typically seen in advanced disease state) is the key to diagnosing "super scan."

● Diagnosing a diffuse skeletal involvement with metastases is critical for patient management.

ADDITIONAL IMAGE

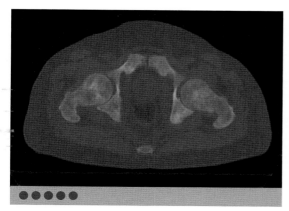

C. Axial CT slice over the pelvis showing diffuse skeletal metastases in the bones.

DIFFERENTIAL DIAGNOSIS IMAGES (D-G)

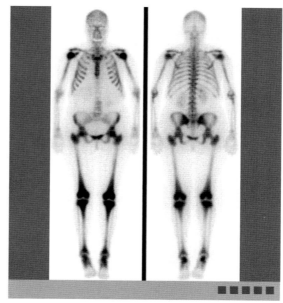

D. Whole body Tc-99m MDP bone scan in a patient with myelofibrosis shows characteristic diffusely increased uptake in the ends of long bones in the lower extremities due to marrow expansion.

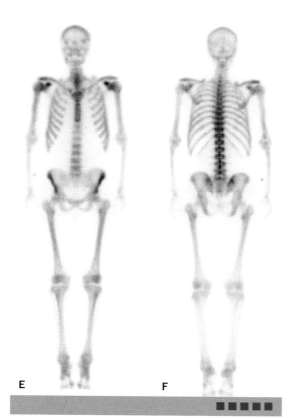

E   F

E. and **F.** Whole-body, Tc-99m MDP bone scan shows diffusely increased uptake without obvious focal abnormality and essentially no uptake in the kidneys. Note the uptake is fairly homogenous in the skeleton, resulting in a "beautiful bone scan."

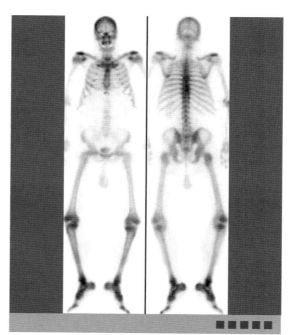

G. Whole-body, Tc-99m MDP bone scan shows diffusely increased uptake without obvious focal abnormality and essentially no uptake in the kidneys (due to chronic renal failure). There is also mildly prominent uptake in the jaws and anterior rib ends. These findings are suggestive of renal osteodystrophy.

Sidharth Damani, MD

PRESENTATION

A 45-year-old male with pain in the left knee for last 3 months off and on and lately increased severity and longer duration.

FINDINGS

The Tc-99m MDP bone scan shows a focus of increased tracer uptake in the medial condyle of the left knee.

DIFFERENTIAL DIAGNOSES

- *Osteomyelitis*: Typically presents with classic signs of fever, pain, and leukocytosis and on Tc-99m MDP bone scan as either an increased blood flow and delayed uptake (hot scan) or a decreased uptake (cold scan) which extend beyond the limits of a joint capsule.

- *Septic arthritis*: Presents with classic signs of infection and on Tc-99m MDP diffusely increased blood flow in the region of the joint limited to the level of the joint capsule. Delayed images usually show normal uptake in the bone.

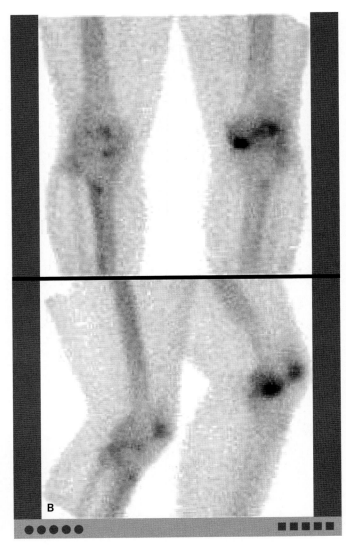

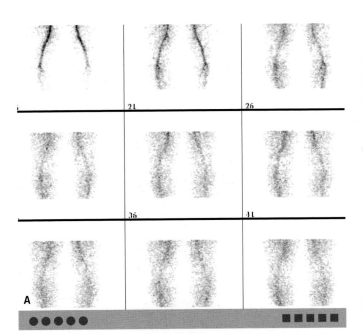

A., and **B.** Tc-99m MDP bone scan shows symmetrical blood flow to both knee regions. Delayed images show a focus of increased uptake in the left knee (medial condyle of the left femur) corresponding to the radiographic abnormality. There are areas of mild, diffusely increased uptake in the joints likely due to degenerative disease. (*Images courtesy of Sidharth Damani, MD.*)

COMMENTS

Brodie abscess, also called subacute osteomyelitis or primary subacute osteomyelitis or chronic osteomyelitis. Sir Benjamin Brodie, a surgeon in St George's Hospital, London, first described subacute osteomyelitis in 1832. Subacute osteomyelitis is characterized by mild-to-moderate

PEARLS

- Low-grade infection of the bone with minimal symptoms and typically caused by hematogenous spread.

- Slow progression and longer clinical course are the hallmarks of this condition.

degree of pain—described usually as a persistent ache, intermittent symptoms, insidious onset, and, often, a long delay between the onset of pain (the commonest presenting symptom) and diagnosis. Usually, symptoms are present for 2 weeks or longer. The course is generally marked by few or no constitutional symptoms and no known previous acute disease. Incidence has increased since antibiotics have been used to treat osteomyelitis. In East Africa, subacute osteomyelitis is the commonest form of osteomyelitis. Subacute osteomyelitis is one of the many clinical presentations of hematogenous osteomyelitis. Subacute osteomyelitis may have elevated WBC count with left shift, normal/slightly elevated ESR and CR, and negative blood cultures. True osteomyelitis has a more aggressive course. Plain radiographs can be equivocal in most cases, but Tc-99m MDP bone scan is positive in most cases but false-negative results are also possible. Gallium 67 (^{67}Ga)- or Indium 111 (In-111)-labeled WBCs imaging can also be used to confirm the diagnosis. The CT and MR are more sensitive and specific, and hence more reliable in establishing the diagnosis.

ADDITIONAL IMAGE

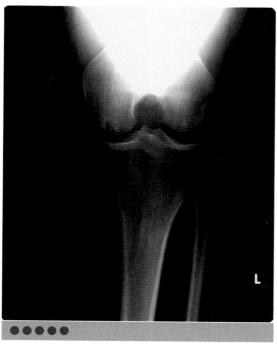

C. Plain radiograph of the left femur showing a lucent focus with sclerotic margin in the medial condyle. (*Image courtesy of Sidharth Damani, MD.*)

DIFFERENTIAL DIAGNOSIS IMAGES (D–E)

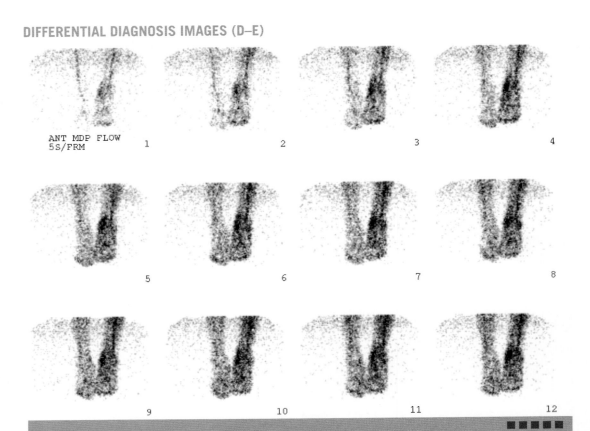

ANT MDP FLOW
5S/FRM   1   2   3   4

5   6   7   8

9   10   11   12

D: Tc99m MDP shows increased blood flow to the distal left lower extremity. There is increased blood pool activity in the distal left lower extremity.

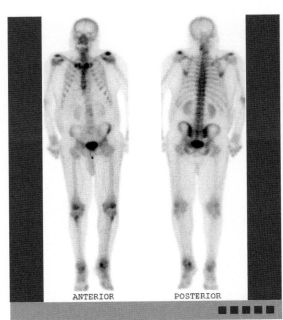

ANTERIOR   POSTERIOR

E. Septic arthritis: Whole body Tc-99m delayed images show a focal area of uptake in the medial left ankle corresponding to the focus of septic arthritis in the left ankle.

Joseph Rajendran, MD

PRESENTATION

A 65-year-old male with known prostate cancer and generalized pain.

FINDINGS

Anterior and posterior images of Tc-99m MDP whole body show diffusely increased uptake in the entire skeleton with normal uptake in the kidneys. The distribution is uniform and symmetrical, predominantly involving the ends of the long bones such as femur and tibia.

DIFFERENTIAL DIAGNOSIS

- *Myelofibrosis*: Also can show diffusely increased uptake in the skeleton as a result of diffusely increased marrow activity due to the pathologic process

COMMENTS

Bone marrow fibrosis also known as myelofibrosis is a rare condition, resulting in the loss of hematopoietic cells and ultimately ending in compensatory extramedullary hematopoiesis. It is primarily caused by malignant transformation of the totipotential stem cells in the bone marrow that will activate fibroblasts. Additional causes include malignant (eg, leukemia), toxin (eg, radiation), and infectious (eg, tuberculosis [TB]) pathologies. Initial presentation is as a result of extramedullary hematopoiesis (splenomegaly) and in late stages due to bone marrow failure and pancytopenia. Presenting symptoms (such as anemia, splenomegaly, and thrush and bleeding) are substantiated by peripheral blood smear and bone marrow aspirates in clinching the diagnosis. Imaging studies are rarely performed for making the diagnosis but occasionally done because of symptoms and include abdominal ultrasonography (for splenomegaly) and MR imaging. Bone scanning is usually not performed for making a diagnosis but may be obtained in patients with unexplained bone pain. Treatment of myelofibrosis is directed at the primary causes, and other approaches include allogeneic bone marrow transplantation, antileukemic therapy, imatinib mesylate, corticosteroids, thalidomide, and so on.

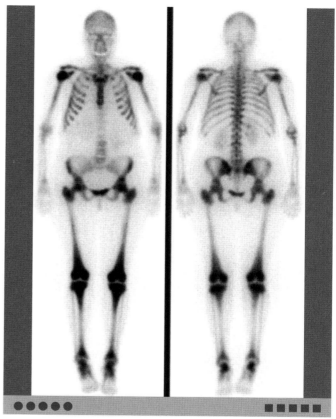

A. Myelofibrosis: Diffusely increased uptake in the ends of long bones of the lower extremities as a result of marrow expansion.

PEARLS

- Bone scan images show greater contrast and appear to be normal uptake in the skeleton. Myelofibrosis usually does not show focal areas of uptake in the skeleton.

- Myelofibrosis results in bone marrow expansion and extramedullary hematopoiesis. There is uptake in the distal end of long bones that typically do not show increased uptake.

- Uptake in the kidneys is normal—differentiating from a "super scan."

DIFFERENTIAL DIAGNOSIS IMAGE

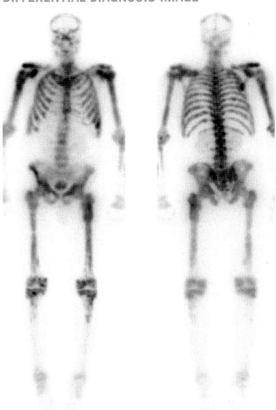

B. Myelofibrosis: Whole body, Tc-99m MDP bone scan in patient with widespread metastatic disease involving the axial and appendicular skeleton showing diffusely increased uptake in these bones with minimal activity in the kidneys characteristic of a "super scan."

Vivek Manchanda, MD

PRESENTATION

Man in late teens with osteosarcoma of left tibia, pre- and post-chemotherapy scans.

FINDINGS

Increased Tc-MDP uptake in the known osteosarcoma in the post-therapy scan in comparison to pretherapy scan.

DIFFERENTIAL DIAGNOSES

* *Worsening of disease*

* *Response to therapy*

Increased tracer uptake in the bone lesions post-therapy can be due to "flare response" and must be correlated with other imaging modalities (MR/PET) and clinical response.

COMMENTS

Bone scan has been the traditional imaging modality to assess chemotherapy response for osteosarcomas.

Response to chemotherapy is elicited by decreased Tc-99m MDP uptake, and nonresponders show increased or similar uptake.

There are instances (within 6 months of therapy or so), where the scan actually looks worse than before and may even show more areas of uptake than before. This is called "flare phenomenon" and is due to healing response to chemotherapy.

The theories behind this phenomenon have been attributed to (a) increased blood flow to the area and (b) increased turnover of hydroxyapetite in the new bone that is laid down as the part of healing process.

Clinical improvement after therapy accompanied with a worsening scan should be interpreted with caution. Newer lesions on the post-therapy scan may not be the deciding factor between the "flare response" and worsening of disease. The new lesions on the bone scan may simply represent healing lesions, which might have not been seen on pretherapy FDG-PET or MR scans, as in the index case.

Both MR and FDG-PET can help differentiate between the flare response and worsening disease. In lytic metastases, osteoclasts stimulated by malignant cells result in imbalance between osteoblasts and osteoclasts. Osteoclastic activity is reduced as the tumor heals and osteoblastic activity ensues.

"Flare phenomenon" has been described in PET with breast cancer on hormonal therapy. On bone scans, it has been described in prostate cancer, primary bone tumors, and

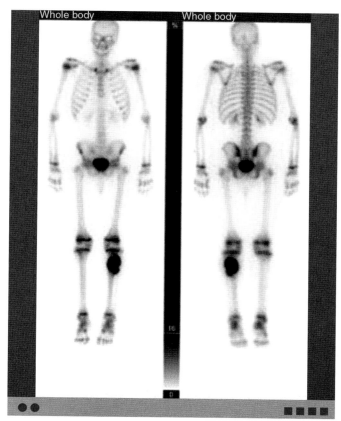

A. Bone scan, pretherapy with intense radiotracer corresponding to left tibial osteosarcoma.

breast cancer. New lesions on a bone scan after 6 months are indicative of progressive disease. Fluorine 18-sodium fluoride PET scan can show similar osteoblastic "flare response."

PEARLS

* A bone scan/X-ray/^{18}F-PET may actually look worse after chemotherapy in osteosarcoma and other malignancies such as breast cancer due to "flare response." It signifies successful systemic therapy.

* FDG-PET is superior to planar bone scintigraphy in assessing response to treatment in primary osteosarcomas.

* With therapy, the osteoclasts stimulated by malignant cells may be reduced as the tumor heals and osteoblastic activity ensues.

ADDITIONAL IMAGES (B-F)

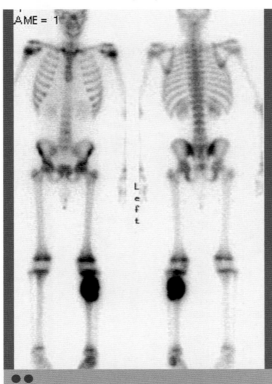

B. Bone scan, post-therapy with more intense tracer uptake, "flare response."

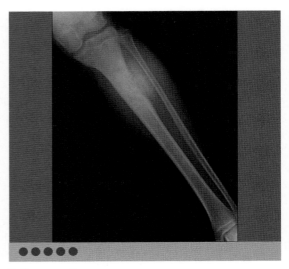

C. X-ray, pretherapy.

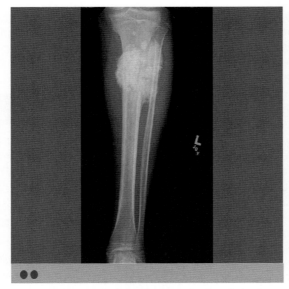

D. X-ray, post-therapy with increased sclerosis in the lesion and focal sclerotic lesion abutting epiphysis.

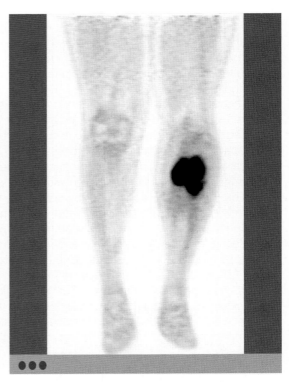

E. Coronal FDG-PET, pretherapy scan with intense FDG activity corresponding to known osteosarcoma.

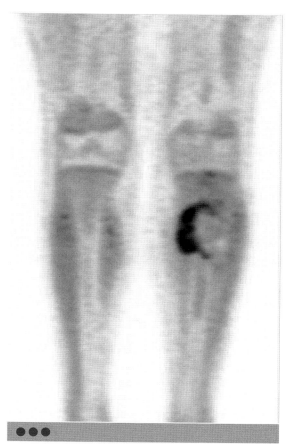

F. Coronal. Post-therapy FDG-PET scan. Note significant decrease in metabolic activity.

Vivek Manchanda, MD

PRESENTATION

Man in late fifth decade of life, with increasing right rib cage pain. Multiple rib fractures as a child.

FINDINGS

Intensely increased FDG activity in right-sided ribs and posterior elements and thoracic vertebrae, corresponding to expansile lytic lesions on the CT. Heterogeneous, mild Tc-MDP activity in the right-sided ribs and mid-thoracic vertebrae.

DIFFERENTIAL DIAGNOSES

- *Fibrous dysplasia (FD)*
- *Aneurysmal bone cysts*
- *Metastases*
- *Multiple hemangiomas/lymphangioma*
- *Multiple myeloma*
- *Malignant degeneration of fibrous dysplasia (extremely rare)*
- *Telangiectatic osteosarcoma*

Patient had multiple right rib fractures in childhood from underlying FD. Over time, multiple secondary aneurysmal cysts developed. FDG activity cannot exclude malignancy/malignant degeneration of FD (rare).

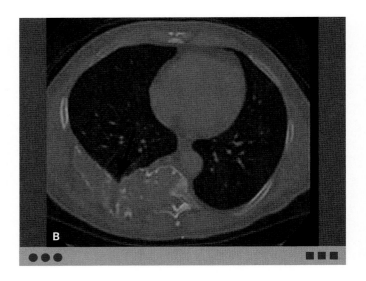

COMMENTS

FD, the commonest benign rib tumor, involves replacement of medullary bone with fibrous tissue (mesenchymal anomaly) which causes expanded and weak bones. About a third of FDs are polyostotic and predominantly unilateral. Two-third patients are symptomatic before age 10 with pathologic fractures. In a series of six fibrous dysplasia patients, the mean SUV on FDG-PET was 2.05 (+/–0.98).

Mean age for aneurysmal bone cysts (ABCs) is 14 to 16 years, with a female preponderance. Thoraco-lumbar vertebrae are most commonly affected. Posterior elements and pedicles are affected first, with extension into the vertebral body. Sudden collapse of vertebral body/associated scoliosis and kyphosis may be present. In one-third cases, the lesion may cross over to an adjacent vertebra.

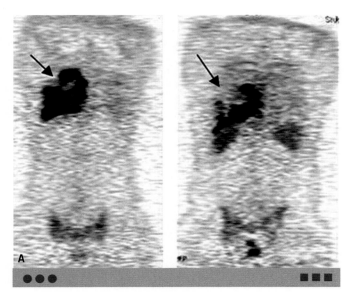

A. and **B.** Intense coronal FDG-PET activity in right mid-thoracic ribs and vertebrae. Corresponding axial CT with expansile lytic posterior rib and vertebral body.

PEARLS

- Both FD and ABC have variable FDG activity. Usually, FD is more Tc-MDP avid and ABC is more FDG avid.
- ABC can be a reparative process superimposed on a preexisting lesion such as FD.
- Paget disease is typically more Tc-MDP avid and variably (usually mildly) FDG avid.
- High FDG uptake in Paget disease is associated with increased alkaline phosphatase levels.
- FD of the vertebra affects the same age group as ABCs, usually includes more than one vertebra, grows slowly until the patient's skeletal growth ceases, and is often painless.

The potential for rapid growth of ABC and bony destruction and neurologic involvement has guided aggressive therapy.

It has been postulated that ABC can arise in a preexisting lesion such as a giant cell tumor or FD and that the diagnosis of primary ABC should be made after the exclusion of other lesions.

ABCs are characterized by the presence of multiloculated cysts containing fluid-fluid interfaces on T2-weighted images (T2-WI). Telangiectatic osteosarcoma is a differential for ABC.

FDG-PET may help assess rare malignant change in prior FD. Both FD and ABC have variable FDG and Tc-MDP activities (FD is usually more Tc-MDP avid and ABC is usually more FDG avid). Bone scans can distinguish monostotic from polyostotic lesions.

ADDITIONAL IMAGE (C-E)

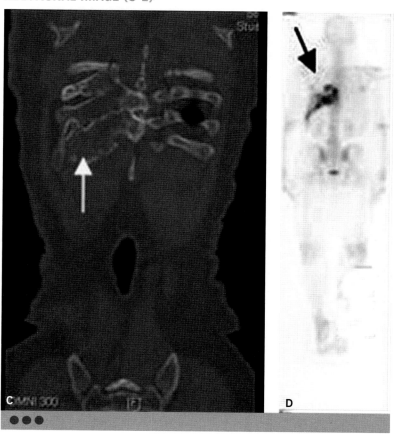

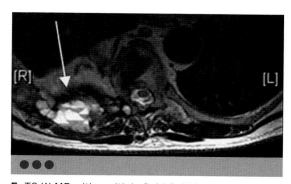

E. T2 W MR with multiple fluid fluid levels (*arrow*).

C. and **D.** Coronal CT with lytic expansile posterior mid thoracic ribs with extension into vertebral bodies and posterior elements. Whole body bone scan showing corresponding heterogeneous Tc MDP uptake in the same region.

DIFFERENTIAL DIAGNOSIS IMAGES (F–J)

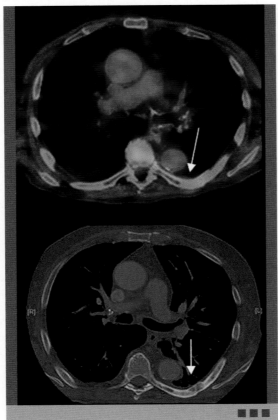

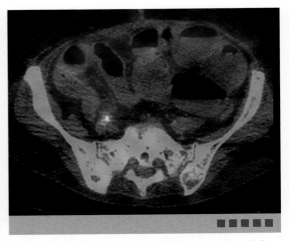

G. Fused PET-CT with minimal FDG activity in pelvic Paget disease.

F. Different patient, CT (ground glass, mildly expansile) and fused PET/CT images (mild FDG activity) of left seventh rib fibrous dysplasia.

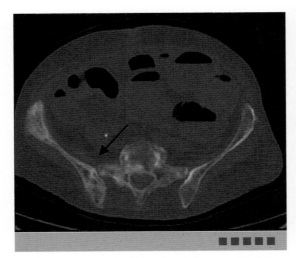

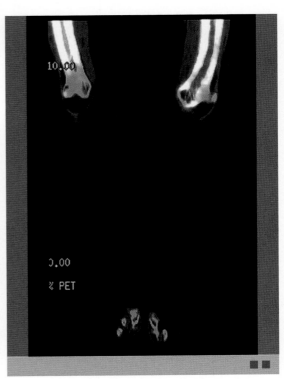

H. Corresponding axial CT of Paget disease with thickened trabeculae.

I. Diffuse Paget disease with diffuse hypermetabolic bones (high alkaline phosphatase levels). Coronal fused FDG-PET/CT.

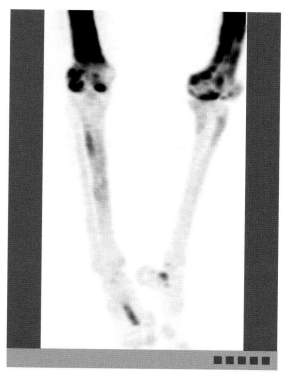

J. Corresponding bone scan with Tc MDP uptake.

Vivek Manchanda, MD

PRESENTATION

Patient with lymphoma, for FDG-PET.

FINDINGS

Diffusely increased FDG activity in the muscles, decreased sensitivity to detect subtle metastases/foci of disease involvement.

DIFFERENTIAL DIAGNOSES

• Exercise before injection of FDG.

• *Shivering*

• *Intrinsic hyperinsulinemia* (glucose-rich diet prior to examination)

• *Extrinsic hyperinsulinemia* (insulin injection)

The index patient drank electrolyte solution ("Gatorade®") an hour and a half before examination and resulted in insulin peak during the uptake phase. Proper history is essential in distinguishing the etiology of diffusely increased muscular FDG uptake.

COMMENTS

In hyperglycemia, excess glucose competes with FDG for access to glucose transporter (GLUT) receptors on the cell membranes. Glucose levels greater than 200 mg/dL may decrease ability to detect subtle metastases/cancers.

Preferably, all patients must fast for 4 to 6 hours. Diabetic patients should be scheduled in the morning with serum sugar goal of less than150 mg/dL.

Urgent diabetics can be admitted for tighter blood sugar control. Diet controlled diabetics or patients on oral medications do not need to stop medications.

One-half to three-fourth of long-acting insulin may be given in the morning. No regular/fast-acting insulin should be given within 2 to 4 hours of the scan. After the uptake period of 45 to 60 minutes, orange juice can be given to prevent hypoglycemia.

Insulin peak drives glucose and FDG into the skeletal muscle. Postprandial blood sugar peaks at around 2 hours (intrinsic hyperinsulinemia), hence fasting for at least 4 hours is essential.

Myocardial uptake of FDG is greater in nonfasting/hyperglycemic states. Prolonged fasting (12 hours or so) switches the metabolism of myocardium from glucose to free fatty acids.

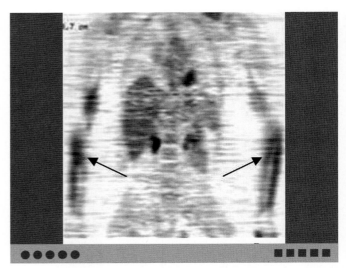

A. Increased muscle FDG activity related to intrinsic hyperinsulinemia (Gatorade® prior to examination).

The peaks of fast-acting insulin (Humulin [insulin isophane]/NovoLog [insulin aspart]): around 1.5 to 2.5 hours; regular insulin (short to intermediate acting): around 2 to 4 hours; NPH (longer-acting insulin): gradual peak around 4 to 9 hours. Similarly long-acting insulin zinc (Lente and Ultralente) peak gradually at 8 to 14 hours. Long-acting insulin analogs glargine (Lantus) and detemir (Levemir) have gradual peaks at 6 hours and 8 hours, respectively and do not significantly affect the muscle uptake.

The other cause of increased muscular FDG activity is exercise, shivering, and tense muscles.

PEARLS

• **Diet-/oral medication-controlled diabetics do not need to stop any oral medication, even on the day of the examination.**

• **Patients may take one-half to three-fourth of their long-acting insulin in the morning.**

• **Regular/fast-acting insulin should be avoided within 2 (preferably 4) hours of the PET scan as insulin peak drives the glucose and analogs (FDG) into muscles.**

DIFFERENTIAL DIAGNOSIS IMAGES (B-G)

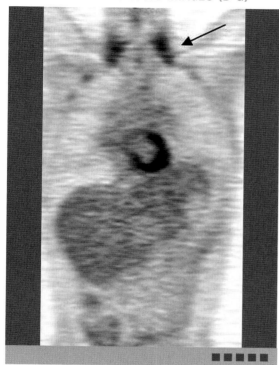

B. Increased muscle activity in the neck related to labored breathing. Coronal FDG PET.

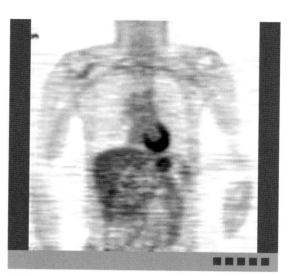

C. No abnormally increased muscle activity in a patient with insulin pump (constant discharge of insulin, without sudden insulin peaks). Coronal FDG-PET.

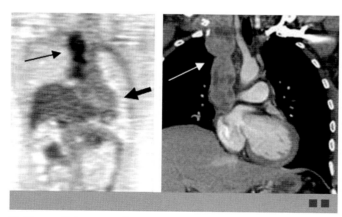

D. Myocardial suppression of FDG activity, achieved by prolonged fasting (24 hours) (*thick black arrow*), in a patient with angiosarcoma of the superior vena cava (*thin black arrow*). Coronal FDG-PET and corresponding CT.

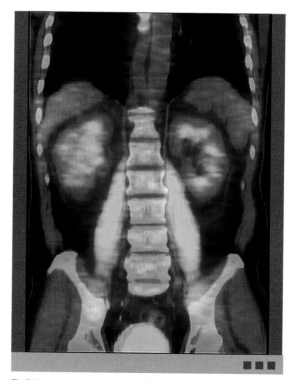

E. Bilateral psoas muscle FDG uptake from shivering.

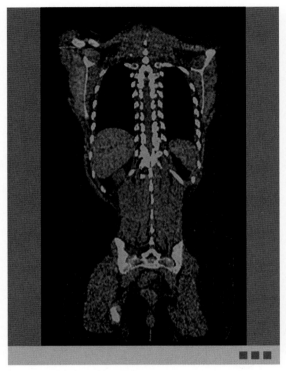

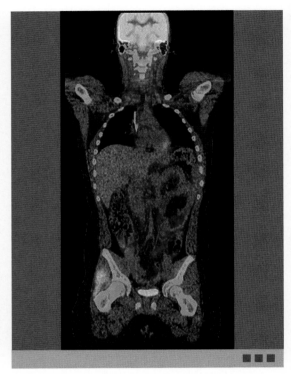

F. Right upper back muscle FDG activity from knitting during uptake phase of scan.

G. Increased FDG activity in right gluteal muscles from altered weight bearing.

Joseph Rajendran, MD

PRESENTATION

A 65-year-old male complaining of diffuse lower limb edema and distension of the abdomen.

FINDINGS

On delayed whole-body Tc99m MDP images show mild diffusely increased uptake in the entire abdomen. The patient has had multiple paracentesis in the past and had moderate amount of ascites at the time of imaging.

DIFFERENTIAL DIAGNOSES

- *Electrical burns*: Usually at the point of contact, history will help with the diagnosis.

- *Myalgias from other etiologies*: Usually generalized and confirmed by the history. Rare complication of statins is rhabdomyolysis; however, imaging is typically not required to diagnose these conditions.

COMMENTS

After IV injection, normal biodistribution of Tc-99m MDP is circulation in the blood pool, passive distribution in the extravascular compartments and third spaces (eg, pleural effusion, edema, ascites). There is also active excretion via the kidneys and uptake in the skeleton, resulting in a biexponential clearance pattern. Therefore, immediately after the IV injection, there is poor contrast between the bones and the soft tissues. In the ensuing several hours and dependence on the normal physiologic function, there is continuous recirculation of the radiotracer into intravascular spaces while at the same time there is active clearance in the urine. This will result in a better contrast between the bones and soft tissues over time and hence the reason for conventional 3- to 4-hour delayed images. However, it takes longer for the activity initially localized in the third spaces to redistribute to the intravascular space for eventual clearing by the kidneys. This delayed clearance from these spaces is typically seen as mildly increased diffuse radiotracer uptake in the location on delayed images. Typically these findings are incidental on bone scans. While this is a nonissue on diagnostic Tc-99m MDP imaging, it might be a significant issue in patients receiving skeletal-targeted therapy with other similar radiopharmaceuticals such as samarium-153 ethylene diamine tetramethylene phosphonate (^{153}Sm EDTMP) since the soft tissue radiation absorbed doses would be significantly increased reducing the therapeutic ratio.

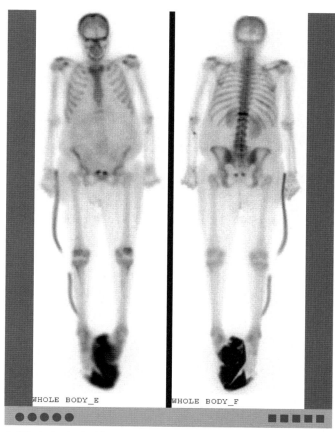

WHOLE BODY_E   WHOLE BODY_F

A. Whole body Tc-99m MDP images show mild diffusely increased uptake in the entire abdomen in the ascitic fluid, better visualized on anterior images.

PEARLS

- Delayed clearance from the soft tissues with activities in the extravascular spaces ranging from mild to significant.

- Maximum radiotracer uptake is seen in 24 to 48 hours and shows resolution within 1 week.

- Bone scanning is rarely used in the primary diagnosis of rhabdomyolysis as history and other findings are usually able to clinch the diagnosis. But it can be used in situations that are difficult to establish the diagnosis.

- Diffuse renal parenchymal uptake may be seen as part of this disease process.

Joseph Rajendran, MD

PRESENTATION

A 41-year-old male with pain in the right thigh and an abnormal, plain radiograph.

FINDINGS

- Tc-99m MDP bone scan shows a solitary focal increased uptake in the right posterior elements of the C7 vertebra.

- CT shows a lytic lesion with thin sclerotic margins, right anterior portion of C7 lamina. Nidus with small calcifications and no evidence of cortical disruption or soft tissue mass.

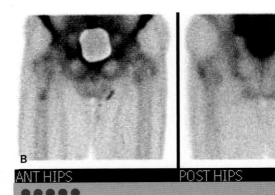
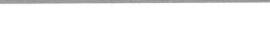

B

ANT HIPS   POST HIPS

DIFFERENTIAL DIAGNOSES

- *Infection/osteomyelitis*: Patients typically present with pain, fever, and leukocytosis.

- *Bone island.*

- *Osteoblastoma.*

COMMENTS

Osteoid osteoma is a benign skeletal neoplasm without known etiology and is composed of osteoid and woven bone. The tumor is typically less than 2 cm in diameter and can occur in any bone, but more commonly in the appendicular skeleton. It is commonly seen in younger patients but can occur in older individuals. As with younger individuals, older patients present with focal bone pain at the site of the tumor. The pain worsens at night and increases with activity and is effectively relieved with aspirin. The lesion initially appears as a small sclerotic bone island within a

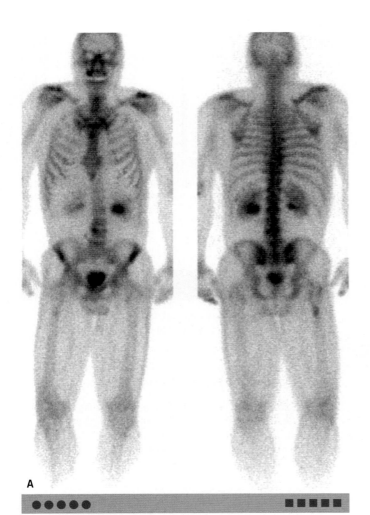

A

A. and B. Tc-99m MDP bone scan: Solitary focus of markedly increased uptake in the proximal right femur (anterior and posterior hips, Image B).

PEARLS

- **Osteoid osteoma is a benign tumor of the bone with many similarities to osteoid blastoma.**

- **Typically seen in younger patients but can present in older patients also.**

- **Double-density sign is seen in typical cases.**

- **Bone scan is highly sensitive and specific and is helpful to clinch the diagnosis when used in conjunction with other imaging methods and can help guide surgical excision.**

circular lucent defect. The tumors may regress spontaneously. Plain radiograph is usually the initial examination of choice and may be the only examination performed. The CT and MRI can be used on occasions to confirm diagnosis in equivocal cases. Single-photon emission computed tomography (SPECT) is useful in the localization of the tumor when the spinal arch or spinous process is involved. Skeletal scintigraphy with Tc-99m MDP uptake shows fairly intense focal uptake at the tumor site, and bone scanning may be used to localize the tumor preoperatively and to guide surgical excision of the tumor/nidus using a hand-held probe. Bone scan is very sensitive and may be positive before radiographic changes are apparent. A double-density sign is seen where a small focus of radioactivity in the nidus of increased vascularity is superimposed on a larger area of radioactivity. SPECT may be useful in areas with complex anatomy, such as the posterior elements of the spine.

ADDITIONAL IMAGE

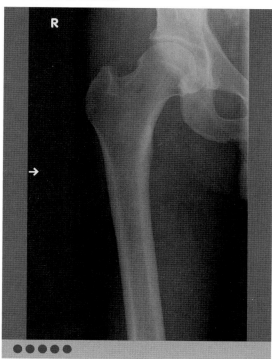

● ● ● ● ●

C. Radiograph: Showing the focus of osteoid osteoma in the right femur with the central nidus.

DIFFERENTIAL DIAGNOSIS IMAGES (D-E)

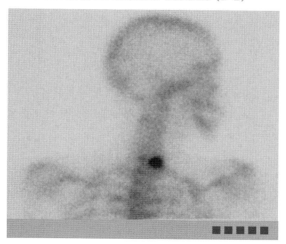

D. Tc-99m MDP bone scan: Solitary focal marked uptake in the right posterior elements at C7 vertebra.

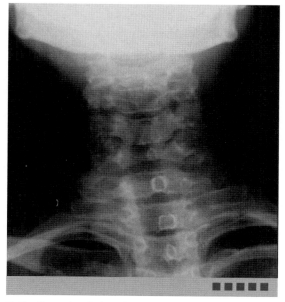

E. Radiographs: Sclerotic right C7 pedicle/lamina.

Joseph Rajendran, MD

PRESENTATION

A 30-year-old female with chronic pain, no history of malignancy, and long-standing history of acne.

FINDINGS

Bone scan: There are multifocal diffusely increased uptakes in several bones.

DIFFERENTIAL DIAGNOSES

- *Bony sclerosis without osseous enlargement, including blastic metastases, myelofibrosis, renal osteodystrophy, fibrous dysplasia, fluorosis, mastocytosis, and tuberous sclerosis.*

- *Calvarial hyperostosis:* Hyperostosis frontalis interna, fibrous dysplasia, and metastatic disease.

- *Metastatic disease* from prostate cancer has similar appearance, but radiographic or CT appearance and serum tumor markers help differentiate the condition.

- *Paget disease.*

COMMENTS

SAPHO syndrome is a spectrum of chronic conditions with synovitis, acne, pustulosis, hyperostosis, and osteomyelitis that share common features. It frequently affects the vertebral column and hence may be related to other chronic conditions of the vertebrae such as ankylosing spondylosis although it can affect other joints such as sacro iliac and sterno clavicular joints. Appearances on bone scans are similar to any sclerotic or hyperostotic condition. More commonly (60%-90%), this condition affects bones in the anterior chest wall involving sternoclavicular joints. Plain radiographs of the bones show findings that range from hyperostosis, sclerosis, and hypertrophy. Tc-99m MDP bone scans show characteristic findings of diffusely increased uptake in the affected bones, and serial bone scans can be used to monitor response to therapy. These bone findings may or may not be associated with dermatologic changes. Bisphosphonate therapy has been recommended as the first line of therapy although treatment with (tumor necrosis factor) TNF-α inhibitors, corticosteroids, nonsteroidal anti-inflammatory drugs (NSAIDs), and the like has been tried with some success.

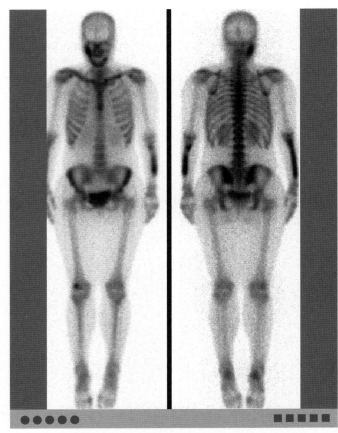

A. Whole-body Tc-99m MDP bone scan images show diffuse, intensely increased uptake in both ulnae involving the bones in entirety.

PEARLS

- **SAPHO syndrome is a group of chronic conditions with synovitis, acne, pustulosis, hyperostosis, and osteomyelitis and of unknown etiology.**

- **Bone scan is helpful in detecting the polyostotic presentations and in the follow-up of treatment response.**

- **Scintigraphic and radiographic findings may or may not be associated with dermatologic findings.**

ADDITIONAL IMAGES (B-C)

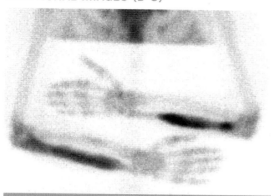

B. Spot image of the forearms shows diffusely increased uptake in both ulnae.

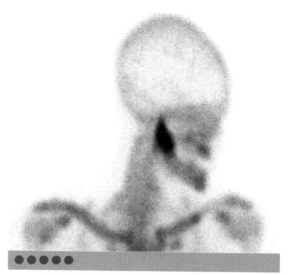

C. Spot image of the lateral head and neck shows the focus of increased uptake in right mandible.

Vivek Manchanda, MD

PRESENTATION

Right paraspinal mass in a woman in late twenties.

FINDINGS

Intensely FDG-avid right paraspinal mass. Peripheral calcification on the corresponding CT.

DIFFERENTIAL DIAGNOSES

- *Myositis ossificans*

- *Sarcomas*: *Parosteal osteosarcoma, synovial sarcoma*

- *Tumoral calcinosis*

- *Metastases*: Melanoma, breast

COMMENTS

- *Myositis ossificans (MO)*: Extraosseous, non-neoplastic heterotopic bone growth

- *MO circumscripta*: New extraosseous bone after trauma

- *Progressive MO*: Fatal inherited disorder with fibrosis and ossification of muscle, tendon, and ligaments

MO is commonest in the second and third decades and typically involves thigh and arm muscles. Associated pain is variable.

Calcification in MO starts peripherally (vs central in parosteal osteosarcoma). Bone scans show enhanced uptake in all three phases in "immature MO." FDG-PET scan shows typically intense FDG activity.

Surgery for MO is contemplated once blood flow and blood pool activity on Tc-MDP scan subsides ("mature" MO). Usually, MO decreases in size in 4 to 6 months and disappears in 1 to 2 years.

Parosteal osteosarcoma: between the second and the fifth decades; FDG-avid sessile mass with smooth or irregular margins attached to thickened cortex. MR and PET/CT help document medullary involvement. Intensely FDG-avid areas of radiolucency within the tumor mass indicate dedifferentiated/high-grade foci.

Synovial sarcoma: painful FDG-avid soft tissue mass between the third and the fifth decades of life; may have peripheral calcification in one-third of the cases and mainly seen in lower extremity.

Periosteal fibrosarcoma: FDG-avid rare tumor from periosteal connective tissue, involving long bones of lower

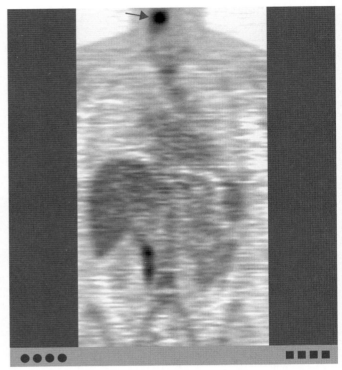

A. Intense focal FDG activity corresponding to right paraspinal mass on CT (*arrow*).

extremity and jaw. Cortical irregularity and periosteal reaction with perpendicular bone formation may be present.

Rhabdomyosarcomas: FDG-avid masses that rarely calcify. Tumoral calcinosis (FDG avidity unknown) is a rare juxta-articular disorder (African ancestry), seen commonly in the second decade with typical painless calcific masses surrounded by fibrous tissue around hips/other joints.

PEARLS

- **MO exhibits intense FDG activity and peripheral extraosseous calcification on CT.**

- **All three phases on bone scan are positive for immature MO and, negative flow and blood pool phase indicates mature MO that can be resected.**

- **The most important differential is parosteal osteosarcoma in which the ossification typically starts centrally.**

ADDITIONAL IMAGES (B-C)

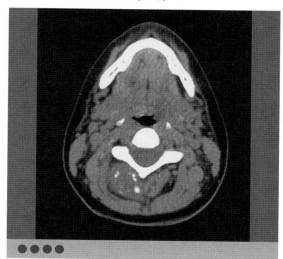

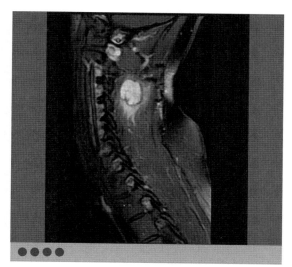

B. Corresponding CT showing peripheral calcification.

C. Corresponding MR, T1-W FS, post-gadolinium (post-Gd) with high signal.

DIFFERENTIAL DIAGNOSIS IMAGES (D-M)

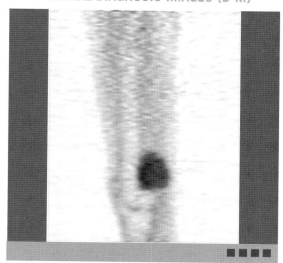

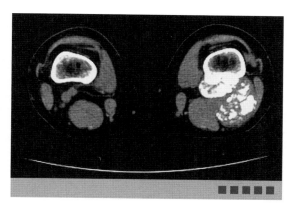

E. Parosteal osteosarcoma, axial CT with central calcifications. 42-year-old female.

D. Parosteal osteosarcoma, moderate FDG activity. Sagittal.

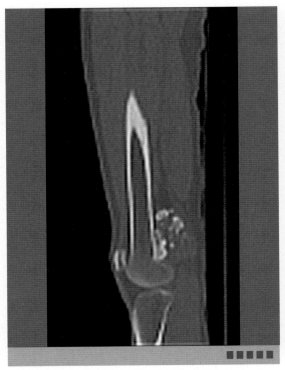

F. Parosteal osteosarcoma, sagittal reconstruct.

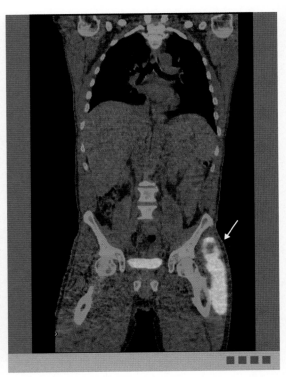

G. Left thigh poorly differentiated sarcoma, 52-year-old man. Coronal fused FDG-PET/CT.

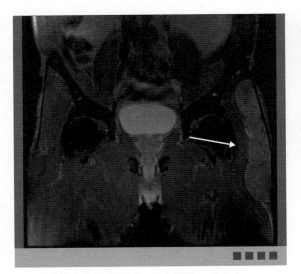

H. T1-W, post-Gd left thigh poorly differentiated sarcoma.

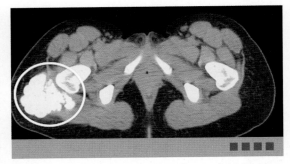

I. Minimal FDG activity corresponding to right thigh tumoral calcinosis.

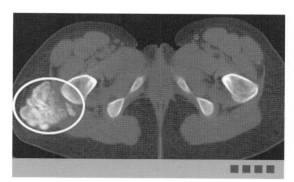

J. Tumoral calcinosis, right thigh. Axial CT.

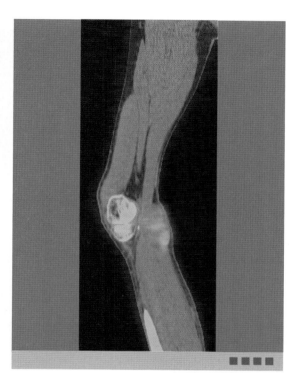

K. Synovial sarcoma, sagittal.

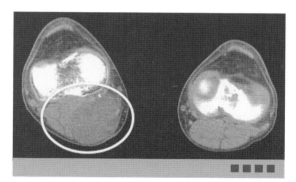

L. Axial noncontrast CT, synovial sarcoma, faint peripheral calcification (*circle*).

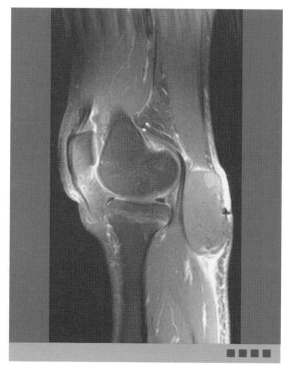

M. Synovial sarcoma, sagittal postcontrast T1 W.

Vivek Manchanda, MD

PRESENTATION

Teenager with left humeral lymphoma.

FINDINGS

Symmetrical, multifocal FDG activity in bilateral neck, bilateral shoulders, and paraspinal region on first day and no such activity on the next day.

DIFFERENTIAL DIAGNOSES

- *Lymphoma*
- *Metastases*
- *Muscle activity*
- *Melanoma* (unlikely given age)
- *Castleman disease*
- *Granulomatous disease*

The disappearance of FDG activity within a span of one day (along with no corresponding CT finding) is unlikely to be due to nodal disease.

COMMENTS

Brown fat uptake is usually seen as multifocal, symmetrical FDG uptake along neck, supraclavicular, interscapular, mediastinal, and paravertebral regions. Other regions include renal hila and near great vessels. It corresponds to areas of fat density on CT images.

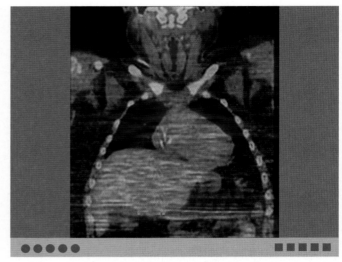

B. The same patient; images acquired next day with blankets; brown fat FDG activity disappeared.

Brown adipocytes in these regions become activated as one of the initial steps in thermogenesis in response to cold. Glycolysis is significantly increased through sympathetic innervation. Higher levels of circulating catecholamines may be responsible for some FDG uptake. Although it is most commonly seen in children and young adults, it has been shown in patients up to 60 years of age.

Brown adipose tissue (BAT) functions as a thermogenic organ by producing heat to maintain body temperature in many mammals. It requires glucose as a source of adenosine triphosphate production. The adenosine triphosphate resulting from glycolysis is required for continued fatty acid oxidation in the mitochondrial uncoupling proteins, which is the main mechanism for heat production. It is innervated

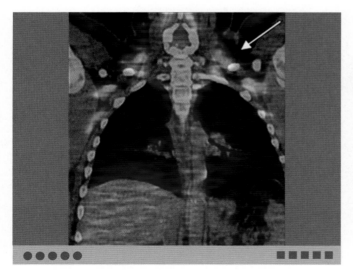

A. Symmetrical brown fat uptake in neck and shoulders.

PEARLS

- Symmetric increased FDG uptake can be seen in cervical, supraclavicular, mediastinal, and paraspinal regions, as well as near great vessels and kidneys from brown fat.

- Unilateral brown fat is not uncommon.

- Brown fat uptake is due to ATP production by brown adipocytes, which utilize glucose.

- Using blankets, increasing injection room temperatures, and beta-blockers can reduce brown fat FDG uptake.

by the sympathetic nervous system and expresses β_1-, β_2-, and β_3-adrenergic receptors, predominantly β_3.

Using blankets and increasing the room temperatures decrease brown fat FDG uptake. Some studies have shown that beta-blockers help as well.

At our center, lorazepam (Ativan) was not helpful in reducing FDG uptake due to brown fat.

Usually, the brown fat is symmetrical; however, unilateral brown fat FDG activity can be seen. The other radiotracers which can show uptake in brown fat are 123-I MIBG and Tc-99m tetrofosmin.

In the index case presented, the patient had to be reimaged to include the arm in the field of view the second day. We used blankets before the second injection and the BAT FDG activity disappeared.

DIFFERENTIAL DIAGNOSIS IMAGES (C-F)

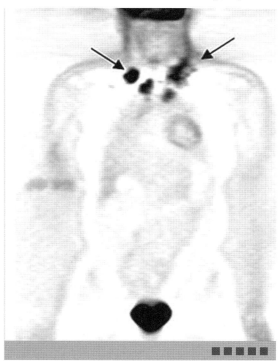

C. Increased FDG uptake in the neck in a patient with nodular sclerosing Hodgkin disease. Coronal NAC image.

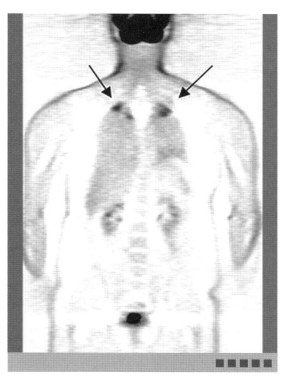

D. Symmetrical FDG uptake upper chest, NAC image, radiation induced.

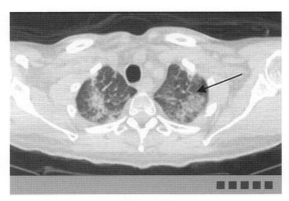

E. Corresponding CT clearly shows radiation-induced inflammation/ fibrosis.

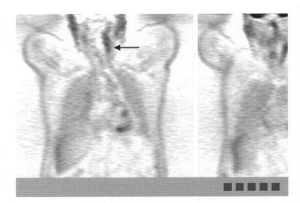

F. NAC image with neck musculature FDG uptake. This is usually linear and bilateral, but unilateral neck muscle uptake can be seen.

Vivek Manchanda, MD

PRESENTATION

Right chest wall mass in a man in early second decade of his life.

FINDINGS

Intensely hypermetabolic right chest wall mass.

DIFFERENTIAL DIAGNOSES

- *Neoplastic*: Mesenchymal, muscle, neural, bone origin; lymphoma

- *Traumatic*: Hematoma (may show peripheral FDG activity)

- *Infection*: Actinomycosis, nocardiosis, blastomycosis, aspergillosis, TB, staphylococcosis, Klebsiella infection

- *Chest wall involvement*: Metastases, peripheral lung cancer (unlikely due to age), lymphoma

Chest wall lipoma would be typically FDG negative.

COMMENTS

The resected mass proved to be an abscess from *Staphylococcus* infection.

Chest wall masses can be benign (such as infection) or malignant and arise from skin, fat, muscle, bone, fibrous connective tissue, breasts, cartilage, and lymphatic and blood vessels. They may occur as an extension of breast, lung, and mediastinal or pleural mass. Metastasis from lung, breast, or other distant carcinoma or sarcoma may occur.

When the chest wall mass extends into the lungs, it usually displaces the pleura and forms an obtuse angle with the chest wall on the CT. Rib remodeling is seen in extrapleural masses.

Primary soft tissue masses of the chest wall are rare. In adults, lipoma (benign) and fibrosarcoma and malignant fibrous histiocytoma (malignant) are the most common. In children, primitive neuroectodermal tumor (PNET), extraosseous Ewing sarcoma, and rhabdomyosarcoma are common.

It is difficult to differentiate between an abscess, sarcoma, and lymphoma by FDG-PET. It can help in the evaluation of distant metastases.

Some other chest wall tumors include neurogenic tumors (posterior chest wall) and schwannomas (very FDG avid). Hemangiomas usually have abundant fat on the CT with phleboliths and bone remodeling. MR shows intermediate (T1) and marked hyperintensity on T2-WI. FDG-PET may show none (common) to mildly increased FDG activity.

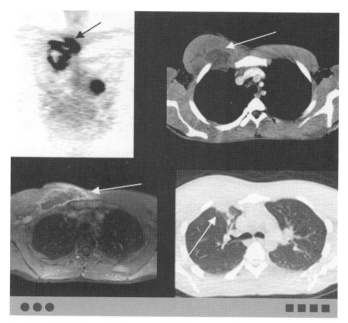

A. (*Top left*) Intensely hypermetabolic, centrally necrotic right chest wall mass (abscess). (*Top right*) Corresponding contrast-enhanced CT (CECT). (*Bottom left*) Fat-suppressed, post-Gd MR image. (*Bottom right*) CT with right apical pulmonary infection.

Osteochondromas are the commonest benign tumor of the cartilage and bone; enchondroma and osteoblastoma are less common. Fibrous dysplasia manifests as an expanding lytic lesion with a ground-glass appearance. Solitary plasmacytomas are seen in adults with "punched-out" lytic lesions in bone.

Chondrosarcomas with chondroid matrix and endosteal scalloping are mainly seen in adults. Chest wall osteosarcomas are rare.

PEARLS

- Chest wall masses can be benign or malignant and arise from skin, fat, muscle, bone, fibrous connective tissue, breasts, cartilage, and lymphatic and blood vessels.

- Increased FDG activity can be seen with abscess, sarcoma, lymphoma, and metastases.

- Since many chest wall infections begin as pulmonary infections, an adjacent pulmonary infiltrate is often associated with chest wall mass.

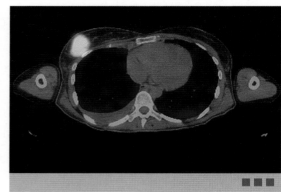

B. Right chest wall melanoma metastasis.

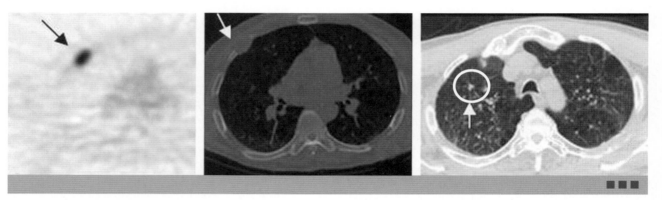

C. (*Left*) Right chest wall hypermetabolic lesion due to metastasis from small adenocarcinoma (*right*) in right apical lung. (*Middle*) Corresponding CT with lytic mass.

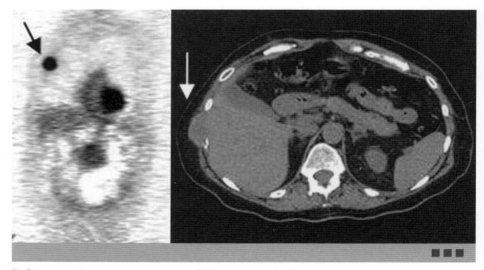

D. Pleomorphic spindle cell sarcoma PET, coronal with CT.

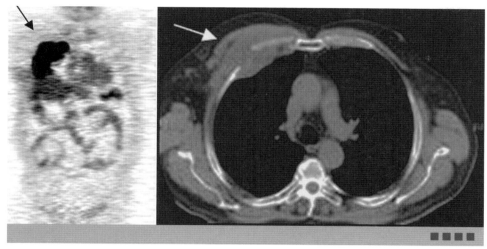

E. Right chest wall B-cell lymphoma. Coronal FDG-PET and CT.

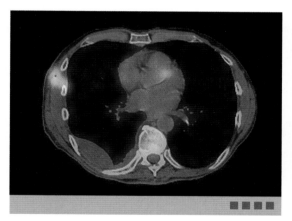

F. Recent (5 days prior to PET) right pleural biopsy, FDG-avid biopsy track. Note FDG negative right loculated pleural effusion.

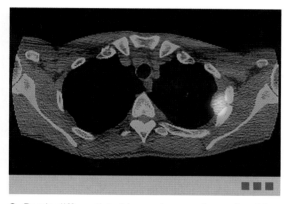

G. Poorly differentiated lung adenocarcinoma involving chest wall.

Naoya Hattori, MD

PRESENTATION

A 54-year-old male patient with right hip prosthesis and persistent right hip pain.

FINDINGS

Three-phase Tc-99m MDP bone scan shows normal and symmetrical blood flow and blood pool. Delayed images show focal uptake near the tip of the femoral component and around the right acetabulum.

DIFFERENTIAL DIAGNOSIS

- *Infected prosthesis*: Usually is positive on all three phases and also in WBC imaging.

COMMENTS

Total hip arthroplasty is performed in patients with late-stage degenerative disease of the hip joint and results in significant improvement in pain and movement. It is very highly successful but has a failure rate of 10% in 10 years from surgery and is influenced by the type of prosthesis and patient characteristics. Over a period of time, there is slow loss of bone around the prosthesis as a result of

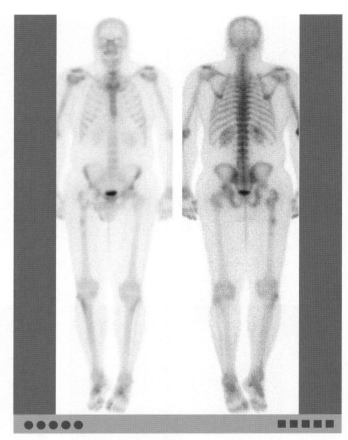

B. Whole-body images show mildly increased uptake in the region of the right hip prosthesis, mainly at the tip of the femoral component and the trochanters.

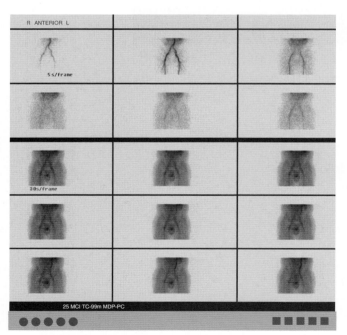

A. Three-phase Tc-99m MDP bone scan images show symmetric blood flow and blood pool activity in both hips.

PEARLS

- It is important to distinguish between infection and loosening as the management will be different. Three phase bone scan is critical in making this distinction.

- Infection specific imaging may be necessary to confirm infection.

- All infections are likely to be associated with loosening.

- Minimal uptake in the early periods after implantation is normal and is due to post-operative changes.

"stress shielding." Apart from acute complications, long-term complications include prosthetic wear and loosening as well as infection. Common causes for chronic pain in patients with total hip arthroplasty may include aseptic loosening and, rarely, infection. It is important to rule out infection in such patients. Findings for loose prosthesis on plain radiographs include loss of bone around the prosthesis especially in the proximal part that transmits less weight (resulting in lack of stress for active remodeling). However, it may require the loss of 40% to 50% of the bone mass for it to be seen on the plain radiographs. Skeletal scintigraphy is frequently used in the evaluation of painful hip prosthesis. Some degree of uptake, as a result of normal postsurgical healing, can be seen for up to 1 year in cemented prosthesis and 2 to 3 years in noncemented prosthesis. In loosening the uptake is typically seen at the tip of the prosthesis and around the lesser and greater trochanters of the femur likely as a result of bone remodeling. Three-phase bone scintigraphy typically does not show increased blood flow or blood pool activity in prosthesis loosening. In infection (osteomyelitis), there is diffusely increased uptake in the bone surrounding the prosthesis and all three phases of bone scan can be positive. A negative bone scan helps rule out osteomyelitis. The differentiation of the diagnosis of infection and loosening is usually made with radio-labeled WBCs. The sensitivity is very high for In-111 and Tc-99m hexamethylpropyleneamine oxime (HMPAO)-labeled WBC scan. One of the important difficulties with the radio-labeled WBC study is the increased uptake in the presence of reactive bone marrow surrounding the prosthesis, when a combination with Tc-99m sulfur colloid scan will help with the diagnosis.

ADDITIONAL IMAGES (C-D)

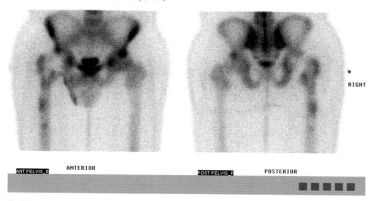

C. Planar spot views confirm the location of this abnormal radiotracer uptake related to the prosthesis (anterior and posterior).

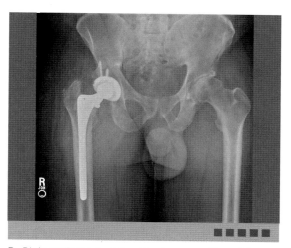

D. Plain radiograph of the hip shows position of the right hip prosthesis.

Vivek Manchanda, MD

PRESENTATION

A woman in her early forties with right arm pain, with known multiple myeloma.

FINDINGS

Intense FDG activity in the right humerus and left rib (arrows).

DIFFERENTIAL DIAGNOSES

- *Multiple myeloma* (MM) involvement of right humerus
- *Metastases*: Melanoma, breast, lung
- *Osteosarcoma*
- *Chondrosarcoma*
- *Lymphoma*
- *Leiomyosarcoma* (rare)

FDG-avid, marrow-based metastases can be seen in other cancers such as breast, lung, and melanoma. Given known history of MM, most likely diagnosis is humeral involvement from MM.

COMMENTS

Multiple myeloma forms a spectrum of diseases ranging from monoclonal gammopathy of unknown significance (MGUS) to plasma cell leukemia. It is characterized by proliferation of malignant plasma cells and monoclonal paraproteins.

The presence and extent of bone marrow and extra-medullary involvement are important factors that influence the prognosis and clinical management. Extramedullary disease indicates poorer prognosis.

Radiological survey, limited MR, and FDG-PET/CT have been recommended for initial staging of MM. PET/CT has been extremely helpful in the evaluation of extramedullary disease.

Both FDG-PET and MRI have reported false negatives pertaining to diffuse bone marrow disease.

MRI and CT do not readily distinguish between active disease and scar tissue, necrosis, bone fracture, or benign disease. FDG-PET also contributes to improve clinical management in patients with solitary plasmacytoma, when a higher sensitivity to detect medullary involvement is essential. Some studies have suggested that the MR signal may remain abnormal for up to 6 to 9 months, whereas FDG-

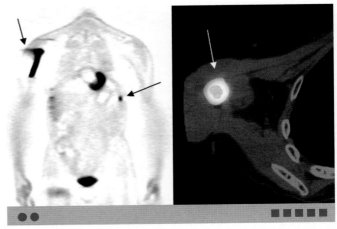

A. Intense right humeral and left rib FDG activity corresponding to active multiple myeloma.

PET can detect changes in active disease earlier. FDG-PET is very valuable in the follow-up of disease and a baseline scan is important for the comparisons.

Whole-body FDG-PET has helped in the evaluation of patients with gammopathy of unknown origin and may contribute to diagnostic or discriminatory criteria.

In general, if the PET scan is negative, stable monoclonal gammopathy of unknown significance is likely. If it is positive, it is likely due to active disease, even if the CT/MR results are negative.

In nonsecretory phase, FDG-PET is especially helpful in localizing the disease.

PEARLS

- Radiological survey, limited MR, and whole-body FDG-PET are being adopted for the initial staging of MM.

- In MGUS, negative FDG activity suggests stable disease. Positive scan indicates active disease, even if the corresponding radiography is negative.

- FDG-PET is important in detecting and follow-up of extramedullary disease.

- Crystal-storing histiocytosis is associated with MM, MGUS, or extramedullary plasmacytoma with intralysosomal accumulation of crystallized secreted immunoglobulins.

ADDITIONAL IMAGES (B-D)

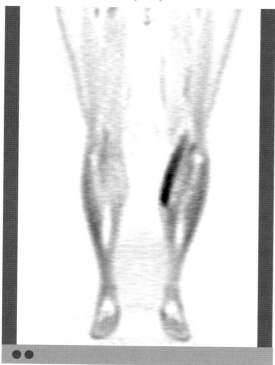

B. Different patient with extramedullary plasmacytoma in left leg muscle. Coronal FDG-PET, nonattenuation corrected image.

C. Extramedullary plasmacytoma in left supraclavicular node. Coronal FDG-PET, nonattenuation corrected image, and corresponding CT.

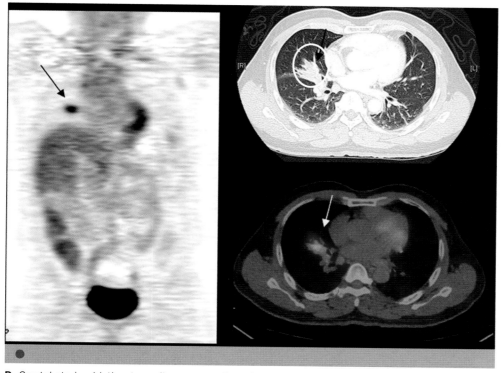

D. Crystal-storing histiocytoma (kappa-secreting plasma cells) in right mid-lung with corresponding CT in a patient with an unknown primary monoclonal gammopathy.

Chapter 3

CHEST

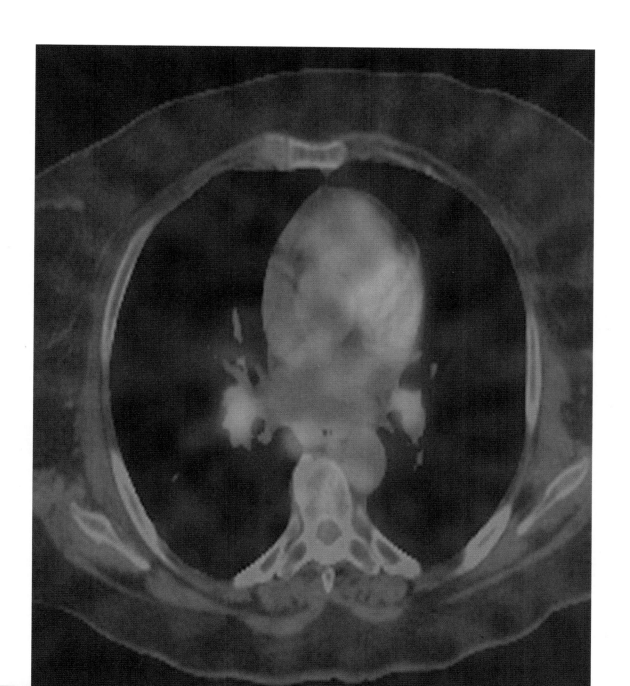

Vivek Manchanda, MD

PRESENTATION

Man in his fifties with mediastinal lymphadenopathy.

FINDINGS

Bilateral hilar and mediastinal hypermetabolic nodes. No abnormal hypermetabolic focus in the lungs or remainder of the imaged body.

DIFFERENTIAL DIAGNOSES

- *Neoplastic adenopathy*

  - *Lymphoma*
  - *Metastases* (lung, breast, melanoma, renal)

- *Inflammatory*

  - *Sarcoidosis* (right paratracheal and bilateral hilar predominant)
  - *Tuberculosis (TB)*/histoplasmosis/coccidiomycosis/ drug reaction/ connective tissue disease/silicosis

Positron emission tomography (PET) cannot distinguish between the etiologies of hypermetabolic nodes; however, inflammatory nodes are usually less FDG avid than metastases from cancers that commonly metastasize to mediastinum. History, CT appearance and nodal distribution should be taken in account.

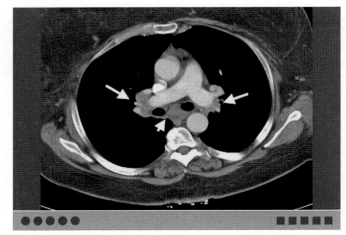

B. Corresponding CT.

COMMENTS

Fluorodeoxyglucose (FDG) uptake in mediastinal nodes can be characterized as mild in leukemias such as chronic lymphocytic leukemia (CLL), inflammation, or subacute sarcoidosis to intense in lymphomas (both Hodgkin and non-Hodgkin), infections such as TB, and cancers such as small-cell lung cancer (SCLC) and active sarcoidosis.

Metastases from lung, breast, and esophageal carcinomas are generally FDG avid. Among extrathoracic primary tumors; kidney, testis, head, and neck neoplasms may be implicated. Castleman disease in patients younger than 30 years can present as hypermetabolic and enhancing mediastinal adenopathy.

FDG activity in lymphadenopathy from amyloidosis, Wegener granulomatosis, cystic fibrosis, and chronic mediastinitis has not been described.

Calcification in mediastinal nodes is uncommon with Hodgkin disease (HD), although NHL may present with calcified mediastinal adenopathy. Majority of mediastinal germ cell tumors

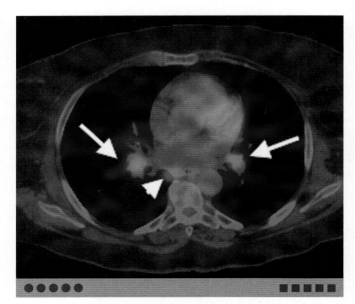

A. Coronal fused FDG-PET with hypermetabolic hilar and mediastinal nodes in sarcoidosis.

PEARLS

- Sarcoidosis is associated with high FDG uptake in paratracheal and bilateral hilar nodes. Degree of FDG uptake may reflect disease activity.

- Bilateral hypermetabolic hilar lymphadenopathy is most commonly due to sarcoidosis.

- Lymph node calcification is very rarely due to neoplastic disease. Calcification in untreated lymphoma is rare, seen more in NHL than HD.

are benign and may not show FDG activity. Malignant seminomas tend to be FDG avid. Nonseminomatous germ cell tumors have variable FDG activity.

Aortopulmonary nodes that are not accessible by cervical mediastinoscopy can be characterized with the help of FDG-PET. MR disadvantages include nonvisualization of calcified nodes (which are rarely malignant) and blurring together of nodes to form a large mass. Mediastinoscopy has not been replaced as staging tool for non–small-cell lung cancer (NSCLC) by FDG-PET owing to the latter's limitations.

Nonspecific mediastinal adenopathy on CT in a patient at high risk for cancer can be assessed with FDG-PET. Non–FDG-avid nodes or metabolic activity less than mediastinal blood pool indicate benign etiology.

FDG activity in mediastinal brown fat is a pitfall and correlation with CT is helpful.

ADDITIONAL IMAGES (C-E)

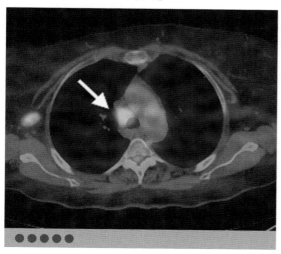

C. Hypermetabolic right paratracheal and axillary node.

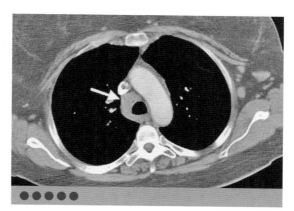

D. Corresponding CT.

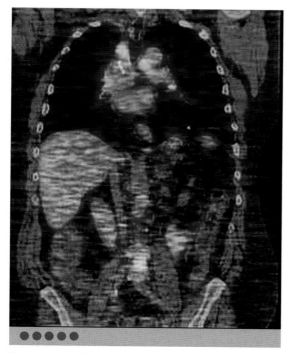

E. Hypermetabolic mediastinal nodes in a 52-year-old man, biopsy showed noncaseating granulomas, negative for infection (sarcoidosis).

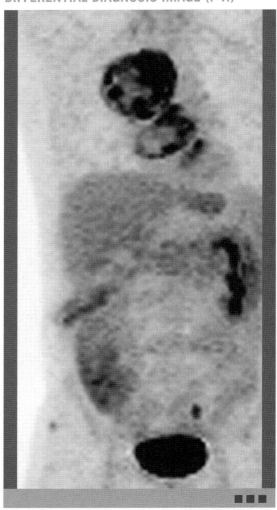

F. Hypermetabolic metastatic mediastinal lymph nodes, renal cell carcinoma (RCC), coronal FDG-PET.

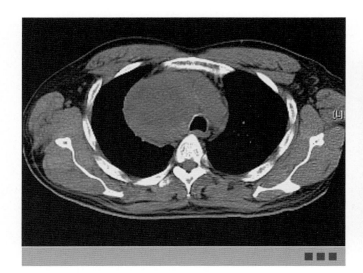

G. Corresponding enlarged nodes on CT, RCC.

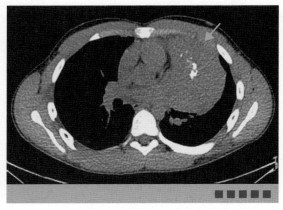

H. Untreated partially calcified anterior mediastnal NHL in a teenager (*arrow*).

Vivek Manchanda, MD

PRESENTATION

A female in midfifties with enlarging painful left breast.

FINDINGS

Intensely increased FDG activity corresponding to the left breast masses and thickened skin (arrow).

DIFFERENTIAL DIAGNOSES

- *Inflammatory breast cancer*
- *Mastitis* (tubercular or other organisms)
- *Duct ectasia* (plasma cell mastitis)
- *Lymphoma*

Hypermetabolic and thickened left breast skin and multiple intense FDG-avid masses in the left breast in a nonlactating patient in age group of 50 to 55 years is most worrisome for inflammatory breast cancer. Plasma cell mastitis is well circumscribed involving less than one-third of the breast area. Infections of the female breast are uncommon (except postpartum).

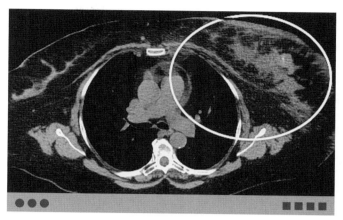

B. Corresponding CT, left breast inflammatory cancer.

COMMENTS

The sensitivity of PET/CT in detecting primary breast cancer is highly dependent on the tumor size and histology. The detection of T1a and b (<1 cm) is low and less than 0.5 cm (T1a) may not be detected. There is increased sensitivity for T2 (2-5 cm) and T3 (> 5 cm).

MR has slightly better sensitivity and specificity than FDG-PET.

In general, primary breast cancers have less metabolic activity than most other tumors (least for invasive lobular).

Dense breasts do not interfere with PET imaging. False-negative results may be seen in small lesions, invasive lobular, tubular cancers, and carcinoma in situ. False-positive results may be seen in abscess, inflammation, TB, sarcoidosis, hematoma (with ringlike uptake), benign neoplasms such as ductal adenoma, and fibroadenoma.

For axillary staging, FDG-PET cannot substitute for sentinel node mapping. Some studies have suggested that patients with positive axillary disease could potentially forego sentinel node biopsy and proceed to axillary lymph node dissection.

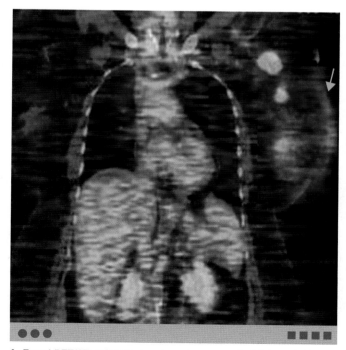

A. Fused PET/CT: Inflammatory breast cancer with thickened skin (*arrow*) and hypermetabolic masses.

PEARLS

- **FDG-PET cannot substitute for sentinel node imaging for breast cancer staging.**
- **FDG-PET has shown promise in characterizing disease extent in newly diagnosed locally advanced and inflammatory breast cancer.**
- **FDG-PET may be falsely negative in invasive lobular cancer.**
- **FDG-PET is excellent in following the tumor burden and treatment response in metastatic disease.**

In studies, FDG-PET was more accurate than CT in the detection of internal mammary and mediastinal nodes. In distant staging, FDG-PET helped in about 10%. Some studies have described the accuracy of FDG-PET to be much higher for lytic bony metastases as compared to blastic metastases (in contrast to the bone scan) and F18 sodium fluoride.

FDG-PET is accurate in both locoregional and distant tumor recurrences, useful in asymptomatic patients with elevated tumor markers, and in patients with clinical suspicion for recurrence and negative tumor markers.

Some studies have described metabolic flare because of inflammation in 7 to 10 days after treatment.

DIFFERENTIAL DIAGNOSIS IMAGES (C-F)

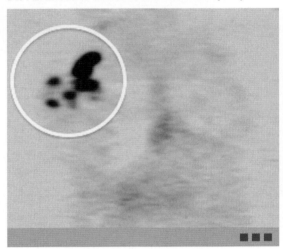

C. Primary right breast non Hodgkin lymphoma, coronal FDG-PET (*circle*).

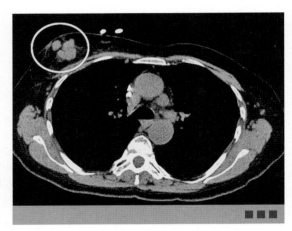

D. Right breast primary NHL, corresponding CT.

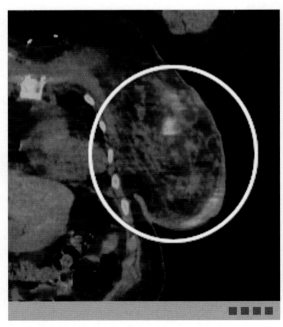

E. Left breast plasmacytomas with underlying multiple myeloma.

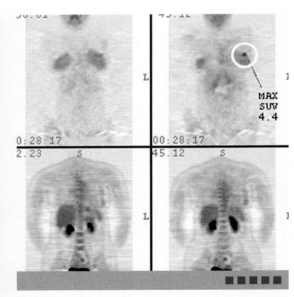

F. Left breast invasive ductal cancer, coronal FDG-PET (*circle*).

Vivek Manchanda, MD

PRESENTATION

Woman in mid sixties with ground glass opacity in left lower lobe.

FINDINGS

No abnormally increased FDG activity corresponding to the left lower lobe ground glass opacity on CT.

DIFFERENTIAL DIAGNOSES

- *Focal inflammation*
- *Bronchoalveolar cell cancer (BAC)*
- *Well-differentiated adenocarcinoma*
- *Mucosa-associated lymphoid tissue (MALT)*
- *Pulmonary infiltrate with eosinophilia*

In the index case, the solitary ground glass opacity had mildly increased in size, without any corresponding FDG activity, over a year.

COMMENTS

Bronchoalveolar cancer is a unique cancer epidemiologically, pathologically, and clinically in comparison to other non–small-cell cancer subtypes. Its relationship with smoking is less strong than other subtypes. It is mostly indolent and less likely to metastasize.

CT features of BAC include solitary ground glass opacity, which is more common than a single mass or diffuse nodular/ground glass opacity. Uncommon features include mediastinal adenopathy, spontaneous pneumothorax, atelectasis, and cavitation.

Nodular ground glass opacity can also be seen in adenocarcinoma and the precursor lesions such as atypical adenomatous hyperplasia. It can also be seen in benign lesions such as inflammation, focal interstitial fibrosis, and hemorrhage.

Eosinophilic pneumonia, bronchiolitis obliterans with organizing pneumonia, lymphomas, thoracic endometriosis, and focal traumatic lung injury may be associated with ground glass opacity. Aspergillosis may appear as nodular ground glass opacity caused by hemorrhage or inflammatory cellular infiltration.

BAC and well-differentiated adenocarcinoma may have no corresponding FDG activity. Some studies have suggested that the non–FDG-avid disease subtypes of BAC are biologically more indolent than FDG-positive ones.

Persistence of ground glass opacity or increasing size or increasing attenuation irrespective of FDG uptake is strongly suggestive of BAC.

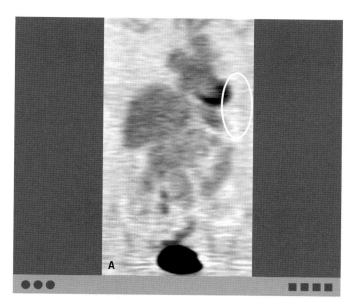

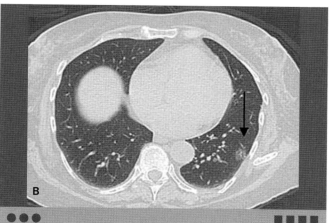

A. and **B.** Non–FDG-avid left lower lobe ground glass opacity with corresponding CT (*arrow*) BAC.

PEARLS

- In the evaluation of pulmonary ground glass opacities, BAC should be considered.

- BAC and well-differentiated adenocarcinomas can be falsely FDG negative.

- Some studies have suggested that the FDG negative BACs are more indolent than the positive ones.

- Persistence of ground glass opacity, increasing size, and attenuation strongly favor malignancy.

MALT lymphoma in the lungs is usually associated with air bronchograms with consolidation and mild FDG activity and can be confused with BAC (diffuse type) which can have a similar presentation.

ADDITIONAL IMAGES (C-D)

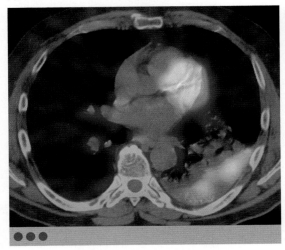

C. Hypermetabolic left lower lobe bronchoalveolar cell cancer in a different patient.

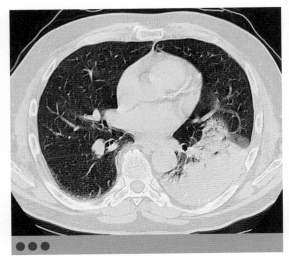

D. Corresponding CT, BAC.

DIFFERENTIAL DIAGNOSIS IMAGES (E-J)

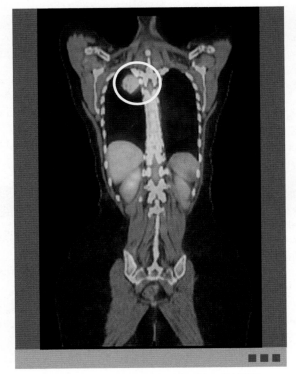

E. RUL MALT (47-year-old female) with mild FDG (standardized uptake value [SUV] 3.6).

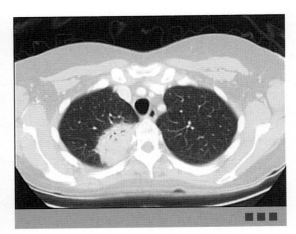

F. RUL consolidation with air bronchogram, MALT.

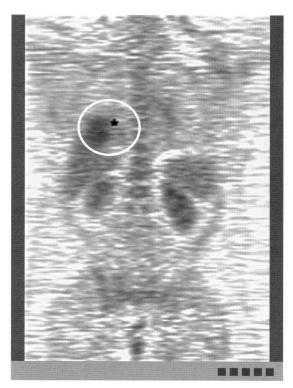

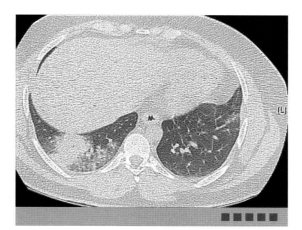

H. RLL pneumonia, CT.

G. Right lower lobe (RLL) pneumonia, (*star with circle*). Coronal FDG-PET.

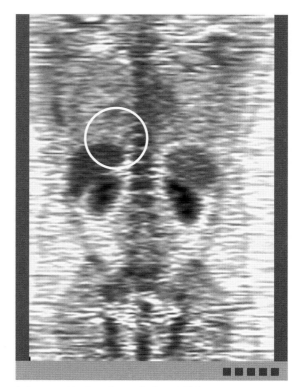

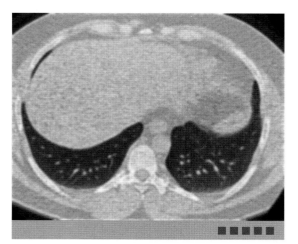

J. Resolution of RLL pneumonia, CT.

I. Same patient as G, resolution of RLL pneumonia, coronal FDG PET.

Case 3–4 Central Lung Mass and FDG-PET

Vivek Manchanda, MD

PRESENTATION

Woman in midforties with right central lung mass.

FINDINGS

Mildly hypermetabolic right central lung mass.

DIFFERENTIAL DIAGNOSES

- *Lung Cancer*: Squamous cell, small cell; usually intense FDG

- *Sarcoma*: Rare; usually intense FDG

- *Lymphoma*: Usually intense FDG

- *Nodal metastases*: Usually intense FDG, histology-dependent

- *Pulmonary hamartoma*: Usually non–FDG-avid

- *Wegener granulomatosis*: Variable FDG

- *Adenoid cystic carcinoma/mucoepidermoid carcinoma*: Salivary gland tumors which may arise in main bronchi; variable, usually mild FDG unless high-grade mucoepidermoid

COMMENTS

Biopsy in the index case showed carcinoid.

Tumors are designated central if they involve a main, lobar, or segmental bronchus and peripheral if they arose distal to a segmental bronchus. Central tumors may result

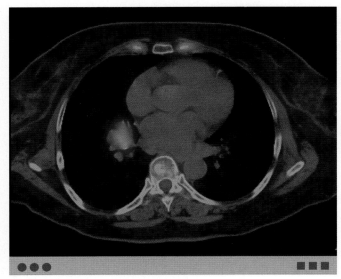

A. Right pulmonary carcinoid, PET.

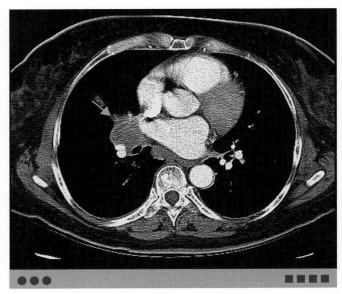

B. Corresponding CT.

in airways obstruction with recurrent infection, lobar collapse, and a central mediastinal or hilar mass.

Bronchial carcinoids are rare low-grade neuroendocrine tumors (1%-2% of total lung cancers), located in the airways of central/middle-third of the lung (in 80%) and present with hemoptysis or lobar obstruction. About 20% occurrences are peripheral and usually asymptomatic.

On CT, the mass may be seen within bronchial lumen, usually with both intra-and extraluminal component. It is typically round or ovoid with smooth or lobulated border with common calcification. Cavitation and hilar adenopathy are rare. Intense homogenous enhancement following contrast injection may be seen. On MR, bronchial carcinoids have high-signal intensity on T2-weighted (T2-W) and short T1 inversion recovery (STIR) images. Somatostatin receptor scintigraphy may help in localization. If the lesion secretes adrenocorticotropic hormone (ACTH), marked nodular adrenal hyperplasia may be seen.

PEARLS

- Both typical and atypical bronchial carcinoids may show FDG avidity.

- In some studies, majority of bronchial carcinoids were FDG negative.

- Hypermetabolic central lung masses differential on FDG-PET includes SCLC, carcinoid, and squamous cell lung cancer.

The sensitivity of FDG-PET for diagnosis of primary pulmonary carcinoids was believed to be reduced due to the low metabolic activity and slow growth. However, many current studies and case reports have shown increased FDG activity corresponding to both typical and atypical carcinoids. Typical and atypical carcinoid tumors were defined based on established World Health Organization (WHO) pathologic criteria with typical carcinoids having less than 2 mitotic figures per 2 mm^2 and no necrosis, while typical carcinoids have 2 to 10 mitotic figures per 2 mm^2 or evidence for necrosis.

The other central primary lung malignancies include squamous cell and small cell, both of which are characteristically intensely FDG avid.

ADDITIONAL IMAGES (C-D)

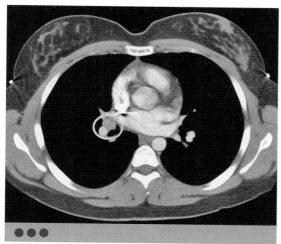

C. Right central carcinoid in 18 F, axial CT (*circle*).

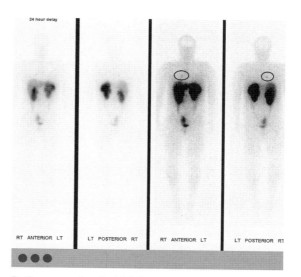

D. Corresponding In 111 Pentetriotide scan with focal carcinoid in right mid lung (*black circle*). Note absent liver lesions.

DIFFERENTIAL DIAGNOSIS IMAGES (E-I)

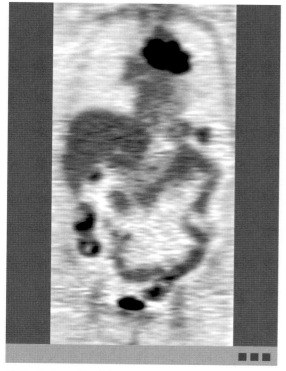

E. Central small cell lung cancer, coronal FDG-PET.

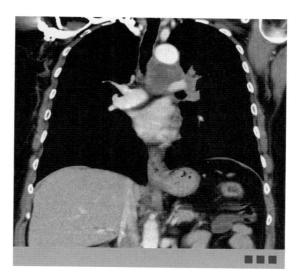

F. Corresponding CT.

131

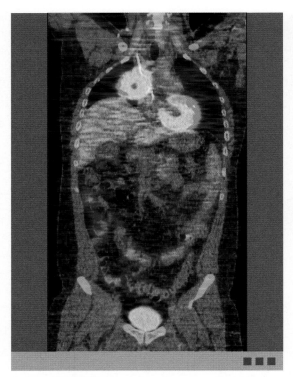

G. Fused PET/CT, right lung primary non-Hodgkin lymphoma.

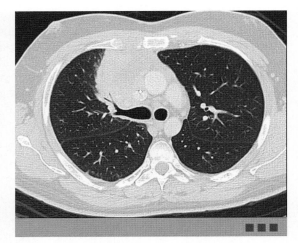

H. Corresponding CT to image H.

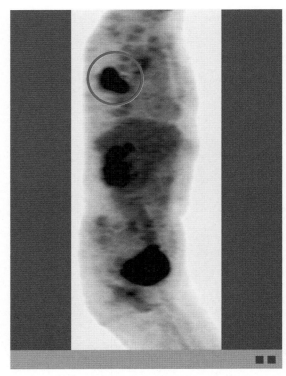

I. High-grade primary pleomorphic sarcoma of lung (*circle*), MIP.

Vivek Manchanda, MD

PRESENTATION

Diabetic man in midfifties with history of 30 pack years of smoking, cough for 1 month, and chest pain.

FINDINGS

Intensely hypermetabolic mass in the superior segment of left lower lobe (maximum SUV of 12.8), corresponding to the mass seen on CT.

DIFFERENTIAL DIAGNOSES

* *Malignancy*: Bronchogenic carcinoma, lymphoma, sarcoma, plasmacytoma

* *Inflammation/infections* such as TB, focal organizing pneumonia, Rheumatoid/Wegener nodule

* *Metastases*: Breast, melanoma, RCC

Wedge dissection showed active airspace pneumonitis with numerous encapsulated cryptococci. Level of FDG activity cannot differentiate neoplastic from infectious causes. Hamartoma and infarct would typically be FDG negative.

COMMENTS

Cryptococcal infection can be due to *Cryptococcus neoformans* var *gattii* or var *neoformans*. This fungus reproduces

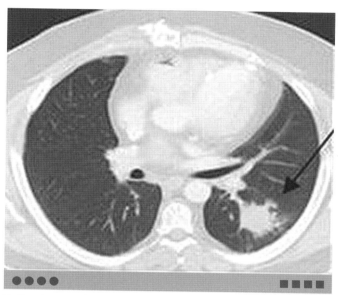

B. Cryptococcal infection with corresponding CT.

by budding and forms round, yeast-like cells. Infection occurs by inhaling the fungus in soil contaminated with pigeon excreta.

Many patients may have no symptoms and others may present with fever, chest pain, cough, and mucus production.

FDG uptake ranges from moderate to intense in cryptococcal infections. FDG activity cannot distinguish cancer from infections such as TB and Cryptococcus. Similarly, distinguishing cryptococcal infection from primary lung cancer is difficult on CT as well.

The CT manifestations of pulmonary nodules in cryptococcosis include small nodules to large masses. They are mainly single (but can be multiple) and have variable location. Immunocompetent patients develop well-defined nodules with or without central necrosis. There are no calcifications and cavitations are rare. Approximately half of the nodules can have "halo sign," which is ground glass opacification related to granulomatous inflammation.

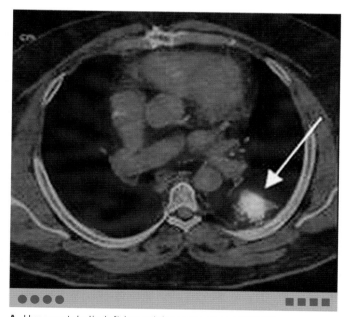

A. Hypermetabolic left lower lobe mass, fused PET/CT.

PEARLS

* *Cryptococcus* is most commonly seen in immunocompromised, including diabetics.

* FDG uptake in infections such as cryptococcosis or TB or *Mycobacterium avium*-intracellulare (MAI) can be moderate to intense and difficult to distinguish from neoplasm.

* CT features can be different in nodules in immunocompetent versus immunocompromised patients.

Cavitation of nodules along with areas of consolidation, pleural effusions, and lymphadenopathy are more commonly seen in immunocompromised patients. Diffuse and systemic dissemination (such as to meninges) is also common in such patients.

Surgical resection is recommended for both diagnosis and treatment of pulmonary cryptococcosis. *Cryptococcus* colonizes the respiratory tract of many patients with chronic disease and can be cultured from the sputum and bronchial washings of patients with lung cancer.

Typical *Mycobacterium avium* presentation involves elderly female with bronchiectasis and centrilobular nodules mainly in right middle lobe and lingula.

DIFFERENTIAL DIAGNOSIS IMAGES (C-I)

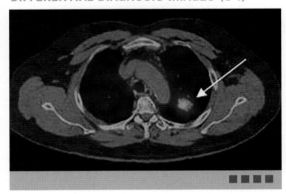

C. Primary NSCLS, fused PET/CT.

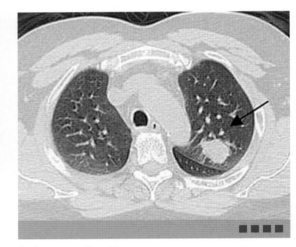

D. Corresponding CT.

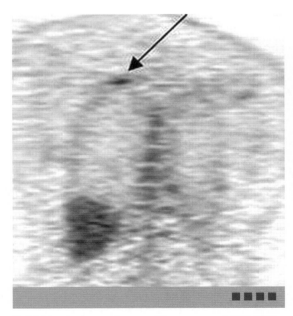

E. Right apical caseating granuloma, coronal FDG-PET.

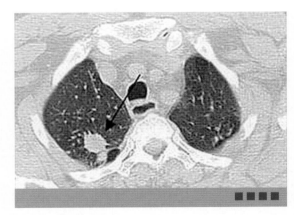

F. Corresponding CT.

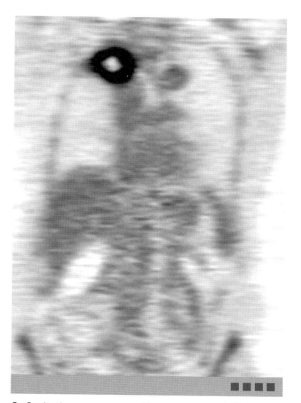

G. Cavitating squamous cell cancer, coronal FDG-PET.

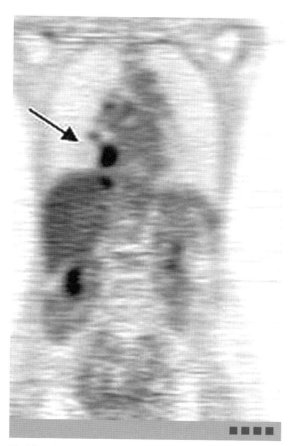

H. *Mycobacterium avium* infection, coronal FDG-PET.

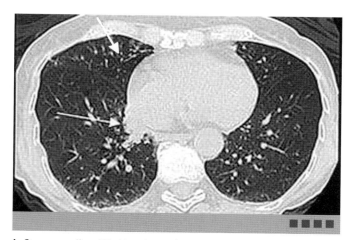

I. Corresponding CT, *Mycobacterium avium* infection (*arrows*).

Vivek Manchanda, MD

PRESENTATION

Woman in her sixth decade of life with lung cancer, for staging.

FINDINGS

Diffuse, moderately increased FDG uptake in the right lung and left upper lung along with nodular thickening of interlobular septa and fissures.

DIFFERENTIAL DIAGNOSES

• *Sarcoidosis*

• *Infection*

• *Interstitial pneumonias*

• *Pulmonary edema*

• *Lymphangitic spread of cancer:* Breasts, pancreas, stomach, colon, prostate, lymphoma

Given the history of lung cancer and CT findings of nodular thickening of interlobular septae and fissures along with increased FDG uptake, the findings are most consistent with lymphangitic carcinomatosis. Pulmonary edema would not be FDG avid.

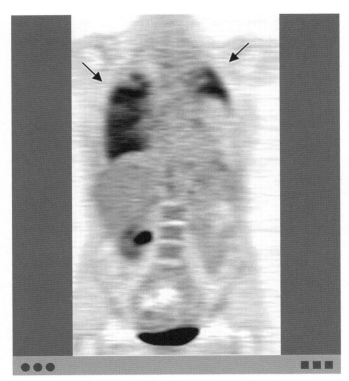

A. Diffuse FDG activity in the right lung and left upper lung, coronal FDG-PET. Lymphangitic carcinomatosis.

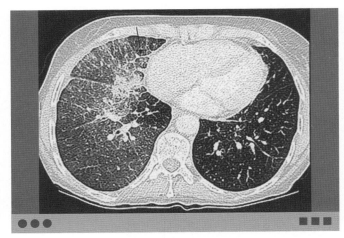

B. Corresponding CT. Lymphangitic carcinomatosis.

COMMENTS

Lungs are a common site of metastases for many cancers. Majority of metastases reach the lungs through arterial system and manifest as multiple nodules.

Metastases from tumors such as melanoma, colon and kidney, and sarcoma may occur as solitary nodules. Miliary nodules are more likely to occur from thyroid, kidney, and melanoma.

Pulmonary lymphangitic carcinomatosis (PLC) is due to hematogenous metastases to small pulmonary capillaries and secondary involvement of peripheral pulmonary lymphatics. Disease extension from hilar or mediastinal nodes or diaphragmatic lymphatics is uncommon. The cancers most often associated with lymphangitic carcinomatosis include lung, breast, gastrointestinal (GI), and prostate

PEARLS

● **Nodular interstitial thickening of interlobular septa from tumor cells, desmoplastic response, and dilated lymphatics characterize PLC.**

● **Variability of FDG-PET in PLC (diffuse vs segmental; intense vs hazy/none) may depend on distribution and concentration of tumor cells in the interlobular septa.**

● **Interlobular septal thickening from pulmonary edema is typically smooth and FDG negative.**

● **In some studies, central PLC was associated with higher FDG uptake in comparison to peripheral PLC.**

as well as melanoma, lymphoma, and leukemia. Incidence of PLC is variably reported to be around 7%.

Differential diagnosis includes sarcoidosis. On CT, sarcoidosis involvement of lungs is typically symmetric, involving the upper lobes more commonly as opposed to PLC, which has predilection for subpleural interstitial spaces. Thickened polygonal lines are hallmark of PLC.

High-resolution CT (HRCT) is the mainstay for diagnosis in which irregular, nodular, and/or smooth interlobular septal thickening and thickening of the fissures may be seen.

Peribronchovascular thickening, mediastinal and/or hilar lymphadenopathy, and pleural effusions are other features associated with PLC. Corresponding to the CT findings, the PET findings may include diffuse, lobar, or segmental FDG uptake in the lungs. In some case reports of limited disease, linear area of FDG uptake extending from the tumor, corresponding to thickening of interlobular septa/fissures has been described.

Idiopathic pulmonary fibrosis (IPF) features include patchy distribution with predilection for basilar and subpleural regions, interlobular septal thickening and subpleural honeycombing.

DIFFERENTIAL DIAGNOSIS IMAGES (C–H)

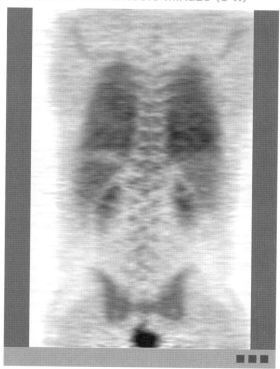

C. Bilateral mild diffuse FDG uptake from Bleomycin chemotoxicity, coronal FDG-PET.

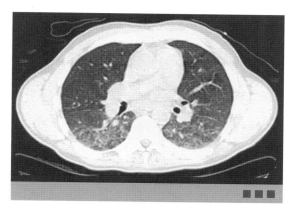

D. Corresponding CT.

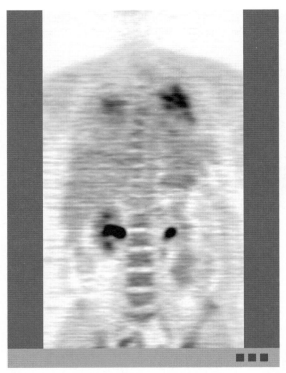

E. Bilateral upper lobe FDG activity, from *Pneumocystis jerovecii* pneumonia, coronal PET.

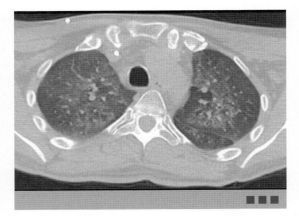

F. Corresponding CT with geographic ground glass upper lobe opacities.

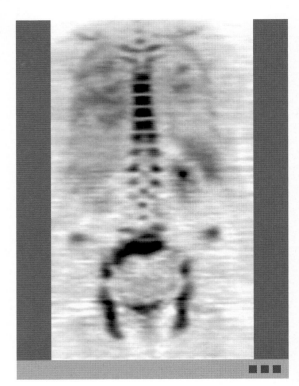

G. Patchy bilateral lung FDG uptake, interstitial lung pneumonia, and GCSF-stimulated marrow.

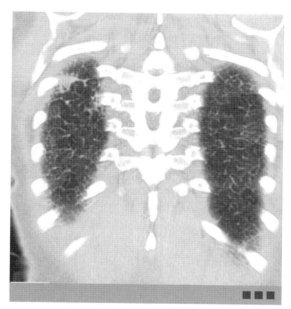

H. Corresponding coronal CT.

Vivek Manchanda, MD

PRESENTATION

Man in midfifties with asbestos exposure and chest pain.

FINDINGS

Moderate to intensely hypermetabolic thickened right pleura with nodularity. Hypermetabolic right epigastric node.

DIFFERENTIAL DIAGNOSES

- *Benign pleural* thickening from TB or old hemothorax, empyema (usually smooth), asbestos exposure (variable contour)
- *Metastases*: Lung cancer, lymphoma, breast cancer, thymoma (usually discrete mass)
- *Talc pleurodesis*
- *Primary pleural liposarcoma, osteosarcoma* (rare)
- *Plasmacytoma, epithelioid hemangioendothelioma* (very rare)

Given asbestos exposure, nodular and noncalcified pleural thickening on CT and hypermetabolism on PET, the findings are most consistent with primary mesothelioma. No prior history of any other primary cancer to suspect metastases.

COMMENTS

Malignant pleural mesothelioma is an uncommon mesothelial cell tumor. Previous occupational exposure to asbestos is associated with a long latent period of 25 to 45 years.

Other than the primary pleural malignancy, metastases from cancers such as lung and breast, lymphoma, and thymoma may involve the pleura. FDG-PET can be used for selecting most metabolically active site for biopsy. Primary pleural liposarcoma and osteosarcoma are rare. Plasmacytoma and epithelioid hemangioendothelioma are other very rare pleural tumors.

Although maximum SUV values (too low or very high) can differentiate malignant from benign pleural thickenings with high degree of confidence, intermediate SUVs may not be helpful in decision making. Dual point imaging and FDG activity greater than liver has been described for differentiating between the two.

It is to be noted that calcified pleural plaques are not a precursor to mesothelioma and FDG uptake corresponding to these plaques is commonly seen (SUVs can be as high as 4.0). Case report of false-negative, slow-growing epithelioid mesothelioma has been reported. On MR, malignant

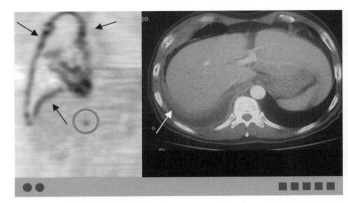

A. Mesothelioma: Hypermetabolic right pleural thickening with corresponding CT. Epigastric nodal metastasis (*green circle*).

mesothelioma is typically hyperintense on T2 and enhances with gadolinium on T1-WI (T1 weighted images), but this appearance is not specific.

The nodular and lobulated pleural thickening is characteristic of mesothelioma. Pleural effusion may be an associated feature. Mediastinal shift in effusions associated with mesothelioma may not be seen due to fixation of mediastinum from disease. Calcification of the tumor is rare. Circumferential pleural thickening and extension into mediastinal pleura and fissures is rare in benign pleural disease. Pleural deposits of thymoma and lymphoma are usually more discrete.

PEARLS

- Noncalcified, hypermetabolic nodular pleural thickening in prior asbestos exposure is most concerning for primary mesothelioma. Metastatic pleural disease may appear identical to mesothelioma.

- Benign pleural thickening from old TB or hemothorax typically has smooth pleural thickening. Active pleural TB/inflammation may result in FDG uptake.

- Calcified plaques are not precursors to mesothelioma. FDG-PET has high accuracy and negative predictive value to rule out a pleural malignancy.

- Talc pleurodesis can remain intensely hypermetabolic for up to 12 years.

ADDITIONAL IMAGE

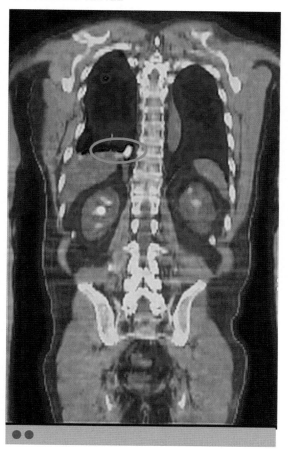

B. Right diaphragmatic pleural epithelioid mesothelioma, coronal FDG-PET/CT.

DIFFERENTIAL DIAGNOSIS IMAGES (C-K)

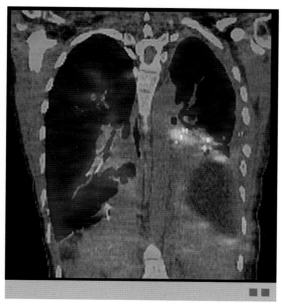

C. Left pleural involvement from rectal cancer. Fused FDG-PET/CT coronal. Note left photopenic effusion.

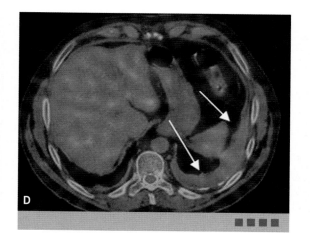

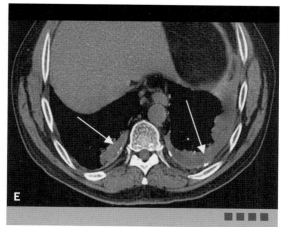

D. and **E.** Mildly hypermetabolic right and left calcified fibrotic (biopsy proven) pleural plaques.

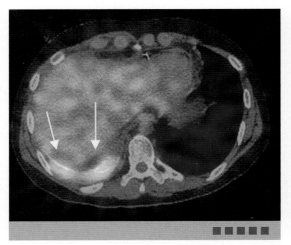

F. Intense FDG activity corresponding to talc pleurodesis.

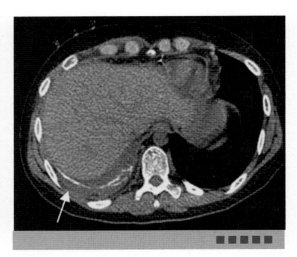

G. Corresponding CT.

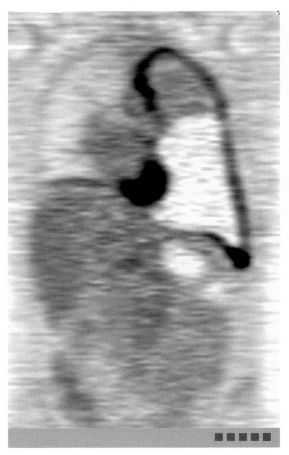

H. Breast cancer–related left pleural metastases, coronal FDG-PET.

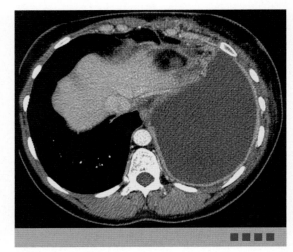

I. Corresponding CT.

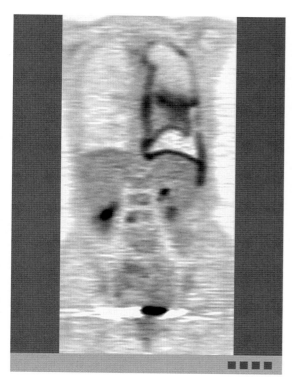

J. Left pleural involvement from non–small-cell lung cancer.

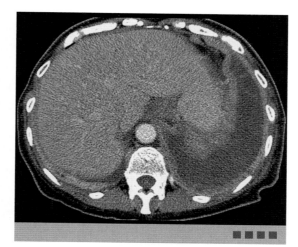

K. Left pleural thickening and pleural effusion from NSCLS.

Vivek Manchanda, MD

PRESENTATION

Teenaged girl with weight loss, fever, and sweating.

FINDINGS

Moderate to intensely increased FDG activity corresponding to anterior mediastinal nodal mass and pericardium.

DIFFERENTIAL DIAGNOSES

- *Leukemia/lymphoma*
- *Malignant thymoma*
- *Malignant germ cell tumor/metastases*
- *Primary pericardial malignancy, myocardial tumors*

COMMENTS

Malignant pericardial effusions occur in about 21% of cancer patients and may be missed until pericardial tamponade develops. Two-thirds of patients have subclinical pericardial effusions with no overt cardiovascular signs/symptoms.

Concomitant pleural effusions and pulmonary parenchymal disease are common in patients with pericardial disease.

About one-third of pericardial metastases are caused by lung cancer. Breast cancer (25%) and hematological malignancies (leukemia, Hodgkin disease, NHL, 15%) and melanoma are usual causes of malignant pericardial effusions.

Malignant involvement of the pericardium results in pericardial effusions, resulting from blocked venous and lymphatic circulation of pericardial fluid. It may be caused by primary malignancy of the pericardium (such as with pericardial mesothelioma), or by myocardial tumors, including angiosarcoma, rhabdomyosarcoma, and malignant fibrous histiocytosis. Direct extension from carcinomas of the lungs or esophagus, thymoma, or lymphoma is possible. Nonmalignant causes include pericarditis, myocardial infarction, uremia, hypothyroidism, AIDS, radiation, or chemotherapy.

A negative cytology of pericardial fluid does not distinguish malignant from nonmalignant etiologies. Pericardial biopsy may increase the sensitivity of diagnosis. At least two studies failed to show a difference in survival in cancer patients with pericardial effusion dependent on the results of fluid cytology.

FDG-PET/CT can accurately show disease involvement of the pericardium and fused images help make such a diagnosis. Nodular thickening of pericardium on CT with FDG

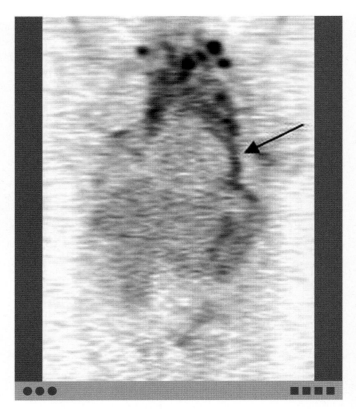

A. Pericardial involvement in Hodgkin lymphoma, coronal PET, filtered back projection.

uptake is characteristic of pericardial disease. However, no FDG uptake in the pericardial fluid does not exclude pericardial disease. FDG-PET can distinguish pericardial scar from pericardial metastases in recurrent lung cancer.

PEARLS

- **Negative cytology and negative FDG uptake in pericardial fluid does not rule out disease involvement.**
- **Nodular pericardial thickening and corresponding FDG uptake is characteristic of disease involvement.**
- **Lymphatic or hematogenous metastases to the pericardium is seen in carcinomas of the breast and lung, lymphoma, and melanoma.**

ADDITIONAL IMAGES (B-D)

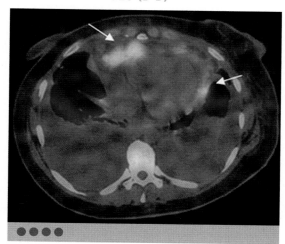

B. Pericardial involvement in Hodgkin lymphoma, fused PET/CT, 16-year-old female.

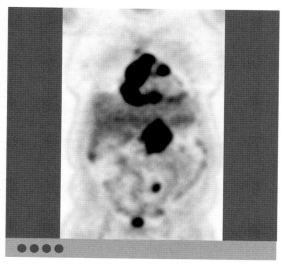

C. Pericardial (and abdominal) involvement in non-Hodgkin lymphoma, 63-year-old female. Coronal FDG-PET.

DIFFERENTIAL DIAGNOSIS IMAGES (E-H)

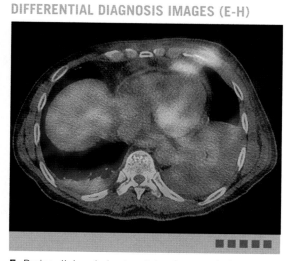

E. Pericardial and chest wall involvement in lung cancer, 60-year-old male, fused PET/CT. Note left pleural effusion.

D. Corresponding noncontrast CT.

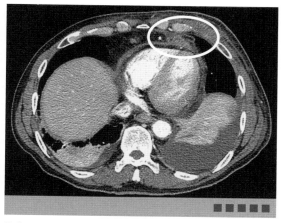

F. Corresponding CT.

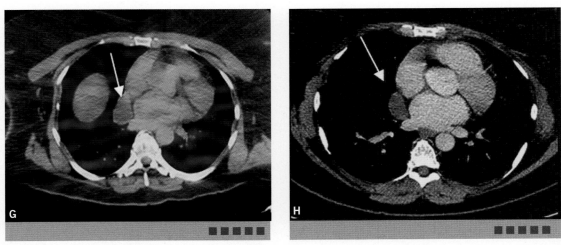

G. and **H.** Right pericardial cyst, fused axial PET/CT and CT (*white arrow*), non–FDG-avid.

Vivek Manchanda, MD

PRESENTATION

Female in late forties with NSCLC for staging.

FINDINGS

Intense focal FDG activity in the right pulmonary recess, with no corresponding CT finding.

DIFFERENTIAL DIAGNOSES

• *Rib trauma*

• *Focal muscular uptake*

• *Pleural metastasis/rib metastasis*

In index case, there was no evidence of trauma or pleural thickening on corresponding CT. Thoracoscopy confirmed dropped pleural metastasis.

COMMENTS

Pleural metastasis and malignant pleural effusions are common in patients with NSCLC. Although most pleural effusions associated with lung cancer are due to tumor, benign effusions may develop in response to the tumor in a few patients.

For evaluation of pleural fluid, multiple cytopathologic examinations or video thoracoscopy and direct pleural biopsies may be needed. When these investigations and clinical judgment dictate that the effusion is not related to the tumor, the effusion is excluded as a staging element.

In the experience of authors, effusions with FDG activity are nonspecific and may be seen in cancers, infections, empyema, and lymphatic blockage. Non–FDG-avid pleural effusions are indeterminate, as small volume tumor cells may get dispersed in the pleural fluid and may not be detected by PET.

Perhaps the most important finding in predicting pleural disease involvement on FDG-PET/CT is focal increased FDG uptake corresponding to nodular thickening on CT.

FDG-avid foci may be seen in the pulmonary recesses, as seen in the index case. These should be considered as dropped metastases, even though no corresponding finding may be seen on CT. Also, even if the cytologic analysis of the pleural fluid in these patients is negative, they should have thoracoscopic examination of the pleura.

Malignant pleural effusion in a patient with lung cancer renders the T stage to be T4 (III B).

Unilateral brown fat and muscular FDG activity can be differentiated from posterior dropped metastasis by coregistering with CT done with the PET scan.

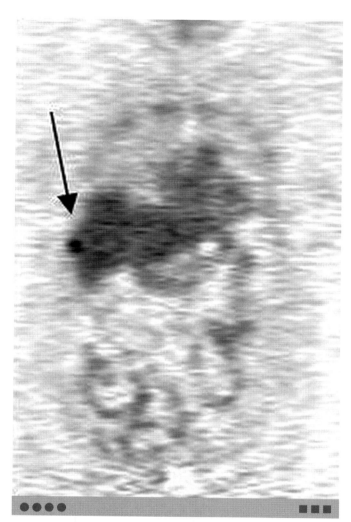

A. Right pleural recess focal FDG deposit with no corresponding CT abnormality (*not shown*), coronal FDG-PET.

PEARLS

• **Patients with malignant lung mass and ipsilateral pleural effusion suggest malignant pleural effusion.**

• **Positive or negative FDG activity in pleural effusion does not substantiate or negate disease involvement.**

• **Focal hypermetabolic pleural lesion corresponding to nodular thickening is perhaps most specific for disease involvement.**

• **Hypermetabolic pleural recess/surface deposits in lung cancer, without corresponding CT findings, are usually from pleural metastases and can be confirmed with thoracoscopy.**

ADDITIONAL IMAGES (B-C)

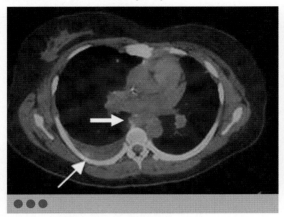

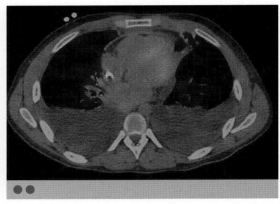

B. Right pleural effusion with malignant cell deposition in breast cancer (*thin arrow*), along with involvement of medial pleura (*thick arrow*). Axial PET/CT.

C. Non–FDG-avid bilateral pleural effusions in patient with NHL, pleural tapping negative for malignancy x 2. Axial PET/CT.

DIFFERENTIAL DIAGNOSIS IMAGES (D-F)

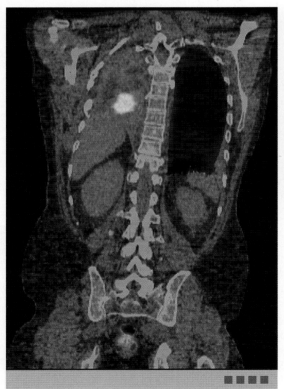

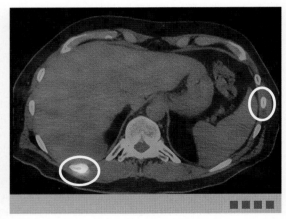

E. Right and left rib involvement in multiple myeloma. Axial PET/CT.

D. Hypermetabolic right thoracic recurrent non–small-cell lung cancer post-pneumonectomy. Coronal fused PET/CT.

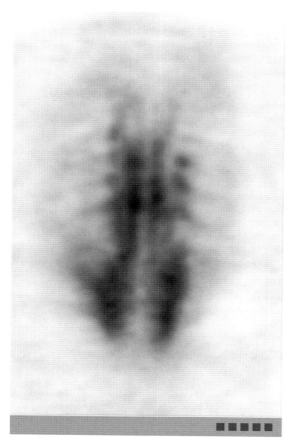

F. Coronal FDG-PET, paraspinal muscular FDG activity, no corresponding CT finding (*not shown*).

Vivek Manchanda, MD

PRESENTATION

Man in the fifth decade of life, left lung non–small-cell lung cancer (NSCLC) for staging by PET.

FINDINGS

Hypermetabolic left lung mass with hypermetabolic right mediastinal node.

DIFFERENTIAL DIAGNOSES

- *NSCLS stage IIIA*
- *NSCLS stage IIIB*

The level of FDG activity in contralateral mediastinum is most consistent with metastases rather than from inflammatory lymph node. Contralateral nodal involvement is categorized as stage IIIB. This was proven by biopsy.

COMMENTS

FDG-PET has been used to improve the detection of distant metastases in lung cancer. The following is the staging system for primary NSCLC. It is important to stage the mediastinum with FDG-PET and correlate the findings with mediastinoscopy/biopsy as both false-positive and false-negative studies have been reported with FDG-PET. There have been a few instances where mediastinoscopy was negative (probable sampling error) in FDG-positive patient, which ultimately on surgery turned out to be truly positive. Level of FDG activity is not a prognostic indicator for stage I or II cancer.

REGIONAL LYMPH NODES (N)

- *N0*: No regional lymph node metastases
- *N1*: Ipsilateral peribronchial and/or ipsilateral hilar lymph nodes, and intrapulmonary nodes including involvement by direct extension of the primary tumor
- *N2*: Ipsilateral mediastinal and/or subcarinal lymph node(s)
- *N3*: Contralateral mediastinal, contralateral hilar, ipsilateral or contralateral scalene, or supraclavicular lymph node(s)

DISTANT METASTASES (M)

- *MX*: Distant metastases cannot be assessed.
- *M0*: No distant metastases.
- *M1*: Distant metastasis present. (Note: M1 includes separate tumor nodule(s) in a different lobe [ipsilateral or contralateral].)

AMERICAN JOINT COMMITTEE ON CANCER (AJCC) STAGE GROUPINGS

- *Stage IA*: T1N0M0 (size <3 cm)
- *Stage IB*: T1N0M0 (size >3 cm)

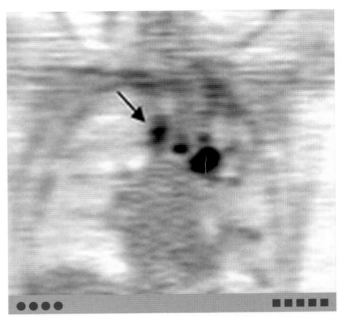

A. Hypermetabolic left lung mass with contralateral (N3) node (*arrow*), stage IIIB.

- *Stage IIA*: T1, N1, M0
- *Stage IIB*: T2, N1, M0; T3, N0, M0
- *Stage IIIA*: T1, N2, M0; T2, N2, M0; T3, N1, M0; T3, N2, M0
- *Stage IIIB*: Any T, N3, M0; T4, any N, M0
- *Stage IV*: Any T, any N, M1

PEARLS

- FDG-PET and mediastinoscopy are complementary and an experienced thoracic surgeon uses both modalities to stage NSCLS. Some studies have suggested that a negative PET at the level of mediastinum may predict a negative thoracotomy with high confidence.

- In mediastinum, both false-positive (mainly inflammation) and false-negative (mainly due to spatial resolution limitation or sampling error) results for FDG activity may occur.

- Because of intense FDG activity in primary lung cancer, the detection of ipsilateral N1 nodes may be suboptimal. The best clinical impact is to distinguish between N2 and N3 nodes (stages IIIA and IIIB) and metastases.

- Treatment of stage IIIA lung cancer involves surgery, unlike stage IIIB, where chemotherapy is the mainstay of treatment.

- Staging of brain metastases by FDG-PET is insufficient due to high physiological brain FDG activity.

DIFFERENTIAL DIAGNOSIS IMAGES (B-G)

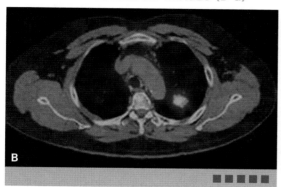

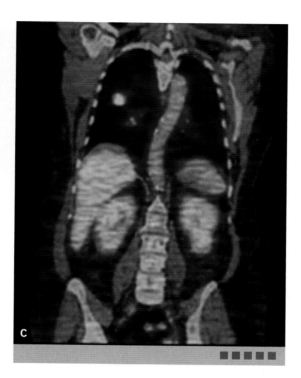

B. and C. Hypermetabolic left apical lung cancer, stage 1A in Figure B, and right stage 1A in Figure C.

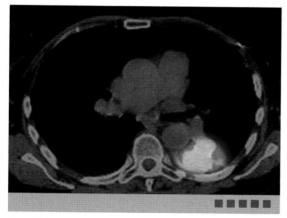

D. Left lower lobe lung cancer (>3 cm), stage IB. No other hypermetabolic lesions.

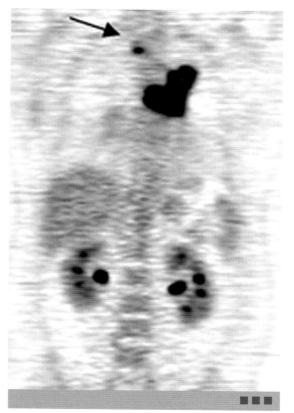

E. Left lung cancer with bony metastases to vertebral body (*arrow*), stage IV. Coronal FDG-PET.

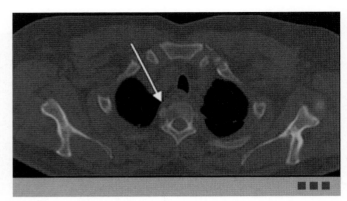

F. Corresponding CT. T2 lytic lesion, stage IV lung cancer.

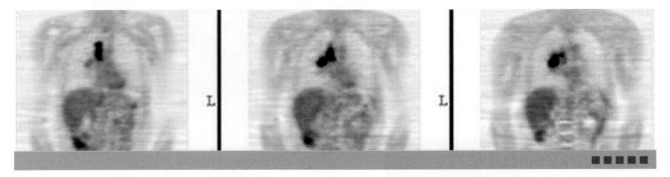

G. Hypermetabolic right lung mass with ipsilateral hypermetabolic nodes, stage IIIA. Coronal FDG-PET.

Vivek Manchanda, MD

PRESENTATION

Enlarging pulmonary nodule in a woman in her fourth decade of life and underlying idiopathic pulmonary fibrosis (IPF).

FINDINGS

Mild focally hypermetabolic nodule in the right lower lobe with underlying idiopathic pulmonary fibrosis. Left transplanted lung.

DIFFERENTIAL DIAGNOSES

- *Infection*
- *Noninfectious granuloma*
- *Carcinoma*

Other differentials for solitary pulmonary nodule remain the same such as metastases, benign tumors such as hamartomas, vascular and inflammatory. But given underlying IPF, the findings are most concerning for primary lung cancer, especially when the nodule is increasing in size. Based on the level of FDG activity, infectious or noninfectious granuloma cannot be excluded.

COMMENTS

Apart from cigarette smoking, chronic lung diseases including chronic obstructive pulmonary disease (COPD) and fibrotic disorders—asbestosis, silicosis, and prior TB have been associated with lung cancer.

On CT, bibasilar reticular abnormalities or honeycombing or both with minimal ground glass opacities are major criteria for diagnosis of IPF. Traction bronchiectasis and/or bronchiolectasis are often seen. Subpleural lines in the

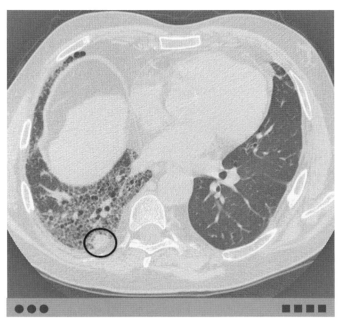

B. Corresponding CT with right lung IPF and nodule (*circle*). Note transplanted left lung.

upper lungs are a common and important distinguishing feature of IPF. Additionally, mediastinal adenopathy may be seen. In advanced cases, pulmonary ossification may occur.

Significant complications of IPF include infection, lung cancer, and worsening of disease itself. Infections include MAI and mycetoma due to *Aspergillus* species.

The development of cancer in these patients is about 15 times higher than that in general population. Majority of these cancers are squamous cell type. Contrary to smoking-related lung cancer, the fibrosis-related lung cancers are typically located peripherally in the lower lobes, in the areas with most prominent fibrosis. On CT, it typically appears as an area of ill-defined consolidation. These cancers tend to be multifocal and usually in patients with moderate and advanced fibrosis.

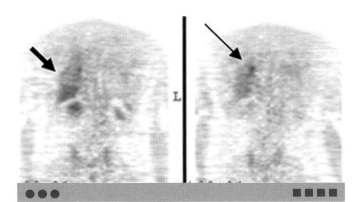

A. Small, mildly hypermetabolic right posterior lower lobe lung nodule (*thin arrow*) with underlying idiopathic pulmonary fibrosis (*thick arrow*). Well-differentiated squamous cell cancer. Transplanted left lung.

PEARLS

- IPF and scleroderma with underlying fibrosis are risk factors for lung cancers and any grade of FDG activity associated with them should be concerning for malignancy.

- Level of FDG activity cannot differentiate cancerous from infectious etiology.

Progressive systemic scleroderma has been associated with scar carcinoma as well. On FDG-PET, IPF and scleroderma show mild to moderate increased FDG activity corresponding to the area of fibrosis/reticulations or honeycombing. CT shows esophageal dilatation and bronchiectasis in most scleroderma patients.

In smokers, pulmonary Langerhans (histiocytosis) can be FDG avid with underlying cystic and nodular lung disease (upper lobes predominant) and mimic carcinoma.

ADDITIONAL IMAGES (C-D)

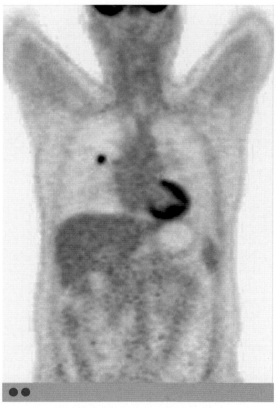

C. Hypermetabolic Langerhans cell nodule in underlying pulmonary histiocytosis.

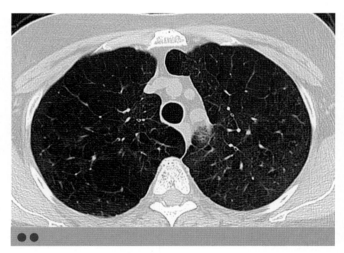

D. Corresponding CT with bilateral upper lobe cystic and small nodular lung disease, pulmonary histiocytosis.

DIFFERENTIAL DIAGNOSIS IMAGES (E-F)

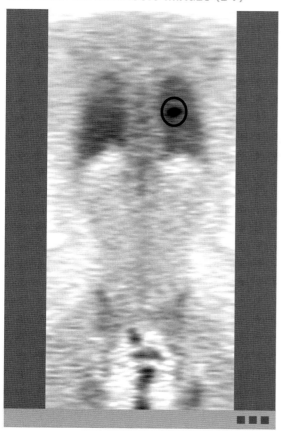

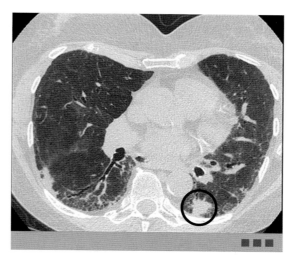

F. Corresponding CT with left adenocarcinoma in underlying scleroderma.

E. Hypermetabolic adenocarcinoma in the left lung (62-year-old female) with underlying diffusely hypermetabolic interstitial lung disease from scleroderma.

Vivek Manchanda, MD

PRESENTATION

Woman in her fifth decade of life with right small-cell lung cancer (SCLC) for staging.

FINDINGS

Increased FDG activity in the right hilum and right posterior lung mass, confined to right hemithorax.

DIFFERENTIAL DIAGNOSES

- *Limited stage SCLC*
- *Extensive stage SCLC*

Since the disease is confined to right hemithorax, the findings are most consistent with limited disease. No evidence of metastases outside the right hemithorax.

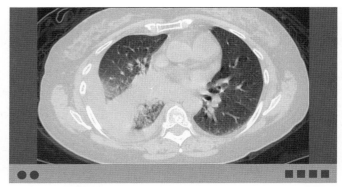

B. Corresponding CT.

COMMENTS

In NSCLC, unexpected distant metastases detection by FDG-PET has resulted in upstaging in up to 15% of patients that were potentially resectable.

SCLC is an aggressive malignancy, which is divided into limited and extensive stages. Limited stage is defined as the disease confined to one hemithorax (within suitable radiation field) whereas extensive stage confirms to disease extending beyond one hemithorax (outside suitable radiation field).

At presentation, about two-third patients with SCLC have extensive stage and about one-third have limited stage disease. Limited stage disease treatment involves radiation and chemotherapy whereas extensive stage disease is treated with chemotherapy alone.

The 5-year survival of patients with treated limited stage disease is 15% to 25% in comparison to 1% to 2% with extensive stage. Most SCLC have poor prognosis.

Extensive stage disease can involve multiple distant sites, including the contralateral lung, pleura, liver, bone, bone

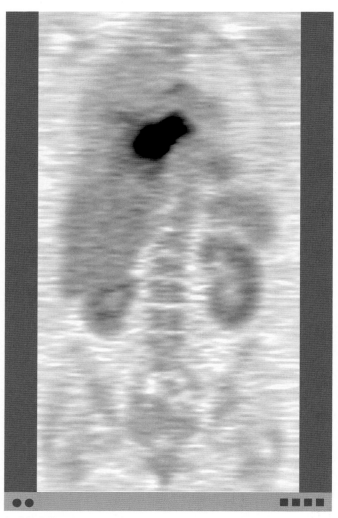

A. SCLC in patient: Limited stage (limited to right hemithorax).

PEARLS

- SCLC is divided into limited and extensive stages.

- Limited SCLC is treated with chemotherapy and radiation, whereas, extensive SCLC is treated with chemotherapy only.

- FDG-PET is an excellent complimentary tool to stage SCLC, and follow up response to therapy.

- MR has been shown to be more sensitive for bony metastases than FDG-PET, per some studies.

marrow, brain, adrenals, retroperitoneal lymph nodes, pancreas, and subcutaneous soft tissue.

Current staging includes CT, bone scan, and CT/MRI of the brain. FDG-PET is becoming a widely used tool for the initial staging and subsequent evaluation of SCLC.

In contrast to conventional staging (including bone scan), FDG-PET can result in a change of stage in about 10% to 25% patients, per some studies. It is also more sensitive in assessing response to therapy and in detecting residual viable disease. PET is also more sensitive for the detection of metastatic mediastinal and hilar lymph nodes.

ADDITIONAL IMAGES (C-D)

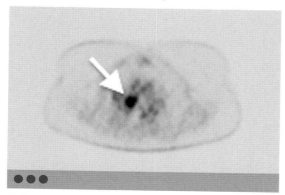

C. Right central small cell lung cancer (*arrow*), axial FDG-PET, different patient.

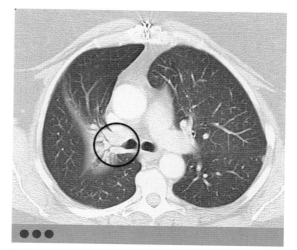

D. Corresponding CT, right small cell lung cancer (*circle*).

DIFFERENTIAL DIAGNOSIS IMAGES (E-H)

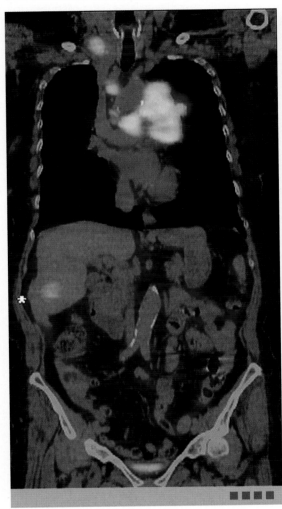

E. Disseminated SCLC with nodal and liver metastases (*white star*). Coronal fused PET/CT.

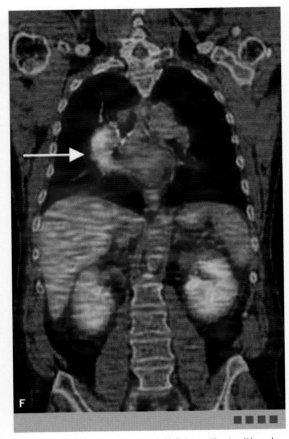

F., G., and **H.** Disseminated SCLC in patient with subtle metastases to right sacrum. Contrast-enhanced MR with metastases to right sacrum (as seen on PET) and additionally left sacrum (not seen on FDG-PET).

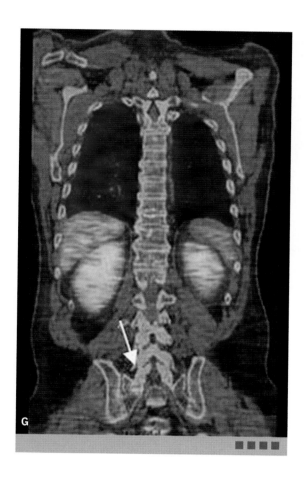

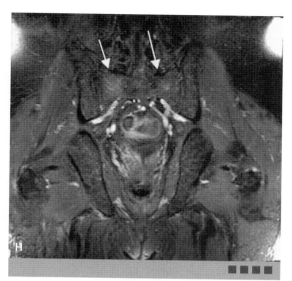

Vivek Manchanda, MD

PRESENTATION

Man in the fifth decade of life, with a strong history of smoking.

FINDINGS

Hypermetabolic right upper lobe nodule. Spiculated nodule on the corresponding CT.

DIFFERENTIAL DIAGNOSES

- *Malignant*: *Primary lung cancer*, metastases, lymphoma (usually intense FDG-avid, varies with histology)

- *Infectious*: Granuloma (TB, fungal), *Nocardia*, round pneumonia (variable FDG)

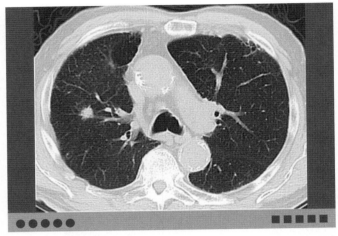

B. Corresponding CT.

- *Immune disorders*: Rheumatoid, Wegener's granulomatosis.

- *Benign*: Hamartoma, fibroma, intrapulmonary node, deposits from splenosis, endometrioma, extramedullary hematopoiesis (mild/non–FDG-avid)

- *Vascular*: Hematoma, organizing infarct (peripheral FDG/non–FDG-avid)

Given history of smoking, a hypermetabolic and spiculated solitary pulmonary nodule (SPN) is most concerning for primary lung cancer. Biopsy proved the same.

COMMENTS

SPN is defined as focal, round, or oval area of increased attenuation which measures less than 3 cm in diameter.

Solid nodular benign lesions typically have well-circumscribed smooth borders. Malignant nodules typically have an irregular, lobulated, or spiculated border. This may

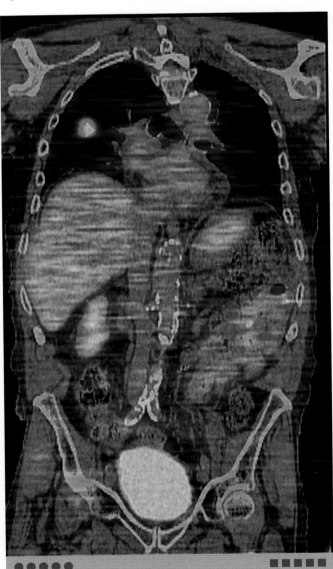

A. Right lung hypermetabolic primary adenocarcinoma, as SPN.

PEARLS

- SPN analysis on FDG-PET/CT is an artful combination of the patient's history, serial size, FDG uptake, and CT appearance of the nodule.

- New lung nodule detected in a young adult with peripheral sarcoma or melanoma is more likely to be a solitary metastasis than primary lung cancer or infection.

- Enlarging SPN, irrespective of FDG activity, should be assessed with percutaneous aspiration biopsy or video-assisted thoracoscopic surgery (VATS).

distort adjacent vessels which gives rise to sunburst appearance. Lobulation may be seen in up to 25% of benign nodules.

Solitary metastasis may account for up to 3% to 5 % of resected nodules.

Homogeneous attenuation may be seen in both benign (majority) and malignant (about 20%) nodules. Pseudocavitation may be seen with BAC and air bronchograms may be seen in lymphoma.

Benign cavitary nodules have generally smooth and thin walls and malignant nodules have typically thick and irregular walls.

Intranodular fat (Hounsfield unit [HU] –40 to –120) is reliably seen in hamartoma.

Diffuse, central, laminar, concentric, and popcorn calcifications are typically benign. Stippled or eccentric calcification is most commonly seen in the malignant lesions. Up to 33.3% to 60% of benign nodules are not calcified and calcification in hamartoma is variable. Punctate calcification may be seen due to engulfment of preexisting calcified granuloma and metastases. Very fast or very slow growing solitary pulmonary nodules are rarely malignant.

SPN with increased FDG uptake should be considered malignant, but false-positive results can be seen in infectious and inflammatory processes such as active TB and histoplasmosis.

DIFFERENTIAL DIAGNOSIS IMAGES (C-M)

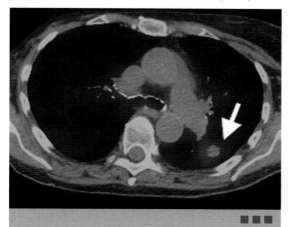

C. Left lung SPN from endometrial cancer.

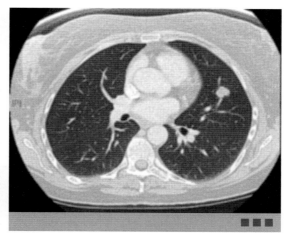

D. Corresponding CT.

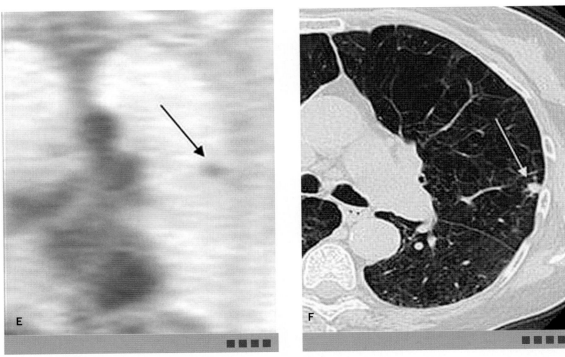

E. and **F.** Mildly hypermetabolic left lung granuloma, FDG-PET and CT.

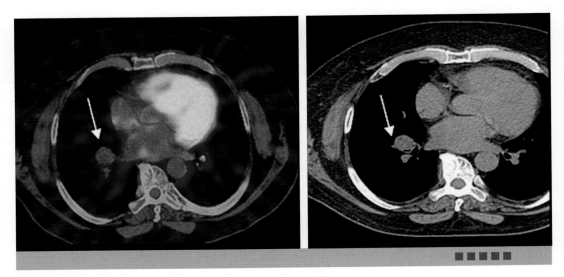

G. Fused PET/CT, right lung hamartoma, and corresponding CT.

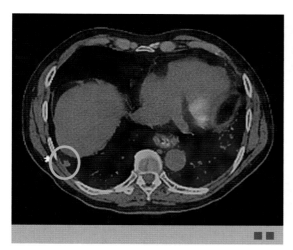

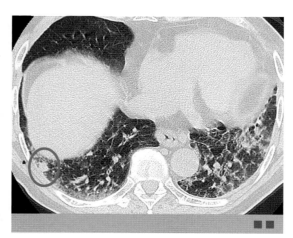

I. Corresponding CT.

H. Plasma cell granuloma of the lung fused PET/CT, minimal FDG avidity.

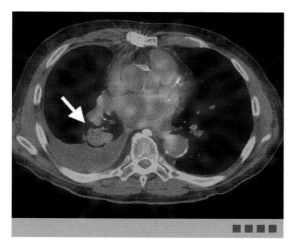

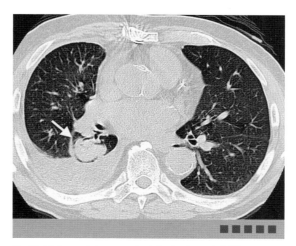

J. Axial fused PET/CT for round atelectasis, right lower lobe, non–FDG avid.

K. Right lower lobe round atelectasis, axial CT.

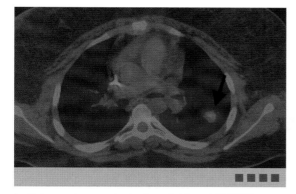

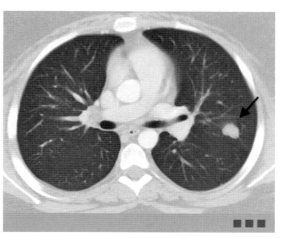

L. Osteosarcoma metastasis, axial fused PET/CT.

M. Osteosarcoma metastasis (*arrow*) axial CT.

Vivek Manchanda, MD

PRESENTATION

Man in late fifties with prior asbestos exposure and known mesothelioma.

FINDINGS

Intense FDG activity corresponding to left pleural mesothelioma with right proximal femoral hypermetabolic lesion.

DIFFERENTIAL DIAGNOSES

• *Stage IV mesothelioma*

Distant metastasis in right proximal femur is consistent with stage IV disease.

COMMENTS

According to AJCC, Stage IV mesothelioma is defined as:
  a) T4 Any N M0

Where T4: Tumor involves same side pleura of the chest wall with at least one of the following features:
  1. Diffuse or multi-focal involvement of the soft tissue of the chest wall
  2. Involvement of the rib
  3. Invasion through the diaphragm to the peritoneal cavity

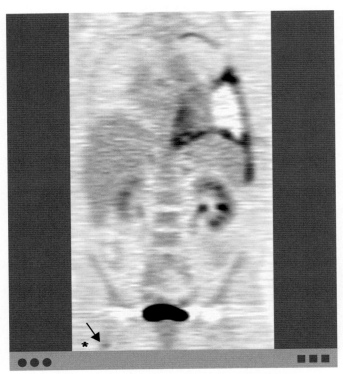

A. Left pleural mesothelioma with metastases to right proximal femur (stage IV) in patient A, at level of black star, indicated by black arrow, coronal FDG-PET.

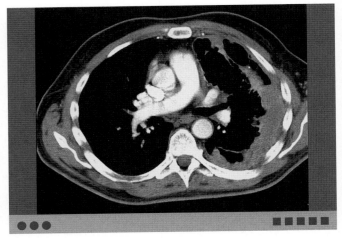

B. Corresponding CT.

  4. Invasion of any mediastinal organ
  5. Direct extension to the pleura on the other side
  6. Invasion into spine
  7. Penetration of the pericardium
  8. Pericardial effusion which is positive for cancer cells
  9. Involvement of heart muscle
 10. Involvement of the nerves of brachial plexus

  b) Any T N3 M0, where N3 indicates involvement of opposite side mediastinal, internal mammary, or hilar lymph node(s) and or same side or opposite side supraclavicular or scalene lymph node(s).

  c) Any T Any N, M1, where M1 indicates distant metastasis.
  Patients with stage I disease have much better prognosis than those with more advanced stages.

  Histologically, these tumors are composed of fibrous or epithelial elements or both. The epithelial mesotheliomas have a better prognosis than those with sarcomatous or mixed histology.

  Early disease stages benefit from radical surgery. It has been suggested that distant mesothelioma metastases that develop soon after extrapleural pneumonectomy are likely present at the time of surgery but are not detected by conventional staging. Advanced disease stages, though prognostically poor, are treated with multimodality treatment. This includes combinations of chemotherapy, radiotherapy, and surgery. In this regard, an accurate pretreatment staging

PEARLS

• **FDG-PET provides an important role in staging mesothelioma, especially in detecting nodal disease and distant metastases.**

• **Low SUV and epithelial histology has favorable prognosis among MPMs.**

with ^{18}F FDG-PET has proven to be able to provide useful information for staging purposes, especially to identify of metastatic spread to lymph nodes and distant sites.

Degree of FDG activity has been described as a prognostic indicator in some studies.

All FDG-avid N3 nodes in patients with MPM should be biopsied, as false positive nodes can occur. Also, enlarged and non–FDG avid N3 lymph nodes should be sampled in patients considered for surgery.

DIFFERENTIAL DIAGNOSIS IMAGES (C-F)

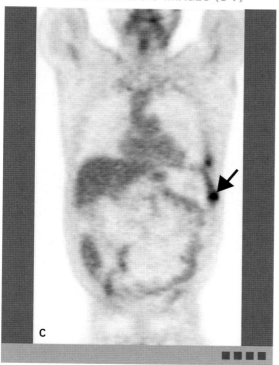

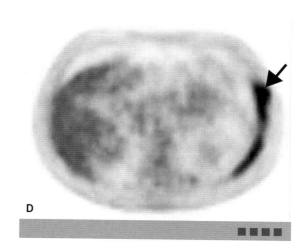

C. and D. Left pleural mesothelioma extending into chest wall (stage III) in another patient.

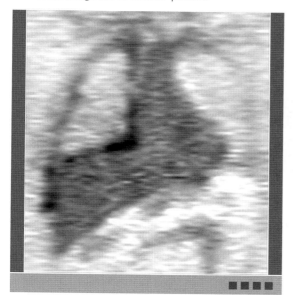

E. Right pleural mesothelioma (stage I) in another patient coronal FDG-PET.

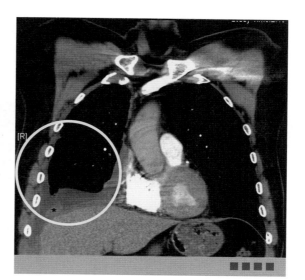

F. Corresponding CT with nodular pleural thickening, stage I.

Vivek Manchanda, MD

PRESENTATION

Teenage girl with repeated episodes of chest infections while growing up.

FINDINGS

Matched ventilation perfusion (VQ) defect in almost entire left lung (green arrow): posterior left lung ventilation and (*black arrow*) posterior left perfusion. Matched VQ defect is also seen in right apex.

DIFFERENTIAL DIAGNOSES

Causes of severe unilateral lung perfusion abnormality:

- *Mucus plug*: Difficult to rule out; a corresponding CT can be conclusive (typically VQ match defect).

- *Pulmonary artery stenosis or atresia* (typically VQ mismatch).

- *Endobronchial tumor*: Difficult to exclude on VQ scan; CT/bronchoscopy can differentiate (matched VQ defect).

- *Congenital hypoplastic lung* (matched VQ defect).

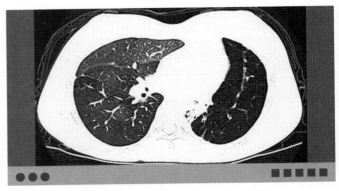

B. Expiration HRCT with significant air trapping in left lung (darker lung).

COMMENTS

Swyer-James syndrome is a type of postinfectious obliterative bronchiolitis.

The insult to the immature lung occurs during the first 8 years of life, as progressive alveolarization is happening. The arrest of progressive growth can result in segmental or lobar hypoplasia and occurs typically unilaterally in the lungs.

Pulmonary tissue is hypoplastic, including pulmonary artery and its branches. Lung distal to the diseased airway is hyperinflated and supplied by collateral air drift.

Patients are typically asymptomatic and commonly present as adults with abnormal radiograph. Less common presentation includes progressive exertional dyspnea or repeated infections.

Characteristic chest radiograph findings include unilateral translucency (caused by reduced lung perfusion), decreased size, and number of mid lung and peripheral vessels. The contralateral lung may show hypervascularity.

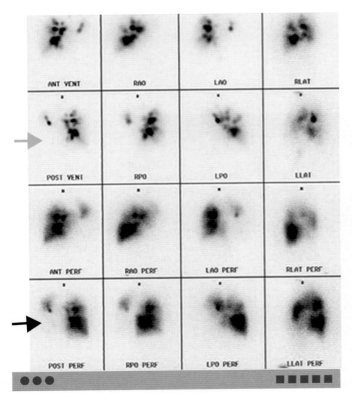

A. Anterior and posterior images of matched VQ defects from air trapping in Swyer-James syndrome. Ventilation (*upper 2 rows*).

PEARLS

- **Differential diagnosis for unilateral, matched ventilation perfusion defect includes Swyer-James syndrome, characterized by (usually) infectious insult to the immature lungs.**

- **Other smaller areas of matched ventilation perfusion defect may be seen in the contralateral lung due to air trapping, corresponding to expiratory CT air trapping.**

- **VQ mismatch results from pulmonary arterial flow obstruction with relatively preserved ventilation, whereas VQ matched defects result primarily from air trapping and resulting reflex vasoconstriction.**

CT, however, shows abnormalities that are more common bilaterally. Multifocal areas of air trapping are usually seen on expiratory phase of CT. Other changes on CT include bronchiectasis, areas of scarring, and collapse.

Ventilation perfusion scan (with technetium-labelled diethylenetriamine pentaacetate [Tc-DTPA] and technetium-labelled macroaggregated albumin [Tc-MAA] respectively) classically demonstrates decreased or absent perfusion in the affected lung and severe corresponding ventilation defect. Smaller areas of matched ventilation perfusion defects corresponding to air trapping may be seen in the contralateral lung.

Angiography, although rarely necessary, shows small hilar vessels on the affected side with narrowed, attenuated arteries coursing through the radiolucent lung (so-called "pruned tree appearance").

A central large airway obstruction causing lung hypoventilation and a compensatory ipsilateral reduction in perfusion is the most worrisome differential diagnosis, which may be resolved by bronchoscopy or by a dedicated CT examination of the central airways.

ADDITIONAL IMAGE

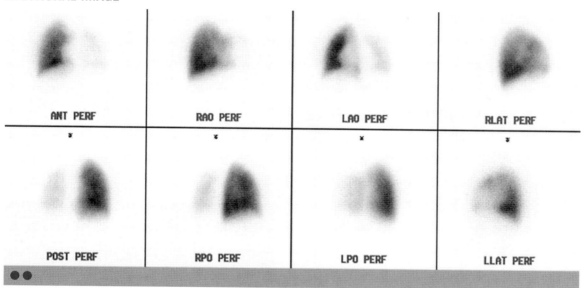

C. Anterior and posterior images of severely reduced left lung perfusion from hypoplastic pulmonary artery, Tc MAA scan. Left lung ventilation (*not shown*) would be relatively preserved.

DIFFERENTIAL DIAGNOSIS IMAGES (D-F)

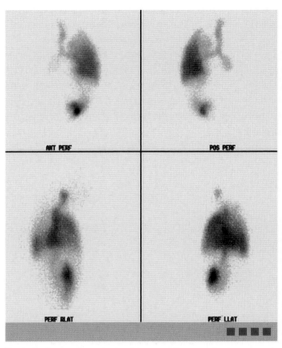

D. Anterior and posterior images of severely decreased perfusion from hypoplastic right lung from scoliosis.

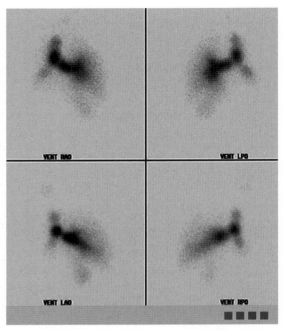

E. Severely decreased ventilation from hypoplastic right lung from scoliosis.

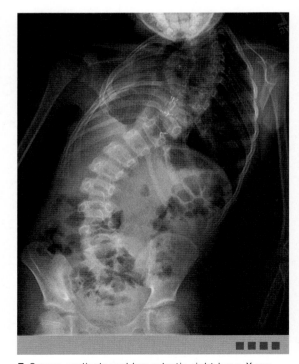

F. Severe scoliosis and hypoplastic right lung, X-ray.

Vivek Manchanda, MD

PRESENTATION

Woman in late twenties with nodular sclerosing Hodgkin disease, status post chemotherapy.

FINDINGS

Diffuse, mildly increased FDG uptake in the anterior mediastinum, corresponding to prominent thymus on CT. No nodularity.

DIFFERENTIAL DIAGNOSES

- *Residual lymphoma*
- *Other thymic tumors*: Thymic carcinoma, sarcoma, lymphoma, and thymomas
- *Thymic rebound*
- *New germ cell tumor*

Thymomas are usually moderately FDG avid and occur in middle-aged women with other associated autoimmune disorders. Thymic cancers are intensely hypermetabolic and the thymic shape is distorted. Thymic rebound is mildly FDG avid, with the shape of the thymus retained, as in the index case. Residual lymphomas have nonhomogeneous, moderate to intensely increased FDG activity.

COMMENTS

The pathophysiology of reactive thymic hyperplasia likely involves initial aplasia (steroid-related apoptosis and inhibited lymphocyte proliferation). It may also be seen after acute infection, stress, intoxication, cortisone, acromegaly, thyrotoxicosis, or radiation. With immunologic rebound, infiltration with plasma cells occurs. With improved immunologic parameters, thymic hyperplasia is generally considered prognostically favorable.

Increased Gallium 67 (^{67}Ga) uptake in thymus after chemotherapy has been described earlier. Although islands of functional residual tissue can be found in the thymus in histologic studies of patients up to 60 years old, reactive thymic hyperplasia occurs mainly in younger patients. Post-iodine 131 (I-131) therapy thymic uptake has been described. Insignificant differences were found in thymic FDG uptake in children before or after chemotherapy.

Thymoma (fourth and fifth decades), is associated with myasthenia gravis and other autoimmune disorders. Moderate FDG activity can be associated with it.

Intense FDG activity corresponding to nodular thymus/ thymus in which the typical triangular shape is abolished is seen in thymic cancer.

Most cases related to rebound thymic hyperplasia secondary to successful chemotherapy occur within a year

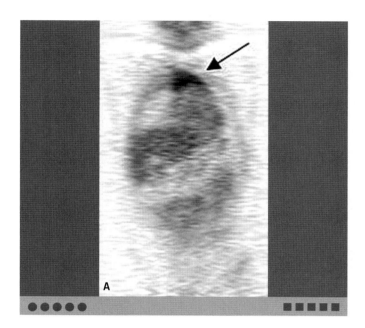

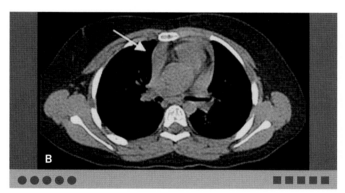

A. and **B.** Mild diffuse FDG activity corresponding to thymic rebound and corresponding CT.

PEARLS

- Most cases of rebound thymic hyperplasia secondary to successful chemotherapy occur within a year and the gland typically returns to normal size.

- Thymic hyperplasia is usually triangular, whereas infiltration is quadrilateral.

- If thymus was not the original site of disease, posttreatment increase in size is likely due to hyperplasia.

- Integrated PET-CT has been shown to be useful in some studies to differentiate subgroups of thymic epithelial tumors and for staging the extent of the disease.

and the gland typically returns to normal size. CT shows normal sized or symmetrically enlarged gland with normal contour, without discrete nodules. The borders of the enlarged thymus are most often concave and occasionally convex. On MR, there is no specific signal pattern for thymic hyperplasia.

Thymic carcinomas are primarily epithelial, lymphocytic, and mixed-cell tumors, in addition to rare lipomas and sarcomas. Pure lymphocytic thymic tumors are classified as primary or secondary lymphomas.

DIFFERENTIAL DIAGNOSIS IMAGES (C-J)

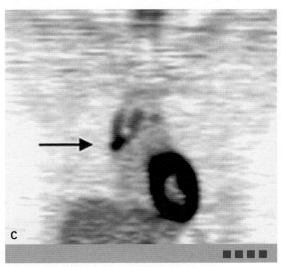

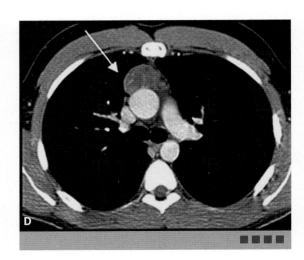

C. and **D.** Thymic nodular activity with residual lymphoma and corresponding contrast enhanced axial CT.

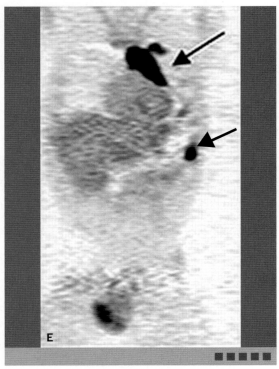

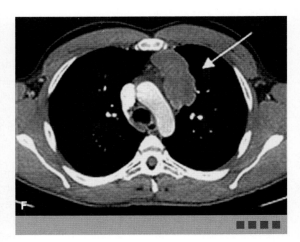

E. and **F.** Coronal FDG-PET with thymic cancer (*upper arrow*) and pleural metastasis (*lower arrow*). Coronal FDG-PET and corresponding CT.

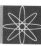

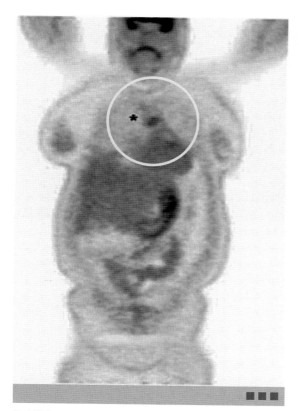

G. Mildly hypermetabolic thymoma in 52-year-old-female, adjacent to black star.

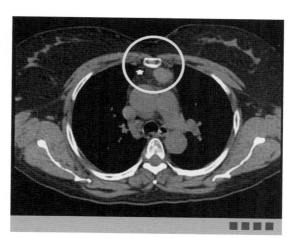

H. Corresponding CT for thymoma, adjacent to white star.

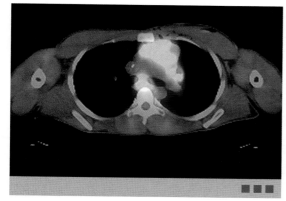

I. Lymphoepithelioma-like carcinoma, variant of thymic carcinoma, 24-year-old male.

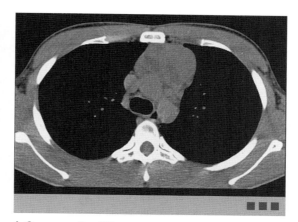

J. Corresponding CT.

Vivek Manchanda, MD

PRESENTATION

Man in his sixth decade of life with mediastinal mass. History of heavy smoking.

FINDINGS

Intensely FDG-avid anterior mediastinal mass.

DIFFERENTIAL DIAGNOSES

The classic differential of anterior mediastinal mass includes:

- *Thymoma*

- *Teratoma*

- *Thyroid tumor/goiter*

- *Lymphoma*

There are multiple other entities in the differential diagnoses discussed in the comment section in relation to FDG avidity.

COMMENTS

Anterior mediastinal masses include nodal mass from lymphoma, metastases, benign nodal hyperplasia, mediastinal lymphadenitis, sarcoidosis, or granulomatous infection. Out of this differential, all entities are moderate to intensely FDG avid, barring benign nodal hyperplasia. Benign nodal hyperplasia is typically non–FDG avid but may show some degree of FDG uptake, equaling or slightly greater than the vascular blood pool.

Cardiovascular anterior mediastinal masses include aneurysms and epicardial fat pads, dilated superior vena cava (SVC), and cardiac tumors. Aneurysms usually have

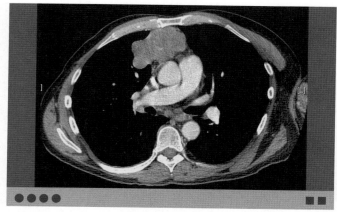

B. Corresponding CT contrast enhanced.

FDG activity similar to the vascular blood pool and epicardial fat pads are FDG negative.

Cysts such as bronchogenic, pericardial, and thymic are typically FDG negative.

Thyroid masses, both benign and malignant can be FDG avid.

Anterior mediastinal masses include thymic lesions, such as thymoma, hyperplastic thymus, thymic cancer, thymic carcinoid, thymic lipoma, thymic cyst, and lymphoma involving thymus. Out of this differential, hyperplastic thymus is only mildly FDG avid, thymoma is usually moderately FDG avid, thymic lipoma and cyst are FDG negative, and the rest are intensely FDG avid.

Amongst solid teratoid lesions, seminomas are typically FDG avid and nonseminomatous germ cell tumors have variable FDG avidity (some are FDG negative). Mature teratomas are typically FDG negative.

Primary lung/pleural tumors invading mediastinum are typically FDG avid. Mediastinal lipomatosis from Cushing syndrome and corticosteroid therapy is typically FDG negative.

Malignant primary sternal tumors include chondrosarcoma, myeloma, and lymphoma; all of which are FDG avid.

Hemangiomas (occasional false-positive case reports) and lymphangiomas are typically FDG negative.

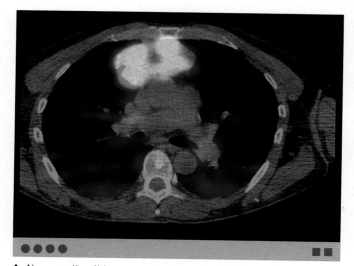

A. Non–small-cell lung cancer axial fused PET/CT.

PEARLS

- The classical differential for anterior mediastinal masses includes teratoma, thymoma, thyroid tumor/ goiter, and lymphoma.

- Some degree of differential diagnosis can be established from the FDG avidity of the masses.

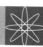

DIFFERENTIAL DIAGNOSIS IMAGES (C-H)

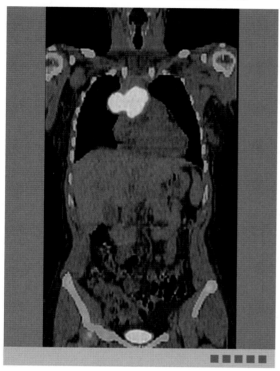

C. Classical nodular sclerosing Hodgkin lymphoma.

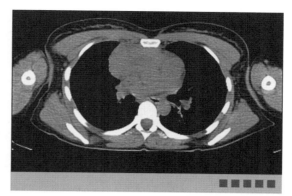

D. Corresponding CT.

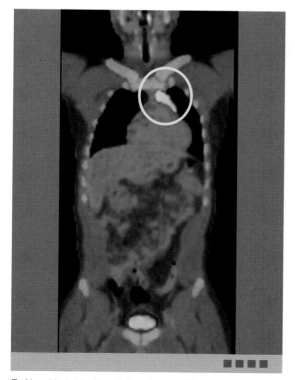

E. Non-Hodgkin B-cell lymphoma, 28-year-old female.

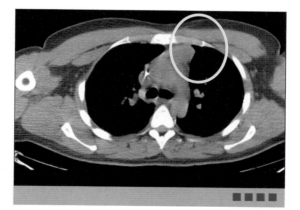

F. Corresponding CT.

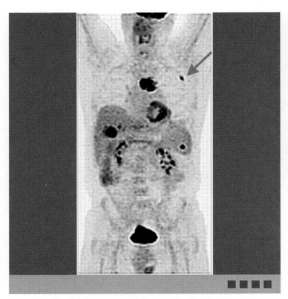

G. Thymic cancer metastasized to pleura (*arrow*), liver, and spleen, 52-year-old male.

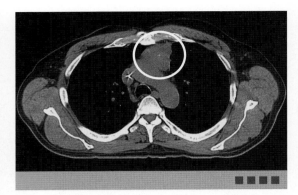

H. Corresponding non-contrast CT, thymoma (*circle*).

Vivek Manchanda, MD

PRESENTATION

Right upper lobe mass in a patient with malignant peripheral nerve sheath tumor (MPNST), growing in size.

FINDINGS

Increased FDG activity corresponding to the right upper lobe pulmonary mass. Plexiform neurofibroma in the right flank.

DIFFERENTIAL DIAGNOSES

- *Infection*

- *Lung primary: Unlikely, but cannot be excluded. No history of smoking.*

- *Metastasis*

In a patient with NF-1 (plexiform neurofibroma) who can develop malignant peripheral nerve sheath tumor (MPNST), metastases from the same is most likely. This was proven on excisional biopsy.

COMMENTS

Neurofibromatosis-1 (NF-1) is an autosomal dominant inherited disorder, characterized by neurofibromas in the skin,

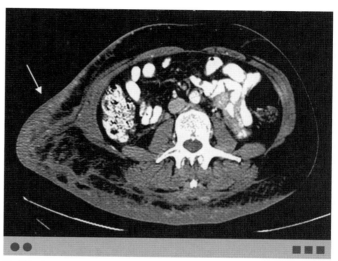

B. CT with plexiform neurofibroma.

subcutaneous tissue, cranial nerves, and spinal root nerves. Rare de novo cases result from genetic abnormality in encoding neurofibromin protein.

The index patient has plexiform neurofibroma, also FDG avid in the right flank.

Rapidly growing tumors/nerve palsies may indicate malignant transformation. NF-1 patients have an increased risk of developing MPNSTs, which are highly aggressive in NF-1. Twenty to seventy percent cases of MPNST arise in association with NF-1. They are locally aggressive and frequently metastasize. They mostly arise from plexiform or nodular neurofibromas and have intermediate chemosensitivity.

Some retrospective NF-1 patient's analysis has demonstrated that ^{18}F-FDG-PET can be used to detect malignant

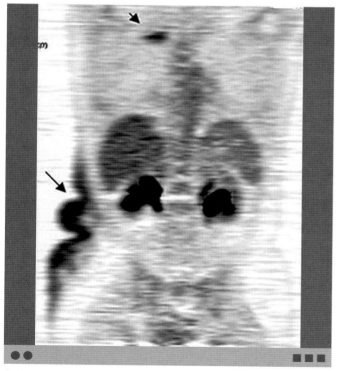

A. Right flank plexiform neurofibroma (*long arrow*) and right apical hypermetabolic focus (*short arrow*).

PEARLS

- MPNST can be a devastating complication of NF-1. They usually arise from nodular or plexiform neurofibromas.

- FDG-PET is a potentially useful, noninvasive method for detecting malignant change in plexiform neurofibromas. However, the distinction between low-grade MPNSTs and benign plexiform neurofibromas would still be difficult.

- FDG-PET/CT has high sensitivity in detecting metastases from MPNST.

- GIST can occur in about 5% to 25% NF-1 patients. They are extremely FDG avid, less common in stomach, usually multiple with variable response to Gleevec.

change in plexiform neurofibromas, but the distinction between low-grade MPNSTs and benign plexiform neurofibromas can not be made. Fluorine 18-thymidine, which detects DNA turnover, may be helpful in distinguishing the two. On CT, benign neurofibromata are well circumscribed with low attenuation. Malignant change results in increased attenuation and vascularity. On MR, the typical "target" sign on T2 is lost, replaced by irregular, highly vascular mass.

Among other tumors that occur in NF-1 patients, GIST has an incidence of 5% to 25%. It tends to be extragastric in origin, multiple, and rarely metastasizes. Gleevec effect on GIST of NF-1 origin has been variable (phenotypic and genotypic distinction from sporadic GIST) and treatment is mainly surgical. FDG-PET usually shows intense FDG uptake and central photopenia in untreated cases. On CT, there may be circumferential thickening and aneurysmal enlargement of the bowel, and strong peripheral enhancement with contrast.

ADDITIONAL IMAGES (C-J)

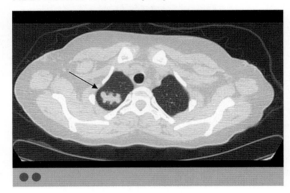

C. CT of right apical lesion.

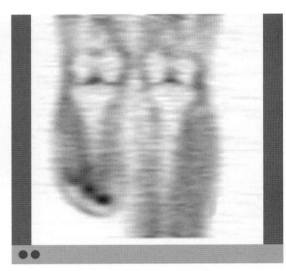

D. Right below knee amputation for MPNST in the right foot (which recurred in the right leg).

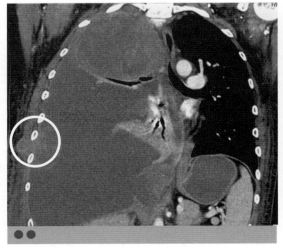

E. Progression of lung disease in 2 months. Note chest wall invasion.

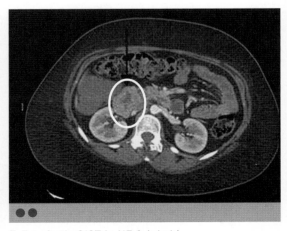

F. Extrafastic GIST in NF-1 (*circle*).

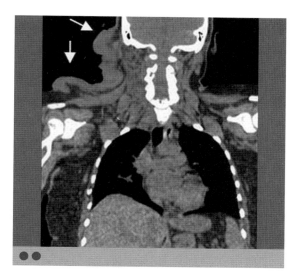

G. Plexiform neurofibroma in the patient with extra-gastric GIST.

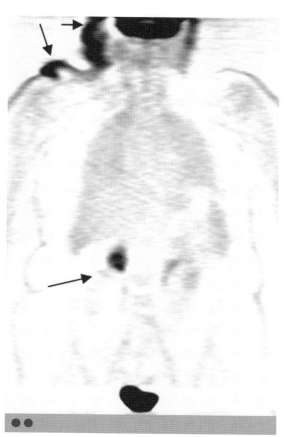

H. Right neck plexiform neurofibroma (*upper arrows*) and duodenal GIST with central photopenia and peripheral hypermetabolism (*lower arrow*).

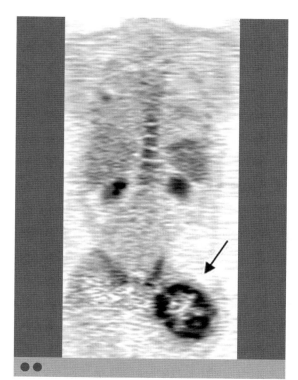

I. Malignant degeneration of neurofibroma (intense, heterogeneous uptake with central necrosis in the left buttock indicating worse prognosis). See corresponding MR (J).

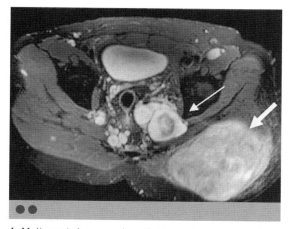

J. Malignant degeneration of Neurofibroma, loss of target sign (*thick white arrow*). Target sign in benign neurofibroma (*thin white arrow*).

Chapter 4

GENITOURINARY

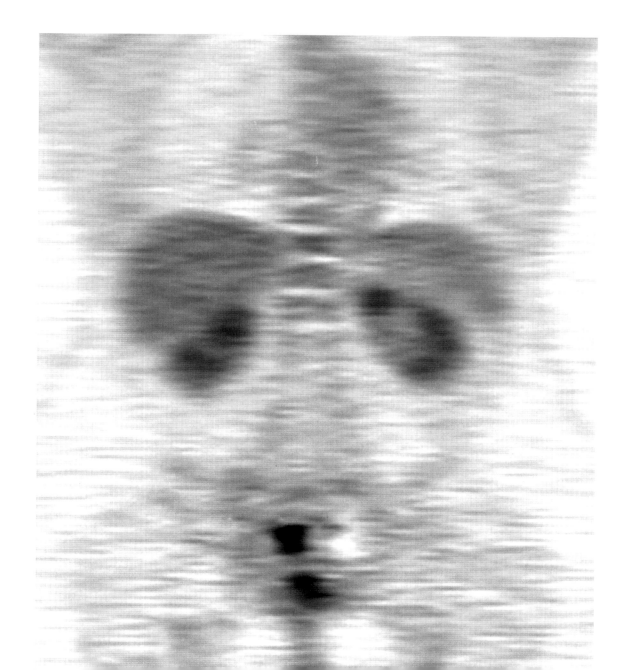

Vivek Manchanda, MD

PRESENTATION

Woman in midfifties with vaginal bleeding.

FINDINGS

Hypermetabolic endometrial and cervical mass.

DIFFERENTIAL DIAGNOSES

- *Endometrial cancer with cervical involvement*
- *Cervical cancer with endometrial involvement*
- *Lymphoma*
- *Metastases*
- *Sarcoma*
- *Polyps* (not much data available for FDG activity)
- *Submucosal leiomyomas*: Variable FDG activity

Postmenopausal bleeding needs investigation. The patient had endometrial cancer with cervical polyp involvement of endometrial cancer.

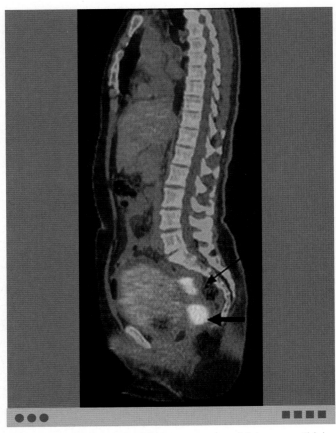

B. Fused PET/CT, superior (*thin arrow*: endometrial cancer; *thick arrow*: cervical involvement of endometrial cancer).

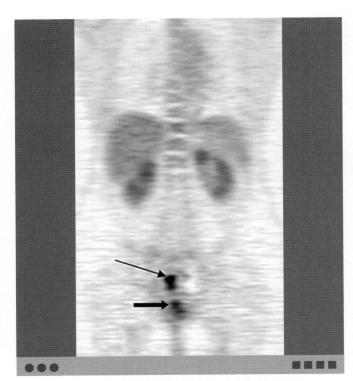

A. Endometrial cancer (*thin arrow*) with cervical involvement (*thick arrow*).

PEARLS

- Hypermetabolic and thickened endometrium should be investigated for primary endometrial cancer. Menstrual blood can cause false-positive results.

- In a subset of high-grade clear cell/papillary cell cancer, FDG-PET has been shown to change staging.

- Surgical staging of endometrial cancer is still the mainstay. Preoperative staging with FDG-PET has moderate sensitivity and high specificity and may allow omission of lymphadenectomy in poor surgical candidates.

- FDG-PET is superior to CT and MRI for detecting recurrences in the follow-up of patients with endometrial cancer.

COMMENTS

Endometrial adenocarcinomas range from well-differentiated (grade 1) to anaplastic (grade 3). They are usually perimenopausal and associated with early onset of symptoms.

Endometrial cancers such as papillary, serous, and clear cell carcinomas are generally postmenopausal with increased risk of metastasis and recurrence. Types of uterine sarcomas include carcinosarcoma (commonest), leiomyosarcoma, and endometrial stromal sarcoma.

No imaging is required for a patient with grade 1 cancer and nonenlarged uterus. Staging of endometrial cancer is primarily surgicopathologic, based on International Federation of Gynecology and Obstetrics (FIGO) criteria. In select cases, FDG-PET coupled with MRI/CT may improve primary cancer staging.

FDG-PET in endometrial cancer has moderate sensitivity and high specificity for regional nodal and distant metastases.

At least one study has suggested that FDG-PET led to upstaging of disease in high-grade clear cell/papillary cell subcategory. The positive predictive value of detecting supraclavicular nodal disease by PET in endometrial cancer has been reported to be very high.

Studies have suggested that FDG-PET has high sensitivity in detecting recurrences and evaluating therapeutic response in the follow-up of patients with endometrial cancer. It has been reported that FDG-PET is superior to CT and MRI for detecting recurrences in the follow-up of patients with endometrial cancer.

The 5-year survival rate for localized disease is about 96% and 25% with metastatic disease. Patients with negative PET results have shown improved disease-free survival.

Increased endometrial uptake can be associated with menstruation and ovulation phases, benign endometrial abnormalities, and oligomenorrhea. Hormonal therapy has not been associated with significant endometrial FDG activity.

ADDITIONAL IMAGES (C-G)

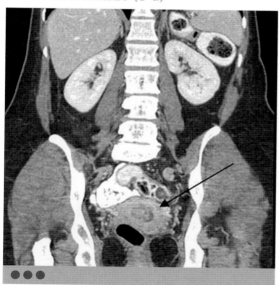

C. CT with endometrial thickening (*thin arrow*).

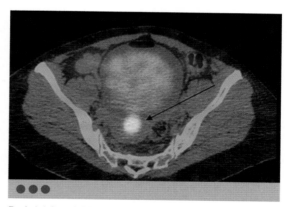

D. Axial fused PET/CT, endometrial cancer (*thin arrow*).

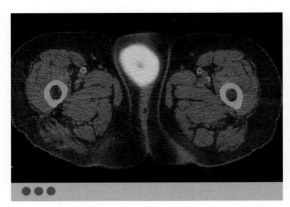

E. Vulvar recurrence of endometrial cancer, axial fused PET/CT.

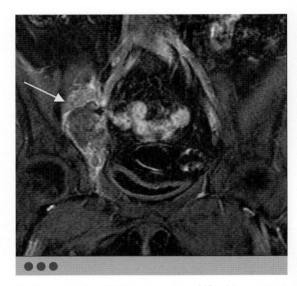

G. Corresponding T1W post-contrast MR with recurrent endometrial cancer (*white arrow*).

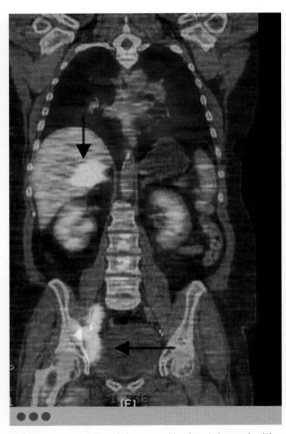

F. Recurrent endometrial cancer (*horizontal arrow*) with liver metastasis (*vertical arrow*). Note retrograde filled hypometabolic bladder. Fused coronal FDG-PET/CT.

DIFFERENTIAL DIAGNOSIS IMAGES (H-J)

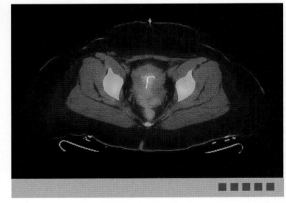

H. Intrauterine contraceptive device and corresponding FDG activity, fused axial PET/CT.

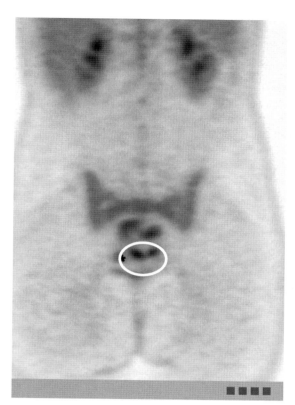

I. Menstrual blood outlining uterine didelphis, coronal FDG-PET, 15-year-old female.

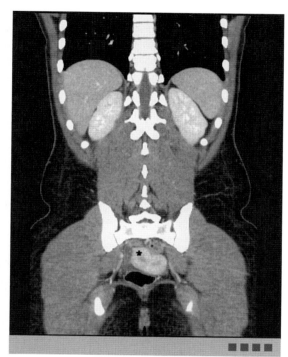

J. Corresponding coronal CT (*black star*).

Vivek Manchanda, MD

PRESENTATION

Woman in midforties with left neck mass and irregular and heavy vaginal bleeding.

FINDINGS

Intensely hypermetabolic cervical mass and hypermetabolic retroperitoneal and left neck nodes.

DIFFERENTIAL DIAGNOSES

• *Metastatic cervical cancer*

• *Cervical cancer with infection such as TB or lymphoma or metastases from other cancers or systemic inflammatory disease*

Although it is difficult to exclude a coexisting systemic condition along with cervical cancer, the asymmetric distribution of hypermetabolic nodes is more indicative of metastatic cervical cancer.

COMMENTS

Cervical cancer, the second commonest cancer of women worldwide, is associated with human papilloma virus (HPV), smoking, and multiple sexual partners.

It can spread directly or via lymph nodes or hematogenously. The direct invasion involves parametria, uterus, and vagina. Spread through lymph nodes involves paracervical, parametrial, and presacral nodal chains initially; followed by external, internal, and common iliac nodal chains. Retroperitoneal and supraclavicular nodal involvement can be seen in late course. Hematogenous spread to the lungs, bone, and liver is unusual.

FDG-PET/CT in a newly diagnosed patient with cervical cancer (FIGO stage ≥ stage IB) has a high sensitivity and specificity and can be a valuable supplement to the FIGO staging procedure. PET can reduce unnecessary surgical interventions, help modify radiation fields, and change the therapeutic approaches. Advanced stage disease on FDG-PET correlates with poor prognosis. Both squamous and nonsquamous histologies show FDG avidity and it helps detect both the presence and absence of pelvic and para-aortic nodal metastatic disease. FDG excretion in the urine can be minimized by retrograde filling of the bladder with saline and use of Lasix (furosemide).

In patients with suspected recurrence of cervical cancer (both pelvic and extrapelvic), ^{18}F-FDG provides excellent localization.

Detailed menstrual history is important in the interpretation of the scan.

Some studies have suggested that detection of new abnormalities noted on PET scan after therapy is the most significant prognostic factor for survival.

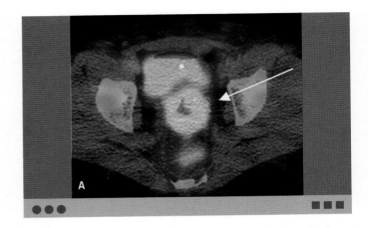

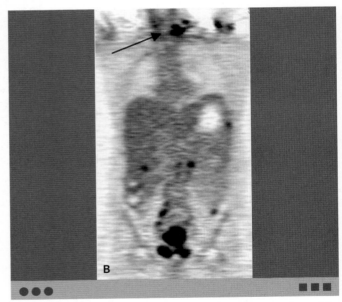

A. and **B.** Cervical cancer (*thin arrow A*) with left supraclavicular nodal metastasis (*thin arrow B*). Note hypermetabolic retroperitoneal nodes as well. Fused axial PET/CT (*above*) and coronal FDG-PET (*below*).

PEARLS

• **FDG-PET has high sensitivity and specificity in cancer staging in a newly diagnosed patient with cervical cancer (FIGO stage > stage IB) and in patients with both pelvic and extrapelvic recurrence of disease.**

• **PET/CT has good sensitivity and specificity related to para-aortic lymph node metastases.**

• **MR is the preferred modality for local staging with loss of perivesical or perirectal fat plane accompanied with nodular bladder/rectal wall thickening. Demonstration of fistula on CT and corresponding FDG activity, meets both CT and PET criteria for bladder or rectal wall involvement.**

In advanced cervical cancer, progression-free survival is significantly related to para-aortic lymph node metastases, for which PET/CT has higher sensitivity and specificity than CT alone.

ADDITIONAL IMAGE

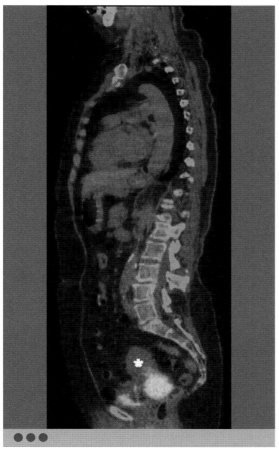

C. Fused PET/CT image of cervical cancer. Note noncatheterized bladder (*white star*).

DIFFERENTIAL DIAGNOSIS IMAGES (D-E)

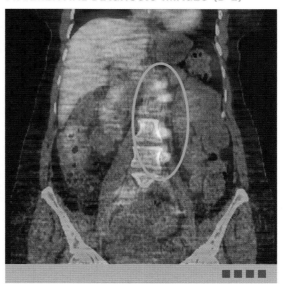

D. Ovarian cancer metastasis to retroperitoneal nodes.

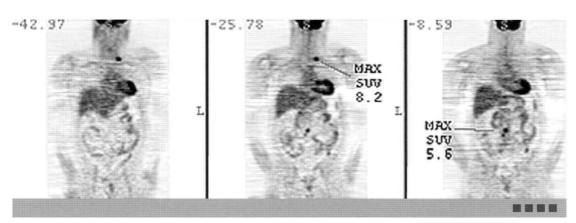

E. Embryonal cell testicular cancer metastases to left supraclavicular and right retroperitoneal nodes. Coronal FDG-PET.

Vivek Manchanda, MD

PRESENTATION

Woman in late forties with intermittent vaginal bleeding.

FINDINGS

Intense FDG activity corresponding to cervical mass.

DIFFERENTIAL DIAGNOSES

- *Cervical lymphoma.*

- *Cervical cancer.*

- *Metastases.*

- *Physiological FDG activity:* Unlikely as a mass is present.

Core cervical biopsy is necessary for definitive diagnosis of cervical lymphoma. Given no primary tumor on FDG-PET, metastases is unlikely.

COMMENTS

About 1% of cervical malignancies are due to cervical lymphoma, the most common site of lymphoma (primary or secondary) in the female genital tract. The age at presentation ranges from 20 to 80 years, mostly postmenopausal. The prognosis of cervical lymphoma is good, even when locally advanced at presentation.

Intermittent vaginal bleeding or spotting, pelvic mass, and/or urinary symptoms can be modes of cervical lymphoma presentation.

Cervical cytology is typically negative/nonspecific as these tumors arise from cervical stroma. A deep cervical biopsy is required for diagnosis. Diffuse cervical enlargement (average 4 cm) is the commonest CT finding. These masses are intensely FDG avid. Most of these lymphomas are of diffuse large B-cell histology. Less commonly, there may be a polypoidal or multinodular mass or a submucosal mass mimicking leiomyoma.

On MR, cervical lymphoma is best defined as high-signal intensity lesion on T2- or contrast-enhanced T1-WI. The mucosa and the low-signal junctional zone are characteristically spared. A large mass, which is mainly homogeneous with scant necrosis, should suggest lymphoma. A large cervical mass with invasion of vagina and parametrium and pelvic lymphadenopathy are more characteristic of squamous or adenocarcinoma of cervix.

FDG-PET is excellent in follow-up and treatment response. In case a pregnant patient develops a cervical lymphoma, treatment can be started while pregnant.

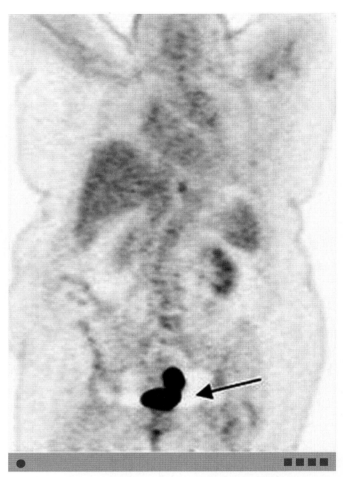

A. Coronal FDG-PET, intensely hypermetabolic cervical lymphoma (*arrow*).

Ovarian lymphoma is less common and carries worse prognosis than uterine lymphoma. Intact endometrium and absence of necrosis have been reported to be characteristic features of uterine lymphoma on MR.

PEARLS

- Diffuse cervical enlargement on CT with corresponding intensely increased FDG activity, is characteristic of cervical lymphoma.

- Secondary involvement of cervix is more common in advanced widespread disease than isolated extranodal non-Hodgkin lymphoma (NHL).

- PET is excellent in follow-up and response to treatment.

ADDITIONAL IMAGES (B-F)

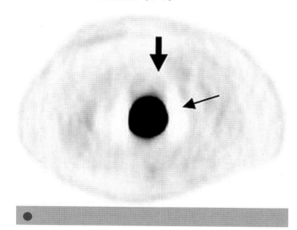

B. Cervical lymphoma (*thin arrow*) with catheter in retrogradely filled hypometabolic bladder (*thick arrow*).

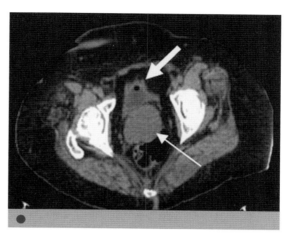

C. Corresponding axial CT with cervical mass (*thin arrow*) and gas in bladder (*thick arrow*).

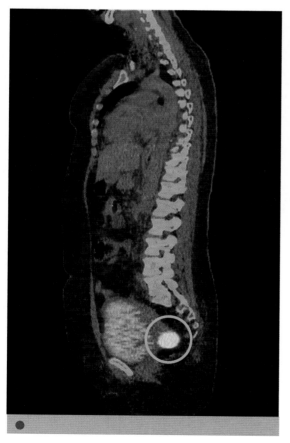

D. Sagittal fused PET/CT with bladder (anterior) and hypermetabolic cervical lymphoma (*circle*) posterior.

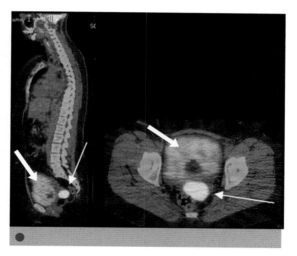

E. Sagittal and axial fused PET/CT, cervical lymphoma (*thin arrows*), and catheterized bladder (*thick arrows*).

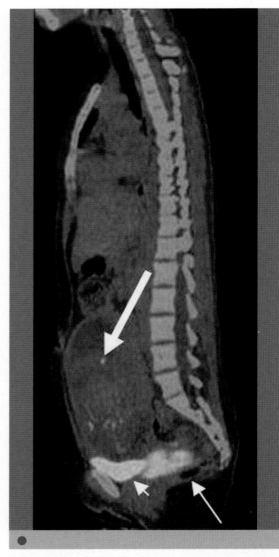

F. Sagittal fused PET/CT with vaginal fornix lymphoma (*thin long arrow*), bladder (*thin short arrow*), and intrauterine pregnancy (*thick long arrow*).

Vivek Manchanda, MD

PRESENTATION

Woman in midfifties with history of IBD (inflammatory bowel disease), total abdominal hysterectomy (TAH), and palpable left inguinal mass.

FINDINGS

Hypermetabolic left pelvic nodes/mass. Hypermetabolic left inguinal nodes.

DIFFERENTIAL DIAGNOSES

- *Lymphoma*
- *Ovarian cancer*
- *Metastases*
- *TB, other infection*
- *Infected aneurysm*
- *Sarcoma*

Ovarian or fallopian tube (FT) remnants in patients with IBD may give rise to cancers in a patient with earlier TAH.

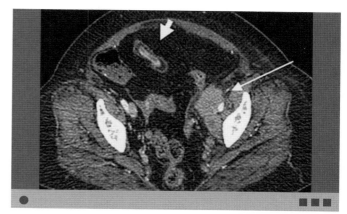

B. Thickened bowel mucosa from Crohn disease (*thick arrow*) and left pelvic nodal mass (*thin arrow*).

Hypermetabolic inguinal nodes favor FT cancer over ovarian cancer. Biopsy proved the same.

COMMENTS

Primary adenocarcinoma of FT is rare and contributes to less than 0.5% of all gynecologic malignancies.

It is similar to ovarian cancer in surgical FIGO staging and disease management. They also share similar age distribution. The FT cancers are more common in nulliparous women.

Most of the primary FT cancers are of serous papillary histology. However, FT cancer is more often diagnosed earlier (tubal dilatation causing pain and abnormal bloody-watery discharge). Staging requires routine lymphadenectomy and inguinal nodes may be involved, as inguinal nodes drain lymph from FTs (unlike ovarian cancer, where inguinal nodal involvement is rare). The involvement of para-aortic and pelvic nodes is, however, equal.

Surgery consists of bilateral salpingo-oophorectomy, TAH, and comprehensive surgical staging. More than 80% patients have elevated pretreatment serum CA-125 levels.

Bulky extratubal disease and postoperative residual disease of larger than 2 cm are indicators of worse prognosis.

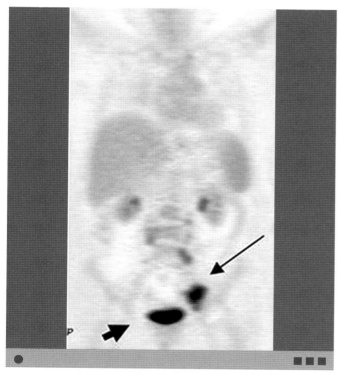

A. Left pelvic hypermetabolic nodes (*thin arrow*), remnant FT cancer in a patient with history of Crohn disease and total abdominal hysterectomy. Coronal FDG-PET. Thick arrow represents bladder.

PEARLS

- **FT cancer or ovarian cancer may arise in the remnants of ovaries or FTs in patients with TAH and underlying endometriosis, IBD, and appendicitis or appendectomy.**

- **Inguinal nodes are more commonly involved in primary FT cancer than in primary fallopian tube cancer.**

The patients who have had TAH may retain remnants from ovaries or FTs and may develop cancer from these remnants. Predisposing risk factors for the remnants include extensive adhesive disease from endometriosis, pelvic inflammatory disease, IBD, appendicitis or appendectomy, history of previous pelvic surgeries, neoplastic lesions, and improper surgical techniques. In patients with hereditary breast-ovarian cancer syndrome, if the surgical procedure does not include hysterectomy, the FT should be amputated as close as possible to the uterine cornua.

PET-CT has unique capability to detect and localize metastatic disease when serum CA-125, laparoscopy, and CT scan alone are unable to detect recurrence.

ADDITIONAL IMAGE

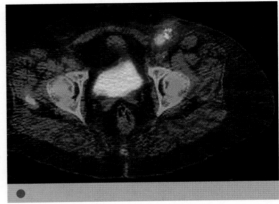

C. Same patient with hypermetabolic left inguinal nodes. Axial fused PET/CT.

Vivek Manchanda, MD

PRESENTATION

Woman in midsixties with weight loss and pulmonary nodules.

FINDINGS

Intense, focal left ovarian uptake.

DIFFERENTIAL DIAGNOSES

- *Benign ovarian uptake* (premenopausal)
- *Ovarian metastases*: Stomach, colon, pancreatic, breast, and lung
- *Ovarian cyst* (typically non-FDG avid, unless complicated)
- *Cystadenoma*
- *Teratoma*: Mature, usually FDG negative
- *Endometrioma*
- *Schwannoma*
- *TB*
- *Salpingitis*
- *Abscess*
- *Hydrosalpinx*

In a postmenopausal woman, any ovarian uptake is abnormal and is most likely from malignancy/metastasis than physiologic. The opposite is true for a premenopausal woman. Surgery proved primary ovarian cancer.

COMMENTS

Ovarian cancer has the highest mortality rate among all gynecologic cancers. The prognosis is worse as the cancers are detected late and there are no reliable screening tests.

FDG-PET has been shown to detect primary, recurrent, and metastatic ovarian cancers. Benign lesions of the ovary such as simple ovarian cysts, cystadenomas (mucinous and serous), benign fibromas, and mature cystic teratomas are usually FDG negative.

Low-grade, well-differentiated serous and mucinous cystadenocarcinomas may be FDG negative.

Other malignant ovarian tumors such as mixed malignant mullerian ovarian tumors, undifferentiated germ cell tumor, and metastatic lesions are FDG avid.

Some of the false positives include tubo-ovarian abscess, corpus luteum cyst and ovarian endometriosis, and benign cystadenomas.

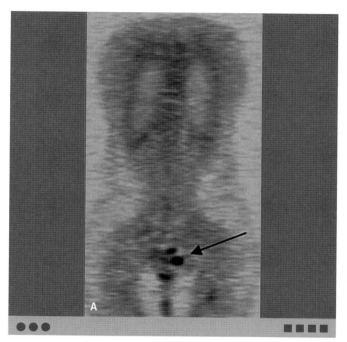

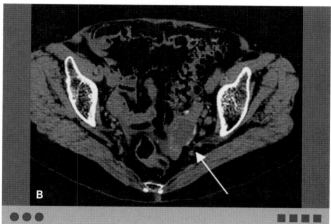

A. and **B.** Left ovarian cancer, incidental detection with corresponding CT in 65-year-old.

PEARLS

- In cases with elevated CA-125, ^{18}F-FDG-PET can determine presence, location, and extent of disease recurrence.

- Benign lesions such as corpus luteum cysts can mimic cancer in premenopausal women.

- Postmenopausal ovarian FDG activity is highly concerning for ovarian malignancy/metastases.

Peritoneal carcinomatosis from ovarian cancer is difficult to diagnose. FDG-PET/CT certainly aids in improving the sensitivity for detection of peritoneal carcinomatosis. However, if negative, it does not exclude the same. Laparoscopic examination is more sensitive.

Bladder catheterization with retrograde filling can help in decreasing FDG activity in the bladder and in getting a clearer image of the pelvis.

FDG-PET/CT has relatively high sensitivity in detecting recurrent ovarian cancer with rising CA-125 levels and negative conventional imaging. The sensitivity of detecting recurrent disease has been reported to be as high as 95% in patients with suspected disease. It is helpful in radiation treatment planning and selection of optimal surgical candidates. Some studies have shown that patients with a negative PET scan have a longer relapse-free interval than with a positive scan.

ADDITIONAL IMAGES (C-F)

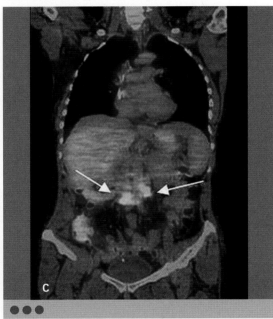

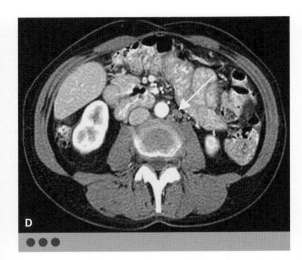

C. and **D.** Ovarian cancer metastasis to nonenlarged para-aortic nodes (*white arrows*).

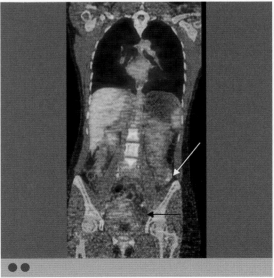

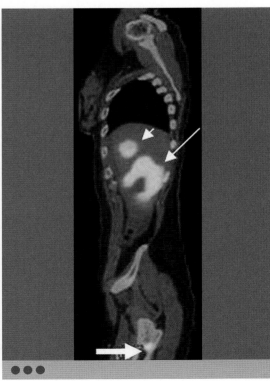

E. Left ovarian transplant in flank (*white arrow*) and lymphocele (*black arrow*) at native ovarian position.

F. Ovarian cancer metastasis to liver (*small thin arrow*), peritoneum (*long thin arrow*), and bone (*thick arrow*). Sagittal fused PET/CT.

192

DIFFERENTIAL DIAGNOSES IMAGES (G-I)

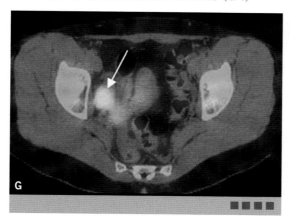
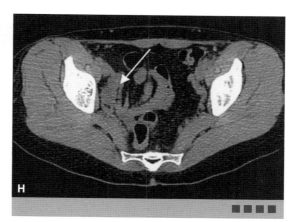

G. and **H.** Benign ovarian FDG uptake in 32-year-old with corresponding CT.

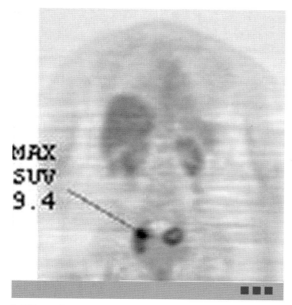

I. Bilateral ovarian metastasis from breast cancer. Coronal FDG-PET.

Vivek Manchanda, MD

PRESENTATION

Male in midtwenties with embryonal nonseminomatous germ cell tumor (NSGCT).

FINDINGS

Intense FDG activity in left supraclavicular and right retroperitoneal nodes.

DIFFERENTIAL DIAGNOSES

- *Lymphoma*
- *Metastases*
- *Multicentric castleman disease*

Given the history of NSGCT, other differentials are less likely and metastases is most likely. The NSGCTs tend to have discontiguous spread.

COMMENTS

PET is valuable in stage II testicular germ cell tumors but may not be of additional value in patients with stage I germ cell tumors. Small retroperitoneal nodes may not be FDG avid.

PET is useful in tumor recurrence evaluation in both seminomatous and nonseminomatous germ cell tumors, although more useful in seminomas. If the baseline scan shows FDG-positive disease in an NSGCT, recurrence can be detected with FDG-PET scan. A negative scan, without baseline, does not rule out disease in NSGCTs.

Mature teratoma is present in more than 40% of resected masses in NSGCTs; however, it makes only about 4% of residual lesions in seminomas.

Seminomas in general have higher SUVs than the NSGCTs. Nodal metastases from seminomas tends to have soft tissue attenuation. On contrary, NSGCTs are heterogeneous with cystic change. Right-sided testicular cancer initially involves aortocaval node or right paracaval node caudal to right renal vein/IVC (inferior vena cava) junction. For left-sided cancers,

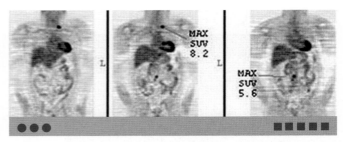

A. Left supraclavicular and right retroperitoneal (discontiguous) nodal involvement in embryonal nonseminomatous testicular tumor.

initial node is usually just below left renal vein. In the absence of ipsilateral nodal disease, contralateral disease is rare. The nodal spread in seminoma is contiguous, whereas in NSGCT it is discontiguous. Pelvic nodal involvement may be seen in retrograde extension from bulky retroperitoneal lymphadenopathy.

Most common hematogenous spread is to the lungs. Aggressive tumors may spread to brain, bone, or liver.

FDG-PET is very effective in differentiating residual tumor from fibrosis and is valuable in defining disease in patients with elevated tumor markers. Cystic masses in areas of nodal chains after lymphadenectomy may represent lymphoceles or recurrent disease, and FDG can differentiate between the two.

PEARLS

- **Seminomas in general are more FDG avid than NSGCTs.**
- **NSGCTs can be FDG negative and a baseline assessment helps in follow-up.**
- **FDG-PET can differentiate between residual tumor, fibrosis, and lymphoceles after nodal resection.**

ADDITIONAL IMAGES (B-H)

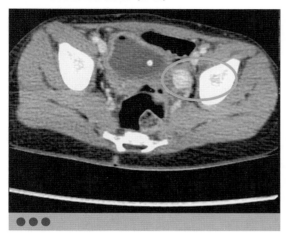

B. CT showing left pelvic recurrence of embryonal germ cell tumor in 5-year-old female.

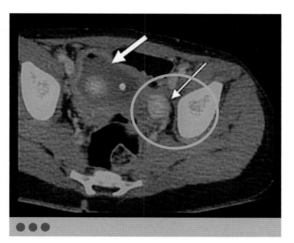

C. Corresponding fused PET/CT with non–FDG-avid recurrence (*green circle and thin arrow*), bladder (*thick arrow*).

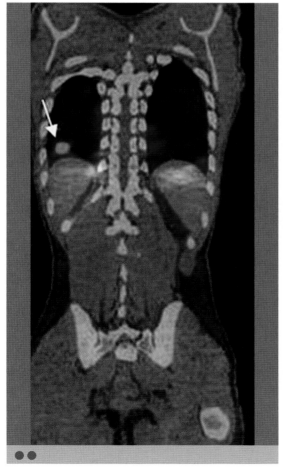

D. Pulmonary metastasis in mixed germ cell tumor. Coronal fused FDG-PET/CT (*arrow*).

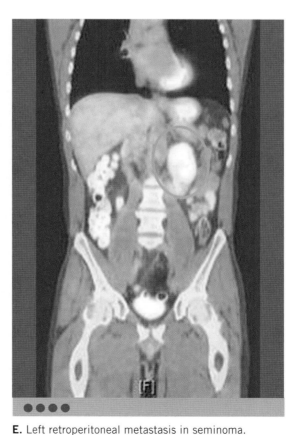

E. Left retroperitoneal metastasis in seminoma.

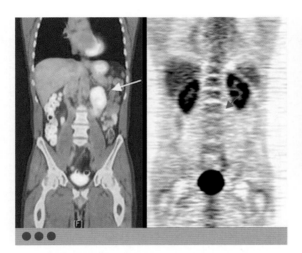

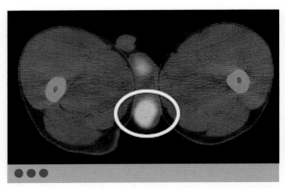

G. Asymmetrical testicular FDG uptake in left testicular embryonal cell carcinoma (*circle*). Note physiological FDG uptake in normal testis.

F. Resolved metastasis after chemotherapy (right nonfused coronal PET, *red arrow*).

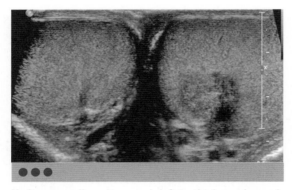

H. Corresponding ultrasound, left testicular embryonal cell carcinoma.

Vivek Manchanda, MD

PRESENTATION

Woman in midforties, being imaged for mantle cell lymphoma.

FINDINGS

Intense FDG activity corresponding to the large uterine mass.

DIFFERENTIAL DIAGNOSES

- *Leiomyoma*
- *Uterine sarcoma*
- *Uterine lymphoma*
- *Uterine adenocarcinoma*
- *Uterine hemorrhage*

Stability of FDG activity over time is indicative of leiomyoma. Level of FDG activity cannot distinguish between the two.

COMMENTS

In premenopausal women, FDG uptake in uterus is variable. It can be much higher in a period of 1 week prior to menstruation to up to a few days after menstruation. Thus, normal endometrial uptake of ¹⁸F-FDG changes cyclically, increasing during the ovulatory and menstrual phases.

Postmenopausal women with increased uterine FDG activity should be investigated to exclude malignancy.

FDG activity has also been demonstrated in menstrual blood, as seen in analysis of tampons. Both postpartum and gravid uteruses have variable FDG activity. Placental FDG activity and fetal brain and myocardial activity can be seen in a viable pregnancy.

Causes of increased uterine FDG uptake include menorrhagia, leiomyoma, endometrial and cervical carcinoma, hematometrocolpos, metastases, and carcinosarcoma.

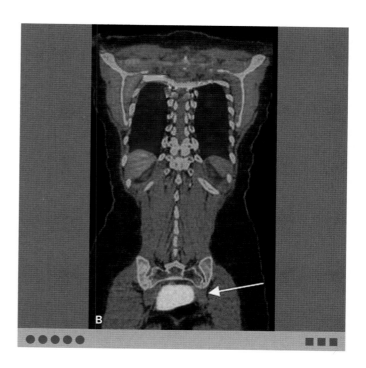

It is difficult to distinguish leiomyoma from leiomyosarcoma on the basis of FDG activity, which may be variable.

Leiomyomas can show intense FDG uptake, that can wax and wane.

PET/CT may be of use in detection of occult choriocarcinoma if the conventional imaging is negative with persistent elevated β-human chorionic gonadotropin (β-HCG).

FDG-PET can be performed safely in a pregnant patient as long as risks are carefully considered and outweighed by the expected benefits. Reducing dose and increasing imaging

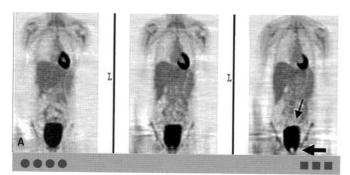

A. and B. Uterine fibroid: Coronal PET/CT. Thin arrow corresponds to fibroid and thick arrow corresponds to catheterized bladder.

PEARLS

- Premenopausal uterus has variable FDG uptake, highest in ovulatory and menstrual phases.

- Postmenopausal uterine FDG uptake should be worked up for disease involvement.

- Leiomyomas, menorrhagia, endometrial/cervical cancer, hematometrocolpos, metastases, and carcinosarcoma are some of the causes of increased uterine FDG activity.

- Both gravid and postpartum uteri myometrium can be FDG avid.

- FDG-PET scan can be safely performed in pregnant patients as long as precautions are undertaken and there is awareness regarding fetal exposure, as described above.

time, IV hydration, and Foley catheter can be used to minimize fetal radiation dose (mostly due to maternal bladder). Lasix (furosemide) should not be used in pregnant women.

The estimated fetal radiation dose from FDG in early pregnancy to 3-month gestation: 67 mrem/mCi; 6-month gestation: 59 mrem/mCi; and term: 57 mrem/mCi.

ADDITIONAL IMAGE

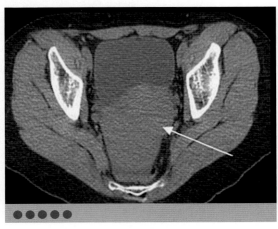

C. Corresponding CT.

DIFFERENTIAL DIAGNOSIS IMAGES (D-I)

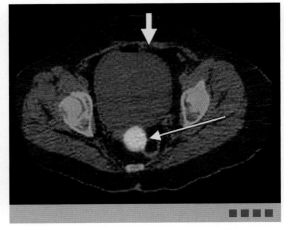

D. Recurrent uterine sarcoma (*thin arrow*) with catheterized bladder with retrograde saline filling (*thick arrow*). Axial fused FDG-PET/CT.

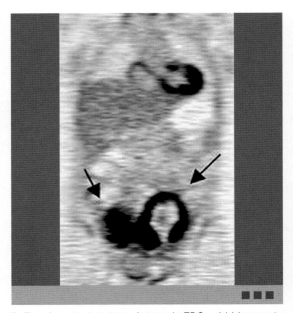

E. Two days post partum, intensely FDG avid bicornuate uterus, 30-year-old female.

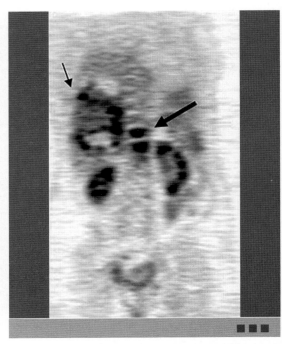

F. Uterine sarcoma metastasis to right thorax (*thin arrow*) and T11 and T12 (*thick arrow*), s/p hysterectomy.

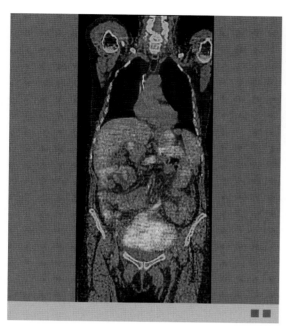

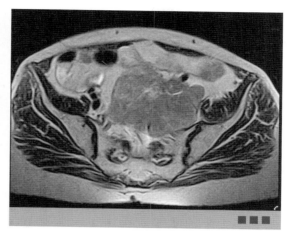

H. Corresponding T2-W MR.

G. High-grade leiomyosarcoma in 66-year-old female. Coronal fused PET/CT.

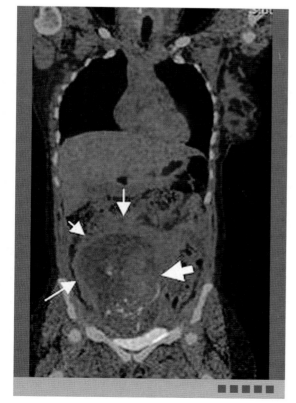

I. Mildly hypermetabolic gravid uterus (*thin arrow*) with intrauterine pregnancy (*thick arrow*), 33-year-old female.

Case 4–8 Vaginal Cancer and FDG-PET

Vivek Manchanda, MD

PRESENTATION

Woman in early seventies with vaginal bleeding.

FINDINGS

Intensely hypermetabolic vaginal mass.

DIFFERENTIAL DIAGNOSES

- *Primary vaginal squamous cell cancer*
- *Metastasis*
- *Lymphoma*
- *Smooth muscle neoplasm (leiomyoma, leiomyosarcoma)*: Rare
- *Connective tissue neoplasm (fibromyoma)*: Rare
- *Paraganglioma*: Extremely rare
- *Hemangioma*: Usually non-FDG avid
- *Nonspecific vaginal FDG activity*

COMMENTS

The biopsy showed vaginal squamous cell cancer.

Vaginal cancer comprises only 1% to 2% of gynecologic malignancies. The majority are squamous cell cancers; others include adenocarcinoma, melanoma, and sarcoma.

In early stages, vaginal cancer is often curable. For local staging, MR is the method of choice.

FDG-PET/CT can be helpful in evaluation of regional nodal disease, which includes pelvic nodes (obturator, internal, external, and common iliac) and inguinal nodes.

Tumors involving upper third of vagina drain to pelvic nodes and those involving the lower one-third drain to the inguinal nodes. Vaginal adenocarcinomas tend to involve pelvic lymph nodes locally and supraclavicular nodes distantly. The commonest distant nodes involved in the squamous cell cancers of vagina include retroperitoneal nodes.

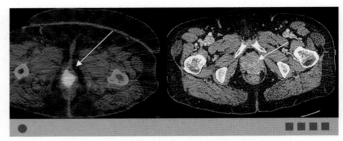

A. Hypermetabolic vaginal mass and corresponding CT.

The non-nodal metastases from both squamous cell and adenocarcinomas include lungs and liver.

Advanced stage, older age, middle and lower vagina tumors, and greater length of vaginal wall involvement indicate poorer prognosis.

Surgery or radiation is highly effective for early stages. In stages III and IVA, radiation therapy alone is the standard of treatment. In patients who have undergone hysterectomy, vaginal cancers are more likely to involve the upper one-third of vagina.

FDG-PET scans have been used for radiation therapy planning and follow-up of treatment. They have also been used to detect distant metastases. FDG activity in menstrual blood may affect interpretation of FDG-PET scan. It is advisable to use retrograde bladder filling with saline for proper assessment of pelvis, but it may be uncomfortable for many patients.

PEARLS

- **FDG-PET is helpful in detecting distant vaginal cancer metastases and involvement of locoregional nodes.**

- **FDG is secreted in the menstrual blood and may be seen nonspecifically in vagina.**

- **Non-nodal metastases from both vaginal squamous cell and adenocarcinomas include lungs and liver.**

DIFFERENTIAL DIAGNOSIS IMAGES (B-C)

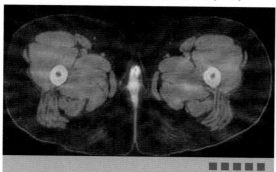

B. FDG excretion in menstrual blood.

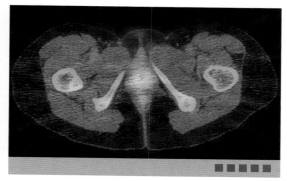

C. Nonspecific vaginal FDG activity in 34-year-old female, no corresponding mass.

Vivek Manchanda, MD

PRESENTATION

Woman in early forties with recently diagnosed vulvar cancer and diffuse lymphadenopathy on CT.

FINDINGS

Diffuse hypermetabolic lymph nodes.

DIFFERENTIAL DIAGNOSES

- *Metastatic vulvar cancer*
- *Lymphoma*
- *Systemic inflammatory disease such as sarcoidosis*

The regional nodes for vulvar cancer include femoral and inguinal nodes and the distant nodes include intrapelvic nodes. Mainly symmetric extrapelvic nodal distribution with mediastinal nodes suggest a systemic inflammatory etiology, such as sarcoidosis. The biopsy of both axillary and inguinal nodes showed noncaseating granulomas.

COMMENTS

Vulvar cancer is a rare gynecologic malignancy. Most vulvar cancers are squamous cell cancers. Early detection

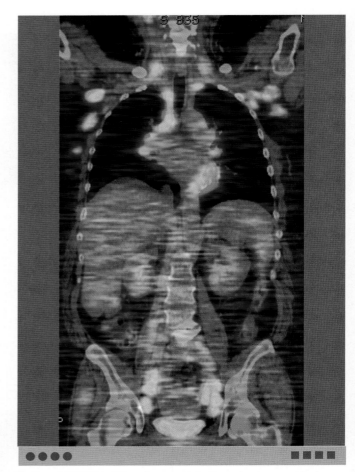

B. Fused PET/CT, diffuse hypermetabolic nodes in sarcoidosis.

has a higher rate of cure. It most commonly affects inner edges of labia majora or labia minora. HPV has been suggested as one of the etiologies.

FDG-PET scan can play an important role in characterizing the local extent of disease and regional nodal disease involvement for planning of treatment. The regional nodes

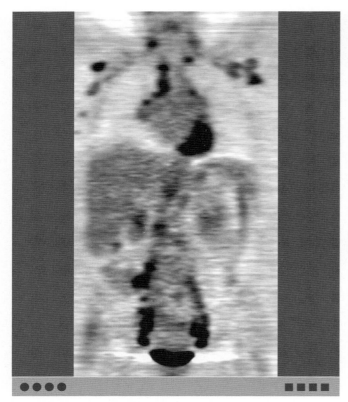

A. Diffuse hypermetabolic lymph nodes. Coronal FDG-PET.

PEARLS

- Regional nodes for vulvar cancer include femoral and inguinal nodes and the distant nodes include all intrapelvic nodes. FDG-PET can help in characterizing nodal extent of disease and help detect distant metastases.

- Unusual diffuse and symmetrical nodal disease pattern on an FDG-PET scan should raise the suspicion for coexisting systemic disease such as sarcoidosis.

for vulvar cancer are femoral and inguinal nodes and the distant nodes include all intrapelvic nodes.

Most important prognostic factors for vulvar carcinoma are nodal status and diameter of the primary lesion.

The 5-year survival for a T1N0 disease is close to 100% and drops to about 30% if three or more unilateral nodes or two or more bilateral nodes are involved.

The standard treatment for vulvar cancer is surgery. External beam radiation therapy is applied along with surgery for stage III or IV cancers.

Again, since majority of the vulvar cancers are squamous cell in origin, they are extremely FDG avid. FDG secretion into menstrual blood can affect the scan interpretation.

Currently, MR is the method of choice for local staging as it can assess both the local extent of disease and regional nodal involvement.

CT is limited by suboptimal soft tissue contrast and FDG-PET is limited by its secretion in the menstrual blood. However, both can be useful for detection of distant metastases. F18 FDG-PET can help in evaluation of treatment response and presence of recurrence.

DIFFERENTIAL DIAGNOSIS IMAGES (C-D)

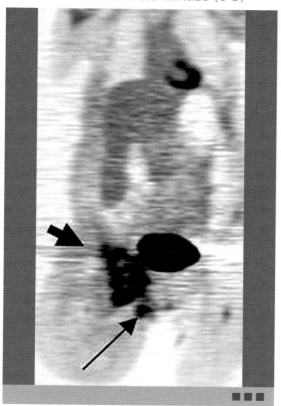

C. Right vulvar cancer (*thin arrow*) with right inguinal metastatic nodes (*thick arrow*). Coronal FDG-PET.

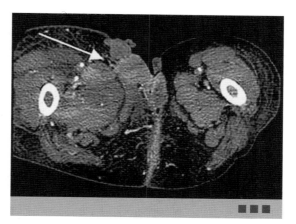

D. Right vulvar squamous cell cancer with centrally necrotic metastases in right groin CT.

Chapter 5

GASTROINTESTINAL

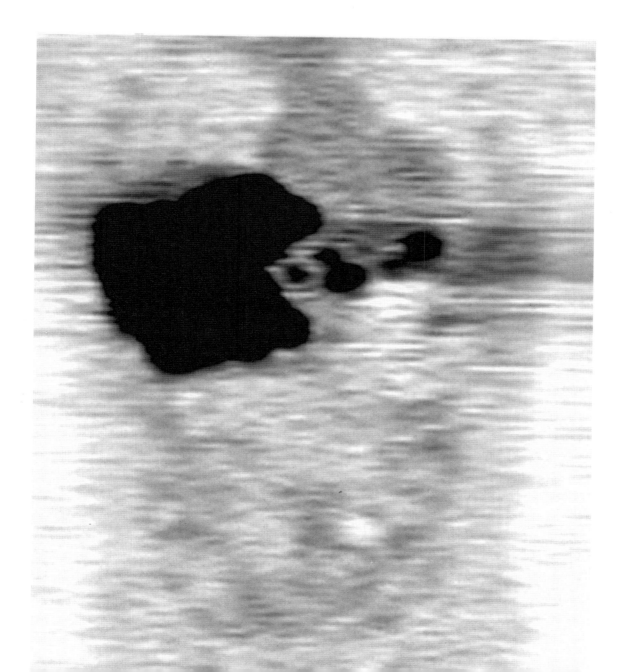

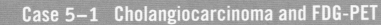

Vivek Manchanda, MD

PRESENTATION

Man in midforties with jaundice.

FINDINGS

Intense heterogeneous fluorodeoxyglucose (FDG) activity corresponding to a large mass and multiple other smaller masses, in liver.

DIFFERENTIAL DIAGNOSES

- *Malignancy*: Metastases, multifocal primary hepatocellular carcinoma (HCC), lymphoma, cholangiocarcinoma

- *Infection*: Multiple abscesses

- *Sarcoidosis*

Given intense metabolic activity, cavernous hemangiomas, adenomas, bile duct hamartomas, and congenital cystic diseases are unlikely.

COMMENTS

In the index case, the biopsy showed cholangiocarcinoma.

Cholangiocarcinomas arise from bile duct epithelium. Peak incidence is in fifth and sixth decades of life with slight male preponderance.

Predisposing factors include choledochal cyst, *Clonorchis sinensis* infection, thorotrast, and primary sclerosing cholangitis.

Intrahepatic cholangiocarcinoma arises from bile duct epithelium, mucinous glands, or fibrous stroma or combination (which affects FDG activity). It is difficult to differentiate from other metastatic adenocarcinomas.

CT shows hypoattenuating/isodense lesion on noncontrast phase with marked homogeneous, delayed enhancement. Dilated intrahepatic bile ducts may be seen which are uncommon in liver metastasis. Calcifications are uncommon. Capsule is not present (unlike hepatocellular cancer).

MR shows heterogeneously hypointense mass on T1-WI with gadolinium enhancement of the lesion.

Cholangiocarcinomas (especially nodular in comparison to infiltrating) are generally very FDG avid. PET may change management in up to 30%. It is useful in the evaluation of recurrent and metastatic disease and for assessment of treatment response.

False-positive FDG activity (for hilar cholangiocarcinoma) may be seen with primary sclerosing cholangitis, biliary stents, and granulomatous disease. Per one small study, carbon 11 (^{11}C)-acetate PET did not show FDG uptake in any cholangiocarcinomas. In a subgroup analysis, peripheral mass-forming cholangiocarcinomas were more FDG avid than hilar

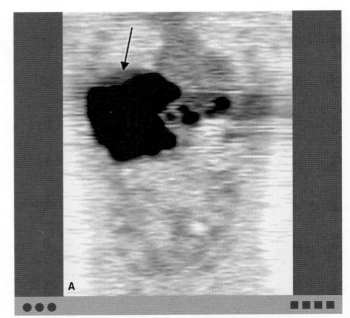

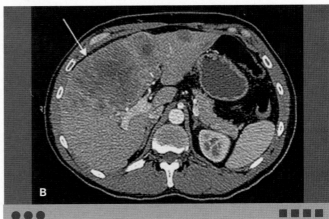

A. and **B.** Peripheral cholangiocarcinoma FDG-PET and corresponding CT.

PEARLS

- FDG-avid liver mass with dilated bile ducts is strongly suggestive of intrahepatic cholangiocarcinoma.

- Peripheral mass-forming cholangiocarcinomas are more FDG avid than infiltrative types.

- Fluorodeoxyglucose-positron emission tomography (FDG-PET) can change management in up to 30% cases of cholangiocarcinomas with detection of diseased locoregional nodes and distant metastases.

- Mucinous cholangiocarcinomas may be falsely FDG negative.

cholangiocarcinomas which were mainly non-mass forming and infiltrative (variable FDG activity).

Early-stage treatment of cholangiocarcinoma is surgical resection/liver transplantation.

Immunohistochemical stain positive for epithelial membrane antigen and tissue polypeptide antigen with staining for cytokeratin subtypes can be helpful in differentiating cholangiocarcinoma from metastatic colorectal carcinoma.

ADDITIONAL IMAGES (C-D)

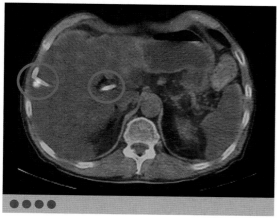

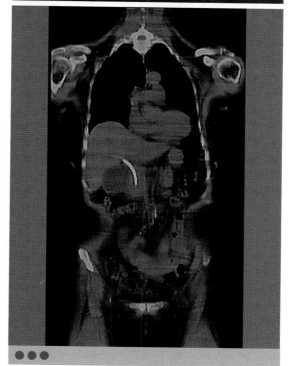

C. FDG-negative mucinous common bile duct (CBD) cholangiocarcinoma. Note FDG activity in stent (circles).

DIFFERENTIAL DIAGNOSIS IMAGES (E-I)

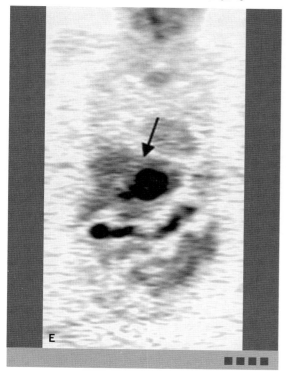

D. FDG-negative hilar cholangiocarcinoma, fused PET-CT (*below*) with corresponding MR (*above*) showing biliary ductal dilation, and ill-defined, enhancing hilar cholangiocarcinoma.

E. and **F.** Hepatocellular carcinoma (HCC) and corresponding CT.

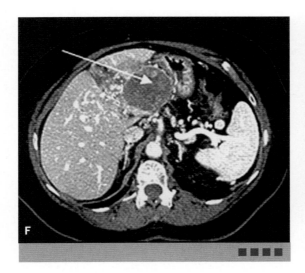

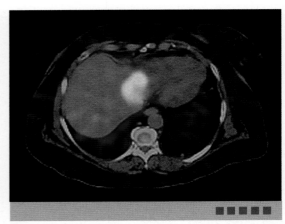

G. Hepatic metastasis from colon cancer. Fused FDG-PET/CT.

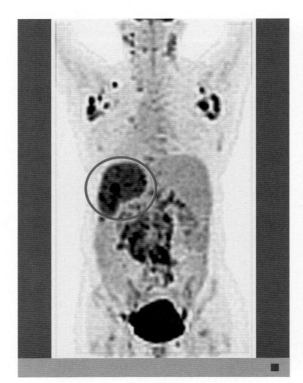

H. Liver involvement, follicular lymphoma, coronal FDG-PET.

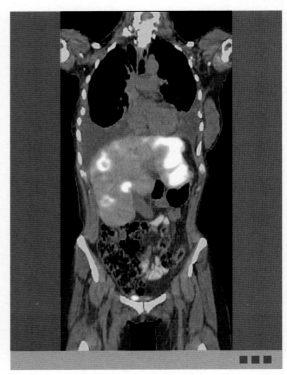

I. Breast cancer metastases to the liver. Fused FDG-PET/CT.

Vivek Manchanda, MD

PRESENTATION

Man in his fourth decade of life with anemia.

FINDINGS

Intense focal FDG activity corresponding to right colonic mass.

DIFFERENTIAL DIAGNOSES

- *Polyp* (typically adenomatous)
- *Focal inflammation*: Inflammatory bowel disease (IBD)/diverticulitis
- *Infection*: TB
- *Metastases*: Breast, stomach, lung, and melanoma
- *Lymphoma*

When focal, intensely increased FDG activity is seen in the bowel, lipoma and lymphangioma can be safely excluded; others like neurofibroma are very unlikely.

COMMENTS

Colon cancer patients present with bleeding and anemia (right side), whereas left-sided tumors tend to be obstructive. Family history of colon cancer, familial polyposis, or ulcerative colitis increases the risk for colon cancer.

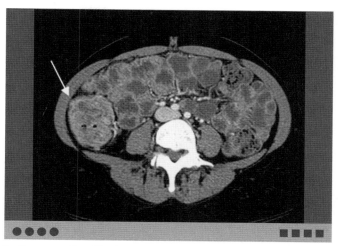

B. Corresponding CT, right colon mass (*white arrow*).

FDG-PET has a high sensitivity and specificity for detection of colorectal carcinomas (primary and liver metastases) and is useful in staging and restaging of primary colorectal carcinoma. Patients with head and neck cancer or lung cancer may show incidental primary colon cancer, related to smoking.

There is a direct correlation between primary colon cancer uptake and cellularity, but negative correlation between amount of mucin and FDG activity (up to 40% mucinous adenocarcinomas may be falsely negative per one study).

Sensitivity and specificity of FDG-PET in detecting recurrent nonmucinous adenocarcinoma is high. In a patient with rising carcinoembryonic antigen (CEA) levels, it provides an important test for detecting distant, residual, or recurrent disease.

PET/CT has high sensitivity, specificity, and accuracy in detecting metastases. In liver, sensitivity varies significantly with the lesion size. Isolated liver metastasis from the colon cancer has the potential of curative resection and FDG-PET plays a crucial role in detection of the same.

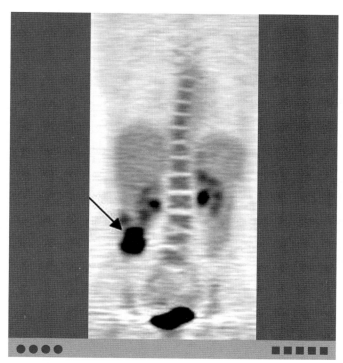

A. Intense coronal FDG-PET FDG activity in right colon in patient A, biopsy-proven adenocarcinoma.

PEARLS

- **FDG-PET is sensitive but not specific in detecting primary colorectal cancers.**
- **FDG-PET plays a role in restaging of the disease with rising CEA level.**
- **Focal bowel FDG activity justifies colonoscopic correlation.**
- **Polyps (mainly adenomatous) are FDG avid, depending on their size.**

Focal incidental FDG uptake in FDG-PET scan justifies colonoscopic examination and should be recommended.

FDG activity in adenomatous polyps, which are precursor to the colon cancer, is directly related to the size of the polyp. In one study, more than 90% of adenomatous polyps larger than 13 mm were FDG avid. Hyperplastic polyps have been shown to be FDG avid as well.

ADDITIONAL IMAGES (C-F)

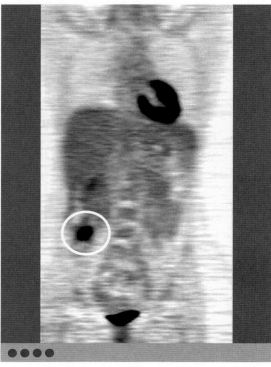

C. Decreased FDG activity after chemotherapy in patient A, consistent with response.

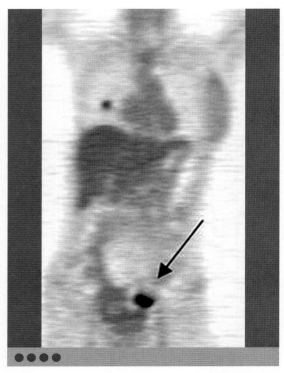

D. Left colon cancer (*black arrow*) with right lung metastasis.

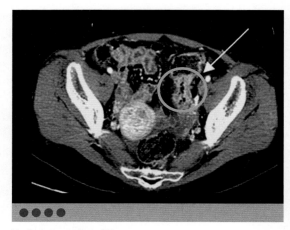

E. Corresponding CT.

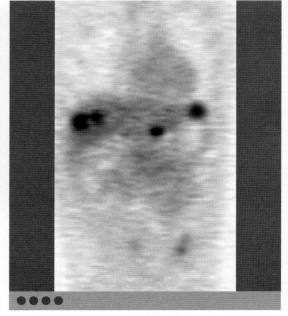

F. Liver metastasis from colon cancer, coronal FDG-PET.

DIFFERENTIAL DIAGNOSIS IMAGES (G-H)

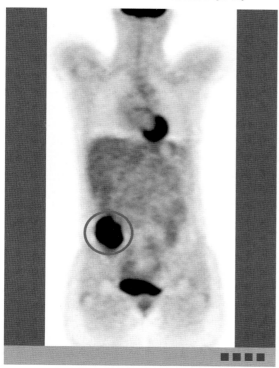

G. 44-year-old female, right colon, diffuse large B-cell (DLBC) lymphoma, coronal FDG-PET.

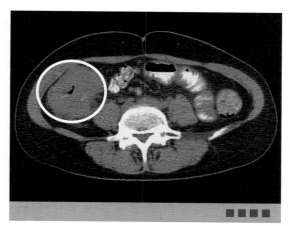

H. Corresponding CT. Note circumferential bowel thickening.

Case 5–3 Crohn Disease and FDG-PET

Vivek Manchanda, MD

PRESENTATION

Woman in midtwenties with diarrhea and abdominal pain.

FINDINGS

Intense segmental FDG activity in bowel with moderately increased focal FDG activity in the mesentery.

DIFFERENTIAL DIAGNOSES

- *Colon cancer*
- *Infection/Ischemia/IBD*
- *Multiple polyps*
- *Physiological*

Segmentally increased FDG activity in colon usually implies inflammation. FDG activity related to colon cancer is typically focal.

COMMENTS

In the index case, segmentally increased FDG activity was due to Crohn disease (CD) with mesenteric phlegmon. Fluorine

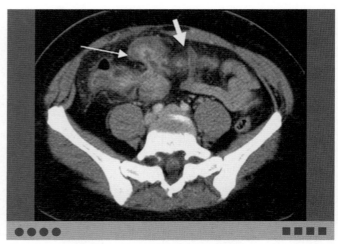

B. Corresponding CT with thickened bowel wall (*thin white arrow*) and phlegmon (*thick white arrow*).

18-FDG-PET/CT correlates with the clinical, endoscopic, and biologic activity of CD, per studies. It has good sensitivity for detection of intestinal segments with moderate to severe mucosal lesions.

Barium studies and colonoscopy are better than CT for superficial mucosal changes. PET/CT may be helpful in early and superficial mucosal changes.

Evaluation of flat areas of high-grade dysplasias or adenomas in patients with IBD is not feasible on PET. However, inflammatory stenosis can be reasonably differentiated from scar stenosis.

Segmentally increased FDG activity with perinuclear antineutrophil cytoplasmic antibodies (p-ANCAs) for ulcerative colitis (UC), anti-*Saccharomyces cerevisiae* antibodies (ASCA), and outer membrane porin to *Escherichia coli* (outer membrane

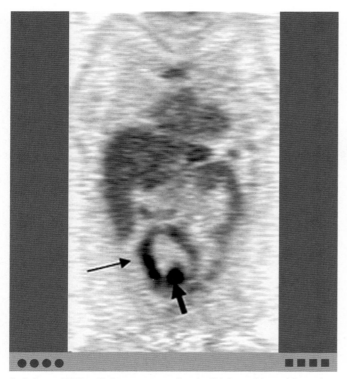

A. Intense FDG activity corresponding to thickened bowel in active CD (*thin arrow*) and phlegmon (*thick arrow*) coronal FDG-PET.

PEARLS

- In limited studies, FDG-PET correlates well with clinical, endoscopic, and biologic activities of CD and provides useful information to differentiate inflammation from scar stenosis.

- FDG-PET has good sensitivity in detection of intestinal and colonic segments with moderate to severe mucosal lesions.

- It should not be used in place of routine surveillance for adenomas or flat areas of high-grade dysplasias arising from long-standing IBD.

- In patients who cannot tolerate biphasic contrast for MR study, PET/CT can be performed without oral contrast for evaluation of active disease.

protein C [Omp C]) antibodies for CD may differentiate IBD from ischemic and infectious colitis.

UC is typically left sided or diffuse, with rectal involvement. CD usually involves right colon and terminal ileum, and may have "string sign" (thickened and narrowed terminal ileum), or "comb's sign" (engorgement of vasa recta) or "fat halo sign" (from thickened submucosal fat). Wall thickening is symmetric and continuous in UC, and eccentric with skip areas in CD. In UC, the rectum typically shows inflammation (unless on steroids). In CD, the rectum may be spared. Ascites (often present in infectious colitis) is usually absent in IBD. In CD, an intensely FDG-avid phlegmon (ill-defined inflammatory mass) may develop in mesentery/omentum. It can resolve with antibiotics or progress to an abscess.

DIFFERENTIAL DIAGNOSIS IMAGES (C-H)

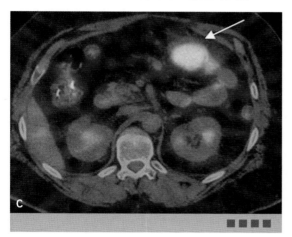

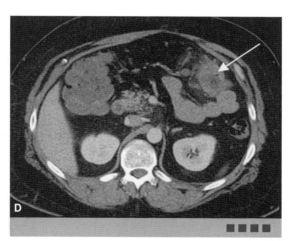

C. and **D.** Focal increased FDG activity in transverse colon cancer axial fused PET/CT and corresponding CT (*white arrow*).

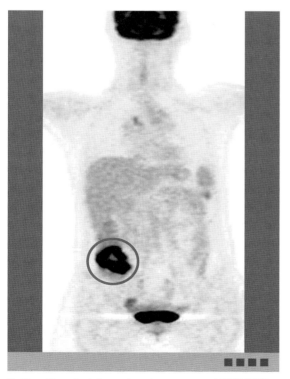

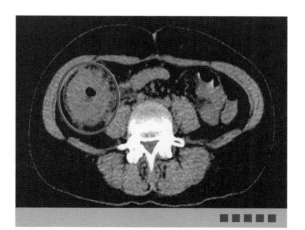

F. Corresponding CT

E. Cecal/terminal ileum lymphoma coronal FDG-PET.

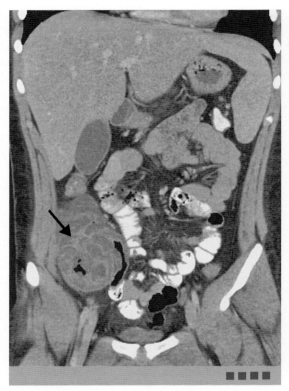

G. CT 4 days before PET. Note typhilitis (*black arrow*).

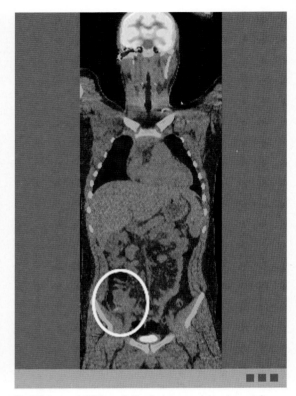

H. Mild cecal FDG activity 4 days post treatment for typhilitis. Coronal fused PET/CT.

Vivek Manchanda, MD

PRESENTATION

Man in midseventies with difficulty breathing while lying down.

FINDINGS

Hypermetabolic mediastinal mass. No other lesions suspicious for metastases.

DIFFERENTIAL DIAGNOSES

- *Leiomyoma/leiomyosarcoma*
- *Primary esophageal cancer*
- *Infected duplication cyst*
- *Melanoma of esophagus* (rare)
- *Gastrointestinal stromal tumor (GIST) of esophagus* (rare)

Unlikely to be simple esophageal duplication cyst, which is usually photopenic. Any of the above can be the differential, given the FDG activity.

COMMENTS

FDG uptake can distinguish benign from malignant esophageal masses. A duplication cyst is typically photopenic, unless it is infected, in which case the patient will have signs and

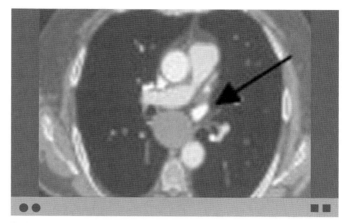

B. Corresponding CT.

symptoms of infection. On the corresponding CT, the duplication cyst will be well defined with fluid density on the noncontrast CT scan examination.

Leiomyoma of esophagus mainly occurs in the distal esophagus. It has variable FDG activity (similar to the leiomyoma of uterus). Increased FDG activity in a lesion that appears to be a leiomyoma on CT does not necessarily mean a malignant degeneration into leiomyosarcoma.

Leiomyosarcomas are extremely rare and mostly intramural. They account for 90% of esophageal sarcomas. Rarely, rhabdomyosarcomas, synovial sarcomas, malignant nerve sheath tumors, osteosarcoma, chondrosarcoma, fibrosarcoma, malignant fibrous histiocytoma, and liposarcoma have been reported.

The second most common stromal tumors after leiomyomas are granular cell tumors. Usually small and asymptomatic, they are most commonly seen in black men in their forties. The endoscopic features include sessile, yellow tumors which are firm to palpation. FDG uptake in granular cell tumors has not been described in the literature.

PEARLS

- Increased FDG uptake in distal esophageal masses may be due to leiomyomas, infected duplication cysts, leiomyosarcomas, GISTs, or primary carcinoma of esophagus.

- Duplication cysts are photopenic on PET, with fluid density on corresponding noncontrast CT scan.

- Most common mesenchymal tumor of esophagus is a leiomyoma with variable FDG activity. Increased FDG activity cannot differentiate leiomyoma from leiomyosarcoma.

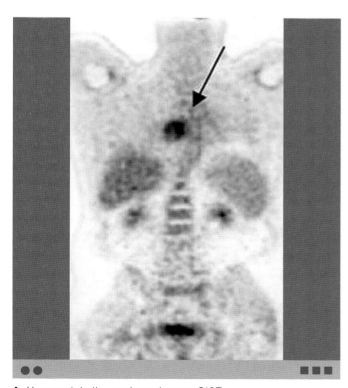

A. Hypermetabolic esophageal mass, GIST.

Other etiologies to consider in case of increased FDG activity include rare entities such as GIST of esophagus and primary melanoma of esophagus. In literature, primary melanomas have been described as intraluminal masses with expanded luminal caliber, which did not cause obstruction.

GISTs of esophagus are usually well circumscribed and may not cause dilation of the esophagus. They are extremely FDG avid and must be differentiated from the other mesenchymal tumors of esophagus, given their usual poor prognosis.

DIFFERENTIAL DIAGNOSIS IMAGES (C-G)

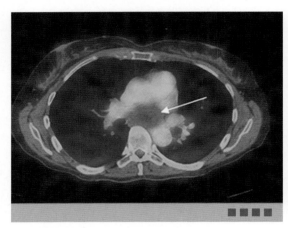

C. Photopenic bronchogenic cyst.

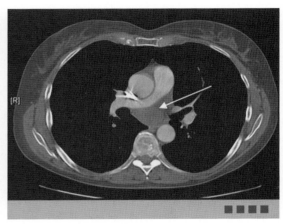

D. CT bronchogenic cyst.

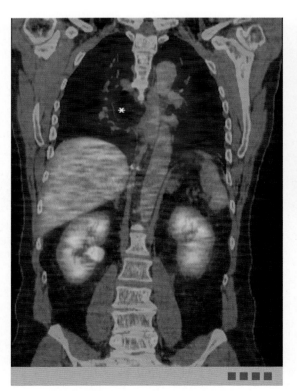

E. Posterior mediastinal pleural lipoma (*white star*), fused PET/CT.

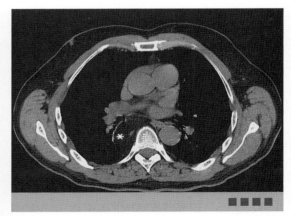

F. Corresponding CT (*white star*).

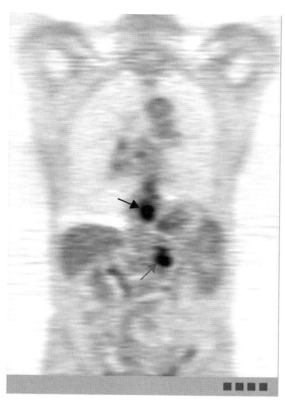

G. Distal esophageal cancer (*black arrow*) with nodal metastasis (*red arrow*). Coronal FDG-PET.

Vivek Manchanda, MD

PRESENTATION

Female in midfifties with breast cancer and right abdominal pain.

FINDINGS

Intense hypermetabolic activity in the right pelvis along with vertebral metastases and lung and mediastinal metastases.

DIFFERENTIAL DIAGNOSES

- *Metastases*
- *Primary colon cancer*
- *Polyp*
- *Lymphoma*
- *Infection*

Although it is difficult to exclude any of the above on the basis of FDG-PET alone, a follow-up CT showed resolution of fat stranding and focal thickening of bowel in the patient.

COMMENTS

Diverticulitis, a common condition in elderly, occurs due to microperforation of a diverticulum, and is usually left-sided. It is characterized by abdominal pain, cramping, low-grade fever, and altered stool habits.

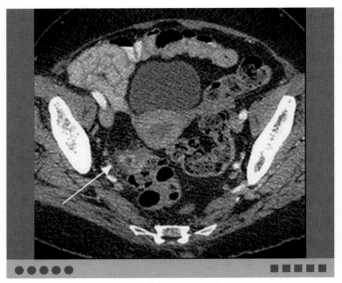

B. Corresponding CT. Note fat stranding around diverticulum (*arrow*).

Acquired colonic diverticula usually form on the mesenteric side, mainly in the descending and sigmoid colon.

On CT, diverticula typically appear as small outpouchings of the colonic wall filled with air.

Diverticulitis appears as intensely FDG-avid focal thickening of the colonic wall associated with pericolonic stranding, engorged mesenteric vessels, and fluid in the mesentery. In sigmoid diverticulitis, fascial thickening close to the pelvic sidewall may occur.

Focal increased FDG activity has also been reported with radiation colitis. Adenomas and colon cancer are other causes of focally increased FDG activity. Colon cancer is suggested by a focal concentric mass and pericolonic nodes. Metastatic breast cancer can involve any site and should be in the differential. A short-term follow-up CT scan after antibiotics trial can help distinguish the two.

CT can accurately depict complications of diverticulitis, such as abscess formation, fistula, and perforation, which also tend to show increased FDG activity due to associated inflammation.

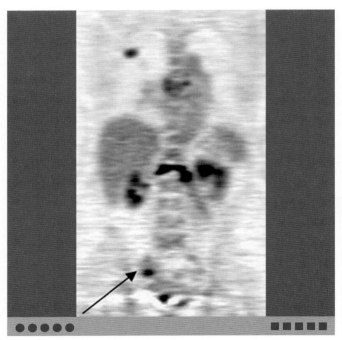

A. Diverticulitis (*black arrow*) in a patient with vertebral metastases and lung and mediastinal nodal metastases from breast cancer.

PEARLS

- Both diverticulitis and colon cancer are extremely FDG avid and short-term follow up CT can help differentiate the two.

- Diverticulitis is characterized by pericolonic fat stranding, engorged mesenteric vessels, and fluid in the mesentery, whereas focal concentric mass and pericolonic nodes suggest colon cancer.

A colovesical fistula is suspected in a patient with air in the bladder and a thickened bladder wall next to the inflamed colonic segment. Colovaginal fistula may occur in women as a complication of diverticulitis. In these cases, positive rectal contrast material or FDG activity may be seen in the vagina.

A contained microperforation may be seen on CT obtained with PET as small extraluminal pockets of air or extravasation of contrast material.

DIFFERENTIAL DIAGNOSIS IMAGES (C-G)

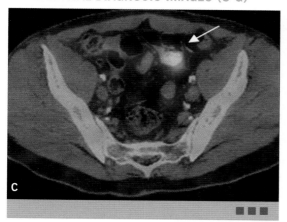
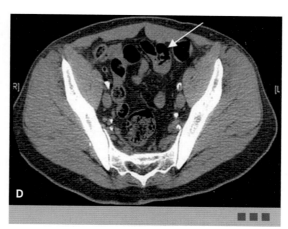

C. and **D.** Hyperplastic polyp, fused axial FDG-PET/CT, no fat stranding on corresponding CT (*arrow*).

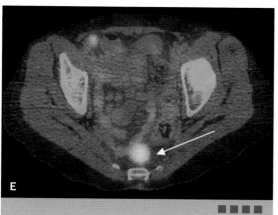
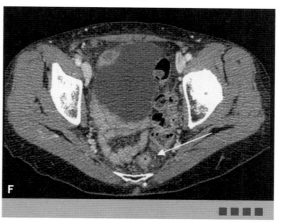

E. and **F.** Sigmoid colon cancer in left pelvis, fused FDG-PET, and corresponding CT (*white arrows*).

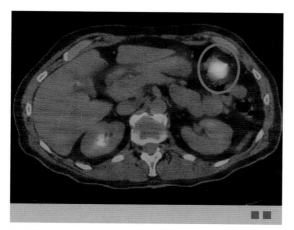

G. Tubulovillous adenoma fused PET/CT image (*circle*).

219

Vivek Manchanda, MD

PRESENTATION

Teenager with right upper quadrant (RUQ) pain after meals.

FINDINGS

Normal gallbladder visualization on Tc-99m mebrofenin scan (*long white arrow*). Severe duodenogastric reflux (*short white arrow*).

COMMENTS

Primary duodenogastric reflux is a rare foregut disorder of unknown origin occurring in late childhood. It is likely to be an important factor in the pathogenesis of gastritis and gastric ulcers, esophagitis, and gallstone dyspepsia. The patients usually present with nonspecific abdominal pain or postprandial abdominal pain for months or years and most other tests are negative. Sometimes and in earlier presentations, esophagogastroduodenoscopic (EGD) findings may be negative.

On a Tc-99m mebrofenin or hepatobiliary iminodiacetic acid (HIDA) scan, the reflux is seen as tracer spurting parallel and immediately below the inferior border of the liver into the stomach. It waxes and wanes and can be differentiated from the tracer excretion into the small bowel, which successively increases as it accumulates over the course of 60 minutes.

With Tc-mebrofenin, the drawbacks encountered with other methods such as gastric intubation are overcome. It is important to recognize that in patients with duodenogastric reflux, the surgical removal of gallbladder may make the reflux even worse. Hence, in evaluating for chronic cholecystitis, appropriate attention should be paid to the rate of administration of cholecystokinin (CCK) and percentage of gallbladder ejection fraction.

In patients with postcholecystectomy symptoms, 99m mebrofenin scintigraphy can again help in identifying duodenogastric reflux as a cause when others have been ruled out. Some duodenogastric reflux is physiological after cholecystectomy, which may assume a pathologic role after cholecystectomy because of loss of gallbladder as a bile

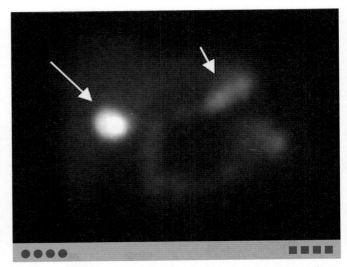

A. Duodenogastric reflux (*short white arrow*). No evidence of acute or chronic cholecystitis.

reservoir, leading to a constant supply of bile into the duodenum even in the fasting state. Prokinetic drugs or erythromycin have been shown to be effective in the treatment of duodenogastric reflux.

PEARLS

- Duodenogastric reflux should always be ruled out as a cause of chronic abdominal pain and postprandial abdominal pain on a hepatobiliary scan.

- Cholecystectomy may make the duodenogastric reflux worse.

- Prokinetic drugs or erythromycin have been helpful in ameliorating symptoms for the same.

ADDITIONAL IMAGE

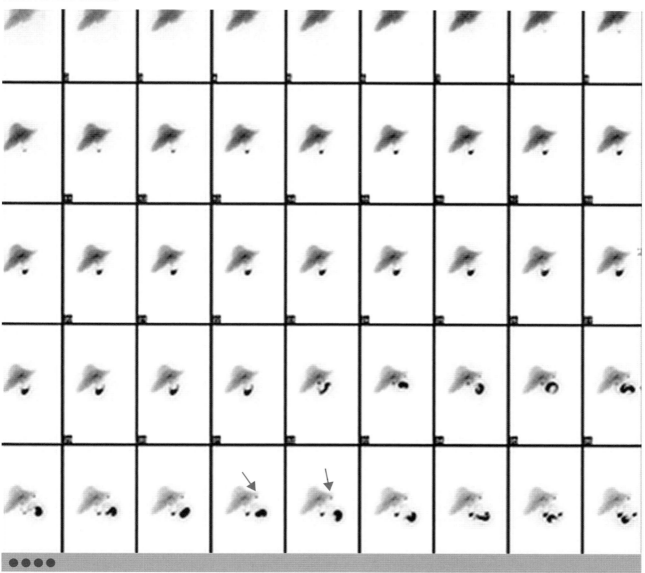

B. Acute cholecystitis (nonvisualization of gallbladder) and mild duodenogastric reflux. Tc mebrofenin hepatobiliary scan.

Vivek Manchanda, MD

PRESENTATION

Man in his early fifties with dysphagia.

FINDINGS

Moderate, focally increased radiotracer activity in the distal esophagus corresponding to thickened esophagus.

DIFFERENTIAL DIAGNOSES

- *Barrett esophagus*

- *Hiatal hernia*

- *Physiological FDG activity*

- *Focal esophagitis*: Medication/infection/reflux

- *Metastases*: Melanoma, stomach, lung, and breast

- *Lymphoma*

- *GIST* (*rare*)

Lipoma, hamartoma, lymphangioma, and noninfected duplication cyst of esophagus can be excluded based on moderately increased FDG activity.

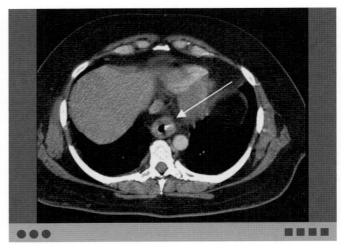

B. Corresponding CT.

COMMENTS

Focal hypermetabolic lesion in the esophagus with corresponding mass on CT is most concerning for primary esophageal cancer, such as in the index case. Mild focal uptake at the gastroesophageal junction could be due to esophagitis or could be a normal variant.

Mild, uniform physiological esophageal FDG activity is likely due to smooth muscle metabolism or saliva. Focal increased FDG activity can also be seen with Barrett esophagus, esophagitis, hiatal hernia, and post surgery and radiation therapies. Leiomyoma-related increased FDG activity has been described in occasional case reports.

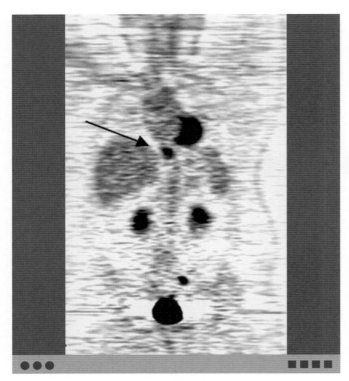

A. Esophageal cancer. Coronal FDG-PET.

PEARLS

- **FDG-PET/CT is mainly used to detect distant metastases. It may not be helpful in detecting N1 nodal disease.**

- **False-positive uptake may be seen with inflammation, Barrett dysplasia, and hiatal hernia.**

- **FDG-PET can identify recurrent disease and predict histologic response and postoperative survival.**

- **Higher SUVs and FDG-positive nodes are independent predictors of poor outcome per some studies.**

- **Mucin-producing signet ring adenocarcinomas may be falsely FDG negative.**

False-negative results may be seen in smaller cancers, cancers close to hypermetabolic myocardium, and signet ring adenocarcinoma that produces mucin. Thoracic spinal photopenia from radiation can be seen in post-therapy scans.

Both primary squamous cell cancer and adenocarcinoma of esophagus are FDG avid. About two-third patients have diseased nodes at initial presentation.

FDG-PET is not the first-line imaging study for esophageal cancer. The depth of tumor invasion is more accurately assessed with endoscopic ultrasound (EUS).

PET has limited resolution to detect N1 nodal disease, because of proximity to the hypermetabolic primary lesion or microscopic disease.

PET scan is primarily used to evaluate for distant metastases (stage IV). After surgery, PET is very sensitive, but not specific for recurrence at the anastomosis site. It is, however, very sensitive and specific in detecting distant recurrence.

In unresectable cancers, decreased FDG activity correlates with favorable chemotherapy response. FDG-PET may be used to identify nonresponders early during neoadjuvant chemoradiotherapy.

ADDITIONAL IMAGES (C-F)

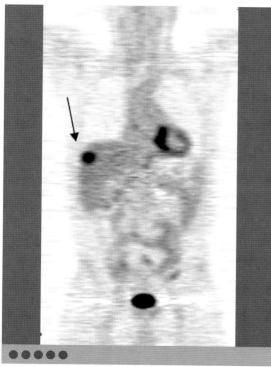

C. Liver metastases from esophageal cancer (coronal FDG-PET).

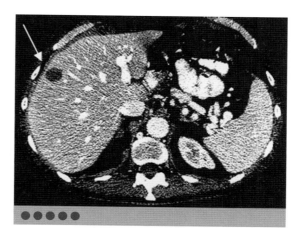

D. Corresponding CT.

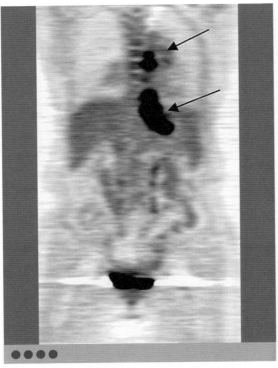

E. Multifocal esophageal cancer (*black arrows*), coronal FDG-PET.

DIFFERENTIAL DIAGNOSIS IMAGE

F. Esophageal cancer: Virchow node (*thin arrow*), esophageal cancer (*thick arrow*), and adrenal metastases (*circle*), coronal FDG-PET.

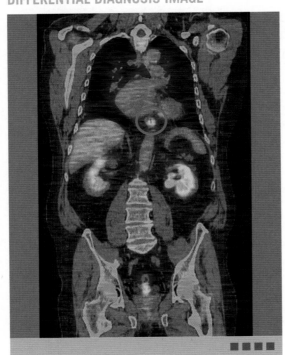

G. Focal physiologic esophageal FDG activity (*circle*), coronal FDG-PET. No corresponding CT abnormality (*not shown*).

Vivek Manchanda, MD

PRESENTATION

Male in midseventies with gallbladder mass extending into liver.

FINDINGS

Mild to moderate increased FDG activity corresponding to gallbladder mass.

DIFFERENTIAL DIAGNOSES

- *Cancer*: Primary gallbladder cancer or cholangiocarcinoma

- *Metastases*: Pancreatic, melanoma, peritoneal carcinomatosis

Other differential diagnoses with gallbladder mass could include polyp, adenomyomatosis and complicated cholecystitis.

COMMENTS

Gallbladder cancer usually affects the elderly (majority 65 and older). It is more common in women and is associated with cholelithiasis.

The most common spread is through direct invasion of liver, but it may spread through regional nodes and other adjacent organs. Focal mass, biliary obstruction at the level of porta hepatis, nodal enlargement, and direct invasion can differentiate gallbladder cancer from complicated cholecystitis. Pericholecystic halo on CT is more suggestive of complicated cholecystitis. Diffuse wall thickening is seen in both. Discontinuity of mucosal echo on ultrasonography (USG) is more indicative of gallbladder cancer.

Gallbladder cancer is associated with poor prognosis due to its ability to spread and nonspecific clinical presentation.

In adenomyomatosis, CT may show thickened gallbladder wall with small cystic-appearing (Rokitansky Aschoff sinus) spaces. There may be increased FDG activity associated with adenomyomatosis of gallbladder, but it is not the rule. These sinuses are cystic spaces filled with bile and are seen as small smooth-walled cysts which enhance on T2-WI without showing contrast enhancement.

FDG-PET has been useful in detecting metastases from primary gallbladder cancer. Smaller gallbladder lesions may not be FDG avid. Also, mucinous adenocarcinomas may be falsely FDG negative. FDG-PET can be useful in differentiating benign versus malignant polyp.

Acute/chronic cholecystitis can result in false-positive results on FDG-PET. In some studies, FDG-PET altered management in up to 20% of cases and is especially useful in detecting distant metastases.

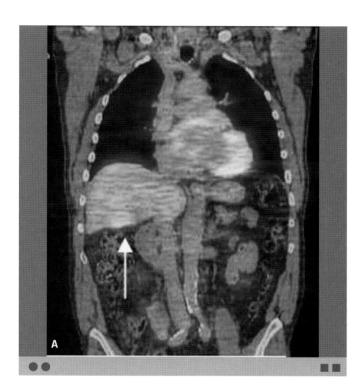

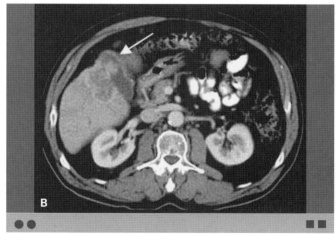

A. and **B.** Well-differentiated gallbladder cancer, PET and CT.

PEARLS

- Gallbladder cancer and adenomyomatosis of gallbladder cannot be differentiated on the basis of FDG-PET.

- FDG-PET is useful in detecting distant metastases and also helpful in recurrent gallbladder cancer.

- FDG-PET may be useful in inconclusive USG or CT findings for gallbladder lesions.

ADDITIONAL IMAGES (C-D)

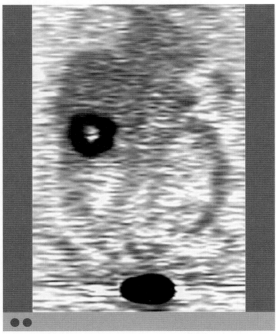

C. Recurrent gallbladder cancer in a different patient. Coronal FDG-PET.

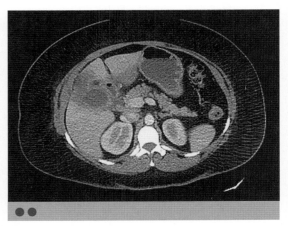

D. Corresponding axial CT.

DIFFERENTIAL DIAGNOSIS IMAGES (E-J)

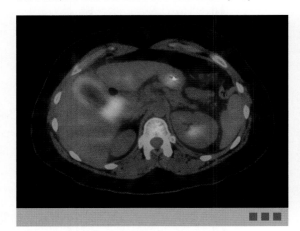

E. Inflamed gallbladder wall and CBD in ascending cholangitis, fused axial PET/CT.

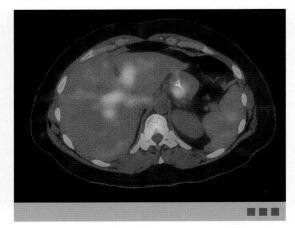

F. Inflamed intrahepatic bile ducts in ascending cholangitis, fused axial PET/CT.

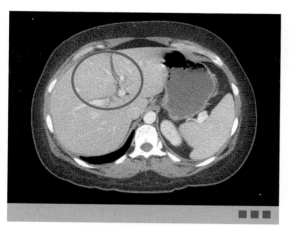

G. Dilated intrahepatic ducts in ascending cholangitis. Axial contrast-enhanced CT (*circle*).

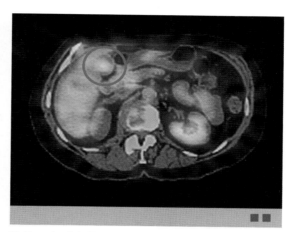

H. Fused axial PET-CT, gallbladder metastases from breast cancer (*circle*).

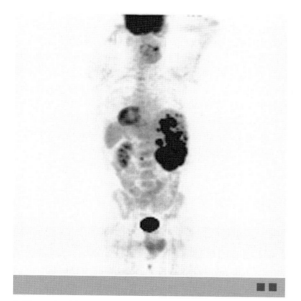

I. Posterior MIP. Poorly differentiated gallbladder cancer with liver invasion, associated with gallstone in 38-year-old male.

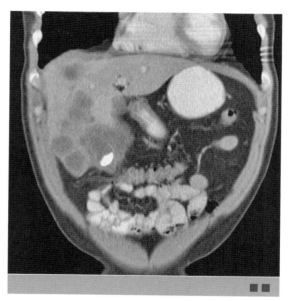

J. Coronal CT, poorly differentiated gallbladder cancer with liver invasion and gallstone.

Vivek Manchanda, MD

PRESENTATION

Korean man in his sixth decade of life with weight loss.

FINDINGS

Intense FDG activity corresponding to gastric mass and adjacent lymph node.

DIFFERENTIAL DIAGNOSES

- *Gastric lymphoma*
- *GIST*
- *Carcinoid*
- *Sarcoma*
- *Metastases*: Melanoma, breast, lung
- *Gastric polyps*
- *Chronic gastritis*

COMMENTS

Hypermetabolic gastric mass in patient with Far East ancestry in the sixth decade of life is most consistent with gastric cancer as seen in the index case, although other differentials as enumerated above could be hypermetabolic.

Stomach cancer, the second commonest cancer worldwide, is seen mainly in the Far East.

FDG-PET sensitivity for the detection of primary gastric cancer depends on the size of the tumor, extent of the tumor, and nodal involvement of disease. PET is not helpful in T staging. Also, signet ring cell gastric adenocarcinomas that produce mucin may be FDG negative.

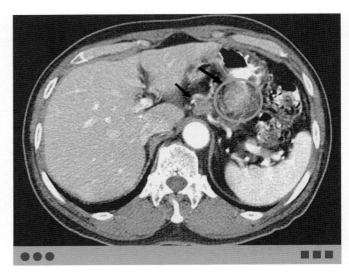

B. Corresponding CT with gastric mass (*green circle*) and involved node (*small arrow*).

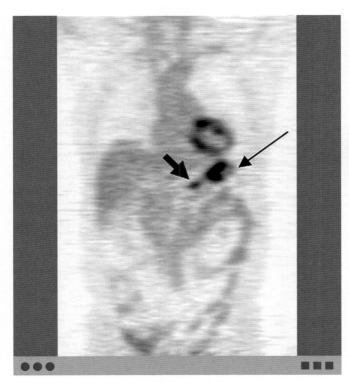

A. Hypermetabolic, poorly differentiated gastric adenocarcinoma (*thin arrow*) with involved node (*thick arrow*), coronal FDG-PET.

PEARLS

- FDG-PET/CT has low sensitivity for detecting N1 nodal involvement in gastric cancer, but good sensitivity and specificity for distant metastases.

- Nodal assessment of compartments III and IV that cannot be removed with routine dissection can be complimented with PET.

- Chronic gastritis can be intensely FDG avid with gastric wall thickening without any mass.

- Gastric adenocarcinomas such as mucinous and signet ring cell types show lower FDG activity than others.

- Large exophytic mass with areas of central necrosis/calcification with peripheral FDG uptake favors GIST over adenocarcinoma.

In the nodal staging, PET is less sensitive in detecting disease in N1(regional) nodes, which comprise compartment I (perigastric) and compartment II nodes (along celiac artery, its branches, and splenic hilum), a classification based on Japanese Research Society for Gastric Cancer due to poor spatial resolution and closeness to the hypermetabolic primary tumor.

Detection of nodal metastases in nonregional nodes of compartments III (hepatoduodenal ligament, head of pancreas, and root of mesentery) and IV (nodes along middle colic vessels and paraaortic nodes) may be possible with FDG-PET and help change the management.

PET is better than CT in detecting distant solid organ metastases; however, small liver metastases may be better seen on contrast CT. In peritoneal metastases, there may be diffuse or nodular FDG activity, with characteristic CT findings.

Many studies have demonstrated that response to preoperative chemotherapy can be predicted with FDG-PET early in the course of disease. Its role in prognostic information has not been substantiated.

ADDITIONAL IMAGES (C-D)

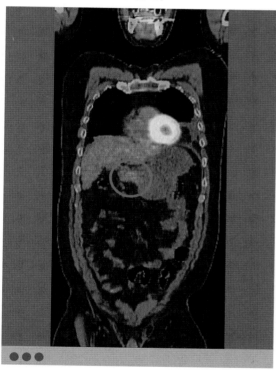

●●●

C. Coronal fused FDG-PET/CT. Mildly hypermetabolic signet cell gastric antral adenocarcinoma (*circle*).

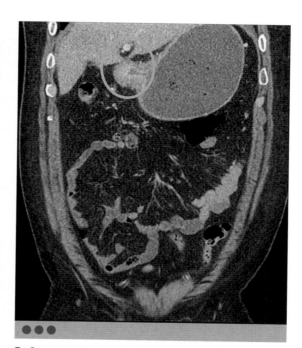

●●●

D. Corresponding contrast CT.

DIFFERENTIAL DIAGNOSIS IMAGES (E–I)

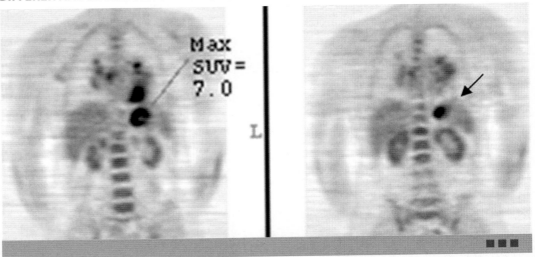

E. Intense FDG activity corresponding to biopsy-proven severe chronic gastritis coronal FDG-PET (*arrows*).

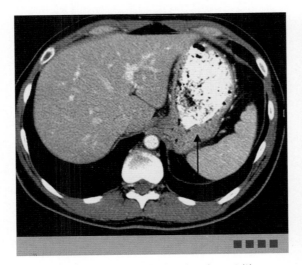

F. Corresponding contrast CT with chronic gastritis (*arrow*).

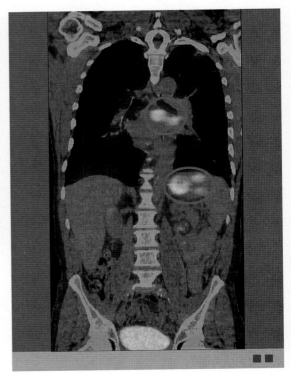

G. Coronal fused PET/CT with gastric and mediastinal involvement in NHL (*circles*).

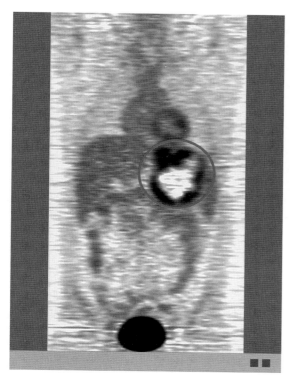

H. GIST of stomach, coronal FDG-PET. Note central photopenia (necrosis) and peripheral hypermetabolism, typical of GIST (*circle*).

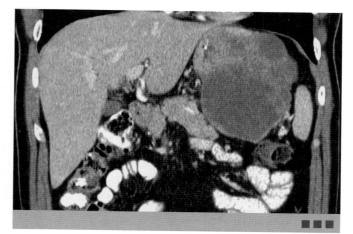

I. Corresponding CT.

Vivek Manchanda, MD

PRESENTATION

Woman in midsixties with history of gastrointestinal stromal tumor.

FINDINGS

Multiple intensely hypermetabolic lesions in the liver with central photopenia.

DIFFERENTIAL DIAGNOSES

- *Gastrointestinal stromal tumor (GIST) metastases*

- *Lymphoma*

- *Liver metastases from other malignancies*

- *Multiple abscesses*

In the absence of fever and chills, abscesses are less likely. In the background of known history of GIST, metastases from the same are most likely.

COMMENTS

GIST is a rare tumor of the gastrointestinal (GI) tract (1%-3% of all GI malignancies), commonly seen in the age group of 50 to 70 years.

They are nonepithelial, nonlymphoid tumors which are thought to arise from intestinal cells of Cajal. Majority (70%) occur in the stomach, 20% in the small intestine, and others in rectum (rarely in the esophagus). Small tumors are generally benign, especially when the growth rate is slow, but large tumors disseminate to the liver, omentum, and peritoneal cavity. (About 10%-30% of the GI tumors are malignant.) They rarely occur in other abdominal organs.

The immunohistochemistry feature of GIST is the c-kit protein (CD-117 antigen), a tyrosine kinase transmembrane receptor. The performances of ¹⁸F-FDG-PET and CT are comparable in staging GISTs before initiation of imatinib mesylate (Gleevec) therapy. However, ¹⁸F-FDG-PET is superior to CT in predicting an early response to therapy. The index patient developed severe allergy to Gleevec and expired from progressive disease.

GIST tumors associated with NF-1 are usually multiple. These tumors tend to be extragastric and multiple. On an FDG-PET scan, they are mostly hypermetabolic with central photopenia. After treatment, the lesions may become entirely cystic. These tumors have a different origin and they may not be influenced by Gleevec.

GISTs associated with esophagus are very rare and may present with nonspecific symptoms. Again, they are very FDG avid and can be differentiated from the more benign conditions of esophagus.

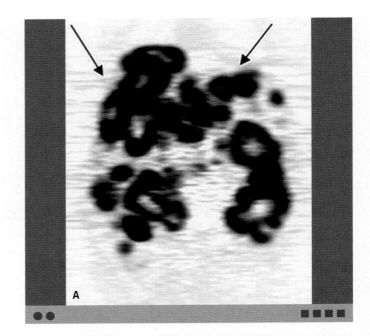

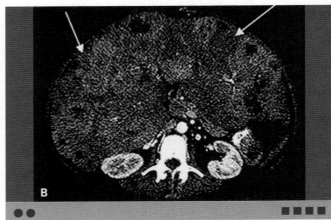

A. and **B.** Multiple, intense hypermetabolic foci with central photopenia, characteristic of GIST metastases, almost a "super PET scan" with corresponding CT.

PEARLS

- GISTs are uncommon GI tumors arising from the connective tissue.

- Most common site of GIST is stomach, followed by small intestine.

- GISTs are extremely FDG avid and FDG-PET can be used to detect response to Gleevec.

- Increased peripheral FDG activity and central photopenia may be a marker for aggressiveness and metastatic potential.

ADDITIONAL IMAGES (C–H)

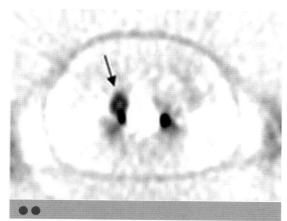

C. Non–attenuation-corrected (NAC) images of a duodenal GIST in NF1. Axial FDG-PET.

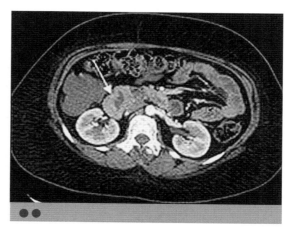

D. Corresponding CT with peripherally enhancing duodenal GIST (*white arrow*).

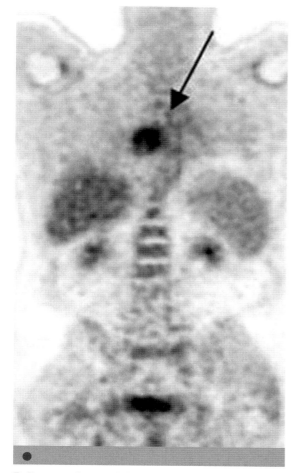

E. Rare esophageal GIST coronal FDG-PET, *arrow*.

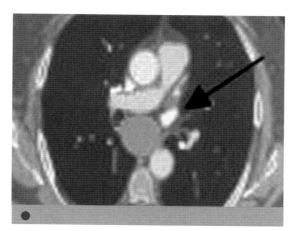

F. Corresponding CT.

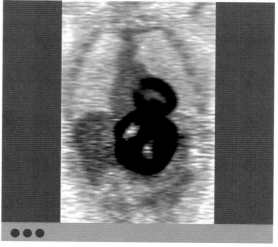

G. Gastric GIST coronal FDG-PET.

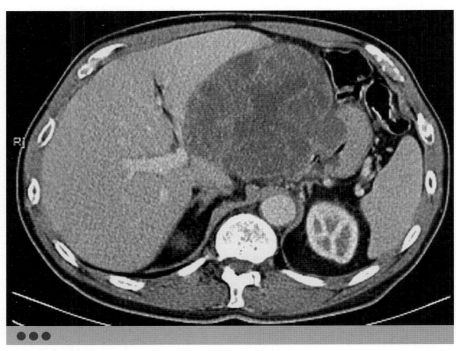

H. Corresponding CT.

DIFFERENTIAL DIAGNOSIS IMAGES (I-K)

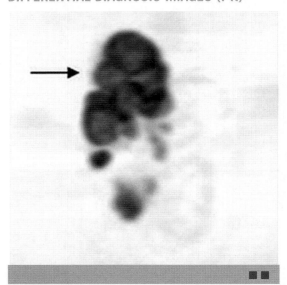

I. Liver involvement in diffuse large B cell (DLBC) lymphoma, coronal FDG-PET.

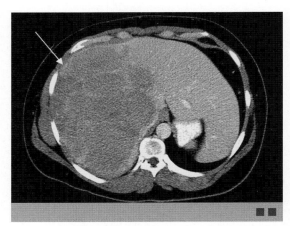

J. Corresponding axial CT with diffuse large B-cell lymphoma.

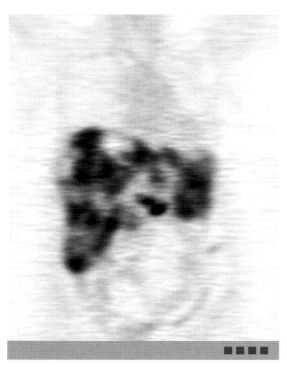

K. Liver metastases from breast cancer, coronal FDG-PET.

Vivek Manchanda, MD

PRESENTATION

Man in midforties with hepatitis B-related cirrhosis, right hepatic mass, and increased AFP (α-fetoprotein level).

FINDINGS

Heterogeneous, moderate to intensely hypermetabolic right hepatic mass.

DIFFERENTIAL DIAGNOSES

- *Metastases*: Usually intense, histology dependent.

- *Cholangiocarcinoma*: Usually intense but well-differentiated/small tumors may be falsely FDG negative.

- *Sarcoma*: Desmoid round cell and angiosarcoma (intense FDG).

- *Focal nodular hyperplasia (FNH)*: Usually isometabolic or decreased, rare increased FDG.

- *Hemangioma*: Usually decreased, photopenic with FDG, rare increased FDG.

- *Hepatic adenoma*: False positive with FDG may occur.

- *Lymphoma*: NHL and typically intense FDG activity.

COMMENTS

Biopsy of the index case showed poorly differentiated HCC.

In general, concentration of glucose-6-phosphatase is high in normal liver which causes rapid clearance of glucose-6-phosphate or FDG-6-phosphate from hepatocytes with consequent mild FDG activity of liver on PET.

HCC develops through malignant transformation of hepatocytes and is commonly seen with cirrhosis.

Measurements of serum α-fetoprotein and liver ultrasound are used for screening. MR imaging and CT are used in inconclusive cases to establish the diagnosis. FDG-PET does not have a role in screening or evaluation of pretransplant cirrhotic patients.

The sensitivity of FDG-PET for HCC is about 50%, with poorly differentiated tumors showing higher FDG avidity. Less differentiated HCC tumors have lower levels of glucose-6-phosphatase and higher levels of hexokinase, likely causing intense FDG uptake of these tumors on PET.

Also, high FDG uptake in HCC has been associated with overexpression of messenger RNA (mRNA) levels for several markers of aggressive tumor behavior, such as vascular endothelial growth factor.

A negative FDG-PET scan in a patient with solitary hepatic lesion does not exclude HCC.

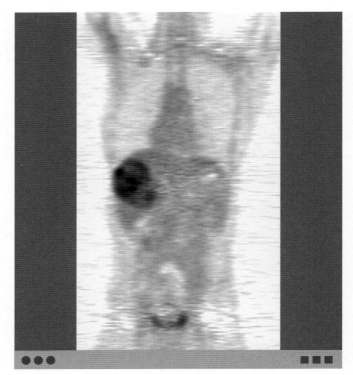

A: HCC: Heterogeneous FDG activity in right liver mass, coronal FDG-PET.

In well-differentiated hepatomas, ^{11}C-acetate has shown higher uptake. If both FDG and ^{11}C-acetate tracers are negative, benign pathology is most likely.

Rare cases of false-positive liver hemangiomas, FNH, and adenomas have been reported with FDG-PET. FDG-PET has been shown to be more sensitive than MRI in detecting extrahepatic metastases from FDG-positive HCC. Washout of contrast from liver lesions in a multiphase CT is highly suggestive of HCC.

PEARLS

- FDG-PET mainly detects poorly differentiated HCCs. In the well-differentiated cancers, ^{11}C acetate has been experimentally shown to be positive.

- Metastases from FDG-avid primary HCCs can influence the staging.

- Rare cases of false-positive hemangiomas, FNH, and adenomas have been reported on PET.

- FDG-PET is more accurate than CT for detecting postchemoembolization tumor viability.

ADDITIONAL IMAGES (B-F)

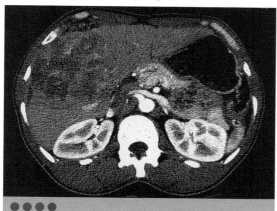

B. HCC: Arterial phase, HCC with heterogeneous enhancement.

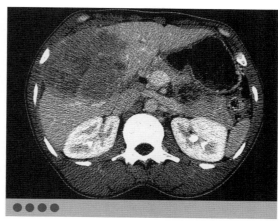

C. HCC: Venous phase.

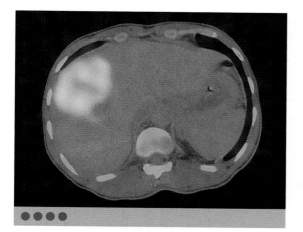

D. Corresponding fused PET/CT.

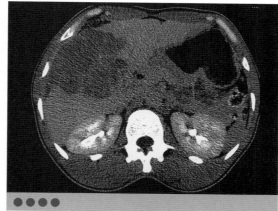

E. HCC: Delayed phase with washout.

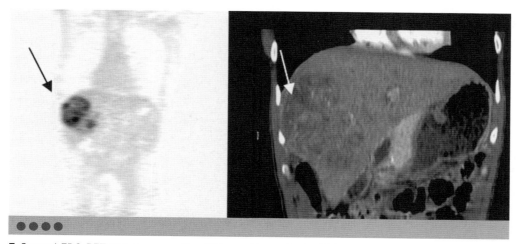

F. Coronal FDG-PET and corresponding CT in another patient with heterogeneous FDG activity in HCC.

DIFFERENTIAL DIAGNOSIS IMAGES (G-L)

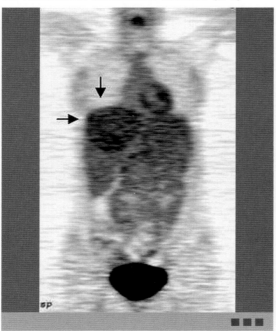

G. Fibrolamellar HCC in a 15-year-old female. Coronal FDG-PET.

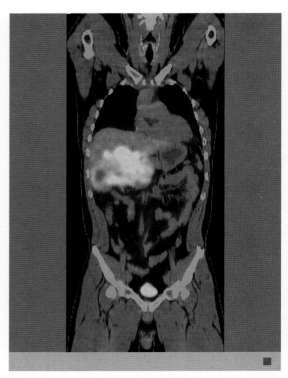

H. Desmoplastic round cell sarcoma of the liver, fused PET/CT.

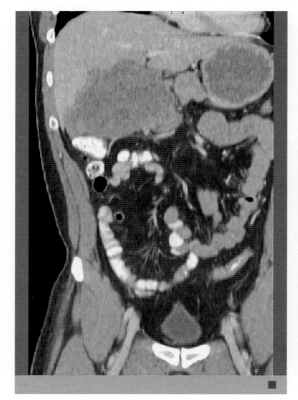

I. Corresponding CT.

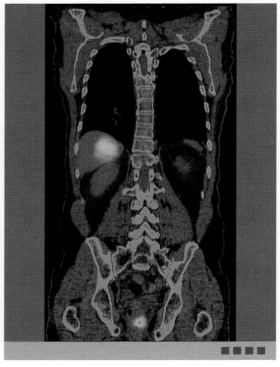

J. Rectal cancer with liver metastases, coronal fused FDG-PET.

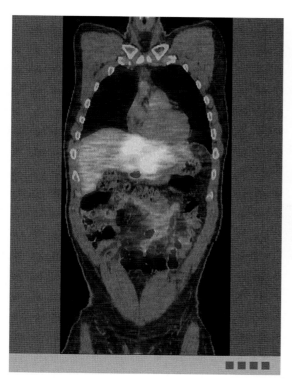

K. Coronal fused PET/CT. Intensely hypermetabolic cholangiocarcinoma.

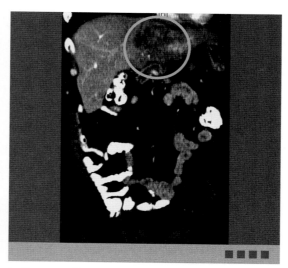

L. Corresponding coronal CT. Note desmoplastic reaction and capsular retraction (*green circle*) associated with the cholangiocarcinoma.

Vivek Manchanda, MD

PRESENTATION

A 21-year-old female with history of sarcoma in childhood and breast cancer (diagnosed with Li-Fraumeni syndrome [LFS]) with pulmonary nodules.

FINDINGS

Hypermetabolic pulmonary nodules and hypermetabolic left pelvic mass.

DIFFERENTIAL DIAGNOSES

- *Colon cancer with lung metastases*
- *Primary colon and lung cancers*
- *Infection*

It is difficult to distinguish between the entities on the basis of FDG-PET. Given spiculated lung nodules (not shown) and absence of FDG avid metastases in liver, it was felt that separate primaries in lung and colon were more likely. The biopsy of lung lesion showed metastasis from colon cancer.

COMMENTS

LFS is a rare autosomal dominant disorder, which greatly increases the risk of cluster of cancers. It results from the mutation in p53 tumor suppression gene (on chromosome 17), which controls the cell growth and causes resistance to the standard chemotherapy.

The types of cancers that occur at an increased risk include breast cancer, sarcomas, ovarian and uterine cancer,

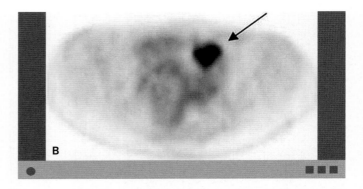

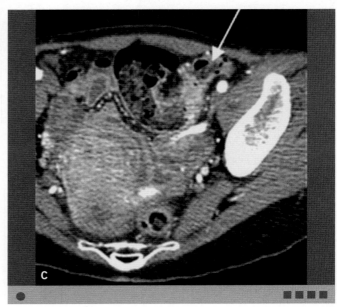

meningioma, gastric cancer, pharyngeal cancer, leukemia, and brain tumors.

Families with this syndrome have an index case younger than 45 years with childhood cancer or sarcoma, brain tumor, or adrenal cortical carcinoma; a first- or second-degree relative with a typical LFS cancer occurring at any age, and another first- or second-degree relative in the lineage younger than 60 years diagnosed with any cancer.

Genetic counseling and genetic testing confirm the gene mutation. Once such person is identified, early and regular screenings for cancer are recommended for him or her. If

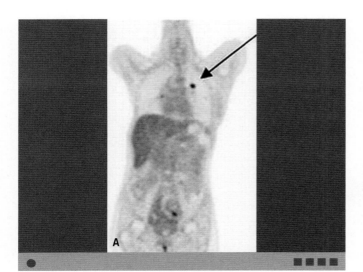

A., B., and **C.** Colon cancer with lung metastases in a 21-year-old female with LFS.

PEARLS

- FDG-PET/CT can detect unknown cancers in patients with LFS.

- There have been reports of PET/CT with use of p53 therapy to follow FDG-avid cancers in LFS patients.

caught early, the cancers can often be successfully treated. Unfortunately, people with LFS are likely to develop another primary malignancy at a future time.

There have been reports of PET/CT with use of p53 therapy to follow FDG-avid cancers in LFS patients.

A major paradox in the treatment of LFS tumors is that conventional cytotoxic therapies (chemotherapy and radiotherapy) that induce DNA damage also contribute to the high incidence of treatment-related secondary malignancies in these patients. In a study of 15 patients with LFS, baseline FDG-PET identified asymptomatic cancers in 3 patients (20%). So far, there are no guidelines for the surveillance of LFS patients with FDG-PET.

ADDITIONAL IMAGES (D-E)

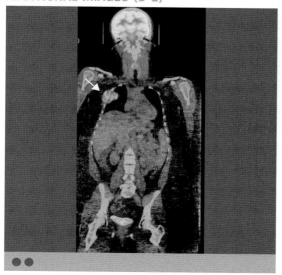

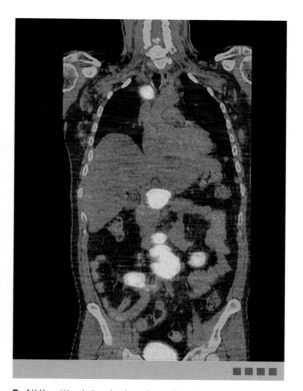

E. Corresponding CT, extraskeletal osteosarcoma.

D. Coronal fused PET/CT. Right chest wall extraskeletal osteosarcoma in another patient with Li-Fraumeni syndrome (*arrow*).

DIFFERENTIAL DIAGNOSIS IMAGES (F-G)

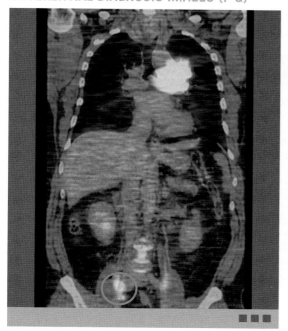

G. NHL with abdominal and mediastinal nodal disease, coronal fused FDG-PET.

F. Left primary lung cancer with right pelvic metastases (*circle*), coronal fused FDG-PET/CT.

Vivek Manchanda, MD

PRESENTATION

Woman in midfifties with breast cancer and liver lesion.

FINDINGS

Focal, moderately increased FDG activity corresponding to the segment 4/8 liver lesion, which on delayed phase contrast CT shows filling in, but enhances more than hepatic veins.

DIFFERENTIAL DIAGNOSES

- *Metastasis*
- *Hemangioma*
- *Cholangiocarcinoma*
- *Abscess*
- *FNH*
- *Adenoma*

On the basis of FDG-PET alone, a liver metastasis cannot be differentiated from primary liver cancer or cholangiocarcinoma.

COMMENTS

The liver provides a fertile soil for metastases because of its rich, dual blood supply and cell growth-promoting factors. After lymph nodes, liver is the second most commonly involved organ by metastatic disease. Most common primary cancers responsible for liver metastases include GI tumors, breast and lung cancers, and ocular melanoma. In pediatric population; neuroblastoma, Wilms tumor, or leukemia are likely to metastasize to the liver.

Most liver metastases are multiple, only a few are solitary. As large metastases outgrow their blood supply, resulting hypoxia and necrosis is seen as photopenia on FDG-PET scan. These patients may be associated with hepatomegaly or ascites.

Some focal lesions may be surgically resectable or treated by means of ablation techniques. FDG-PET plays a vital role in determining residual disease after ablation or resection in previously hypermetabolic metastases.

Causes of calcified liver metastases include ovarian serous lesion, mucinous adenocarcinoma of GI tract, neuroblastoma, and ocular melanoma.

Liver cysts and hemangiomas are typically non-FDG avid. There have been sporadic case reports of some liver

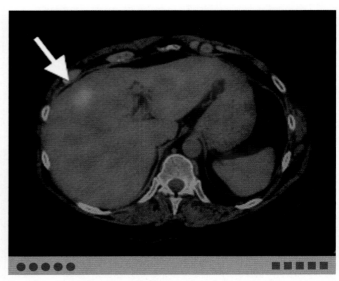

A. Fused PET/CT. Metastatic breast cancer (*arrow*).

hemangiomas being mildly FDG positive. In a patient with a single FDG-avid focus, it may be prudent to exclude rare FDG-positive hemangioma with multiphase contrast-enhanced CT (CECT) scan. On contrary, metastases from mucinous GI cancers may not be very FDG avid and must be accompanied with contrast CT.

Most metastases are hypovascular, but some metastases such as from carcinoids, leiomyosarcomas, neuroendocrine tumors, renal carcinomas, and thyroid carcinomas may be hypervascular. Occasionally, cancers of the pancreas, ovary, or breasts can produce hypervascular metastases.

PEARLS

- Metastases to liver are typically hypermetabolic, but mucinous cancer metastases may be FDG negative.

- Simple hepatic cysts are invariably photopenic on FDG-PET.

- CECT of liver is important in GI malignancies to rule out small metastases.

- Peripheral rim enhancement is a typical feature of malignant lesions and only discontinuous nodular peripheral enhancement that matches bloodpool on all phases is a typical feature of hemangioma.

ADDITIONAL IMAGES (D-F)

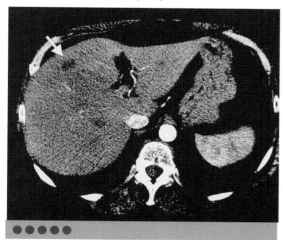

B. Right hepatic lobe metastasis, arterial phase (*arrow*).

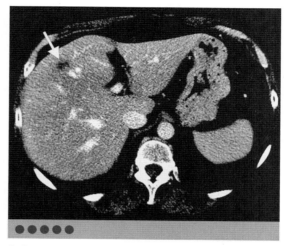

C. Contrast CT venous phase, right lobe lesion (*arrow*).

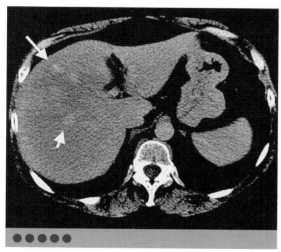

D. Delayed contrast-enhanced CT with enhancement and filling in of right hepatic lobe lesion (*longer arrow*), denser than hepatic vein (*small arrow*).

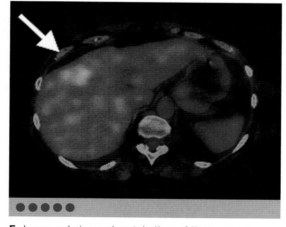

E. Increased size and metabolism of liver metastases after 1 year (*arrow*). Note capsular retraction.

DIFFERENTIAL DIAGNOSIS IMAGES (G-L)

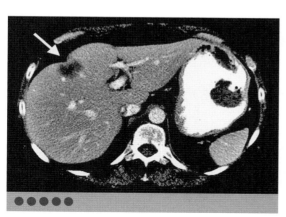

F. Corresponding contrast CT with right liver metastases, increased size post 1 year with capsular retraction.

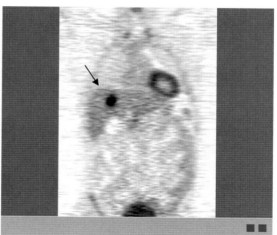

G. Hypermetabolic lymphomatous lesion in T-cell lymphoma. Coronal FDG-PET.

243

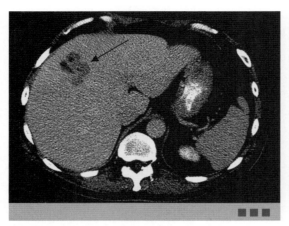

H. Corresponding CT.

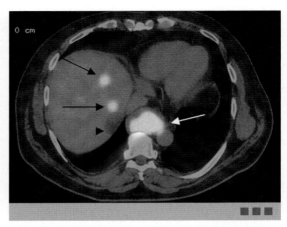

I. Esophageal cancer (*white arrow*) metastases to liver (*black arrows*) and incidental liver cyst (*black arrowhead*).

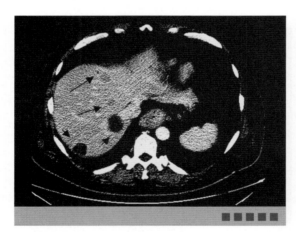

J. Corresponding CT (*black arrows*).

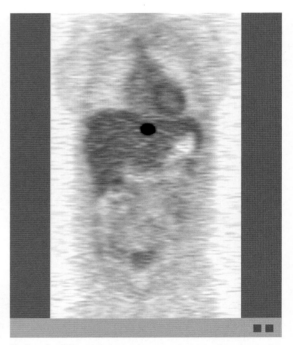

K. Poorly differentiated adenocarcinoma of endocervix metastasis to liver. Coronal FDG-PET.

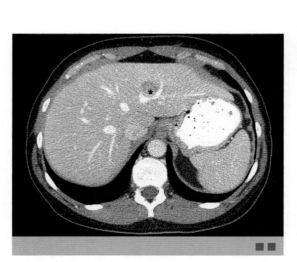

L. Corresponding axial contrast CT scan (*black star*).

Vivek Manchanda, MD

PRESENTATION

FDG-PET in a man in midfifties with lung cancer.

FINDINGS

Diffuse FDG uptake in both small and large bowel.

DIFFERENTIAL DIAGNOSES

- *Inflammatory bowel disease*
- *Infectious colitis*
- *Ischemic colitis*
- *Physiological variant*
- *Drugs*: Metformin
- *Graft versus host disease*

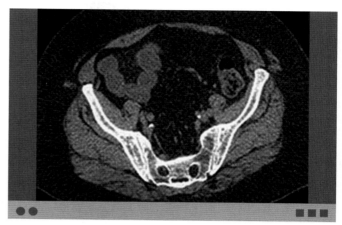

B. Corresponding non-contrast CT.

COMMENTS

Even though some FDG activity may be seen in the bowel physiologically, diffusely increased FDG activity should be correlated with history. In the index case, patient had persistent long-term diarrhea and biopsy showed lymphocytic colitis.

Other causes of diffusely increased FDG activity include drugs. Diabetic patients on metformin have been shown to have diffusely increased FDG uptake. Similar increased activity can be seen in collagenous colitis and autoimmune diseases.

FDG activity is variable and usually more intense in large bowel than in small bowel. Causes of physiological FDG uptake in GI tract include peristalsis, lymphoid tissue, and colonic bacteria.

FDG-PET is not used to diagnose colitis or distinguish various types of colitis. However, different patterns of FDG uptake, clinical and CT findings may help distinguish between etiologies.

Segmental increased FDG uptake with fat stranding may suggest inflammatory bowel disease (IBD), with left colon and rectal predominance in ulcerative colitis (UC) and right colon and small bowel predominance in Crohn disease (CD). Submucosal fat deposition is more commonly seen in UC

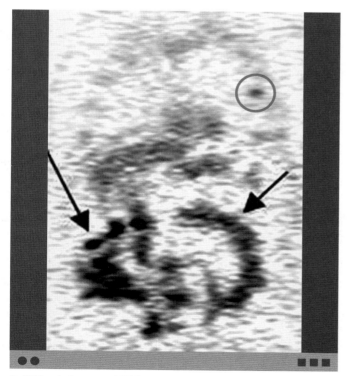

A. Diffusely increased FDG activity in both small and large bowel in lymphocytic colitis (*arrows*), coronal FDG-PET. Note left lung cancer (*circle*).

PEARLS

- **Patients with diffusely increased FDG activity in the colon in a symptomatic patient may be concerning for colitis.**

- **Diffusely increased FDG activity in both small and large bowels may be seen in lymphocytic colitis, collagenous colitis, or metformin therapy.**

- **Evaluation of NAC images may help in distinguishing artifact caused by positive oral contrast on attenuation-corrected images.**

in comparison to CD. Exclusive involvement of right colon and small bowel is most frequently seen with CD and infectious colitis.

Pseudomembranous, ischemic, and acute infectious colitis usually shows ascites, which is rare in IBD. Pancolonic increased FDG activity and bowel wall thickening is more suggestive of infectious than ischemic colitis (which is typically limited to either left or right side). Wall thickening in pseudomembranous and cytomegalovirus (CMV) colitis is typically greater than any IBD, except CD.

DIFFERENTIAL DIAGNOSIS IMAGES (C-F)

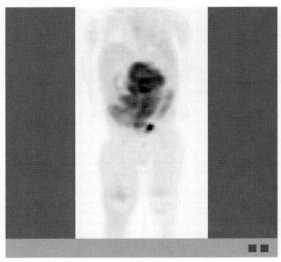

C. Rhabdomyosarcoma in abdomen, 2-year-old boy, mimicking bowel FDG uptake.

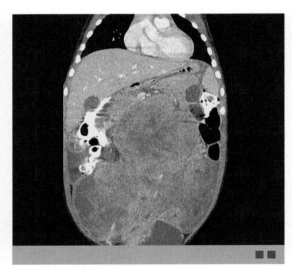

D. Corresponding CT.

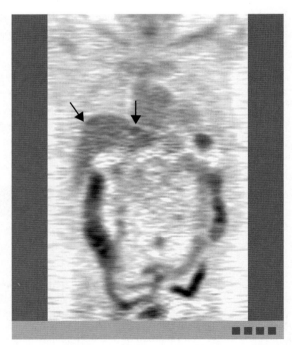

E. Diffuse FDG activity in the colon, *Clostridium difficile* colitis, coronal FDG-PET. Also seen are liver metastases (*arrows*).

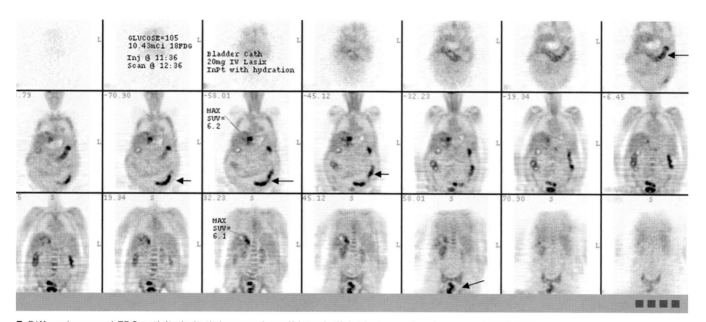

F. Diffuse increased FDG activity in both large and small bowel, diabetic on metformin, coronal FDG-PET.

Case 5–15 Pancreatic Cancer and FDG-PET

Vivek Manchanda, MD

PRESENTATION

Pancreatic mass in fifth decade of life with jaundice.

FINDINGS

Intense, focal increased FDG activity corresponding to the pancreatic mass.

DIFFERENTIAL DIAGNOSES

- *Neoplastic*: Adenocarcinoma, islet cell tumor, lymphoma
- *Metastases*: RCC, lung, breast, sarcomas, colon, melanoma
- *Focal pancreatitis*
- *Pancreatic abscess*
- *Infected pseudocyst*

Pancreatitis is usually associated with clinical signs and symptoms and diffusely increased FDG activity. Pancreatic cancer and metastasis typically have a focal hypermetabolic appearance. In the index case, biopsy showed pancreatic adenocarcinoma.

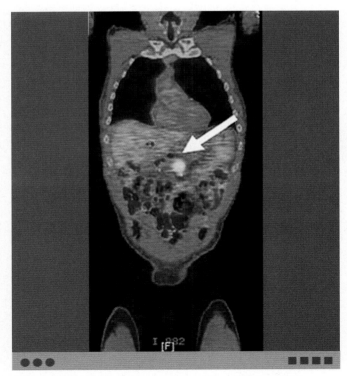

A. Pancreatic adenocarcinoma. Coronal fused FDG-PET/CT (*white arrow*).

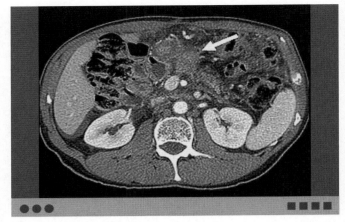

B. Corresponding CT (white arrow).

COMMENTS

FDG-PET has been shown by several investigators to provide an accurate imaging tool for evaluating patients with known or suspected pancreatic carcinoma.

Pancreatic adenocarcinoma has a poor prognosis and many patients present late in the course of disease with weight loss, anorexia, or painless jaundice. Serum tumor marker CA 19-9 is insensitive and nonspecific for screening.

Per studies, FDG-PET can effectively differentiate pancreatic adenocarcinoma from benign lesions with high accuracy. Sensitivity for periampullary carcinoma is less than that for other sites. SUV values cannot be used to distinguish cancer from pancreatitis. Also, dual time imaging is not absolutely specific in distinguishing benign from malignant pancreatic lesions.

PEARLS

- PET/CT has high sensitivity and specificity in detection of primary pancreatic cancer and unsuspected metastases.

- In patients with suspected recurrent pancreatic cancer and rising CA 19-9, PET/CT can help in disease localization.

- Pancreatic neuroendocrine tumors that show increased FDG activity may have worse prognosis.

- Early-stage tumors and elevated glucose can result in false-negative reports.

- FDG-PET has high accuracy in identifying malignant pancreatic cystic lesions.

If CT does not show a discrete mass, an FDG-avid lesion is highly predictive of malignancy. PET/CT is much better in evaluating treatment response than CT alone. It is suggested that PET scan can distinguish between responders and nonresponders and thus predict prognosis.

Majority of chronic pancreatitis cases are not FDG avid. In patients with chronic pancreatitis and positive PET, possibility of malignancy should be investigated.

In patients with suspected primary pancreatic carcinoma, PET is complementary to abdominal CT for detection of unsuspected distant metastases. In patients with suspected recurrent pancreatic cancer and rising CA 19-9, PET/CT can help in disease localization.

Metastases to pancreas, although uncommon, can also be detected by FDG-PET with great accuracy. Per some studies, FDG-PET has been used successfully to monitor patients after intraoperative radiation therapy in unresectable pancreatic cancer.

ADDITIONAL IMAGES (C-E)

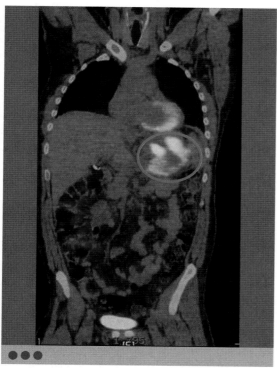

C. Direct extension of squamous cell pancreatic tail cancer into stomach, fused PET/CT.

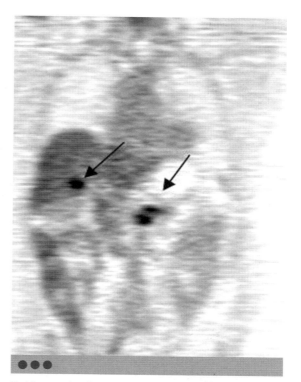

D. Liver and celiac nodal metastases from pancreatic cancer. Coronal FDG-PET.

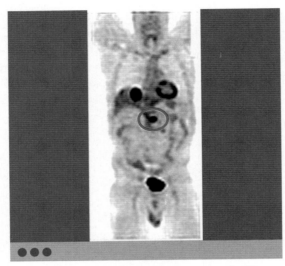

E. Coronal FDG-PET, pancreatic cancer (*oval*) with liver metastasis.

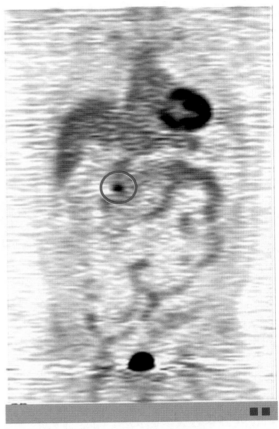

F. Pancreatic adenoma. Coronal FDG-PET.

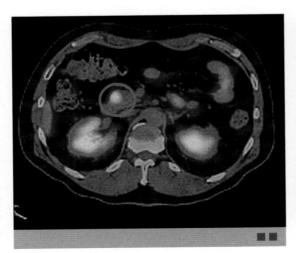

G. Axial fused PET/CT in pancreatic adenoma.

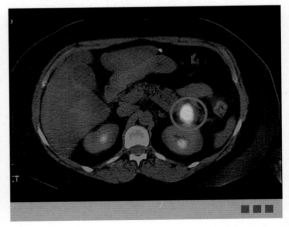

H. Focal pancreatic metastasis from leiomyosarcoma. Axial fused PET/CT.

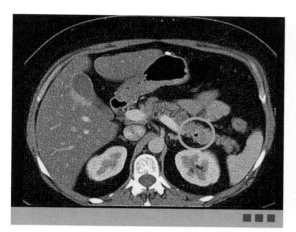

I. Corresponding axial contrast-enhanced CT (*green circle*).

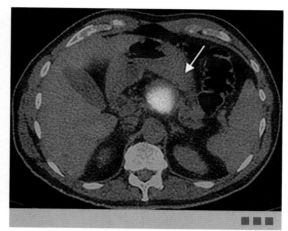

J. Pancreatic neuroendocrine tumor in 71-year-old male, fused PET/CT.

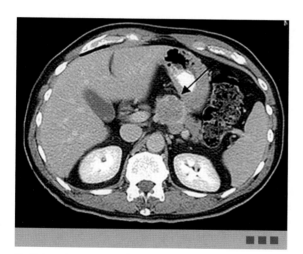

K. Delayed corresponding contrast CT.

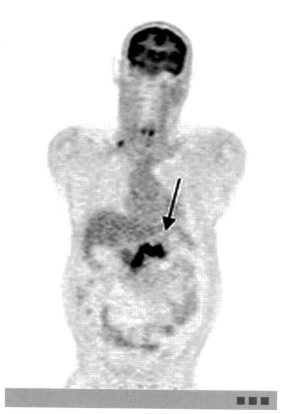

L. Diffusely hypermetabolic pancreatic metastases from Merkel cell cancer. Coronal FDG-PET. Note right supraclavicular FDG uptake.

Vivek Manchanda, MD

PRESENTATION

Man in his fifth decade of life with gastric cancer.

FINDINGS

Focal FDG activity on peritoneal surface of liver and spleen and hypermetabolic gastric mass.

DIFFERENTIAL DIAGNOSES

- *Infection*: TB
- *Peritoneal mesothelioma*
- *Papillary serous carcinoma*
- *Desmoplastic round cell tumor*
- *Malignant mesenchymal tumors*: GIST, leiomyosarcoma
- *Lymphoproliferative disorders*: Leukemia, peritoneal lymphomatosis, plasmacytoma

COMMENTS

Tumor cells from cancers such as stomach, colon, ovary, pancreas, and endometrium, and cholangiocarcinomas may be shed into the peritoneal cavity, follow the ascitic pathways, and get deposited in areas such as pouch of Douglas, right subphrenic space, posterior right subhepatic space or right paracolic gutter, and sigmoid colon and its mesentery.

Cancers such as ovarian, colon, stomach, and pancreatic may spread directly through the peritoneum to involve other organs. Hematogenous dissemination may occur in primary breast and lung cancers and melanomas.

On CT, ascites is one of the commonest findings. Other CT findings include a nodular, plaque-like, or infiltrative soft tissue lesion in the peritoneal fat or on the surface, parietal peritoneal thickening or enhancement, and small bowel wall thickening/distortion.

There are three patterns of FDG uptake in the peritoneum: (1) diffuse FDG activity which spreads uniformly throughout the abdomen and pelvis obscuring visceral outlines; (2) discrete foci of uptake randomly and anteriorly within the abdomen or dependently within the pelvis and unrelated to solid viscera or nodal stations; or (3) hypermetabolic foci which cause a concave or scalloped defect on the adjacent hepatic and splenic parenchyma.

The FDG activity may depend on the metabolic activity of the primary tumor and the size of the soft tissue deposit.

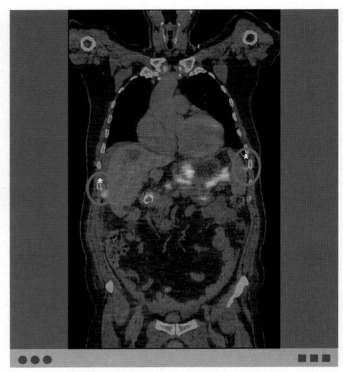

A. Peritoneal metastases (*white stars and circles*) on liver and splenic surface from gastric cancer.

Fat suppressed and gadolinium-enhanced delayed (5-10 minutes) images are most helpful for detecting small peritoneal carcinomatosis on MR scans.

Diagnostic laparoscopy and laparoscopic ultrasonography are better, but invasive. In our limited experience, a negative PET scan does not rule out peritoneal metastases but a positive PET scan with or without corresponding CT abnormality is highly accurate.

PEARLS

- Patterns of FDG uptake in peritoneal metastases include diffuse FDG activity obscuring visceral outlines or discrete hypermetabolic foci with or without CT findings.

- Cancers such as stomach, colon, ovarian, pancreatic, and endometrial, and cholangiocarcinomas may shed tumor cells in the peritoneum.

- A negative PET scan cannot rule out peritoneal metastases as the tumor cells may be dispersed in ascitic fluid.

ADDITIONAL IMAGES (B-G)

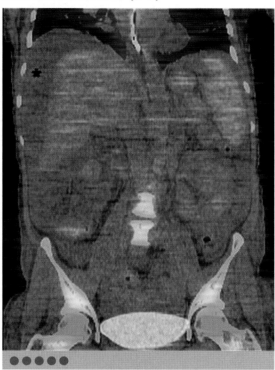

B. Ascites in 47-year-old male with cirrhosis. Coronal FDG-PET/CT (*black star*).

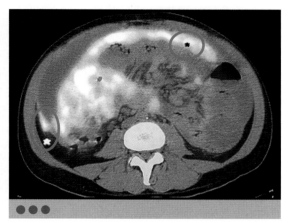

C. Peritoneal (*white star*) and omental hypermetabolic lesions (*black star*), acute myeloid leukemia (AML).

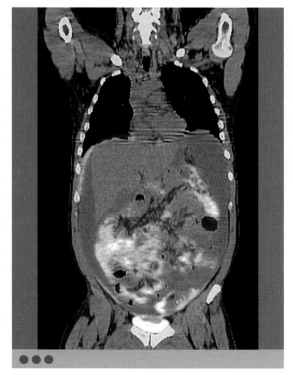

D. Coronal peritoneal and omental metastases, AML.

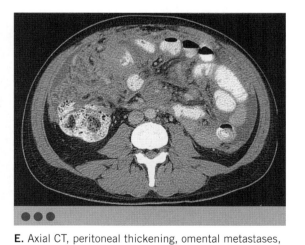

E. Axial CT, peritoneal thickening, omental metastases, AML.

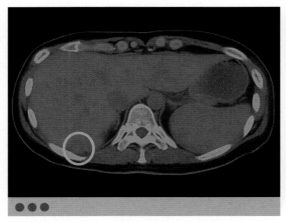

F. FDG-PET, peritoneal metastases on liver surface, leiomyosarcoma.

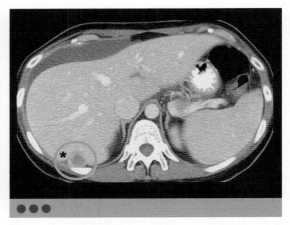

G. Corresponding CT (*green circle*). Note ascites.

DIFFERENTIAL DIAGNOSIS IMAGE

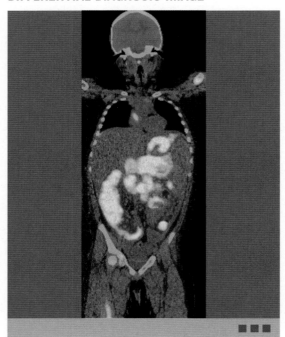

H. Coronal fused FDG-PET/CT. Diffuse peritoneal bowel, mediastinal, and marrow disease in Burkitt lymphoma in 12 year-old-male.

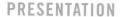
Vivek Manchanda, MD

PRESENTATION

Man in his fifth decade of life with left pelvic pain.

FINDINGS

Moderately increased FDG activity corresponding to mass off the tip of coccyx, abutting the posterior aspect of rectum.

DIFFERENTIAL DIAGNOSES

- *Chordoma*
- *Metastasis*
- *Giant cell tumor*
- *Ependymoma and schwannoma*

Chordomas are the most common primary sacral neoplasm in adults. Given no evidence of primary tumors on FDG-PET, metastasis is less likely. Giant cell tumors usually involve bones. Ependymomas and schwannomas cannot be excluded on FDG-PET.

COMMENTS

Chordoma is the commonest primary sacral neoplasm in adults (second-fourth decade), which arises from notochord remnants. It usually arises in the midline and involves fourth and fifth sacral vertebrae. The tumor can cause destruction of adjacent sacrum and present as a presacral mass. Chordomas have moderately high-signal intensity on both T2-weighted and contrast-enhanced T1-weighted MR sequences and are hypermetabolic on FDG-PET scans.

Giant cell tumor is the second most common sacral (usually eccentric) tumor, which may extend across the sacroiliac joint. Mostly lytic and destructive, they do not contain calcifications or septa. Rarely, they may present as soft tissue masses in the sacral canal. Aneurysmal bone cysts typically involve posterior elements of the sacrum in the first two decades of life, with multiple blood-filled spaces separated by septa. Osteogenic sarcomas may occur in the pelvis after radiation therapy. Extraosseous Ewing sarcoma can present as sacral mass in children.

Ependymomas and schwannomas are the neural tumors that originate in the sacral canal. Ependymomas (malignant) arise from ependymal cells in filum terminale. Schwannomas are usually benign.

Metastases to sacrum is from hematogenous or subarachnoid space, and can be seen in RCC, melanoma, thyroid cancer, or multiple myeloma. Patients with pelvic malignancies (such as rectal cancer) can develop presacral masses

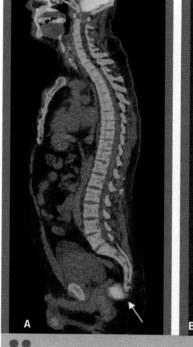
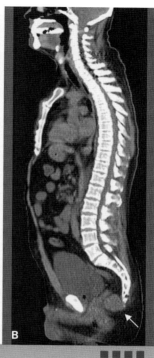

A. and **B.** Chordoma. Sagittal fused PET/CT and sagittal CT (*white arrows*).

after therapy and FDG-PET/CT can help distinguish between recurrent disease or fibrosis, which is difficult to distinguish on the basis of CT or MR.

Sacrococcygeal teratomas, the commonest presacral masses in children, are rare in adults. Rhabdomyosarcomas and undifferentiated sarcomas are also childhood tumors that may involve presacral region.

PEARLS

- **Chordomas are the commonest primary sacral neoplasms in adults, and FDG avid.**

- **FDG-PET can help differentiate between fibrosis and recurrent disease in pelvic malignancy after therapy.**

- **Sacrococcygeal teratomas are the commonest presacral masses in children, which are usually FDG negative. A malignant transformation of such teratoma is usually FDG avid.**

DIFFERENTIAL DIAGNOSIS IMAGE (C-D)

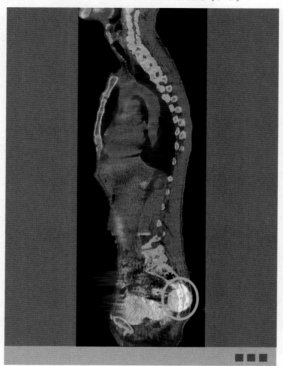

C. Thyroid cancer metsatasis, sagittal fused FDG-PET/CT (*green circle*). Note anterior bladder.

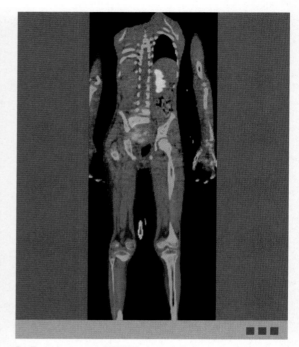

D. Fused coronal PET/CT. Sacral Ewing sarcoma in 13-year-old.

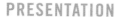

Vivek Manchanda, MD

PRESENTATION

Rectal mass in 39-year-old male.

FINDINGS

Hypermetabolic rectal mass seen on PET/CT.

DIFFERENTIAL DIAGNOSES

• *Rectal cancer*

• *Physiological rectal activity*

• *Infection/inflammatory bowel disease*

Physiological FDG activity can be seen in rectum; however, when associated with a mass on CT, rectal cancer must be ruled out. UC can involve only rectum and be hypermetabolic and can be associated with thickened rectal wall.

COMMENTS

Most rectal cancers are adenocarcinomas (up to 98%). Carcinoid, lymphoma, sarcoma, and squamous cell carcinoma of the rectum are rare.

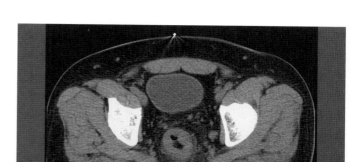

B. Corresponding CT.

The pattern of spread of rectal cancer involves local spread and nodal spread (usually from the level of tumor upward within mesorectum). Downward spread from lymphatic blockage may occur. In lower rectal tumors, inguinal nodes may be involved.

Rectal cancer has a higher risk of local recurrence as its bony pelvic location limits wide resection margins. Small cancers are treated surgically and advanced locoregional disease is treated with neoadjuvant chemotherapy and/or radiation followed by surgery.

Venous invasion, nodal status, and local tumor extension affect prognosis. Rectal cancers can show pulmonary metastases before liver metastases because of dual vascular supply of the rectum.

Although local staging of rectal cancer with transrectal ultrasound or MR has high accuracy in T staging, pretreatment PET/CT can change proposed treatment plan especially in low rectal cancer.

PET/CT has good sensitivity and specificity in detection of recurrent or metastatic colorectal cancer, including retroperitoneal nodes and liver metastases. It offers good sensitivity in detecting recurrence with rising carcinoembryonic antigen (CEA) in the absence of a known source.

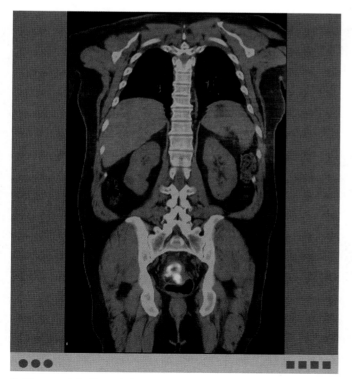

A. Hypermetabolic rectal cancer.

PEARLS

• **FDG-PET/CT is useful in pretreatment, detection of recurrent or metastatic colorectal cancer, and assessment of residual tumor in preoperative scans after neoadjuvant chemoradiation therapy.**

• **True rectal cancers may metastasize to lungs before liver. Lower rectal cancers can spread to inguinal nodes.**

Serial FDG-PET/CT scans are effective in assessment of tumor downstaging, complete metabolic response of those with residual tumor after preoperative neoadjuvant chemoradiation. Post-therapy inflammation may result in decreased specificity for pelvic recurrence. Studies have suggested that the reliability of FDG-PET in distinguishing pelvic recurrence of rectal cancer and postradiation inflammation improves with time. On FDG-PET, the recurrent disease is mainly seen as a focal mass, whereas inflammation shows more diffuse FDG activity.

ADDITIONAL IMAGES (C–H)

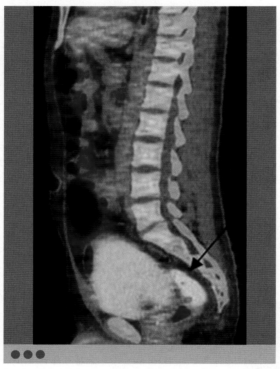

C. Fused PET/CT sagittal image with moderately differentiated rectal adenocarcinoma (*arrow*).

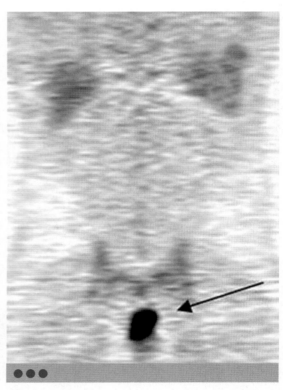

D. Coronal image.

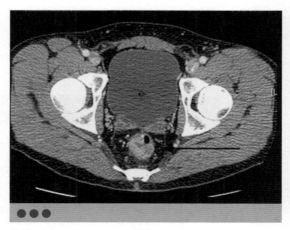

E. Rectal mass, contrast CT.

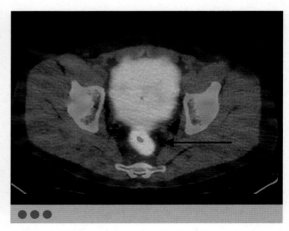

F. Fused PET/CT axial.

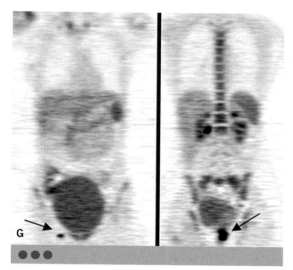

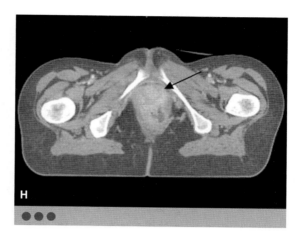

G. and **H.** Right inguinal metastasis and rectal cancer in a different patient. Contrast CT with rectal mass.

DIFFERENTIAL DIAGNOSIS IMAGE (I-J)

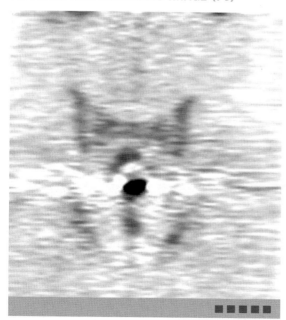

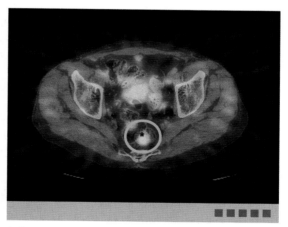

J. Corresponding fused PET/CT. Physiological FDG activity in rectum.

I. Physiological rectal activity, no corresponding mass on CT.

Vivek Manchanda, MD

PRESENTATION

Woman in her early fourth decade of life with right leg numbness and back pain.

FINDINGS

Heterogeneously hypermetabolic mass in right retroperitoneum with right obstructive hydronephrosis.

DIFFERENTIAL DIAGNOSES

- *Sarcoma*

- *Malignant fibrous histiocytoma (MFH)*

- *Neurogenic tumors*: Malignant peripheral nerve sheath tumor (MPNST), paragangliomas, schwannomas, ganglioneuromas

- *Germ cell tumors*

- *RCC*

- *Lymphoma*

Given intense FDG activity, ganglioneuroma is unlikely.

COMMENTS

Retroperitoneal sarcomas are rare tumors. Primary retroperitoneal tumors have traditionally been divided into (1) those arising from mesenchyme (soft tissue sarcomas) and (2) those arising from germ cells (extragonadal germ cell tumors).

Primary retroperitoneal soft tissue sarcomas are the most common primary malignant retroperitoneal tumor (up to 90%). They are classified histologically according to the adult tissue they most resemble: skeletal muscle, fibrous tissue, fat, peripheral nerves, blood vessels.

Soft tissue sarcomas can grow large in the retroperitoneum, without producing symptoms. Nonspecific symptoms, such as abdominal pain and fullness may be associated.

Staging of retroperitoneal soft tissue sarcomas is more affected by histology than anatomical extent.

Most retroperitoneal sarcomas have similar clinical behavior and radiological appearance. On PET, sarcomas present as large heterogeneous masses with FDG uptake corresponding to grades of differentiation (well-differentiated sarcomas have lower FDG uptake). In comparison, at the other end of the spectrum are dedifferentiated tumors which are extremely FDG avid. More dedifferentiated areas can be recognized on PET and biopsied, guiding treatments and follow-ups. Areas of photopenia are due to necrosis within the tumor. Also, on follow-up examinations, increased size due to necrosis/hemorrhage can be differentiated from tumor by PET.

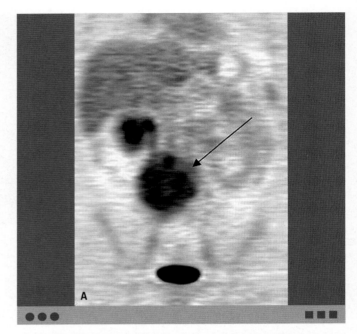

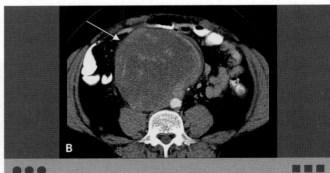

A. and **B.** Right retroperitoneal spindle cell sarcoma with right hydronephrosis and corresponding CT.

PEARLS

- Liposarcomas are the most common histological retroperitoneal tumors, mostly dedifferentiated and pleomorphic, which are FDG avid. Spindle cell sarcomas and MPNSTs are also FDG avid.

- Rhabdomyosarcomas are most common in children.

- FDG-PET can be used to predict grade, guide biopsy for most metabolically active sites, evaluate for metastases, and follow up for response or recurrence.

- Ganglioneuromas and ganglioneuroblastomas may have mild FDG activity occurring in adolescents and younger children respectively.

MPNSTs (between ages 20 and 50) have equal prevalence in men and women. Nerve involvement with pain and neurologic symptoms may be seen. They can be radiation induced (like MFH). They are high grade and FDG avid, and local recurrence is seen in about 40%. Metastases are seen in 65%, most common sites being the lungs, bone, pleura, and lymph nodes.

DIFFERENTIAL DIAGNOSIS IMAGES (C-L)

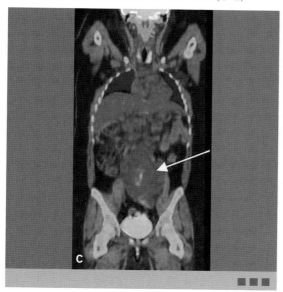

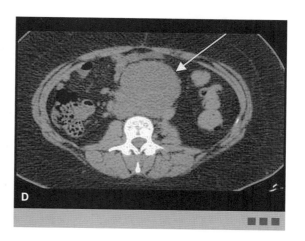

C. and **D.** Mildly FDG-avid ganglioneuroma (*white arrow*) coronal fused-FDG-PET/CT and axial noncontrast CT (*white arrow*).

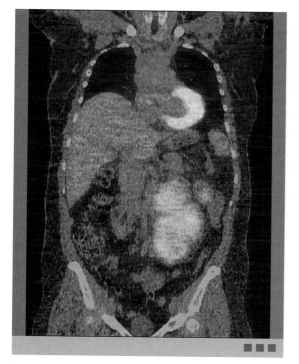

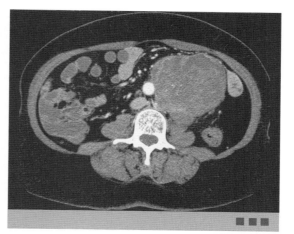

F. Corresponding contrast CT.

E. Left retroperitoneal schwannoma (max. SUV of 6.6) in 58-year-old female. Coronal fused PET/CT.

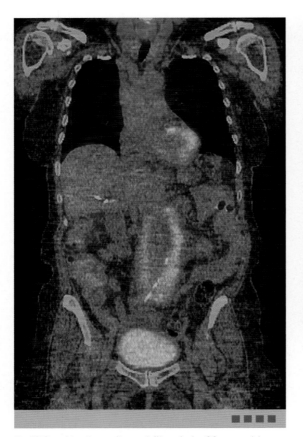

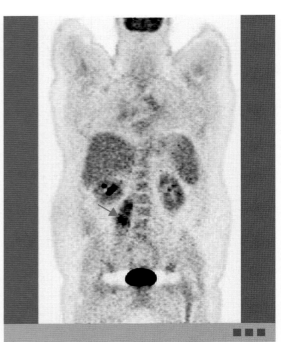

H. Right psoas sarcoma, coronal FDG PET (*red arrow*).

G. FDG-avid retroperitoneal fibrosis in 63-year-old female.

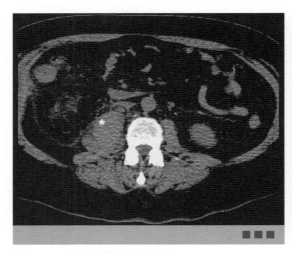

I. Corresponding CT (*white star*).

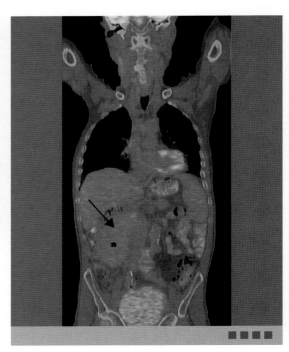

J. Isometabolic right RCC (*black star and arrow*), coronal fused PET/CT.

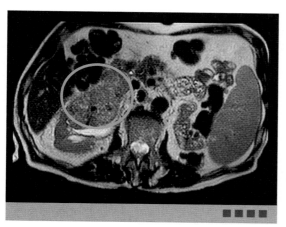

K. Corresponding T2-W MR, RCC with hydronephrosis (*green circle*).

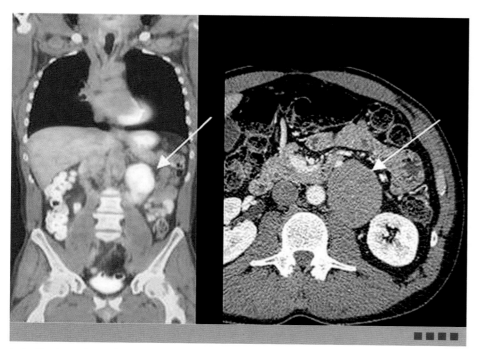

L. Left retroperitoneal seminoma metastasis (fused coronal PET/CT) and axial contrast-enhanced CT (*white arrows*).

Vivek Manchanda, MD

PRESENTATION

Retroperitoneal soft tissue mass. Scar versus colon cancer recurrence.

FINDINGS

Intense focal FDG activity corresponding to retroperitoneal mass.

DIFFERENTIAL DIAGNOSES

• *Scar*

• *Recurrent cancer*

The scar would be typically non-FDG avid or show mild diffuse FDG activity and the recurrent cancer would be focally metabolically active, which was proven in the index case.

COMMENTS

Pelvic recurrence and liver metastases are the commonest sites of relapse after colorectal cancer resection. Patients with anterior resection have higher asymptomatic recurrence.

Patients after undergoing abdominoperineal resection may develop a fibrotic mass in the presacral operative bed, which is a diagnostic challenge. Inflammatory reaction from radiation therapy may result in thickening of perirectal fascia.

Appropriate hydration, prescan voiding, bladder catheterization, and retrograde filling of bladder with saline help in proper localization. The reported range of local recurrence after resection of rectal cancer ranges from 4% to 50%, and surgical resection is the main curative therapy. Additional resection is based on patient's general condition, local extent of tumor, and distant metastases. In patients with locally advanced disease, extended resection (eg, pelvic exenteration and sacral resection) may be indicated.

FDG-PET/CT has an additional diagnostic value in the detection of pelvic tumor recurrence over CT and transrectal ultrasound. It can differentiate a benign fibrous scar from cancer recurrence with high sensitivity and specificity.

There may be heterogeneous uptake of FDG in the presacral mass, with the FDG-avid portion suggesting tumor and the non–FDG-avid area suggesting scar. PET/CT findings can change the treatment approach in patients with such findings.

Alterations in the normal pelvic anatomy can result in false-positive FDG activity in the displaced organs posteriorly. Usually, focal FDG uptake is worrisome for disease and diffuse or segmental FDG uptake is less likely associated with tumor recurrence. It can distinguish postoperative and

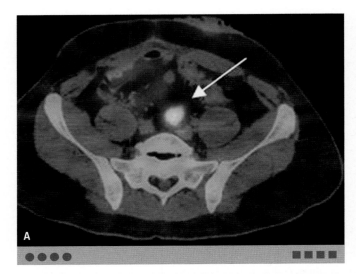

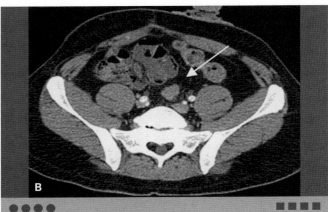

A. and **B.** Intense focally increased FDG activity in the retroperitoneal mass, recurrent colorectal cancer, and corresponding CT.

postradiation scarring from residual or recurrent tumor. FDG-PET has a higher sensitivity than contrast-enhanced CT for the same. In postoperative period, however, FDG activity may be seen at the surgical site for several months due to postsurgical inflammation or granulation tissue.

According to some studies, PET and MR complement each other in the detection of scar versus recurrent colon cancer.

PEARLS

• **FDG-PET/CT can distinguish between scar and recurrent colorectal cancer, as the scars show none to mild diffusely increased FDG activity, whereas tumor recurrence is typically focal and intensely FDG avid.**

ADDITIONAL IMAGE

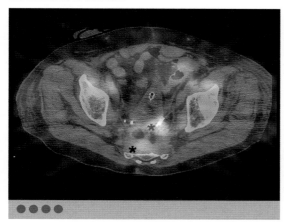

●●●●

C. Intense focal hypermetabolic recurrent cancer (*purple star*) and diffuse mildly hypermetabolic scar tissue (*black star*).

DIFFERENTIAL DIAGNOSIS IMAGE

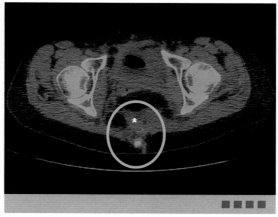

■ ■ ■ ■

D. Presacral scar tissue (*green circle and white star*), fused PET/CT. Note retrogradely filled bladder anterior to scar.

Case 5–21 Splenic Metastases and FDG-PET

Vivek Manchanda, MD

PRESENTATION

Patient with non-Hodgkin lymphoma (NHL).

FINDINGS

Intensely hypermetabolic foci in the spleen and retroperitoneum.

DIFFERENTIAL DIAGNOSES

- *Leukemia/lymphoma*
- *Metastases*
- *Infection*: TB, *Brucella*, fungal
- *Sarcoidosis*
- *Extramedullary hematopoiesis*

Given the level of FDG activity; splenic cysts and splenic infarcts can be safely excluded.

COMMENTS

Splenomegaly in NHL is not a criterion for disease involvement. Splenic involvement in NHL can be focal, diffuse, or multifocal and easily detected on FDG-PET.

Melanoma, adenocarcinomas (breast, lung, colorectal, gastric), and germ cell tumors are common tumors that metastasize to spleen.

Isolated splenic metastasis, in the absence of metastases elsewhere, is rare and is most commonly seen in ovarian cancers followed by colon and lung cancers.

Disease on the splenic surface (FDG avid with indentation of splenic surface) is more common than in the parenchyma. It is most commonly associated with ovarian cancer. Spontaneous splenic rupture from the metastatic disease burden is rare. Parenchymal lesions are often circular. Cystic metastases may be seen with ovarian, breast, and endometrial cancers, and melanoma. Calcification may be seen with mucinous adenocarcinomas and treated infections.

Splenic angiosarcoma, fibrosarcoma, leiomyosarcoma, malignant teratoma, and malignant fibrous histiocytoma are very rare and all may be hypermetabolic on FDG-PET.

Hemangioma, the commonest primary benign splenic neoplasm, may rarely be FDG avid.

Lymphangiomas (minimally FDG avid) are usually subcapsular. Splenic cysts are typically nonenhancing, non-FDG avid and well defined. Splenic hamartomas are isointense on T1 and hyperintense on T2-WI. On CT and MR, they show

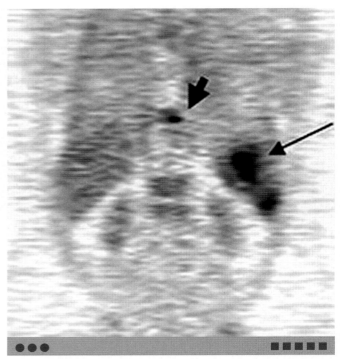

A. Coronal FDG-PET. Intensely hypermetabolic foci from NHL in spleen (*thin arrow*) and retroperitoneum (*thick arrow*).

slow enhancement and filling after contrast administration.

Fungal abscesses in neutropenic patients are small and multifocal and can be intensely FDG avid. Splenic infarcts appear sharply demarcated, low-density wedge-shaped areas and photopenic on FDG-PET.

Other focal causes of FDG uptake in the spleen include sarcoidosis, primary malignant lymphoma of spleen, and extramedullary hematopoiesis.

PEARLS

- FDG uptake in the spleen can be parenchymal (focal, multifocal, or diffuse) or on the splenic surface, which may or may not cause indentation.

- In a series, FDG-negative splenic lesions remained stable on clinical and imaging follow-up.

- Hypermetabolic splenic foci can be seen in infection, sarcoidosis, metastases, and lymphoma.

- Infection typically has smaller, more uniform splenic nodules.

266

ADDITIONAL IMAGE (B-E)

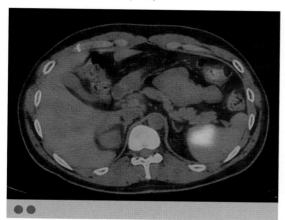

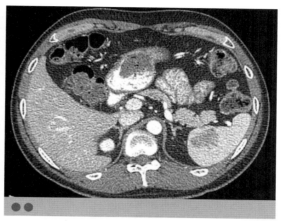

B. Hypermetabolic nasopharyngeal cancer metastasis to spleen in 34-year-old male.

C. Corresponding CT.

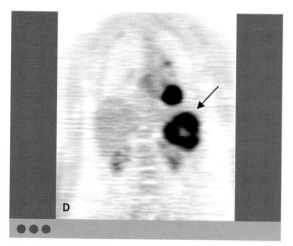

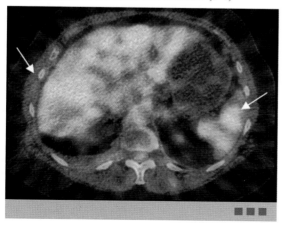

D. and **E.** FDG, melanoma metastasis to spleen with contrast CT.

DIFFERENTIAL DIAGNOSIS IMAGE (F-I)

F. Fused PET/CT with splenic and multiple liver metastases in small-cell lung cancer.

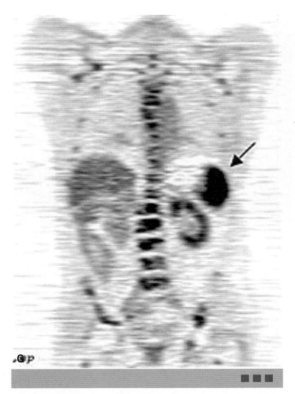

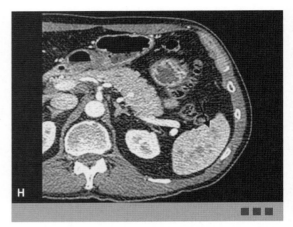

G. and **H.** FDG-PET, confluent sarcoidosis lesions in spleen with vertebral lesions and corresponding CT.

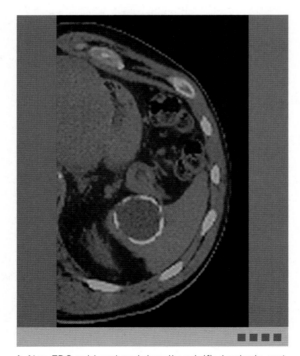

I. Non-FDG avid and peripherally calcified splenic cyst.

Bhasker R. Koppula, MD

PRESENTATION

Neonates presenting with increasing jaundice and worsening liver function tests since birth (neonatal jaundice).

DIFFERENTIAL DIAGNOSIS

- *Neonatal hepatitis*: Due to infections, including TORCH, and due to metabolic conditions like α-antitrypsin deficiency, galactosemia, and hypothyroidism. Prolonged clearance of tracer by hepatic cells from blood pool and the bowel activity can be faint and delayed up to 24 hours.

- *Choledochal cyst*: On HIDA scan, the choledochal cysts are seen as photopenic areas which fill within 60 minutes into the study and there is stasis of tracer within the cyst. There will be prominent hepatic biliary ductal activity with lack of tracer excretion into the bowel.

- *Alagille syndrome*: Abnormal facies, butterfly vertebrae, pulmonary stenosis, and complex congenital heart disease.

- *Hemolysis syndromes*.

COMMENTS

Biliary atresia is characterized by progressive damage of extra- and intrahepatic biliary ductal system secondary to inflammation, leading to fibrosis, biliary cirrhosis, and eventual liver failure. Patients with biliary atresia can be of two distinct groups: The fetal-embryonic (perinatal) form accounts

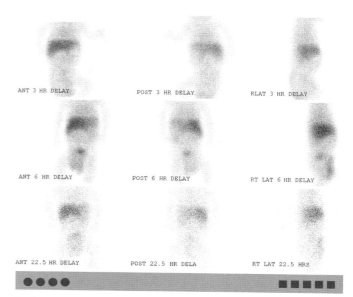

B. Anterior and posterior images obtained at 3, 6, and 24 hours show persistence of tracer activity with no evidence of excretion into the biliary tree. No definite evidence of bowel tracer activity is identified. This appearance of absent tracer activity in the biliary tree and in the bowel, at the end of 24 hours, is highly suspicious for the diagnosis of biliary atresia. (*Image courtesy of Bhasker R. Koppula, MD.*)

for 10% to 35% of cases, and is associated with other congenital defects/abnormalities, including situs inversus, polysplenia/asplenia, malrotation, intestinal atresia, and cardiac anomalies, among others. Patients typically present within the first 2 weeks of birth. The postnatal form of biliary atresia accounts for 65% to 90% cases and typically presents during

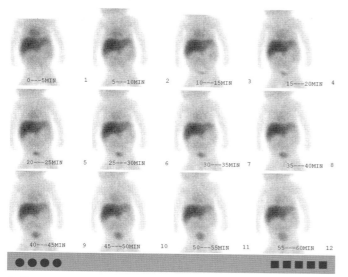

A. Early sequential images from HIDA scan show prompt uptake of the tracer from blood pool. However, there is no excretion of the tracer into the biliary tree at the end of 60 minutes. No evidence of tracer activity in the bowel is identified during this time. There is renal excretion of the tracer, an alternative excretory pathway. (*Image courtesy of Bhasker R. Koppula, MD.*)

PEARLS

- Pretreatment with hepatic enzyme inducing drug, phenobarbital, orally, for 3 to 7 days before the HIDA scan improves the sensitivity of the scan, by activating hepatic enzymes and stimulating biliary secretion.

- Early differentiation of extrahepatic biliary atresia from medical causes of hepatic dysfunction is important because earlier surgical intervention (Kasai procedure or portoenterostomy) is directly associated with better outcomes. Ideally, patient should undergo surgery within the first 2 months. Success rates after 3 months of age are poor.

- In severe hepatic dysfunction in neonatal hepatitis, there may be absent bowel activity and it would be difficult or impossible to differentiate the condition from biliary atresia. Liver biopsy would be helpful in these cases.

the first 2 to 8 weeks after birth and do not present with other congenital abnormalities. Kasai classification system describes three types of biliary atresia, depending on the location of atresia and degree of pathology. In type I, the common bile duct is obliterated while the proximal bile ducts are patent. In type II, atresia of the hepatic duct is seen, with cystic bile ducts found at the porta hepatis. In type IIa, the cystic and common bile ducts are patent, whereas in type IIb, the cystic, common bile duct and hepatic ducts are all obliterated. Type III atresia refers to discontinuity of both right and left hepatic ducts to the level of the porta hepatis and unfortunately accounts for more than 90% of cases. Neonatal jaundice may be due to a variety of causes, including hemolysis, sepsis, and metabolic disease, among others. However, when jaundice persists longer than 14 days, biliary atresia and idiopathic neonatal hepatitis must be considered. Ultrasound plays an important role in the study of biliary tract in the neonates and provides detailed anatomic information to the cause of the problem. Cholescintigraphy with a Tc-99m-labeled IDA (immunodiacetic acid) agent provides functional imaging of the biliary tract and evaluates the patency of the tree and helps differentiate from neonatal hepatitis and cholestasis. Patients should be pretreated with phenobarbital (5 mg/kg for 5 days) to activate enzymes in the liver associated with excretion, thus increasing the sensitivity. Typical dose of Tc-99m IDA is 200 μCi/kg and at least 1 mCi and 24-hour images may be required to complete the diagnosis. Good hepatic uptake with absent biliary clearance and into bowel is characteristic of biliary atresia. Severe hepatic dysfunction can be identified with gross degree of blood pool activity with greater renal excretion.

Bhasker R. Koppula, MD

PRESENTATION

Typically seen in 2-year-old children who present with lower GI bleeding.

FINDINGS

Abnormal focus of activity that appeared at the same time with the initial uptake in the stomach and persisted in the right lower quadrant (RLQ) suspicious for a Meckel diverticulum.

DIFFERENTIAL DIAGNOSES

- Active gastrointestinal bleeding from a non-Meckel source at the time of injection can occasionally give a similar scintigraphic appearance.

- Intestinal duplication cyst with heterotopic gastric mucosa.

COMMENTS

Meckel diverticulum is the most common form of congenital abnormality of the small intestine, resulting from

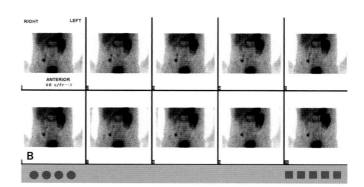

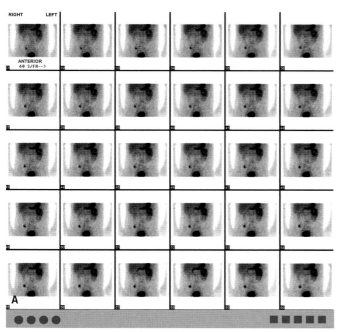

A. and **B.** Serial dynamic anterior images from Meckel scan with Tc-99m pertechnetate show an abnormal focus of radiotracer accumulation in the RLQ. Note that the appearance of this focus in the RLQ coincides with that of appearance within the stomach. This finding is consistent with presence of gastric mucosa in the Meckel diverticulum. There is progressive accumulation of the tracer over the period of image acquisition lasting for 45 minutes. Also, note the tracer activity within the stomach entering into the small bowel. Presence of Meckel diverticulum was confirmed at surgery. (*Images courtesy of Bhasker R. Koppula, MD.*)

an incomplete obliteration of the vitelline duct (ie, omphalomesenteric duct). The heterotopic mucosa is likely to be gastric in origin in 80% of cases of Meckel diverticulum, and peptic ulceration of this or adjacent mucosa can lead to pain, bleeding, and/or perforation. RULE of 2's: incidence of 2%, location being 2 ft from the ileocecal junction, size of 2 cm, usual presentation less than 2 years, and complications in 2% of cases. Complications result from attached bands and ectopic tissue and include bowel obstruction (most common complication), hemorrhage (because of the presence of ectopic gastric mucosa), diverticulitis, intussusception (may act like a leading point for an ileocolic or ileoileal intussusception), and umbilical fistula. Plain radiographs of the abdomen may show signs of

PEARLS

- To be visualized, the Meckel diverticulum must be actively bleeding at a minimum rate of 0.1 mL/min at the time of the study.

- The sensitivity of Meckel scan varies from 75% to 100%, with an accuracy of 95% for detection of gastric mucosa.

- False-positive results occur in up to 15% of patients, which can be due to duodenal ulcer, small intestinal obstruction, ureteric obstruction, aneurysm, and angiomas of small intestine.

- False-negative results is up to 25%, which can occur when gastric mucosa is very slight or absent in the Meckel diverticulum, or if necrosis of Meckel diverticulum has occurred.

- Accuracy of the scan may be enhanced with administration of cimetidine, glucagon, and pentagastrin.

intestinal obstruction or perforation. When a patient presents with bleeding and with suspicion of Meckel diverticulum, the diagnostic evaluation should include a Tc-99m pertechnetate scintiscan (commonly known as Meckel scan), which is especially helpful in infants who present with lower GI bleeding. The ectopic gastric mucosa takes up the radioactive free pertechnetate and shows up as a hot spot in the lower abdomen. The main advantages of this scan are the noninvasive nature with less radiation exposure compared to other diagnostic studies such as upper gastrointestinal and small-bowel follow-through series. During workup of patients, the barium study should never precede the Tc-99m scan because barium may obscure a focal increased uptake on the scan (because of attenuation of photons). Selective arteriography may be helpful in patients in whom the results from scintigraphy and barium studies are negative or inconclusive.

DIFFERENTIAL DIAGNOSIS IMAGES (C-D)

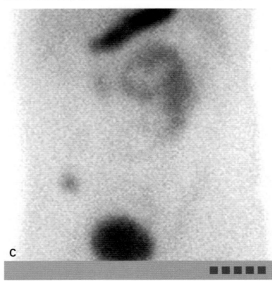 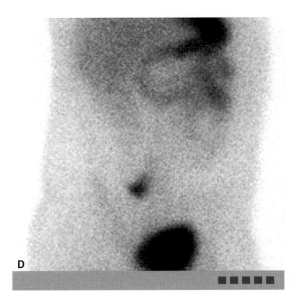

C. and **D.** Spot views of the abdomen and pelvis in anterior and oblique positions confirm the presence of abnormal focus of tracer activity in the RLQ. Activity within the stomach, small bowel, and the urinary bladder is an expected normal finding on Meckel scan. (*Images courtesy of Bhasker R. Koppula, MD.*)

Joseph Rajendran, MD

PRESENTATION

A 31-year-old male, status post 15 feet fall from ladder, hitting his right chest and flank on the way down.

FINDINGS

Tc-99m mebrofenin sequential planar static images (1 minute per frame) of anterior abdomen show normal excretion in the biliary tract and collection in the gallbladder. There is also an irregular focus of increasing accumulation in the superolateral right lobe.

DIFFERENTIAL DIAGNOSES

- Normal variant of biliary tree anatomy may show accumulation of the tracer in unexpected locations in the liver, but history and other imaging studies will help differentiate the diagnosis.

- Postcholecystectomy biliary leak typically is located near the junction of cystic duct and common bile duct (CBD). History also will direct to the diagnosis.

COMMENTS

Common causes for biliary leak are—iatrogenic disruption of the CBD during open cholecystectomy (0.2%), laparoscopic cholecystectomy (up to 2%), acute cholecystitis with perforation, inflammation, posttraumatic, and neoplasm resulting in infiltration and perforation. Hepatic trauma can be as a result of direct injury to the liver or blunt trauma to the liver. Traumatic injuries to the liver are usually associated with injuries to other organs or tissues in the abdomen or elsewhere. Delay in diagnosing hepatobiliary injury can be fatal in the majority of cases as a result of both hemorrhage and biliary peritonitis. Possibility of associated biliary leak should always be kept in mind in patients with trauma to the hepatobiliary system. Patients may present with pain either localized to the RUQ or the entire abdomen. Jaundice and fever usually develop after 3 to 5 days. Physical examination is usually

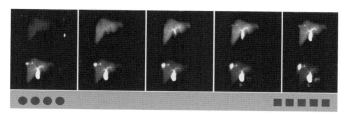

A. Tc-99m mebrofenin sequential planar static images (1 minute per frame) of anterior abdomen show normal excretion in the biliary tract and collection in the gallbladder. There is also an irregular focus of increasing accumulation in the superolateral right lobe corresponding to the CT abnormality of contusion.

not very sensitive in making the diagnosis of biliary leak. Anatomic studies such as ultrasound and CT scanning are sensitive to identify the location and extent of the trauma and the presence of fluid collection, but they cannot adequately differentiate the type of fluid in the collection. Hepatobiliary scanning with an IDA agent is a noninvasive and very specific test in confirming the exact nature of the leak. Liver activity should exceed cardiac blood pool by 5 minutes, biliary activity typically seen by 15 minutes, and in more than 90% of normal studies the gallbladder is seen within 30 minutes.

PEARLS

- In traumatic biliary leak, normal uptake and function is seen in the liver parenchyma.

- Focus of radiotracer activity that is located outside of normal biliary tract that is persistent and increases in size and intensity with time.

- Delayed images would be helpful in case of slow biliary leak and if associated with poor hepatic function.

- Oblique images may be needed to identify the exact location.

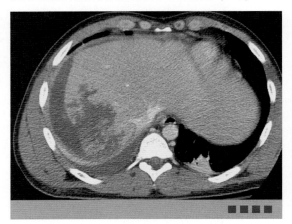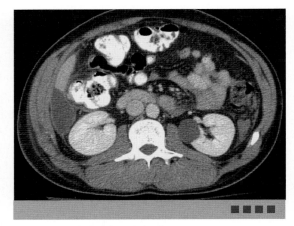

B. and **C.** Axial slices of CT images show the contusion abnormality in the right lobe of the liver.

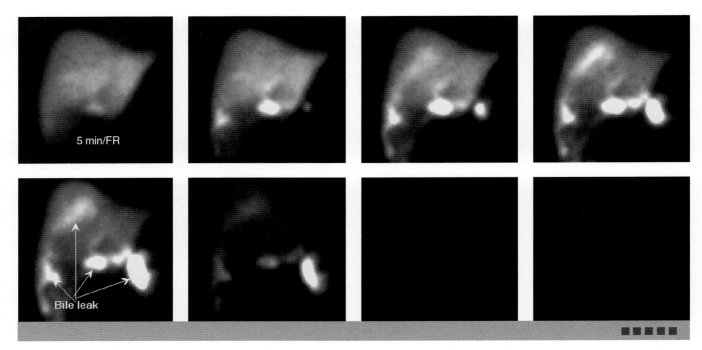

5 min/FR

Bile leak

D. Biliary leak into the right gutter, peritoneal cavity, and over right liver lobe from an open cystic duct following cholecystectomy 9 days prior to this scan. (*Image courtesy of G.T. Krishnamurthy, MD.*)

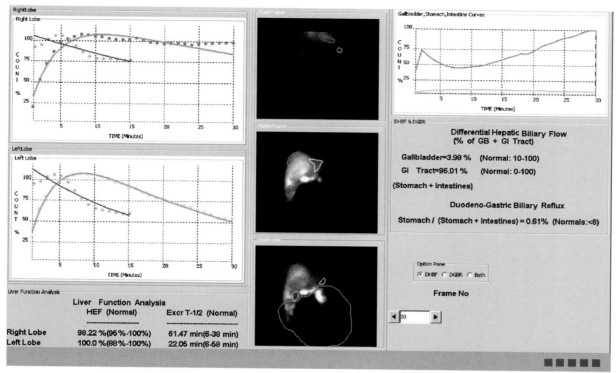

E. Hepatic extraction fraction of both liver lobes is normal, but the excretion T-1/2 of the right lobe (dotted) is prolonged because bile spills over it from the leak. (*Image courtesy of G.T. Krishnamurthy, MD.*)

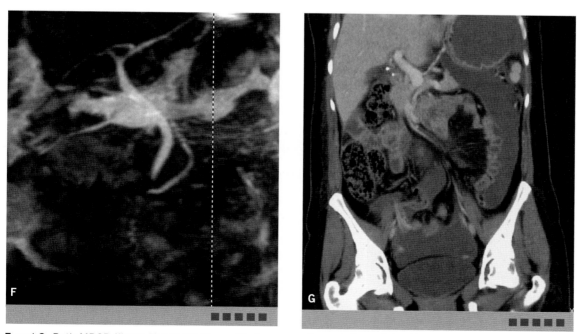

F. and **G.** Both MRCP (figure F) and CT (figure G) show normal morphology of the CBD. Origin of ascites is not clear from CT. (*Image F courtesy of G.T. Krishnamurthy, MD.*)

Case 5–25 Chronic Cholecystitis

Joseph Rajendran, MD

PRESENTATION

A 54-year-old with history of intermittent upper abdominal pain and nausea and vomiting.

FINDINGS

Tc-99m mebrofenin sequential planar static images (1 minute per frame) of anterior abdomen show normal excretion in the biliary tract and collection in the gallbladder. There is delay in the emptying of the gallbladder even after CCK infusion. The calculated gallbladder ejection fraction (EF) is 20% below the normal values.

DIFFERENTIAL DIAGNOSIS

Acute cholecystitis: There is nonvisualization of the gallbladder at the end of the study or even with morphine augmentation along with the classic signs and symptoms.

COMMENTS

Chronic cholecystitis is a long-standing low-grade inflammation of the gallbladder and can be caused typically in the absence of gallstones. The thick bile and stasis, as a result of gallstones or impaired biliary flow, results in chronic, low-grade inflammation of the gallbladder mucosa and eventual infection. This condition has a protracted course and patients present with repeated episodes of pain in the RUQ or the entire abdomen. There can be episodes of acute inflammation that cannot be easily differentiated from acute cholecystitis. Fever and leukocytosis is usually absent in chronic cholecystitis and liver function tests may

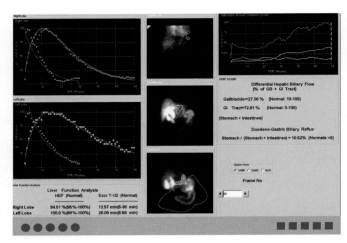

B. Hepatobiliary analysis using the KHBS (Krishnamurthy Hepatobiliary Software) software shows normal filling and delayed emptying of the gallbladder with a calculated gallbladder EF of 20% being below the normal value (> 30%). (*Image courtesy of G.T. Krishnamurthy, MD.*)

not be elevated unless there is obstruction or parenchymal dysfunction. Physical examination may reveal RUQ tenderness. Plain radiograph of the abdomen is usually the first screening test and can reveal the presence of gallstones or the presence of porcelain gallbladder. Hepatobiliary scanning with an IDA agent is a noninvasive and very specific test in confirming the presence of chronic cholecystitis. Currently the most commonly used IDA agent in most facilities is mebrofenin and has the ideal characteristics. Liver activity should exceed cardiac blood pool by 5 minutes, biliary activity is typically seen by 10 minutes, and in more than 90% of normal studies the gallbladder is seen within

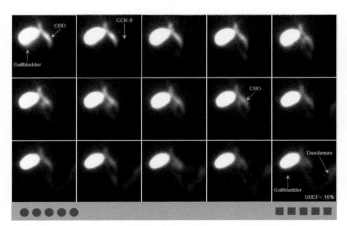

A. Tc-99m mebrofenin sequential planar static images (1 minute per frame) of anterior abdomen show normal filling of the gallbladder with delayed excretion into the biliary tract. There is significant delay in emptying of the gallbladder even after CCK infusion. (*Image courtesy of G.T. Krishnamurthy, MD.*)

PEARLS

- In chronic cholecystitis, typically there is normal extraction and function in the liver parenchyma except in late stages with chronic biliary obstruction when there can be significant delay in extraction.

- In the classic case, there is delay in the filling of the gallbladder, which stays filled for a protracted period without appreciable emptying.

- CCK infusion should be started when the gallbladder has filled to its maximum.

- Oblique images may be needed to identify the exact location of the gallbladder.

30 minutes. In patients with chronic cholecystitis, the time to visualize the gallbladder may be longer than that as also emptying time. The gallbladder may also remain filled for longer periods without much emptying depending on the severity of the dysfunction. Infusion of cholecystokinin (0.02 μg/kg) over 20 to 30 minutes helps in calculating the gallbladder EF (normal > 30%) using regions of analysis (ROI). Typically, CCK infusion starts when the gallbladder filling has reached the maximum. Most patients complain of symptoms ranging from nausea and mild abdominal discomfort to severe pain and vomiting that mimic their presenting symptoms. Typically, rapid infusions are associated with more severe symptoms. Reproduction of patient's symptoms with CCK infusion is helpful to the clinicians in narrowing down the etiologies. Additional analysis can be performed with the data and include quantification of duodenogastric reflux, transit to small bowel etc, using software analysis.

DIFFERENTIAL DIAGNOSIS IMAGES (C-D)

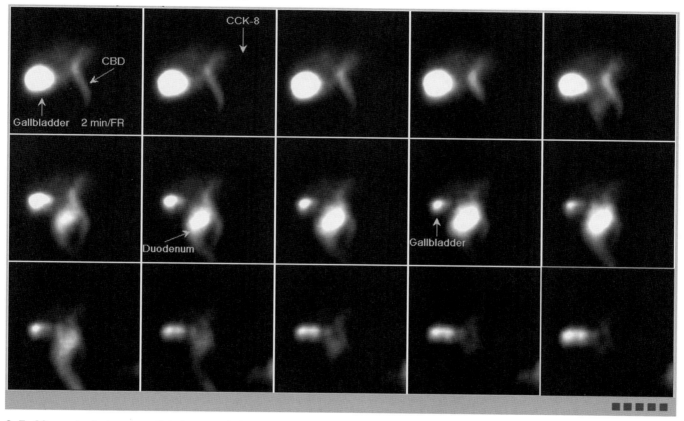

C. Tc-99m mebrofenin sequential planar static images (1 minute per frame) of anterior abdomen show normal filling of the gallbladder and excretion in the biliary tract as well as collection in the gallbladder. There is prompt and adequate response after CCK infusion. (*Image courtesy of G.T. Krishnamurthy, MD.*)

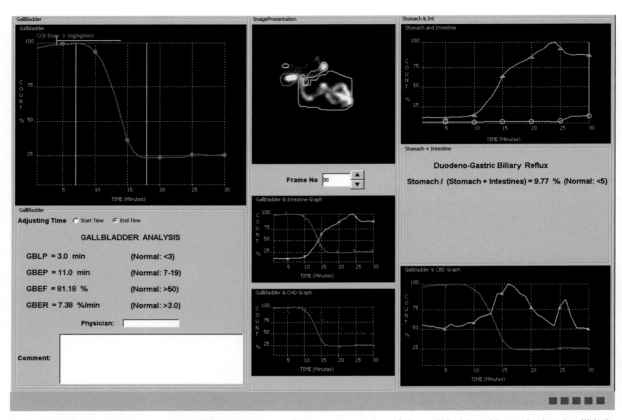

D. Hepatobiliary analysis using the KHBS shows normal filling and emptying of the gallbladder with a calculated gallbladder EF of 81%. (*Image courtesy of G.T. Krishnamurthy, MD.*)

Joseph Rajendran, MD

PRESENTATION

A 58-year-old male with history of colon cancer found incidentally on colonoscopy (polypectomy demonstrated invasion).

FINDINGS

Planar tagged Tc-99m-labeled RBC images: Single focus of increased radiotracer activity in the right lobe of the liver. Single-photon emission CT (SPECT) images: Single focus in the right lobe of the liver (segment IV). New focus of activity in the left lobe of the liver (segment II). These foci correlate with hemangiomas seen on the contrast-enhanced CT scan.

DIFFERENTIAL DIAGNOSIS

- *Metastatic disease*: Often the difficulty is in making the right diagnosis of metastatic disease as biopsy is contraindicated in hemangioma because of the danger of bleeding post biopsy.

COMMENTS

Cavernous hemangioma is the most common primary liver tumor with incidence up to 20%. These tumors arise from the endothelial cells lining the hepatic vasculature. Most often they are asymptomatic and incidentally discovered at imaging, surgery, or autopsy. Typically seen as solitary focal lesions, they can be multiple as well and can widely vary in size. Hemangiomas are generally rare in the presence of cirrhosis of the liver. Cavernous hemangioma of the liver is seen equally in males and females as well as children. Most hemangiomas of the liver are incidentally detected at imaging studies performed for other indications. While ultrasonography is cost-effective for the diagnosis of

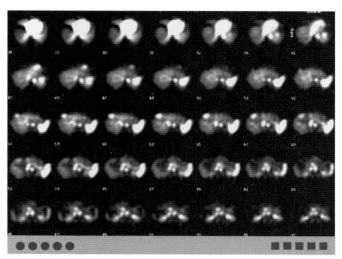

B. Tc-99m-labeled RBC axial SPECT images show a focus of increased uptake in the right lobe of the liver corresponding to the focus of abnormal activity seen on planar images and on axial CT scan.

hemangioma, CT and/or MRI are helpful to characterize and confidently diagnose the presence of hemangioma. Tc-99m-labeled RBC imaging is very helpful in making the diagnosis. There is reduced flow on early and blood pool images but shows gradually increasing uptake in the hemangioma, resulting in delayed uptake more than that of rest of the liver parenchyma. It can often show heterogeneous uptake. Lesion size is critical for the detection—in general 3 cm for planar imaging and 1.5 cm for SPECT imaging. Positive predictive value for tagged RBC scanning

PEARLS

- Both perfusion and immediate images can be performed but might not add more information than delayed images.

- *Delayed images*: Hemangiomas have increased activity compared with the adjacent liver. Uptake is often equal or greater than the blood pool activity in the heart and spleen.

- Giant cavernous hemangiomas often have heterogeneous uptake of the radiotracer with central photopenia (thrombosis, necrosis, and/or fibrosis).

- Often the dilemma is to differentiate metastatic disease from hemangioma. Confirmation of hemangioma is critical prior to attempting needle biopsy and to avoid severe hemorrhage.

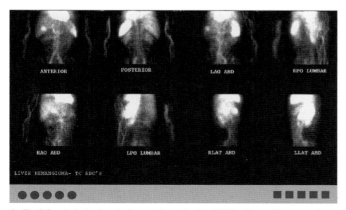

A. Tc-99m-labeled anterior and posterior RBC planar images show a focus of increased uptake in the right lobe of the liver.

approaches 100%. Potential false positives are extremely rarely seen in angiosarcoma and hepatoma while false-negative cases are seen in hemangiomas with extensive fibrosis or thrombosis. Sensitivity is size dependent—ranging from 100% for more than 1.4 cm to only 20% for 0.5 to 0.9 cm. SPECT imaging, superior to planar imaging, can detect lesions as small as 0.5 cm as well as additional lesions (as seen in this case).

DIFFERENTIAL DIAGNOSIS IMAGES (C-H)

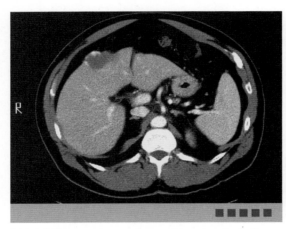

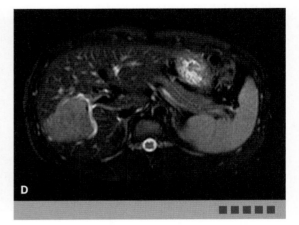

C. Axial CT scan shows a focus of low density in the right lobe of the liver. The focal uptake in the right hepatic lobe seen on tagged RBC scan corresponds to this abnormality. (*Image courtesy of Orpheus Kolokythas, MD.*)

D-G 1-4. Imaging series show well-defined lobulated mass with (D) moderate hyperintensity on inversion recovery sequence; (E) nodular contrast enhancement around focal central stellate hyperintensities; (F) homogeneous strong contrast enhancement on portal-venous phase with similar sparing focal hypointensities; (G) slightly less intense contrast enhancement and stronger enhancement of previously hypointense portions suggestive of several scars. Findings were suggestive of atypical FNH and hemangioma could not be excluded. (*Images courtesy of Orpheus Kolokythas, MD.*)

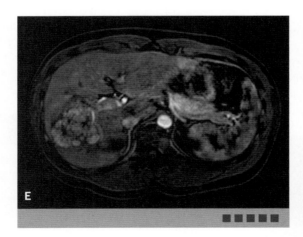

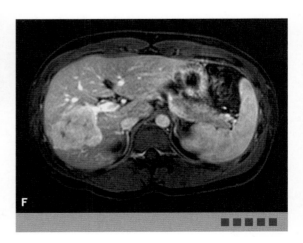

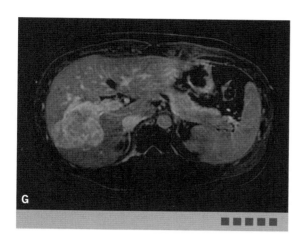

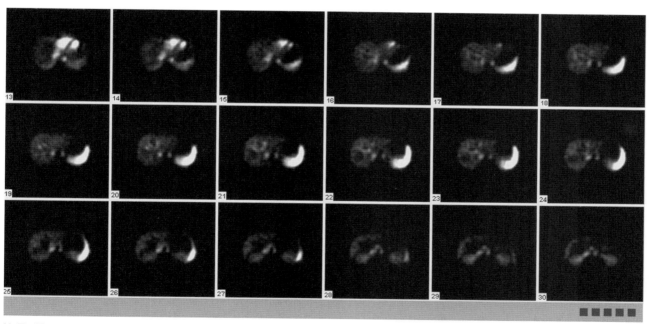

H. Tc-99m-labeled RBC axial SPECT images show a photopenic area in the right lobe corresponding to the contrast enhancement seen in the arterial phase of CT scan, suggesting that it was not hemangioma. The possibilities include metastases and FNH.

Vivek Manchanda, MD

PRESENTATION

Weight loss in 46-year-old male with sacral pain. Sacral biopsy of metastasis shows poorly differentiated cancer of unknown origin.

FINDINGS

Multiple hypermetabolic skeletal lucencies with mildly hypermetabolic left renal mass.

DIFFERENTIAL DIAGNOSES

• Primary renal cancer with skeletal metastases.

• Unknown primary cancer with skeletal metastases.

At least one-third of renal cell cancers (RCC) are hypometabolic, which may be missed on PET. RCC skeletal metastases are typically lytic in appearance.

COMMENTS

Cancer of unknown primary origin (CUP) is the diagnosis when metastatic disease is found, but the primary cancer cannot be determined by physical examination, laboratory testing (eg, for tumor markers), or conventional imaging.

About 2% to 4 % of all cancer patients have a cancer whose primary site is never identified.

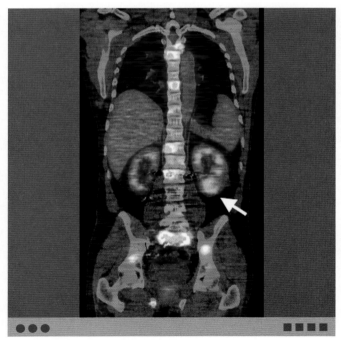

A. Coronal fused PET/CT, hypermetabolic skeletal metastases with hypermetabolic inferior renal pole mass.

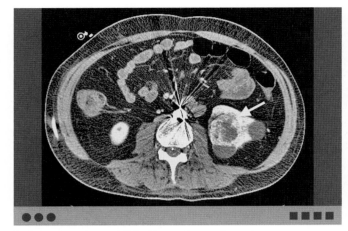

B. Contrast-enhanced CT with renal mass (*arrow*).

FDG-PET can be successful in localizing the primary cancer when the original diagnosis is CUP. In one series, up to one-third of the patients investigated for CUP had localization of the primary on FDG-PET. It also assisted in guiding biopsies and selecting appropriate treatment protocols. In a meta-analysis, the overall sensitivity, specificity, and accuracy rates of FDG-PET in detecting unknown primary tumors were 91.9%, 81.9%, and 80.5%, respectively. Previously unrecognized metastases were recognized in 37% and lung cancers represented majority of unknown primaries. High false-positive rate (58.3%) was seen in tumors of the lower digestive tract.

Metastases in upper part of the body is suggestive of the original site to be above the diaphragm, such as the lungs and breasts, and metastases in the lower part of the body is suggestive of primary origin below the diaphragm, such as in the pancreas and liver.

Many patients with an unidentified primary tumor have adenocarcinoma of unknown origin. The largest number of PET studies in CUP have been for secondary lesions in cervical lymph nodes, with high sensitivity and specificity of primary cancer detection by FDG-PET.

It has been recommended that FDG-PET should be performed sufficiently early in cases of neurologic paraneoplastic syndrome, because established lesions become irreversible.

PEARLS

• **FDG-PET is a good modality with a high success rate to detect primary site in the case of cancer of unknown origin.**

• **It is recommended that FDG-PET be performed sufficiently early in cases of neurologic paraneoplastic syndrome.**

ADDITIONAL IMAGES (C-E)

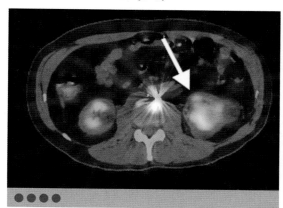

C. Axial fused PET/CT, hypermetabolic left renal cancer (*arrow*).

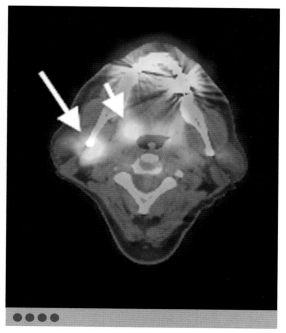

D. Fused axial PET/CT with right palatine tonsil squamous cell cancer (*short arrow*) and right level 2 metastatic node (*long arrow*) in a different patient.

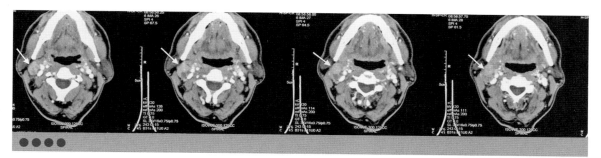

E. Corresponding contrast enhanced CT scan done before FDG-PET, with enlarged right level 2 metastatic node (*arrow*) but no identification of primary site.

Vivek Manchanda, MD

PRESENTATION

A man in his sixth decade of life with jaundice. Normal serum lipase and amylase.

FINDINGS

Intensely hypermetabolic FDG activity in pancreas, right supraclavicular and para-aortic nodes.

DIFFERENTIAL DIAGNOSES

- *Pancreatic cancer*
- *Metastases*: RCC, lung, breast, sarcoma, melanoma, colon cancer
- *Pancreatitis*
- *Lymphoma*
- *Abscess*

COMMENTS

Biopsy in the index case showed metastases from Merkel cell cancer.

Merkel cell cancer is a rare, aggressive primary skin cancer which shows neuroendocrine differentiation.

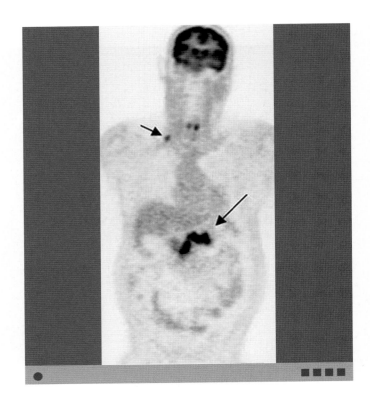

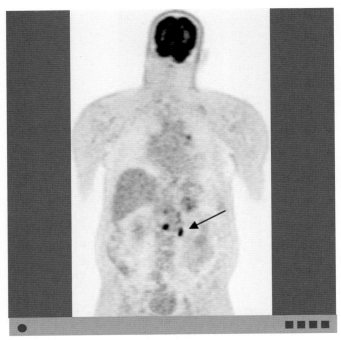

A. and **B.** Intense hypermetabolic foci in right supraclavicular, para-aortic nodes and pancreas, Merkel cell involvement.

The proposed staging for Merkel cell cancer includes stage I (localized disease), stage II (lymph node involvement), and stage III (distant metastases).

For initial assessment, sentinel lymph node biopsy is done. FDG-PET is not sensitive to detect micrometastases in a sentinel node and is useful for staging when the sentinel node is positive and distant spread is suspected.

There is a tendency for local and nodal recurrence, exceeding that of malignant melanoma. If a patient presents with stage III disease, the mean survival is about 8 months.

Once Merkel cell cancer spreads beyond regional nodal basin, it can spread in an unpredictable manner. The lymph

PEARLS

- Merkel cell cancer is an aggressive skin cancer which shows neuroendocrine differentiation and is extremely FDG avid.

- Detection of disease in small-sized nodes, distant metastases, surveillance, and post-therapy assessment by FDG-PET is of great clinical value.

- FDG-PET scan cannot replace sentinel node mapping in Merkel cell cancer for detecting micrometastases in initial staging workup.

node metastases are extremely FDG avid and appear hyper- or isoattenuating to muscle on the contrast-enhanced CT.

Subcutaneous and muscle metastases can also be identified with FDG-PET scan. Similar to melanoma, both solid organ and hollow visceral diseases can be seen in the abdomen and pelvis.

Merkel cell cancers can involve the thorax as (a) nodal disease, (b) intrapulmonary nodules, or (c) masses which can invade bone or chest wall. CNS involvement is less common.

Indium 111-labeled pentetreotide can be used to detect the extent of disease, although involvement of liver, spleen (and kidneys) cannot be detected due to physiologic uptake.

FDG-PET is an excellent tool to detect distant metastases, recurrence, and response to treatment. Male sex, lesions greater than 5 mm, subcutaneous invasion, increased mitosis, and small cell size are all associated with poorer prognosis. In one study, disease stage was the only independent factor in predicting survival rate at 5 years.

DIFFERENTIAL DIAGNOSIS IMAGES (C-D)

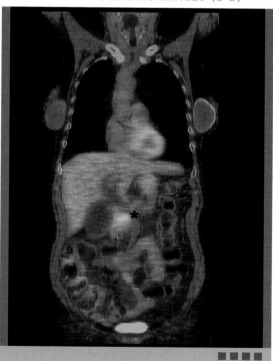

C. Pancreatic adenocarcinoma (*black star*). Coronal fused PET/CT. Note hypometabolic breast implants.

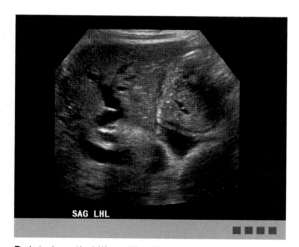

D. Intrahepatic biliary dilatation on ultrasound.

Vivek Manchanda, MD

PRESENTATION

Nausea and vomiting in a woman in her late forties with history of melanoma 10 years ago.

FINDINGS

Intensely hypermetabolic mesenteric mass and small bowel mass.

DIFFERENTIAL DIAGNOSES

- *Carcinoid*
- *Adenocarcinoma*
- *Lymphoma: Typically NHL*
- *Gastrointestinal stromal tumor (GIST)*
- *Metastases: sarcoma, lung and breast*
- *Neurogenic tumor*
- *Leiomyoma, adenoma, lipoma, hemangioma*
- *Lymphangioma*
- *Fibrosarcoma*

Given the intense FDG activity; hemangioma, lymphangioma, lipoma, and carcinoid are unlikely. Large bowel adenomas have variable FDG activity. Given prior history of melanoma, metastases from melanoma is most likely, proved by biopsy.

COMMENTS

Malignant melanoma, a malignant tumor of melanocytes, initially involves regional lymph node basin. Once beyond the regional nodes, it can involve any organ in the body.

Newly diagnosed cutaneous melanoma should be staged by sentinel lymph node biopsy. Microscopic disease in sentinel nodes cannot be detected by PET.

Routine FDG-PET scanning is not recommended for the initial staging evaluation of stage I and II melanomas (including those that were >4 mm in thickness) as it has not been shown to affect patient care.

In stage III (N1, N2, or N3 node positive) or stage IV (M1) patients, FDG-PET is clinically useful. Investigators in several series have reported that FDG-PET demonstrates better disease detection than conventional imaging in patients with advanced melanoma, prompting changes in clinical management decisions.

Lymph nodes are the commonest site for metastases. Melanoma metastases are extremely FDG avid and nodes as small as 4 to 5 mm in size that harbor disease can be detected.

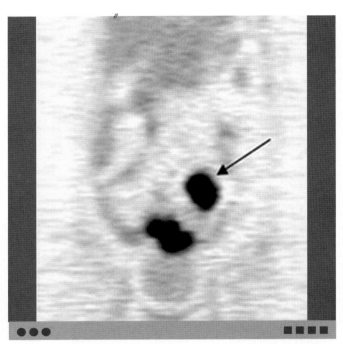

A. Melanoma metastases involving small bowel and mesentery. Coronal FDG-PET (*arrow*).

A single pulmonary nodule in a patient with melanoma is more likely to be metastatic than a primary lung cancer. Metastasectomy in these patients can produce prolonged remission.

Skin and subcutaneous tissues are the most common soft tissue sites of metastases. Lesions as small as 3 mm have been identified by FDG-PET.

The most frequent blood-borne metastases to GI tract is from melanomas. The commonest site is small intestine, where the deposits can trigger intussusception and small bowel obstruction.

PET/CT scan provides additional value in the staging of recurrent melanoma.

PEARLS

- **FDG-PET is not indicated in stage I or II melanoma.**

- **Sentinel lymph node biopsy is still the gold standard in local staging as PET may miss microscopic disease in sentinel node. PET is useful in both stages III and IV and in staging recurrent melanoma.**

- **The most common metastases to the GI tract is from melanoma.**

ADDITIONAL IMAGES (B-F)

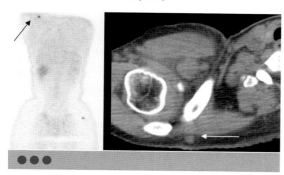

B. Subcutaneous metastasis (3 mm) from melanoma. Coronal FDG-PET and corresponding CT.

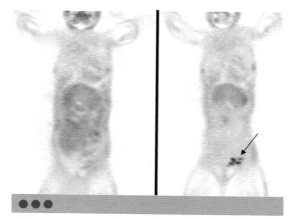

C. Recurrent melanoma in a different patient, nonattenuation corrected images, coronal FDG-PET.

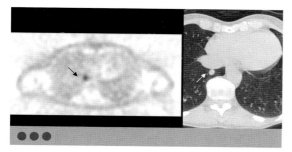

D. Single smooth-margined nodule in melanoma patient, NAC image and corresponding CT (*arrow*), metastasis.

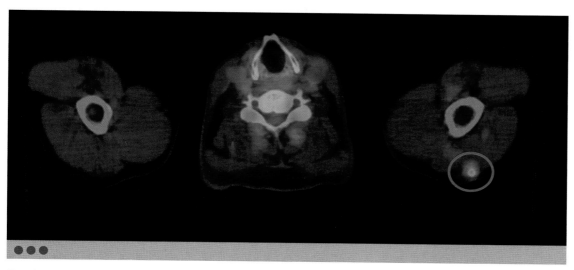

E. Left shoulder skin metastases, melanoma. Axial fused PET/CT (*circle*).

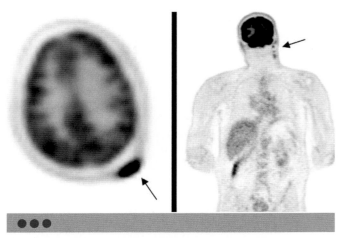

F. Scalp melanoma and left neck nodal metastases. Axial and coronal FDG-PET.

DIFFERENTIAL DIAGNOSIS IMAGES (G-L)

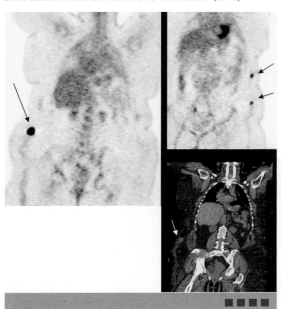

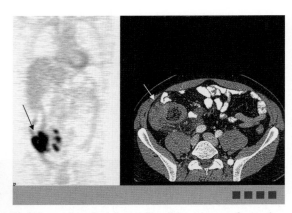

H. Primary terminal ileum B-cell lymphoma. Coronal FDG-PET (*arrow*) and axial CT. Note circumferential bowel thickening.

G. Cutaneous lymphoma, coronal FDG-PET and coronal CT.

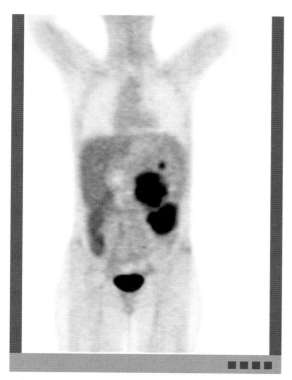

I. Follicular lymphoma, coronal FDG/PET.

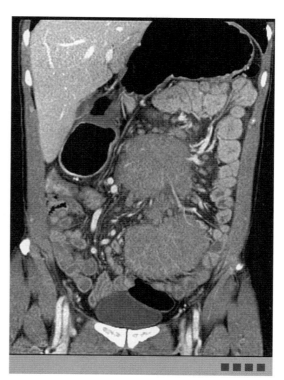

J. Corresponding CT.

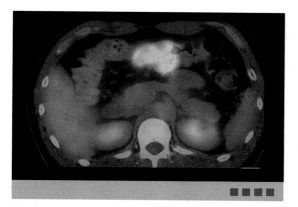

K. Adenocarcinoma, transverse colon, fused PET/CT.

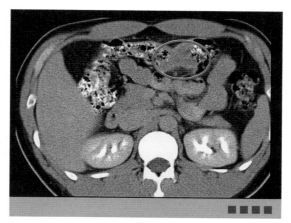

L. Corresponding CT.

Vivek Manchanda, MD

PRESENTATION

Multiple calcified liver hypodensities in woman in her mid-forties. History of uveal melanoma 9 years ago.

FINDINGS

Hypermetabolic calcified liver lesions and periportal nodes.

DIFFERENTIAL DIAGNOSES

Calcified metastases to liver:

- *Mucinous carcinoma* of gastrointestinal (GI) tract (colon, stomach, and rectum)
- *Pancreatic (endocrine) cancer*
- *Osteosarcoma*
- *Breast cancer*
- *Lung cancer*
- *RCC*
- *Medullary thyroid cancer*
- *Papillary serous ovarian cystadenocarcinoma*
- *Testicular cancer*
- *Lymphoma*

COMMENTS

Liver is the commonest metastatic site after regional lymph nodes, and metastases are more common than primary carcinoma. In this case, metastases from uveal melanoma developed after 9 years of diagnosis.

Melanoma of the uveal tract is among the commonest primary tumors of the eye among Caucasians.

It is highly malignant with systemic metastases and high mortality. The commonest site of uveal melanoma metastasis is the liver and less likely the lungs. Approximately half of the patients will develop metastases within 15 years. The average life span after diagnosis of liver metastases is 8 to 10 months.

Modorati et al, studied the usefulness of FDG-PET in intraocular melanoma and reported 7 out of 12 tumors detected with a diameter greater than 7.5 mm. PET/CT can allow differentiation between tumor tissue and subretinal exudates. Extraocular growth can be evaluated with FDG-PET.

Some studies have suggested that the sensitivity of FDG-PET to detect primary uveal melanoma is lower in comparison to cutaneous malignant melanoma. As far as detection and localization of hepatic and extrahepatic (particularly osseous) metastatic choroidal melanoma is concerned, FDG-PET has a high sensitivity and specificity.

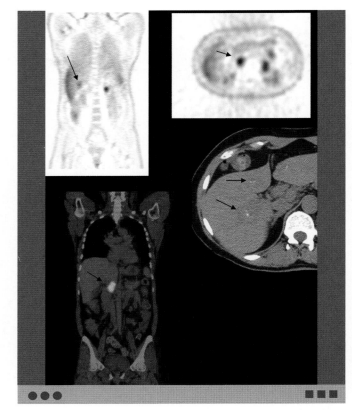

A. Uveal melanoma metastases to liver and periportal region. Note calcified metastases on CT. NAC image (*top left*), axial NAC (*top right*), fused PET/CT (*bottom left*) and noncontrast axial CT (*bottom right*).

Although undetected metastatic spread at the time of diagnosis and treatment of ciliary body melanoma is a major concern in every patient, adjuvant systemic treatment is not advocated currently. In cases of distant metastases in initial systemic workup, management of the intraocular melanomas becomes palliative.

PEARLS

- Uveal melanoma is the commonest primary intraocular tumor in adults.

- The commonest site of metastases is the liver, which may occur after more than 10 years.

- FDG-PET has good sensitivity and specificity for detection of metastases from uveal melanoma. It, however, has lower sensitivity for detection of the primary tumors.

DIFFERENTIAL DIAGNOSIS IMAGES (B-D)

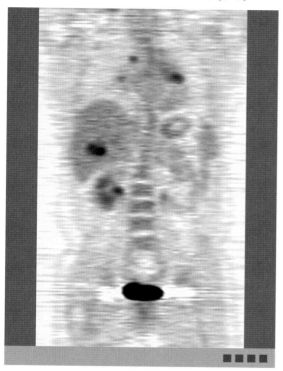

B. Liver metastases from cutaneous nonuveal melanoma with other mediastinal metastases.

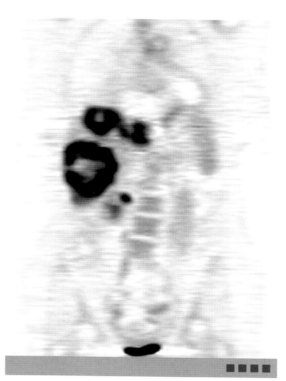

C. Hypermetabolic mucinous colon cancer metastases to liver, coronal FDG-PET.

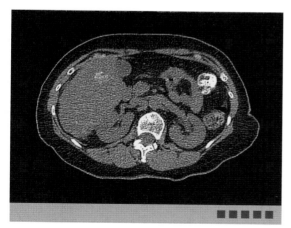

D. Corresponding calcified liver metastases on the noncontrast axial CT.

Chapter 6

LYMPHATIC

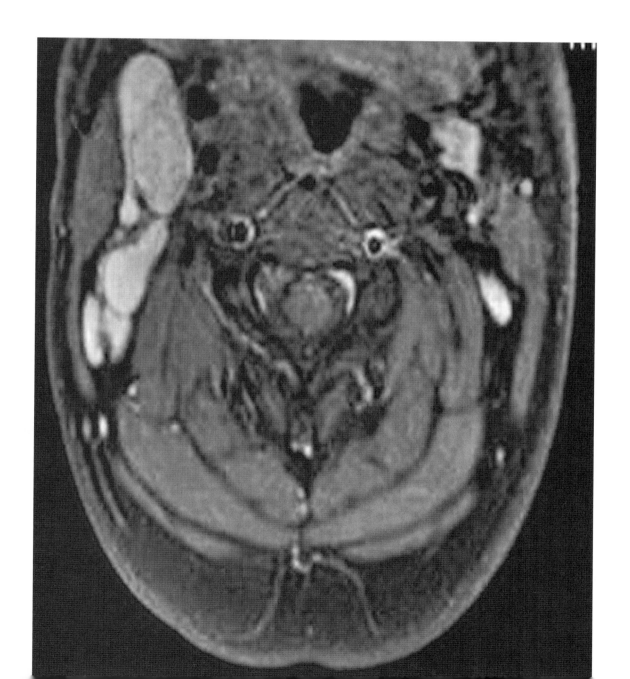

Vivek Manchanda, MD

PRESENTATION

Man in late second decade of his life with right neck mass.

FINDINGS

Right parapharyngeal hypermetabolic mass (maximum [standardized uptake value] SUV of 6.7).

DIFFERENTIAL DIAGNOSES

- *Lymphoma*

- *Metastases from head and neck cancer*

- *Sarcoidosis/granulomatous disease*

- *Reactive lymph nodes*

- *Tuberculous (TB) adenitis*

In a relatively younger age-group, metastases is less likely than lymphoma/Castleman disease. Given the level of FDG activity, it is unlikely to be simply reactive nodes.

COMMENTS

Angiofollicular lymph node hyperplasia (Castleman disease) is a nonneoplastic lymphoid and vascular proliferation, generally seen before age 30. Etiology is unknown.

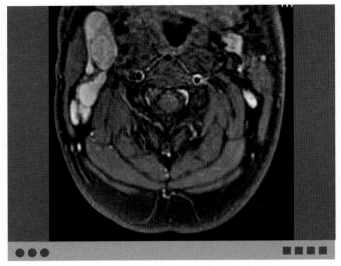

B. T1-W contrast-enhanced MR, right neck Castleman disease, in the same patient.

Most common site of involvement is mediastinum, although retroperitoneum, cervical lymph nodes, pulmonary parenchyma, axillary lymph nodes, and skeletal muscle can be involved.

Commonest subtype is hyaline vascular (mostly unicentric), characterized by vascular proliferation and hyalinization with small follicle centers penetrated by capillaries and capillary proliferation in the interfollicular areas. It is asymptomatic in 97% of the cases.

The plasma cell variant has sheets of plasma cells between normal/enlarged follicles and tends to involve multiple lymph nodes (multicentric) and extrathoracic sites. It is aggressive with elevated erythrocyte sedimentation rate (ESR), hypergammaglobulinemia, and increased risk for lymphoma.

CT features include mass of muscle density, spotty central calcification, enhancement in vascular capsule, marked enhancement in hyaline vascular type, and mild

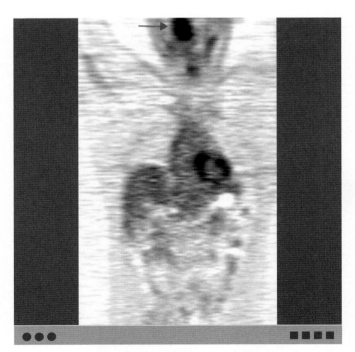

A. Castleman disease: Right neck hypermetabolic mass. Coronal FDG-PET.

PEARLS

- FDG-PET can be used to characterize unicentric (likely hyaline vascular) versus multicentric (plasma cell, more aggressive) Castleman disease and help in follow-up of the treatment.

- It is difficult to predict the histologic subtypes of Castleman disease or distinguish it from lymphoma on the basis of level of FDG activity.

- Plasma cell variants have a much aggressive course.

enhancement in plasma cell type. MR shows isointense signal on T1-WI and a hyperintense signal (compared with muscle) on T2-WI, with homogeneous strong enhancement.

Surgery results are excellent for unicentric Castleman disease. Radiotherapy is helpful in selected patients. Multicentric Castleman disease is more aggressive and most effectively treated with combination chemotherapy. Role of radiotherapy is unclear.

Role of FDG-PET/CT is in detection of unicentric versus multicentric disease and in follow-up after treatment. It is difficult to predict the histologic subtypes with FDG-PET. However, in the case reports, hyaline vascular types have higher SUVs than the plasma cell types.

It is important to keep Castleman disease in the comprehensive differential diagnosis of pediatric lymphoproliferative disorders.

ADDITIONAL IMAGES (C-E)

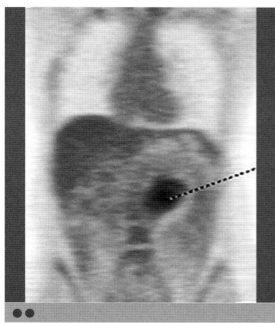

C. Left retroperitoneal lymphadenopathy in 26-year-old female, plasma cell type Castleman disease. Coronal FDG-PET.

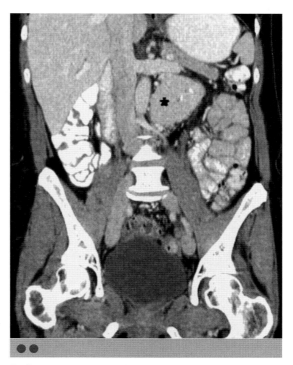

D. Contrast-enhanced CT (*black star*).

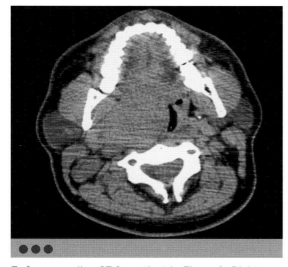

E. Corresponding CT for patient in Figure A. Right parapharyngeal Castleman disease.

DIFFERENTIAL DIAGNOSIS IMAGES (F-H)

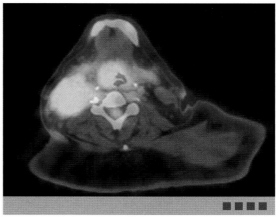

F. Right neck hypermetabolic adenopathy from base of tongue cancer in 62-year-old male. Fused axial PET/CT.

295

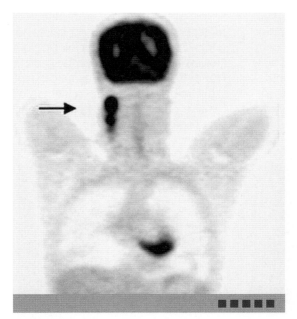

G. Hodgkin disease: Right neck nodal disease in 16-year-old male. Coronal FDG-PET.

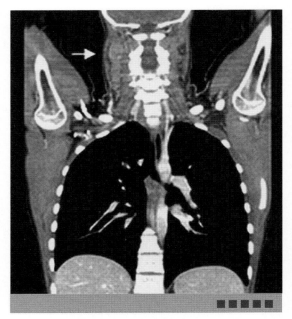

H. Hodgkin disease: Corresponding CT.

Vivek Manchanda, MD

PRESENTATION

Man in his sixth decade of life with generalized lymphadenopathy splenomegaly.

FINDINGS

Mildly hypermetabolic generalized lymphadenopathy splenomegaly. (Maximum SUVs in the range of 2.5-3.0.)

DIFFERENTIAL DIAGNOSES

- *Sarcoidosis*

- *Infections*: TB, human immunodeficiency virus (HIV), syphilis, infectious mononucleosis

- *Autoimmune disorders*: Systemic lupus erythematosus

- *Medication side effects*: Hydralazine, quinidine, captopril

- *Low-grade lymphoma*

Active sarcoidosis is usually intensely FDG avid. Mild FDG activity in generalized lymphadenopathy can be seen in multiple other etiologies as above.

COMMENTS

The biopsy showed chronic lymphocytic leukemia (CLL).

CLL usually manifests as faint metabolic activity related to generalized lymphadenopathy.

PET/CT should be considered in: (a) CLL with fever without infection, elevated lactate dehydrogenase (LDH) level, and rapidly enlarging lymph nodes; (b) bone marrow biopsy with large cells, indicating accelerated phase of CLL. PET/CT is especially important in identifying sites of increased ^{18}F-FDG uptake that are suitable for biopsy and surveillance.

CLL may undergo transformation to malignancies other than large B-cell lymphoma (so-called Richter variants, such as Hodgkin lymphoma). Patients with CLL also have a high incidence of second malignancies, such as that of skin, breasts, prostate, or lungs. PET/CT can demonstrate sites of increased ^{18}F-FDG uptake corresponding to an accelerated phase of CLL rather than frank lymphomatous transformation. This accelerated-phase turnover represents a higher rate of cell turnover. Patients with CLL are susceptible to recurrent infections which can manifest as false-positive findings on PET/CT.

Aggregation of granulocytic tumor cells in patients with myelogenous leukemias is termed chloromas that are extremely FDG avid. Their identification is significant as the preferred treatment of localized chloroma is radiation instead of chemotherapy.

FDG-PET can detect Richter transformation of CLL to large B-cell lymphoma with high sensitivity, specificity, and negative

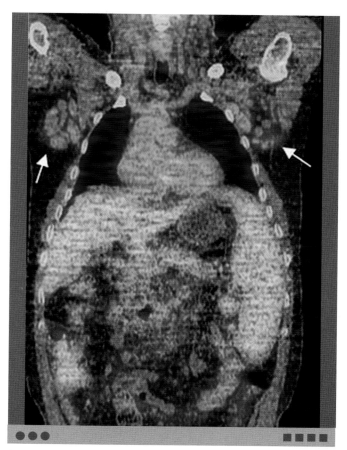

A. Mild FDG activity in bilateral axillary nodes in CLL. Coronal fused FDG-PET/CT. Note mildly hypermetabolic splenomegaly.

predictive value. The rationale is the detection of elevated metabolic rate in large cell lymphomas and the relatively low ^{18}F-FDG accumulation in cells with a low turnover rate, such as the small lymphocytes of CLL.

PEARLS

- **CLL/small lymphocytic lymphoma (SLL) is a low-grade lymphoma characterized by innumerable nodes throughout the body with minimal FDG activity.**

- **PET/CT has a high sensitivity for detection of transformation to high-grade lymphoma and chloromas. It can identify sites of increased FDG uptake suitable for biopsy.**

- **PET/CT can detect low-grade lymphomas with high proliferation index (tumors which clinically behave like high-grade tumors) and accelerated phase of CLL.**

ADDITIONAL IMAGES (B-C)

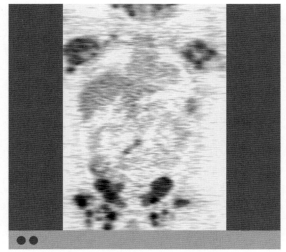

B. Suspected Richter transformation in CLL. Biopsy was negative for such transformation. Coronal FDG-PET.

DIFFERENTIAL DIAGNOSIS IMAGES (D-E)

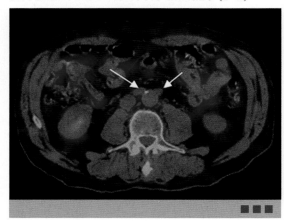

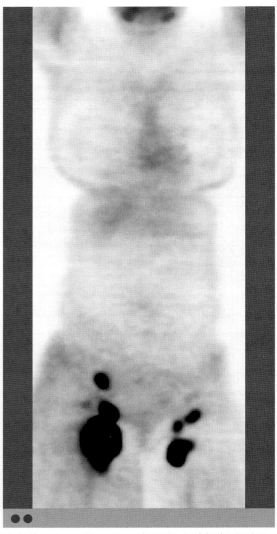

D. Mild FDG activity in marginal zone lymphoma, anterior to aorta (*white arrows*), axial fused PET/CT.

C. Diffuse large B-cell transformation of follicular lymphoma. Coronal FDG-PET.

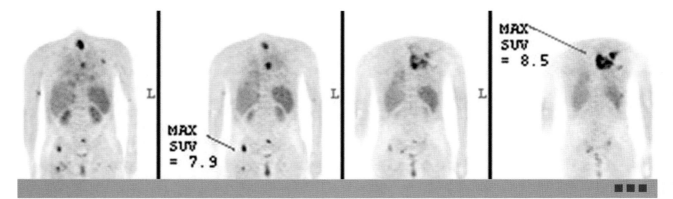

E. Multiple chloromas in 37-year-old male with chronic myelogenous (or myeloid) leukemia (CML). Coronal FDG-PET.

Vivek Manchanda, MD

PRESENTATION

Man in his sixth decade of life with incidental lytic lesions in the pelvis and splenic lesions.

FINDINGS

Multiple hypermetabolic lymph nodes, skeletal lesions, and spleen.

DIFFERENTIAL DIAGNOSES

- *Metastases*: Melanoma, breast, lung

- *Lymphoma*

- *Multiple myeloma*

- *Brown tumors of skeleton* (hyperparathyroidism)

All of the above entities can have moderate to intense FDG activity. The diagnosis of sarcoidosis was suggested based on pulmonary findings of multiple peribronchovascular/subpleural nodules and proven by biopsy.

COMMENTS

Although bilateral hilar lymphadenopathy is the commonest radiologic finding in thoracic sarcoidosis, extrathoracic sarcoidosis can be an initial presentation in about one-half of symptomatic patients.

The extrathoracic organs that can be involved in sarcoidosis include peripheral nodes, skin, eyes, bone marrow, liver, spleen, upper respiratory tract, kidneys, central nervous system (CNS), joints, and endocrine and gastrointestinal (GI) system.

The histological hallmark of sarcoidosis is a nonnecrotizing granuloma with central core of histiocytes, epithelioid and giant cells surrounded by lymphocytes, fibroblasts, and collagen.

Pulmonary findings on CT include multiple peribronchovascular/perilymphatic and subpleural nodules, as seen in the index case.

On CT and MR, minimal hepatomegaly or splenomegaly may be seen. The common manifestation includes multiple hypoattenuating/hypointense nodules. Spleen is more often involved than liver. Gastric antrum is the commonest region to be involved in GI system.

About 5% to 10 % of patients may have skeletal involvement. The most commonly involved bones are the phalangeal bones. Cystic radiolucent regions and lacelike honeycomb appearances are common. In vertebrae, sarcoidosis can cause osteolytic lesions with preserved disc spaces. In the index case, more bone lesions were identified on PET than could be seen by CT alone.

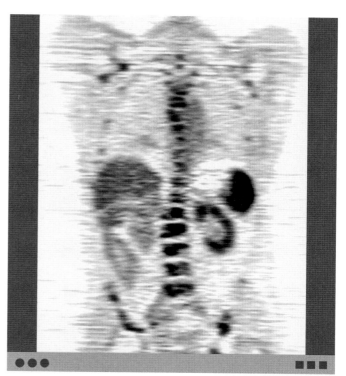

A. Extrapulmonary sarcoidosis involving spine, spleen, and multiple lymph nodes; 62-year-old male with corresponding CT.

It is difficult to recognize cardiac sarcoidosis on FDG-PET, as glucose is the substrate for normal myocardial metabolism. Extended fasting may be helpful in such cases.

Some studies suggest that ^{18}F-FDG-PET can detect pulmonary lesions to a similar degree as ^{67}Ga scintigraphy. However, ^{18}F-FDG-PET appears to be more accurate and contributes to a better evaluation of extrapulmonary involvement in sarcoidosis patients.

PEARLS

- Multisystem hypermetabolic lesions with no underlying risk factors for cancer may suggest systemic inflammatory disorder such as sarcoidosis.

- FDG-PET can be used for follow-up of sarcoidosis.

- FDG-PET seems to be better than gallium for evaluation of extrapulmonary sarcoidosis.

ADDITIONAL IMAGES (B-C)

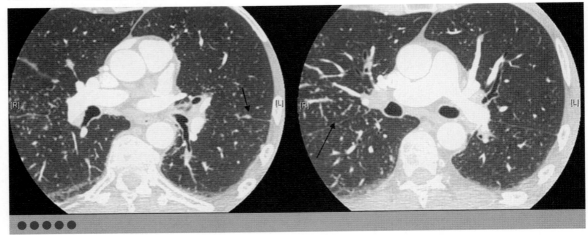

B. Multiple tiny perilymphatic nodules, axial CT, sarcoidosis.

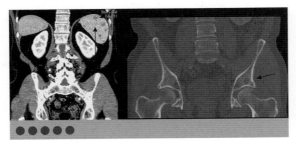

C. Coronal CT, right splenic hypodensities (*black arrow*) and left iliac lucent lesion (*black arrow*).

DIFFERENTIAL DIAGNOSIS IMAGES (D-K)

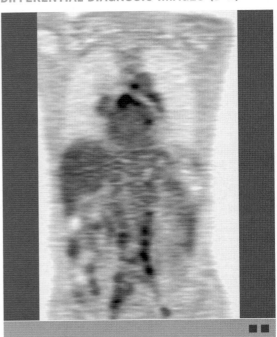

D. Reactive mediastinal and retroperitoneal nodal hyperplasia in 71-year-old female, unusually FDG avid. Coronal FDG-PET.

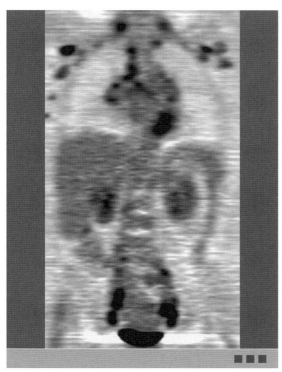

E. Extensive nodal sarcoidosis in PET for cholangiocarcinoma. Coronal FDG-PET.

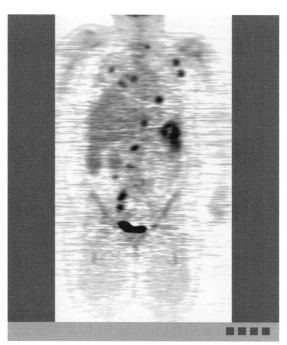

F. Extensive nodal, splenic, and lung involvement with non-Hodgkin lymphoma (NHL). Coronal FDG-PET.

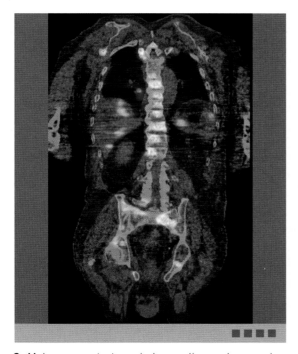

G. Melanoma metastases in bones, liver, spleen, and lungs; coronal fused FDG-PET/CT.

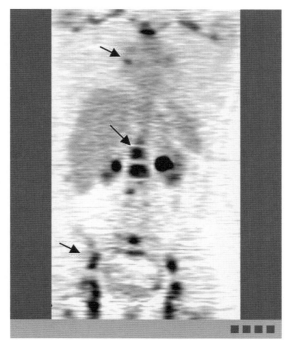

H. Nodal and bony metastases in breast cancer, coronal FDG-PET.

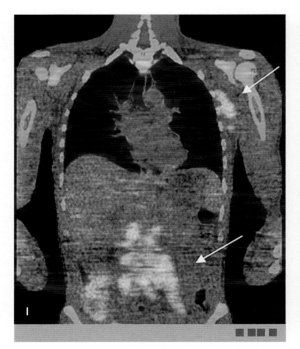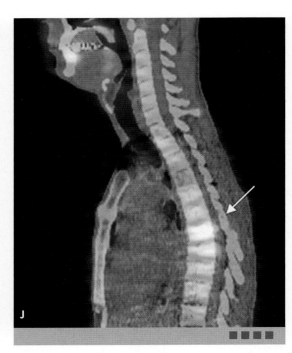

I. and **J.** Left axillary, retroperitoneal, and bony involvement in stage IV Hodgkin lymphoma.

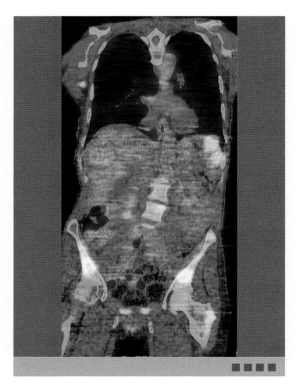

K. Splenic, skeletal, and right axillary nodal disease, NHL. Fused FDG-PET.

Vivek Manchanda, MD

PRESENTATION

A teenager with palpable left neck nodes. Biopsy showed Hodgkin disease (HD).

FINDINGS

Intensely increased metabolic activity related to left neck and mediastinal nodes.

DIFFERENTIAL DIAGNOSES

- *Stage I HD*
- *Stage II HD*
- *Stage III HD*
- *Stage IV HD*

COMMENTS

Ann Arbor staging of lymphoma can be substantiated with FDG-PET as follows:

Stage I: Involvement of a single lymph node region (I) or localized single extralymphatic organ or site (IE).

Stage II: Disease with two or more lymph node regions on the same side of the diaphragm (II) or localized single extra-lymphatic organ or site and its regional lymph node(s) with or without involvement of other lymph node regions on the same side of the diaphragm (IIE).

Stage III: Disease involving nodes on both sides of the diaphragm (III), which may also be accompanied by local-ized extralymphatic organ or site (IIIE), spleen (IIIS), or both (IIIE + S). Stage III disease may be subdivided as: (1) with disease limited above the renal vein; (2) with disease involvement of pelvic and/or para-aortic nodes.

Stage IV: Multifocal involvement of one or more extralym-phatic organs, with or without associated nodes or isolated extralymphatic organ with nonregional nodal involvement.

Studies have shown that FDG-PET is not reliable for excluding disease involvement of bone marrow. Even then, whole-body PET has proved to be a cost-effective and accurate method of staging HD.

Among the histological subtypes of HD, nodular scleros-ing is the commonest with typical mediastinal involvement.

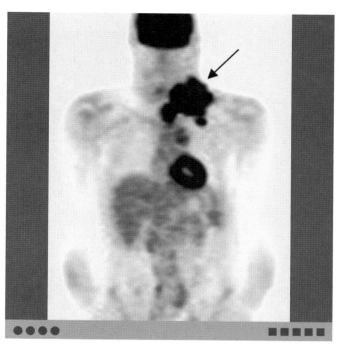

A. Stage II: Nodular sclerosing HD by FDG-PET with mediastinal and neck nodal involvement on the same side of diaphragm.

Majority of lymphocytic predominant and mixed cellularity lymphomas skip mediastinum and involve neck and abdomen. Most common extralymphatic relapse and vascular invasion occurs in lymphocytic depleted patients.

PEARLS

- Stages I and II HD involves disease on the same side of the diaphragm. Stage III involves disease on both sides of diaphragm and stage IV involves disease in extra-lymphatic organs, including bones.

- Nodular sclerosing is the commonest histological type of HD, which most commonly involves mediastinum.

- FDG-PET examination does not substitute for bone mar-row biopsy for staging purposes.

ADDITIONAL IMAGE

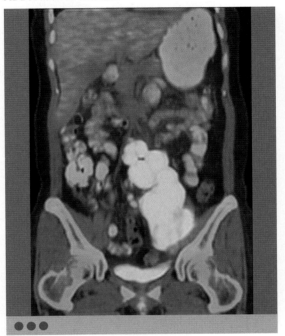

B. Stage II: Mixed cellularity HD with abdominal disease only.

DIFFERENTIAL DIAGNOSIS IMAGES (C-E)

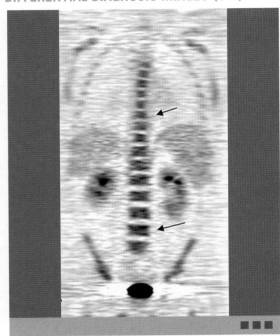

C. Stage IV: Nodular sclerosing HD, involvement of bone marrow on PET.

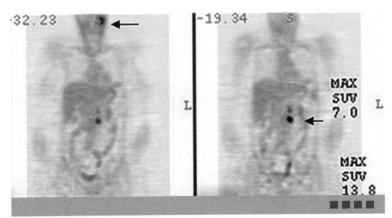

D. Stage III: Mixed cellularity HD with neck and abdominal disease, skipping mediastinum.

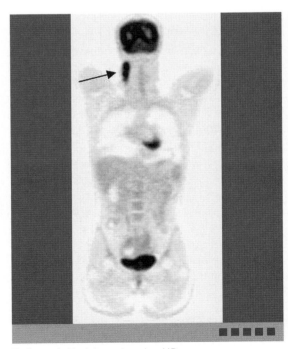

E. Stage I: Nodular sclerosing HD.

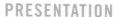

Vivek Manchanda, MD

PRESENTATION

Woman in her sixth decade of life with diffuse large B-cell lymphoma. Assess response to treatment.

FINDINGS

Complete resolution of FDG uptake, consistent with complete metabolic response, except for a single hypermetabolic thyroid nodule.

DIFFERENTIAL DIAGNOSES

- Partial metabolic response with residual disease in thyroid

- Complete metabolic response with primary thyroid cancer/thyroid adenoma

Since metastases to the thyroid gland are rare, the findings are most likely due to complete metabolic response to the treatment and a separate primary thyroid etiology. Biopsy showed papillary thyroid cancer in the patient with earlier diagnosis of diffuse large B-cell lymphoma.

COMMENTS

Diffuse large B-cell lymphomas are typically FDG avid and serial FDG scans can be used to assess treatment response.

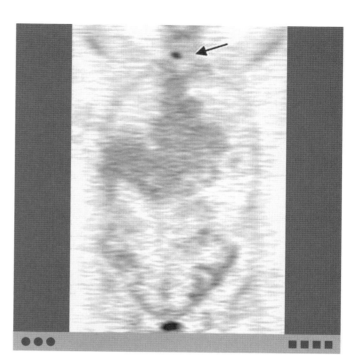

B. Complete metabolic response in the patient (*black arrow*), but persistent focal hypermetabolic activity in thyroid, biopsy-proven primary thyroid cancer. Coronal FDG-PET.

In complete metabolic response, there are no signs or symptoms of disease and there is no evidence of FDG-avid disease. Studies have suggested that bone marrow transplant in a patient who has demonstrated ongoing FDG-avid disease is more prone to a failed transplant in comparison to the patients with negative pretransplant FDG-PET scan.

A complete metabolic response would include resolution of previously seen FDG activity and no new FDG activity. Complete remission would include patients with negative FDG-PET and normal bone marrow by morphology and, if indeterminate, negative by immunohistochemistry, flow cytometry, and/or molecular genetics.

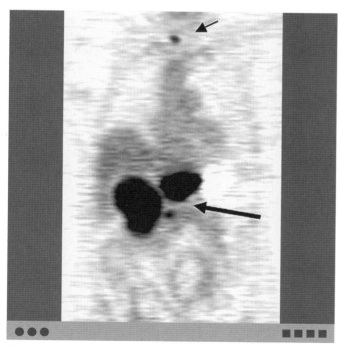

A. Hypermetabolic and large abdominal nodes, diffuse large B-cell lymphoma with focal hypermetabolic lesion in the thyroid. Coronal FDG-PET.

PEARLS

- FDG-PET/CT results in lymphoma can be summarized into complete metabolic response, partial metabolic response, no response, and worsened response.

- Transplanting a patient with PET-positive disease carries much worse prognosis than a patient with non–FDG-avid disease.

- FDG-PET cannot be used to assess treatment response in low-grade lymphomas which may not be FDG-avid to begin with.

A partial metabolic response would include residual PET-positive disease at previously noted site and no new site of metabolic activity.

No metabolic response would be no change to mild change in the level of FDG activity in previously noted nodes (<25% per some studies) and no new disease.

A worsening of metabolic response would include worsening of metabolic activity in previously noted disease and/or new sites of FDG-avid disease.

Some studies have included the size of lesions in the PET/CT report along with the metabolic responses, as part of the response criteria; with 50% increase or decrease in the longest diameter of the lesion being considered as relapse or partial response respectively and complete return of size to the baseline as complete response.

ADDITIONAL IMAGES (C-E)

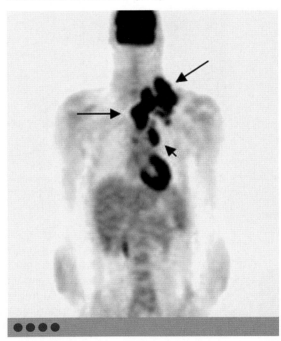

C. Hypermetabolic left neck and mediastinal nodes, Hodgkin disease (HD). Coronal FDG-PET.

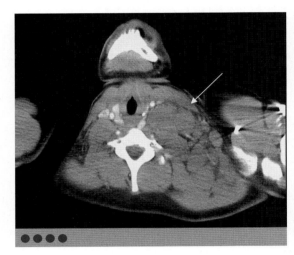

D. Corresponding CT.

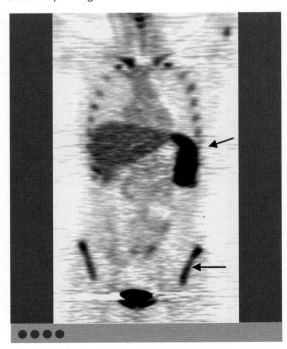

E. Follow-up PET after chemotherapy and granulocyte colony-stimulating factor (GCSF). Complete metabolic response. Coronal FDG-PET. Note FDG uptake in spleen and marrow (*arrows*), post GCSF.

DIFFERENTIAL DIAGNOSIS IMAGES (F-G)

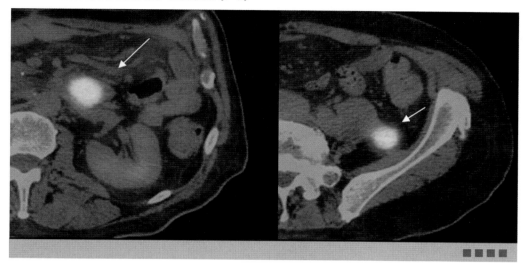

F. Pretransplant PET for NHL and arrows with disease in left renal hilum and left pelvis.

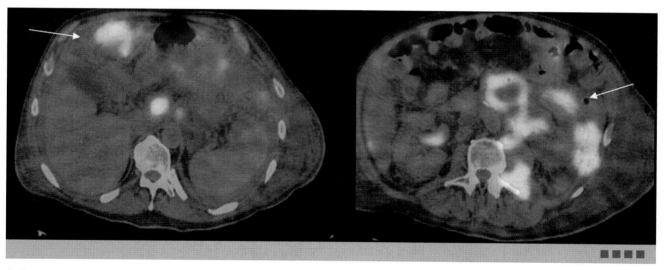

G. Post-transplant PET with clear progression of disease.

Joseph Rajendran, MD

PRESENTATION

A 56-year-old male presented with relapsed non-Hodgkin lymphoma (NHL) with multiple small lymph nodes in the axillae and mediastinum.

FINDINGS

Whole-body images obtained at 24 and 48 hours after the injection of 5 mCi of In-111 ibritumomab tiuxetan show normal biodistribution of the radioimmunoconjugate in the blood pool, liver, spleen, and kidneys.

DIFFERENTIAL DIAGNOSES

- *Abnormal liver uptake*: There is intense uptake in the liver with very minimal uptake in rest of the body. Therapy is contraindicated, as there is potential for severe hepatotoxicity.

- *Abnormal kidney uptake*: Both kidneys show uptake equal to that of the liver precluding therapy.

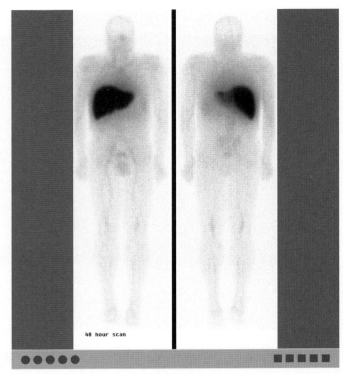

48 hour scan

B. Whole-body anterior and posterior planar images after the infusion of In-111 ibritumomab tiuxetan show intense uptake in the liver with very minimal uptake in rest of the body.

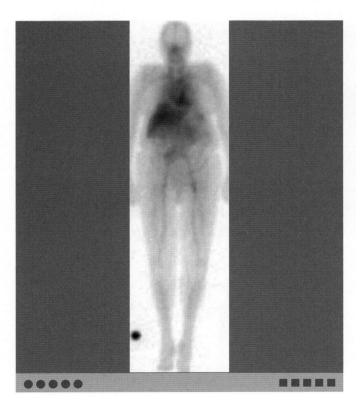

A. Whole-body anterior and posterior planar images after the infusion of In-111 ibritumomab tiuxetan show normal biodistribution in the body with blood pool, liver, spleen, and renal activity. Note uptake in the liver is the maximal.

PEARLS

- **Normal biodistribution of In-111 ibritumomab tiuxetan includes the blood pool, liver, spleen, and the kidneys with liver showing the highest uptake on all the images and is used as the reference organ. In-111 ibritumomab tiuxetan images should always be reviewed prior to deciding therapy with ^{90}Y ibritumomab tiuxetan.**

- **Lungs may show slightly higher uptake on early images but it usually decreases later. Lung uptake needs to be separated from that of mediastinal blood pool and uptake in any mediastinal and/or hilar lymph nodes when deciding on lung uptake.**

- **If the uptake in any organ is higher than that of the liver, then it is considered abnormal biodistribution. Similarly, if there is abnormal localization of uptake in any other vital organ such as the brain, it is considered abnormal biodistribution and the patient cannot be treated.**

- **The case examples presented here illustrate the importance of obtaining images after In-111 ibritumomab tiuxetan to identify patients who are at high risk for toxicity.**

COMMENTS

Radiolabeled ibritumomab tiuxetan (Zevalin) is one of the two radiopharmaceuticals approved by the FDA for radioimmunotherapy of NHL. For evaluating biodistribution, it is labeled with In-111 and for therapy it is labeled with Yttrium-90 (^{90}Y). The radiopharmaceutical targets CD20 antigens expressed in more than 80% of B cells in NHL. In addition to antibody-mediated effects, radiation results in cumulative therapeutic benefit by direct effects. There is also the advantage of cross-fire effect with the beta particles traversing and irradiating adjacent B cells irrespective of the expression levels. Even though unlabeled rituximab is infused prior to the labeled antibody, because of the uptake of this radiopharmaceutical on normal B lymphocytes, there is activity seen in the blood pool and normal organs such as liver, spleen, kidneys, lungs, bone marrow, etc. It is important to exclude abnormal biodistribution to reduce significant toxicities related to these organs. For this purpose, liver uptake is considered as the reference and is important to ensure that uptake in other organs is not higher than that of the liver in order to proceed to therapy. Usually tumor uptake is barely visualized, although on occasions prominent tumor uptake can be seen but it is not a requirement. Whole-body images (one set at 24 or 48 hours or both) following the infusion of 5 mCi of In-111-labeled antibody are obtained mainly to look at the biodistribution of the antibody. Other requirements for therapy include less than 25% marrow involvement, platelet count of greater than 100,000/mm^3, absolute neutrophil count (ANC) of greater than 1500/mm^3, and no known hypersensitivity. In one of our case examples, the entire uptake was seen in the liver indicating abnormal biodistribution meaning if therapy was administered, almost the entire quantity of the therapy dose would have localized in the liver, resulting in severe toxicity. Hence, these patients were not treated with ^{90}Y-labeled ibritumomab tiuxetan. Similarly the second case example shows uptake in both kidneys equal to that of the liver indicating caution in treating that patient.

DIFFERENTIAL DIAGNOSIS IMAGES (C-D)

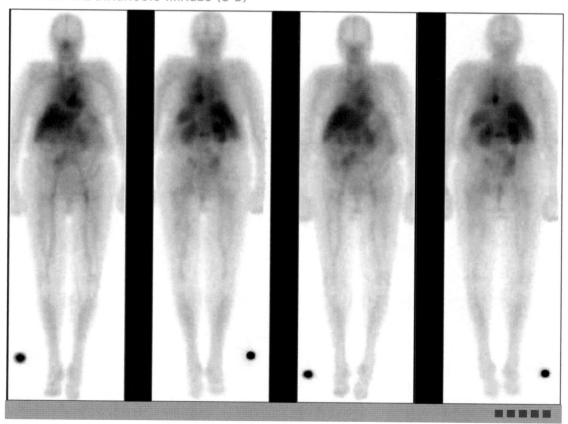

C. Whole-body anterior and posterior planar images after the infusion of In-111 ibritumomab tiuxetan show uptake in the kidneys equal to that of the liver.

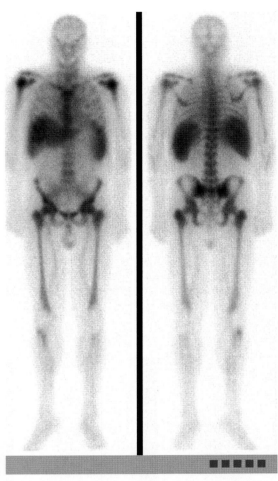

D. Anterior and posterior whole-body images after the infusion of In-111 ibritumomab tiuxetan show diffusely increased uptake in the bone marrow that is abnormal.

Vivek Manchanda, MD

PRESENTATION

Teenager after chemotherapy for Hodgkin disease.

FINDINGS

Intense diffusely increased FDG activity in spleen and bone marrow.

DIFFERENTIAL DIAGNOSES

- *Physiologic stimulation from marrow-stimulating drugs*
- *Leukemia*
- *Diffuse sarcoidosis*
- *Diffuse metastases*

COMMENTS

Splenic FDG uptake is normally less than that of liver. Diffusely increased FDG uptake in comparison to liver should be accounted for by exploring the history.

Diffuse, mildly increased FDG uptake in the spleen can be seen with hemolytic or iron deficiency anemia. It is commonly seen in patients who are undergoing chemotherapy, as a consequence of supportive therapy with cytokines. Bone marrow stimulants, such as granulocyte colony-stimulating factor (filgrastim, G-CSF), granulocyte/ macrophage colony-stimulating factor (GM-CSF), and occasionally erythropoietin can cause diffusely increased FDG uptake in bone marrow and in the spleen on PET. Isolated increased FDG activity in spleen without hypermetabolic activity in bone marrow from supportive cytokine therapy would be unusual.

Even though increased spleen size is no longer a criterion for disease involvement in patients with lymphoma, diffusely increased FDG activity in an enlarged spleen is more likely from lymphoma or leukemia or myelofibrosis rather than physiologic uptake. This pattern is more common in Hodgkin lymphoma as compared to non-Hodgkin lymphoma (which could be diffuse or focal). When the spleen is involved in lymphoma, extrasplenic disease is usually present.

Diffuse increased FDG activity in spleen from metastases (typically focal/multifocal) should be correlated with other imaging modalities/biopsy, especially if spleen is the only site of increased metabolic activity in the FDG-PET scan.

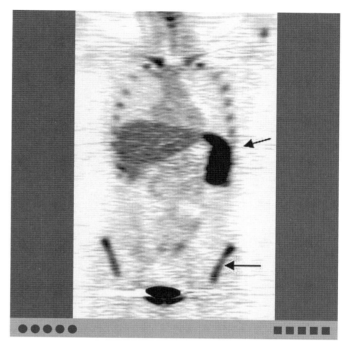

A. Diffuse FDG activity in the spleen and marrow due to G-CSF stimulation. Coronal FDG-PET.

Some other causes of diffusely increased FDG activity in the spleen include extramedullary hematopoiesis, in which focal hypermetabolic lesions can also be seen.

PEARLS

- Causes of diffuse intensely increased FDG uptake in the spleen include marrow-stimulating drugs and lymphoma (Hodgkin lymphoma > NHL). These drugs may be stopped for about 2 weeks before the scan.

- Mild diffuse increased FDG activity can be seen in anemias and extramedullary hematopoiesis and marrow-stimulating drugs.

- Diffuse increased FDG uptake in both lymphoma and leukemia could be variable (from mild to intense).

- Spleen size is not a determinant of disease involvement in lymphoma.

DIFFERENTIAL DIAGNOSIS IMAGES (B-E)

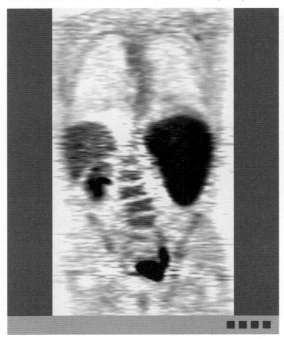

B. Diffuse FDG in an enlarged spleen, prolymphocytic leukemia. Coronal FDG-PET.

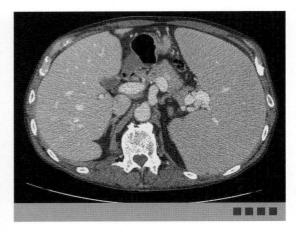

C. Corresponding CT.

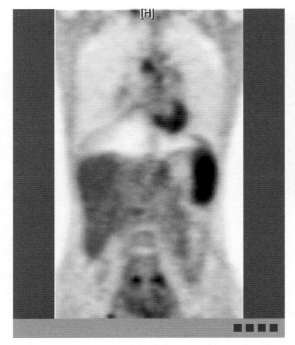

D. Diffusely hypermetabolic spleen and mediastinal node, mantle cell lymphoma. Coronal FDG-PET.

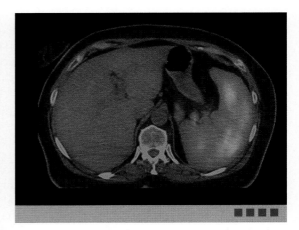

E. Diffusely hypermetabolic spleen in HD in 53-year-old female. Axial fused PET/CT.

Chapter 7

CNS

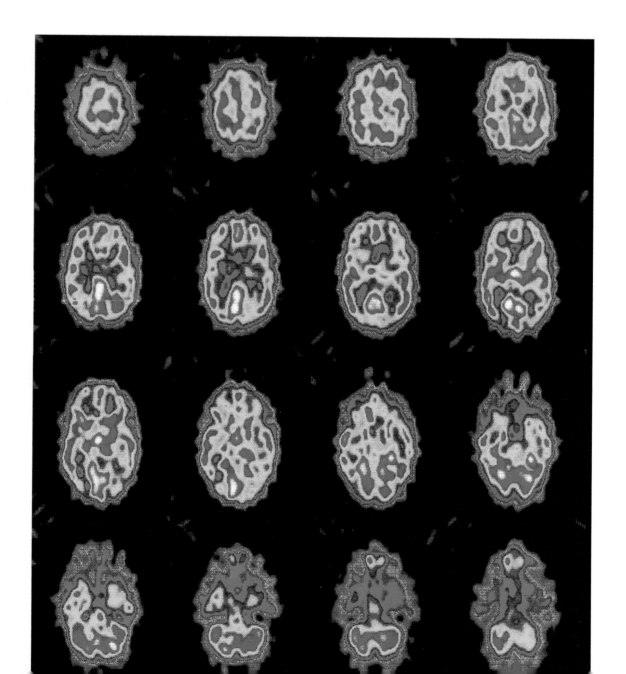

Bhasker R. Koppula, MD

PRESENTATION

Patients present with a history of full-blown AIDS and progressive neurocognitive and behavioral changes.

FINDINGS

Multiple patchy areas of hypoperfusion involving bilateral cerebral cortices including the cerebellum.

DIFFERENTIAL DIAGNOSES

• *HIV-related opportunistic infection.*

• Chronic cocaine or polydrug use shows a similar pattern of perfusion abnormalities with patchy distribution of hypoperfusion, involving cortical as well as the subcortical structures.

• *Multi-infarct dementia*: Brain single-photon emission computed tomography (SPECT) and PET images show multiple, bilateral asymmetric regions of hypoperfusion and hypometabolism, scattered throughout the cortex and deep structures.

• *Frontotemporal dementia*: MRI and CT imaging show a shrunken cortex with loss of volume in the frontal lobes and anterior poles of temporal lobes, with relatively normal parietal lobes. Functional imaging such as SPECT or PET may show reduced perfusion and hypometabolism in the frontal and temporal regions.

COMMENTS

AIDS dementia complex (ADC) is characterized by neurocognitive and motor features in adults with advanced AIDS and significantly decreased CD4+ lymphocyte counts. With the advent of highly active antiretroviral therapy, ADC is now not commonly seen in patients with AIDS. The cause of ADC is manifold, ranging from direct viral infection of neuronal cells to autoimmune process. Diagnosis is often from the history and clinical findings with help from laboratory tests including cerebrospinal fluid (CSF) analysis. However, imaging studies such as CT and MRI play key roles in the diagnosis of these conditions and show diffuse cortical atrophy. Brain SPECT and FDG-PET show changes in cerebral perfusion and metabolism in areas showing cortical atrophy on anatomic imaging. The changes are predominantly seen in the frontotemporal regions but can involve the entire cortex in late stages. With effective treatments now available for AIDS patients, functional imaging can be useful

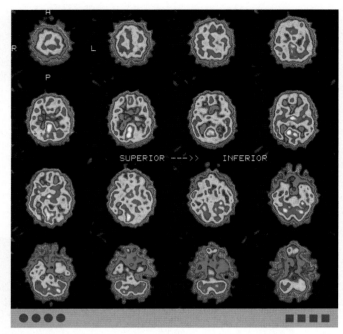

A. Tc99m HMPAO cerebral perfusion images show scattered, multifocal, patchy areas of hypoperfusion involving bilateral cerebral cortical regions. Also, there is hypoperfusion involving the cerebellum bilaterally. This is the typical pattern of perfusion abnormalities that is observed in patients with AIDS dementia. (*Image courtesy of David H. Lewis, MD.*)

in assessing treatment response in patients treated with antiretroviral therapy, even though the incidence of ADC has declined with modern therapy. Differential diagnoses include Alzheimer disease, HIV-associated opportunistic infections, and other neurodegenerative conditions and multiple sclerosis.

PEARLS

• **Patchy, multifocal cortical and subcortical regions of hypoperfusion, most frequently seen in the frontal, temporal, and parietal lobes and sometimes in the basal ganglia.**

• **Similar pattern of perfusion changes are also seen in chronic cocaine use and polydrug users.**

• **The perfusion pattern and the cognitive function improves with therapy with anti-HIV treatment, hence early detection is helpful in management.**

Bhasker R. Koppula, MD

PRESENTATION

Patients are typically in their sixth decade of life or older with a gradually worsening clinical history concerning for dementia with memory loss predominating.

FINDINGS

Significantly reduced perfusion to bilateral parietal lobes and minimally reduced perfusion to temporal lobes. Perfusion to occipital lobes is preserved as is to sensory motor cortex.

DIFFERENTIAL DIAGNOSES

- *Frontotemporal dementia*: MRI and CT imaging show the characteristic findings of a shrunken cortex with loss of volume in the frontal lobes and anterior poles of temporal lobes, with relatively normal parietal lobes. Functional imaging such as SPECT or PET may show reduced perfusion and hypometabolism in the frontal and temporal regions.

- *Multi-infarct dementia*: Brain SPECT and PET images show multiple bilateral asymmetric regions of hypoperfusion and hypometabolism, scattered throughout the cortex and deep structures.

- *Dementia with Lewy bodies (DLB)*: SPECT scanning or PET scanning shows decreased occipital lobe blood flow or metabolism in DLB but not in Alzheimer disease (AD).

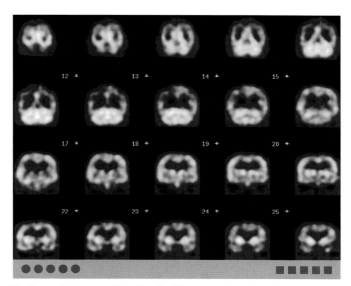

B. Coronal views confirm the findings noted on the axial images. These images also show preservation of perfusion to the basal ganglia and thalami. (*Image courtesy of Bhasker R. Koppula, MD.*)

COMMENTS

AD is the commonest of all dementias, and is an acquired cognitive and behavioral impairment of significant severity that interferes with social and occupational functioning. AD affects about 5 million people in the United States and is a major socioeconomic strain. The major hallmark of AD is neurofibrillary tangles (NFTs); senile plaques (SPs) at the microscopic level; and cerebrocortical atrophy, which predominantly involves the association regions and particularly the medial aspect of the temporal lobe. The incidence of AD is most prevalent in people older than 60 years, although forms of familial early-onset AD can appear as early as in the third decade. In assessing AD, brain MRIs or CT scans typically show diffuse cortical and/or cerebral atrophy. Cerebral blood flow (CBF) with Tc-99m hexamethylpropyleneamine oxime (HMPAO) SPECT, or ethylene-cysteine dimer (ECD)

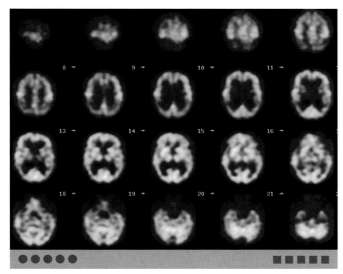

A. Axial images of Tc-99m ECD show significantly reduced perfusion to the bilateral parietal lobes and minimally reduced perfusion to temporal lobes. Perfusion to occipital lobes and the sensorimotor cortex is preserved. (*Image courtesy of Bhasker R. Koppula, MD.*)

PEARLS

- AD is typically seen in people who are 60 years and older and a majority of the cases are diagnosed on the basis of clinical and social history.

- Both FDG-PET and Tc-99m brain SPECT have similar sensitivities in making the diagnosis.

- Typical cases show symmetric hypoperfusion in the parietal, posterior cingulate gyrus regions with maintained perfusion to sensorimotor and visual cortices.

SPECT when used, helps characterize atypical presentations, such as language disorders (eg, progressive aphasia), visuospatial dysfunction syndromes, or other conditions that may be confused with cerebrovascular disease or other neurodegenerative conditions. The characteristic pattern of changes with parietotemporal reduction in blood flow helps in pinpointing the diagnosis but may be limited in distinguishing early cases of AD. Visual and sensorimotor cortices are relatively spared. Characteristically, there is reduced perfusion to posterior cingulate gyrus. The role of SPECT imaging is to help make the diagnosis in equivocal cases.

DIFFERENTIAL DIAGNOSES IMAGES (C-F)

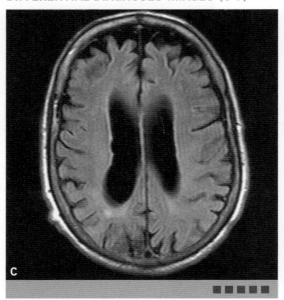 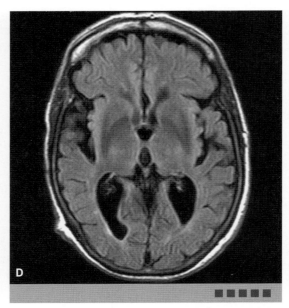

C. and **D.** Selective axial MRI images show diffuse volume loss which is nonspecific. The characteristic pattern of perfusion abnormalities as seen on the brain SPECT images is consistent with the diagnosis of AD. (*Images courtesy of Bhasker R. Koppula, MD.*)

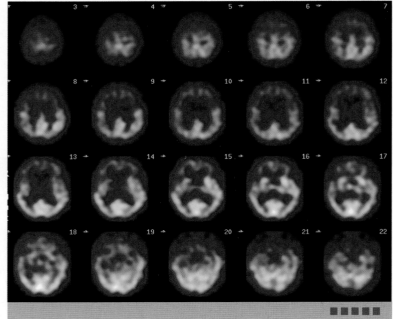

E. Axial brain SPECT images performed using Tc-99m ECD show significantly reduced perfusion to the frontal lobes bilaterally. Also, bilateral temporal lobes show decreased perfusion though not as severely as the frontal lobes. (*Image courtesy of Bhasker R. Koppula, MD.*)

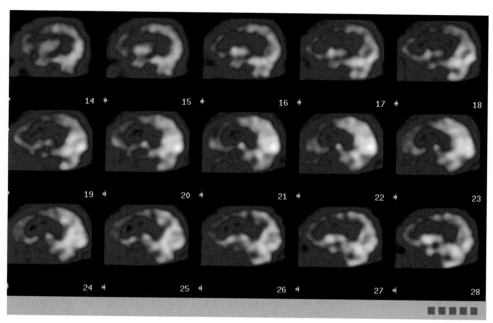

F. SPECT images obtained in sagittal orientation confirm the findings of decreased perfusion to bilateral frontal and temporal regions. Perfusion to the parietal lobes and the occipital lobes is well preserved. (*Image courtesy of Bhasker R. Koppula, MD.*)

Bhasker R. Koppula, MD

PRESENTATION

Patients are typically in post–severe cardiovascular event, resulting in multiorgan failure and kept on life support. Referral for this study is to evaluate brain function to confirm the diagnosis of brain death to corroborate clinical and other findings.

FINDINGS

Planar images from brain death study show no evidence of radiotracer accumulation in the brain parenchyma, consistent with brain death.

COMMENTS

Brain death diagnosis is primarily clinical. Accuracy and speed in making the diagnosis is very important when organ donation is considered and life support systems must be continued. Clinical diagnosis may be difficult because of the specific criteria necessary to make the diagnosis of brain death, as follows: The patient must be in deep coma with total absence of brain stem reflexes of spontaneous respiration. Potentially reversible causes such as drug

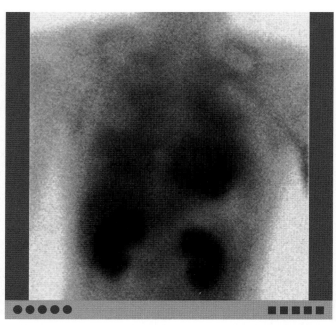

B. Planar images of the chest and abdomen show no uptake in the thyroid gland or stomach, excluding the presence of free pertechnetate and ensuring efficient labeling. (*Image courtesy of Bhasker R. Koppula, MD.*)

intoxication, metabolic derangement, or hypothermia must be excluded and other causes of the brain dysfunction must be established. The radionuclide brain death study is usually performed when the EEG and clinical criteria are equivocal. It is simple, rapid, and can be performed at the bedside with a portable camera. Scintigraphy is not affected by drug intoxication or hypothermia. An abnormal radionuclide

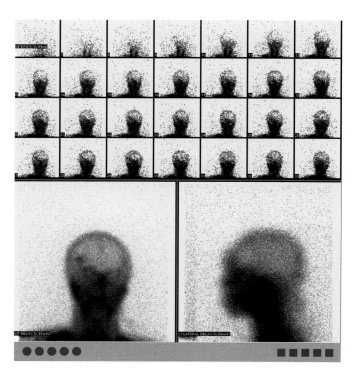

A. Sequential images of radionuclide angiogram (top) and planar anterior and left lateral images of the head show no radiotracer activity in the brain parenchyma, consistent with brain death. (top) and planar anterior and left lateral images. (*Image courtesy of Bhasker R. Koppula, MD.*)

PEARLS

- Hot nose sign is nonspecific and can also be seen in internal carotid artery occlusion without brain death. This sign can be seen with a generalized decrease of cerebral perfusion from various causes, including severe cerebrovascular or carotid occlusive disease or increased intracranial pressure of any cause.

- Radionuclide techniques are independent of interfering conditions and do not require withdrawal of medical therapy, and are very helpful in conditions described above.

- Even though brain perfusion study is highly sensitive to establish brain death, radionuclide cerebral perfusion study alone should not be used to diagnose brain death.

angiogram showing no cerebral perfusion is more specific for brain death than an isoelectric EEG. Brain death can be diagnosed using a radionuclide flow study alone because the lack of intracerebral blood flow is diagnostic. Technetium-labeled radiopharmaceuticals like Tc-99m-diethylene triamine pentaacetic acid (DTPA) are used to assess dynamic flow. Tc-99m-DTPA is rapidly cleared from the blood allowing a repeat study if necessary. Tc-99m-HMPAO and Tc-99m-ECD studies are easier to interpret and are now preferred to Tc-99m-DTPA. Flow images can be obtained but are not necessary because delayed images will show the fixed presence or absence of brain uptake, requiring flow to the brain. If no CBF is present, no cerebral uptake will occur. Planar images are adequate, and SPECT is not necessary to diagnose brain death. Diagnostic findings of brain death include the lack of intracranial arterial flow or major venous sinuses on subsequent static images. Flow to both common carotid arteries is seen to the level of the base of the skull. No visualization of the brain is seen with Tc-99m-HMPAO. Often the hot nose sign is seen as an increasing intracranial perfusion that diverts intracranial blood flow into external carotid circulation, resulting in relatively increased flow to the face and nose. Faint visualization of the venous sagittal or transverse sinus in the absence of intracranial perfusion is also sometimes seen on Tc-99m-DTPA scans. Hot nose sign can be seen with a generalized decrease of cerebral perfusion from various causes, including severe cerebrovascular or carotid occlusive disease or increased intracranial pressure of any cause. Because of such factors as variable anatomy, delayed images may be difficult to interpret. Furthermore, flow images may be inadequate due to poor bolus technique or computer malfunction. Therefore, Tc-99m-DTPA is clearly less desirable than Tc-99m-HMPAO. Although actual diagnosis of brain death should not be made using nuclear imaging techniques alone, these techniques are important supportive evidence of such a diagnosis in the proper clinical setting corroborating other methods of diagnosis. Radionuclide techniques are independent of interfering conditions and do not require withdrawal of medical therapy. They may be especially helpful in the settings of hypothermia, intoxication with fentanyl, barbiturates, or pancuronium, and hypovolemic shock, when EEG recordings are not possible because of significant head injury or in instances in which clinical examination is not conclusive.

Bhasker R. Koppula, MD

PRESENTATION

Patients in their sixth decade or above, present with behavioral symptoms or language disorders. Neurocognitive functions such as memory are typically preserved. Visual hallucination predominates in many patients.

FINDINGS

Brain SPECT images show significantly decreased perfusion to the frontal as well as the temporal lobes.

DIFFERENTIAL DIAGNOSES

- *Alzheimer disease*: The symptoms of memory loss predominate presentation. SPECT shows the characteristically reduced perfusion in the bilateral parietal lobes. Frontotemporal decreased perfusion can be seen in rare cases.

- *Depression*: Can occur at any age and symptoms of mood depression predominate and typically the temporal lobes show normal perfusion.

- *Huntington disease*: Psychotic changes predominate in this condition and there is movement disorder.

COMMENTS

Frontotemporal dementia (FTD) that accounts for about 10% of all dementias in the elderly population is a clinical

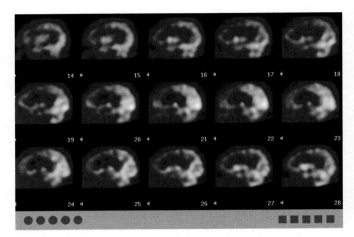

B. SPECT images obtained in sagittal orientation confirm the findings of decreased perfusion to bilateral frontal and temporal regions. Perfusion to the parietal lobes and the occipital lobes is well preserved. (*Image courtesy of Bhasker R. Koppula, MD.*)

syndrome associated with shrinking of the frontal and temporal anterior lobes of the brain. It was previously known as Pick disease. The symptoms of FTD are of two clinical patterns that involve either (1) changes in behavior, or (2) problems with language, all as a result of the predominant location of the pathology. The first type features behavior that can be either impulsive (disinhibited) or bored and listless (apathetic) and includes inappropriate social behavior; the second type of symptoms are primarily due to language disturbance, including difficulty making or understanding speech, and are frequently combined with the behavioral symptoms. Neurocognitive functions such as spatial skills and memory remain preserved. There is a strong genetic component to the disease and FTD often runs in families. MR imaging plays a key role in establishing the diagnosis along with neuropsychiatric assessment. In FTD, MRI shows a shrunken cortex with volume loss and sometimes asymmetric frontal lobes as well as temporal lobes, with relatively normal parietal

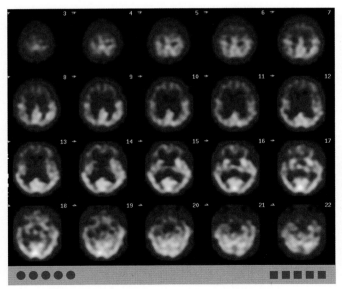

A. Axial brain SPECT images performed using Tc-99m-ECD show significantly reduced perfusion to the frontal lobes bilaterally. Also, bilateral temporal lobes show decreased perfusion though not as severely as the frontal lobes. (*Image courtesy of Bhasker R. Koppula, MD.*)

PEARLS

- **Brain SPECT imaging helps confirm the diagnosis and in the follow-up of patients.**

- **Typical presentation is decreased blood flow to frontal and temporal lobes as well as visual cortex. The latter is responsible for much of the visual hallucination reported in these patients.**

- **Memory loss is secondary and may be absent in sharp contrast to Alzheimer disease.**

lobes. Functional imaging such as SPECT or PET may show reduced perfusion in the frontal and temporal regions in the axial and sagittal projections. Tc-99m-HMPAO or ECD

is typically used for brain SPECT imaging. In addition to visual assessment of perfusion, semiquantitative analysis would help in confirming the diagnosis when subtle changes are present.

DIFFERENTIAL DIAGNOSIS IMAGES (C-E)

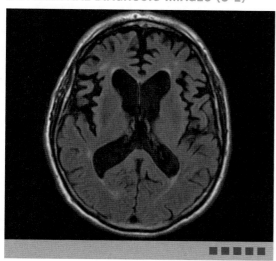

C. Selective transverse axial MRI image shows volume loss with prominent sulcal spaces in bilateral frontal and temporal regions. The posterior sulcal spaces are well preserved in parietal and occipital regions. This finding along with the characteristic brain SPECT findings confirms the diagnosis of frontotemporal dementia. Also, note prominent lateral ventricles bilaterally related to volume loss. (*Image courtesy of Bhasker R. Koppula, MD.*)

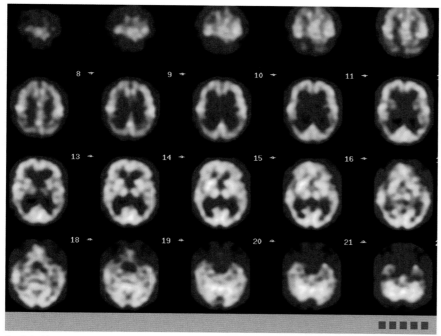

D. Axial images of Tc-99m-ECD show significantly reduced perfusion to the bilateral parietal lobes and minimally reduced perfusion to temporal lobes. Perfusion to occipital lobes and the sensory motor cortex is preserved. (*Image courtesy of Bhasker R. Koppula, MD.*)

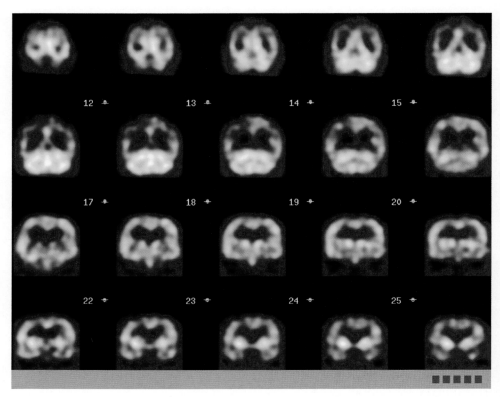

E. Coronal views confirm the findings noted on the axial images. These images also show preservation of perfusion to the basal ganglia and thalami. (*Image courtesy of Bhasker R. Koppula, MD.*)

Bhasker R. Koppula, MD

PRESENTATION

Patients in their sixth decade or above present with confusion and visual hallucinations and movement disorders that typically start simultaneously in contrast to Parkinson disease.

FINDINGS

Severely decreased perfusion in bilateral posterior occipital cortices, and bilateral parietotemporal association cortices.

DIFFERENTIAL DIAGNOSES

- *Alzheimer disease*: Most common cause of senile dementia with the typical finding on brain SPECT of symmetric bilateral posterior temporal and parietal perfusion defects (posterior association cortices). Occipital lobes, sensory motor cortex, and cerebellum are typically spared.

- *Frontotemporal dementia*: MRI and CT imaging show the characteristic findings of a shrunken cortex with loss of volume in the frontal lobes and anterior poles of temporal lobes, with relatively normal parietal lobes. Functional imaging such as SPECT or PET may show reduced perfusion and hypometabolism in the frontal and temporal regions.

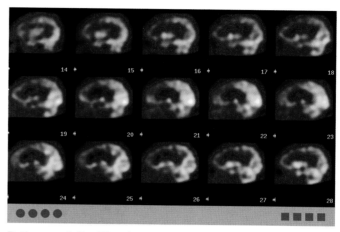

B. Representative T1-weighted axial MRI images show diffuse atrophic changes, most prominent in bilateral temporal regions. Also note periventricular ischemic white matter changes. No diffusion abnormality is identified on the diffusion-weighted images. (*Image courtesy of Bhasker R. Koppula, MD.*)

- *Parkinson disease*: Late stages of Parkinson disease can present with the same findings as dementia with Lewy bodies (DLB), but the long-standing history of movement disorder precedes the onset of dementia as opposed to absence of such history in DLB.

- *Multi-infarct dementia*: Brain SPECT and PET images show multiple, bilateral asymmetric regions of hypoperfusion and hypometabolism, scattered throughout the cortex and deep structures.

COMMENTS

DLB is a primary neurodegenerative dementia characterized by the presence of Lewy bodies in cortical, subcortical, and brain stem structures and is the second most common degenerative dementia after Alzheimer disease. Clinically,

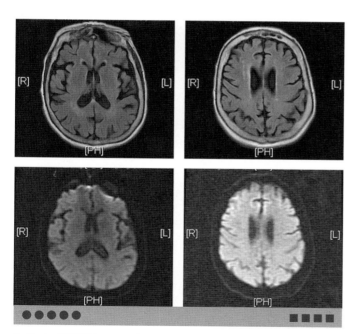

A. Brain SPECT images show severely decreased perfusion in bilateral occipital cortices, and bilateral parietotemporal association cortices. Also, note mildly decreased perfusion in frontal association cortex and posterior cingulate gyrus, left more than right. (*Image courtesy of Bhasker R. Koppula, MD.*)

PEARLS

- Brain SPECT shows characteristic posterior hypoperfusion including the occipital lobes, particularly visual cortex.

- Patients may present with movement disorders at the same time as dementia.

- Late stages of Parkinson disease can present with the same findings as DLB, but the long-standing history of movement disorder precedes the onset of dementia.

DLB is difficult to distinguish from Parkinson disease (which is most likely in the same spectrum of illnesses) or from Alzheimer disease. Patients present with fluctuating dementia, multiple falls, and parkinsonian symptoms and visual hallucinations. In DLB, the onset of movement disorder is at the same time as that of dementia. Major clinical criteria include fluctuation in cognition, visual hallucinations, spontaneous parkinsonism. Minor criteria include recurrent falls, syncope, delusions, other hallucinations, rapid eye movement (REM) sleep disorder, and depression. Functional imaging with PET and SPECT shows hypoperfusion or metabolism in the posterior cortex similar to that of AD but has a greater tendency to involve occipital lobes. Hippocampal uptake may be preserved in DLB. Occipital lobe is not affected histopathologically but metabolic or perfusional reduction is present in the occipital lobe particularly visual cortex, whereas the medial temporal limbic area is minimally affected histopathologically.

DIFFERENTIAL DIAGNOSIS IMAGES (C-F)

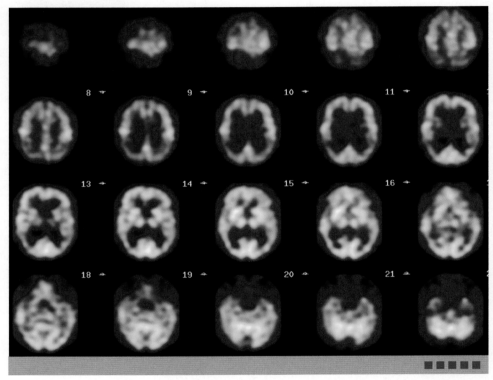

C. Axial images of Tc-99m-ECD show significantly reduced perfusion to the bilateral parietal lobes and minimally reduced perfusion to temporal lobes. Perfusion to occipital lobes and the sensory motor cortex is preserved. (*Image courtesy of Bhasker R. Koppula, MD.*)

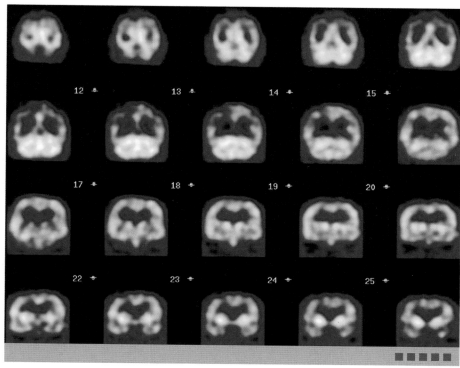

D. Coronal views confirm the findings noted on the axial images. These images also show preservation of perfusion to the basal ganglia and thalami. (*Image courtesy of Bhasker R. Koppula, MD*)

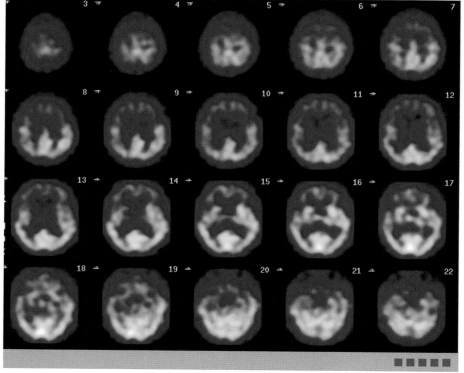

E. Axial brain SPECT images performed using Tc-99m-ECD show significantly reduced perfusion to the frontal lobes bilaterally. Also, bilateral temporal lobes show decreased perfusion though not as severely as the frontal lobes. (*Image courtesy of Bhasker R. Koppula, MD.*)

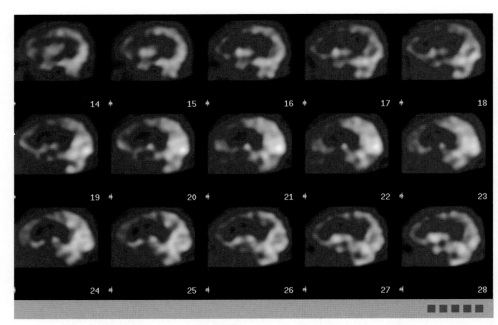

F. SPECT images obtained in sagittal orientation confirm the findings of decreased perfusion to bilateral frontal and temporal regions. Perfusion to the parietal lobes and the occipital lobes is well preserved. (*Image courtesy of Bhasker R. Koppula, MD.*)

Joseph Rajendran, MD

PRESENTATION

Symptoms and clinical course show wide variation from transient events to severe neurologic deficits. Adults present with acute hemorrhagic events compared to more ischemic events seen in children.

FINDINGS

Cerebral infarction on CT and MRI. Decreased cerebral blood flow reserve on acetazolamide (Diamox) challenge test and characteristic "puff of smoke" appearance on angiography—the features consistent with diagnosis of Moyamoya disease (MMD).

DIFFERENTIAL DIAGNOSES

- *Sickle cell disease, radiation arteriopathy*: Cause progressive obliteration of intracranial carotid arteries but clinical history would be diagnostic.

- *Other disease states*: Autoimmune vasculitis syndromes like systemic lupus erythematosus (SLE), meningitis,

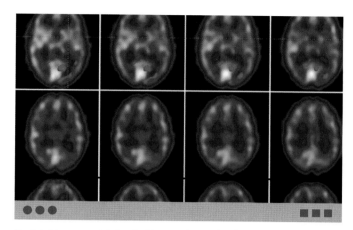

B. Axial images obtained after semiquantitative processing using HERMES software confirm and highlight the difference in perfusion that was noted on the SPECT image.

Downs syndrome, von Recklinghausens disease and head trauma.

These can have similar findings but the history and associated findings clinch the diagnosis.

COMMENTS

MMD is a progressive cerebrovascular disease characterized by stenosis or occlusion at the distal internal carotid arteries and the proximal anterior cerebral and/or the middle cerebral artery with compensatory development of abnormal Moyamoya vessels at the base of the brain. The term "moyamoya" in Japanese means "puff of smoke," describing the characteristic angiographic appearance of extensive abnormal vascular collateral networks that develop.

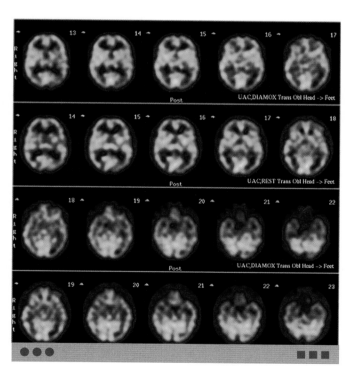

A. Tc-99m-ECD brain SPECT posterior images in axial orientation with acetazolamide challenge (rows 1 and 3) and without acetazolamide challenge (rows 2 and 4) show reduced perfusion in the left posterior parieto-occipital region on acetazolamide challenge images. This region shows improved perfusion on images obtained without acetazolamide challenge.

PEARLS

- **Differential perfusion on acetazolamide challenge. The difference in perfusion can be subtle and might require semiquantitative analysis.**

- **Brain SPECT imaging is a noninvasive method and helps confirm the diagnosis and in the follow-up of patients after surgical intervention.**

- **Allergy to sulpha drugs can cause cross reactivity to acetazolamide and should be borne in mind prior to administering the drug.**

- **Patients may feel distaste from acetazolamide injection.**

Pathologically, MMD is characterized by intimal thickening in the walls of the terminal portions of the internal carotid vessels bilaterally. The anterior, middle, and posterior cerebral arteries arising from the circle of Willis may show varying degrees of stenosis or occlusion, resulting in numerous small vascular channels around the circle of Willis. Patients present with hemiparesis, monoparesis, sensory impairment, involuntary movements, headaches, dizziness, or seizures. All of these are common to both children and adults, but adults present with sudden onset of intraventricular, subarachnoid, or intracerebral hemorrhage. Although there is no cure for MMD, early identification of the disease process will help treat the complications of the disease. Brain perfusion SPECT images obtained with and without acetazolamide help clinch the diagnosis and identify the blood flow reserve.

Acetazolamide increases the regional cerebral blood flow (rCBF) in normal vasculature by approximately 55% to 70% by inhibiting the carbonic anhydrase enzyme, thus reducing the pH. In MMD, there is decreased reactivity to acetazolamide due to a decreased cerebral vascular reserve secondary to vasodilation in the resting state as a compensatory mechanism for proximal stenosis and/or occlusion. This results in relatively low perfusion compared to blood flow in normal tissue on images obtained after administration of acetazolamide. Reduced perfusion to the affected regions is clearly identified after acetazolamide administration and is the result of shunting of blood away from diseased blood vessels, showing altered perfusion compared to another brain SPECT perfusion study obtained without acetazolamide challenge.

ADDITIONAL IMAGES (C-E)

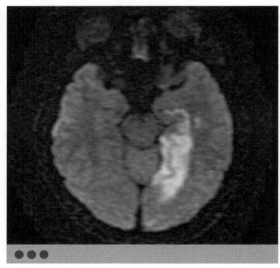

C. Axial diffusion-weighted MR image shows diffusion restriction in temporal and occipital cortices consistent with infarction.

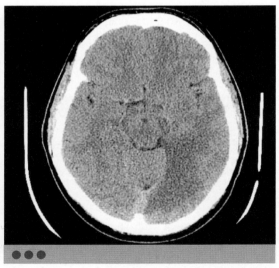

D. Noncontrast-enhanced CT (NECT) scan of the head shows the abnormality in the left posterior parietal/ temporal and occipital cortices, with hypodensity consistent with infarction. Note obliteration of the sulcal spaces related to brain edema.

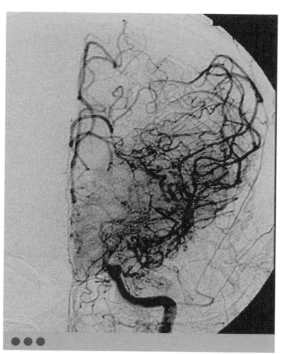

E. Carotid angiogram shows the characteristic "puff of smoke" appearance, diagnostic of MMD.

Bhasker R. Koppula, MD

PRESENTATION

An 81-year-old female with confusion, gait disturbances with frequent falls, and urinary incontinence.

DIFFERENTIAL DIAGNOSES

- *Cerebral atrophy (age-related or ex vacuo ventriculomegaly)*: Sulcal enlargement in proportion to ventricular enlargement. The gyri are rounded in contrast to normal pressure hydrocephalus (NPH) where they are flattened against the inner table of the calvarium due to pressure by the enlarged ventricles pushing the cerebral cortex toward the calvarium.

- *Alzheimer disease*: Most common cause of dementia presenting with progressive loss of memory. Brain SPECT shows the characteristically reduced perfusion in the bilateral parietal lobes with sparing of the visual and sensorimotor cortices and the cerebellum.

- *Noncommunicating hydrocephalus*: Associated with elevated CSF pressures and papilledema. Enlarged ventricles with obliteration of the sulcal spaces. Radionuclide scintigraphy shows normal pattern of flow of the radiotracer without any evidence of ventricular reflux of the tracer.

- *Parkinsonism*: Results from lack of dopamine-producing cells in the basal ganglia. Characterized by resting tremor, cog-wheel rigidity, bradykinesia, and postural instability. Gait of patients with NPH is bradykinetic, broad-based, and shuffling.

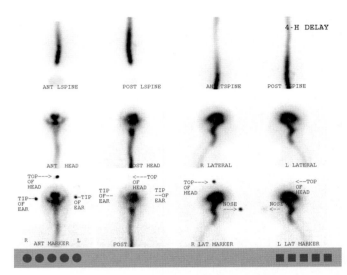

B. Anterior and posterior images obtained 4 hours after the tracer injection again show increasing reflux of the tracer into the lateral ventricles. Note the normal "trident" appearance of tracer accumulation at the basal cisterns is replaced by the "heart"-shaped configuration, which results from the tracer reflux into the lateral ventricles. (*Image courtesy of Bhasker R. Koppula, MD.*)

COMMENTS

NPH is characterized by triad of gait disturbances, dementia, and urinary incontinence, in the presence of normal CSF pressure and absence of papilledema. Approximately, 50% of cases of NPH are idiopathic, probably related to a

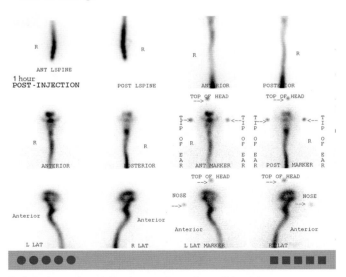

A. Anterior and posterior images by radionuclide cisternogram obtained 1 hour after injection of In-111 DTPA confirms thecal injection of the tracer and shows ascent of the tracer into the basal cisterns. There is early reflux of the tracer into the lateral ventricles. Ventricular reflux of the tracer is confirmed on the lateral images. (*Image courtesy of Bhasker R. Koppula, MD.*)

PEARLS

- Although NPH is a relatively rare cause of dementia, accounting for approximately 5% of cases, identifying NPH is important because it is one of the few treatable causes of dementia.

- NPH closely resembles Parkinson disease (PD) with similar gait disturbances. However, lack of tremor and rigidity differentiates PD from NPH as is the lack of response to carbidopa/levodopa.

- Patients with persistent ventricular reflux and no activity over the convexities are most likely to benefit from interventions like CSF shunting procedure.

- No true ataxia or weakness is present in NPH; hence, the gait disturbance in NPH is described as gait apraxia.

- Traditionally, the success of CSF shunting in NPH is reported as follows: one-third of patients improve, one-third experience arrested symptom progression, and the remaining one-third continue to deteriorate.

deficiency of arachnoid granulations. In the other 50% of patients, there is antecedent history of subarachnoid hemorrhage, trauma, meningitis, infection, carcinomatosis, or surgery, which alters the CSF flow dynamics. The periventricular white matter is stretched and becomes dysfunctional, resulting in decreased perfusion without actually being infracted. The resulting anatomic distortion results in the classic symptoms of this condition. Dementia, in this condition, is subcortical in nature and results from distortion of the periventricular limbic system. Disruption of periventricular white matter tracts and distortion of the central portion of the corona radiata by the enlarged ventricles, which innervates the bladder and legs, explains the gait disturbances and incontinence. Decreased perfusion without infarction is attributed to partial success of CSF shunting, which reduces the stretching of the periventricular white matter tracts and restores some perfusion. CT scan or MRI alone is not sufficient for diagnosis and may show disproportionate ventricular enlargement in relation to sulcal atrophy, thinning and elevation of the corpus callosum, rounding of the frontal horns, and prominent periventricular hyperintensity due to transependymal flow of CSF. Prominent flow void in the aqueduct and the third ventricle, the so-called "Jet sign," can also be seen on MRI, which presents a dark aqueduct and third ventricle on T2-weighted images, where the remainder of the CSF appears bright. On radionuclide cisternography, normally the tracer reaches the basal cisterns by 2 to 4 hours, sylvian fissure by 6 hours, and cerebral convexities by 12 hours with most of the activity clearing into the sagittal sinus by 24 hours. There should not be any reflux into the ventricles. In NPH, which is a communicating type of hydrocephalus, there is absent flow or delay of activity appearing over the cerebral convexities associated with early and persistent reflux of tracer into the lateral ventricles. Reflux of the tracer could also be transient. Clearance of the tracer activity from over the cerebral convexities is very much delayed well beyond the normal 24 hours. Cerebral atrophy can also cause delayed tracer movement through the enlarged subarachnoid space, sometimes associated with transient reflux into ventricles. However, the tracer activity clears by 24 hours over the cerebral convexities.

ADDITIONAL IMAGES (C-D)

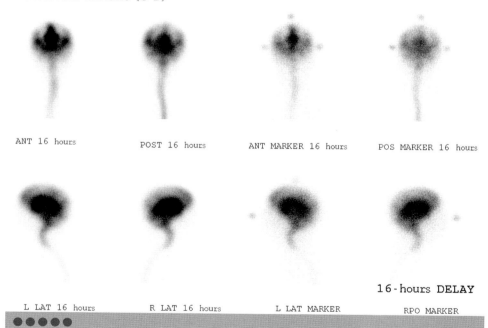

ANT 16 hours   POST 16 hours   ANT MARKER 16 hours   POS MARKER 16 hours

16-hours **DELAY**

L LAT 16 hours   R LAT 16 hours   L LAT MARKER   RPO MARKER

C. Delayed anterior and posterior images after 16 hours show persistent tracer activity in the lateral ventricles. Note the tracer activity along the cerebral convexities. (*Image courtesy of Bhasker R. Koppula, MD.*)

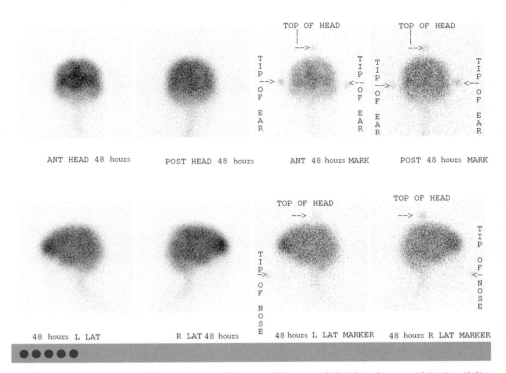

ANT HEAD 48 hours   POST HEAD 48 hours   ANT 48 hours MARK   POST 48 hours MARK

48 hours L LAT   R LAT 48 hours   48 hours L LAT MARKER   48 hours R LAT MARKER

D. Anterior and posterior images obtained 48 hours after tracer injection show persistent activity over the cerebral convexities. The combination of features including the persistent reflux of the tracer into the ventricle and delayed clearance of activity from the cerebral convexities is consistent with the diagnosis of normal pressure hydrocephalus. (*Image courtesy of Bhasker R. Koppula, MD.*)

Bhasker R. Koppula, MD

PRESENTATION

Patients in their young adulthood presenting with intractable seizures since childhood.

FINDINGS

Focus of hyperperfusion in the medial temporal lobe on the ictal images.

DIFFERENTIAL DIAGNOSES

- *Frontal lobe epilepsy*: They appear in clusters of many brief seizures with rapid onset and ending in minimal, postictal state with features which include bizarre behavioral changes including vocalizations and complex motor and sexual automatisms.

- *Occipital lobe epilepsy*: This type of epilepsy may propagate to the temporal lobe and be clinically indistinguishable from a temporal lobe seizure.

- *Panic disorder*: This may be associated with autonomic phenomena and anxiety similar to those observed in the simple partial phase of a temporal lobe seizure (TLE). However, unlike TLE, which lasts for seconds to 2 minutes, panic attacks last several minutes (usually longer than 10 minutes).

- *Psychogenic seizures*: Approximately 10% to 30% of patients with psychogenic seizures also have epileptic seizures.

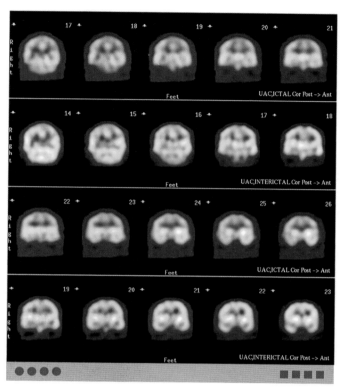

A. Comparison of the brain anterior and posterior SPECT images, in coronal orientation, obtained during ictal and interictal phases show increased perfusion in the region of left temporal lobe on the ictal phase images. This finding is diagnostic of temporal lobe epilepsy in appropriate clinical setting. The interictal phase images are essentially within normal limits. (*Image courtesy of David H. Lewis, MD.*)

COMMENTS

TLE is a condition characterized by recurrent unprovoked seizures originating from the medial or lateral temporal lobe. TLE is the most common type of complex partial seizure and accounts for 55% of all adult seizures and nearly one-third of them are refractory to medical treatment. However, majority of them can benefit from surgical management. The seizures associated with TLE consist of simple partial seizures without loss of awareness with or without aura and complex partial seizures with loss of awareness. Clinically, patients present with intractable partial complex epilepsy with onset in childhood with EEG evidence of unilateral temporal lobe seizure onset. Medial temporal sclerosis is the most common finding in temporal lobe epilepsy and also encompasses changes in the hippocampus, amygdala, and the adjacent entorhinal cortex. Histopathologically, there is neuronal loss, gliosis, and sclerosis of the involved areas. Approximately two-thirds of patients with TLE treated surgically have hippocampal sclerosis as the pathologic substrate.

There may be other etiologies implicated that include infections, trauma including difficult traumatic deliveries like forceps deliveries, brain tumors including hamartomas, and vascular malformations. Imaging evaluation commonly consists of MRI and SPECT and FDG-PET. T1-weighted images of the hippocampus reveal hippocampal volume loss. Increased T2 signal of the hippocampus is presumably due to gliosis.

PEARLS

- MRI is the neuroimaging modality of choice for patients with TLE and the clinical correlate on neuroimaging on MRI is called mesial temporal lobe sclerosis.

- SPECT is useful for surgical candidates; the accuracy of seizure localization is about 90% on ictal phase imaging while interictal imaging has a sensitivity of approximately 70%.

Additionally, there may be loss of internal architecture of the hippocampus and unilateral atrophy of the mammillary body, columns of the fornix, amygdala, and white matter bundle in the parahippocampal gyrus. SPECT is also an adjunctive imaging modality useful only for surgical candidates; the accuracy of seizure localization is about 90% on ictal phase imaging while interictal imaging has a sensitivity of approximately 70%. Epileptic focus is seen as a focus of hyperperfusion on ictal images. PET scan with ^{18}F-FDG shows hypometabolism of a wide area that includes lateral temporal neocortex, and may extend outside the temporal lobe. However, it is almost impossible to perform an ictal PET scan because of logistic reasons.

ADDITIONAL IMAGES (B-C)

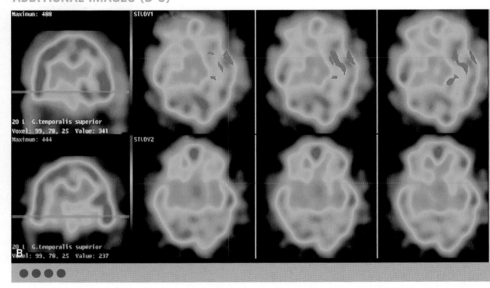

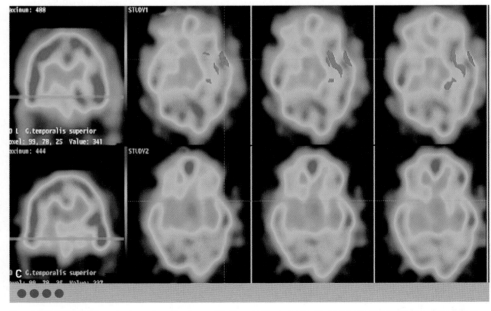

B. and **C.** BRASS analysis using the quantitative software shows increased perfusion, involving the left superior temporal gyrus extending into the left hippocampus, left insula, and the left basal ganglia. (*Images courtesy of David H. Lewis, MD.*) (BRASS is a registered trade mark of Hermes Medical Solutions, Stockholm, Sweden)

Bhasker R. Koppula, MD

PRESENTATION

- *Patient 1*: A 73-year-old male with chronic back pain, post-multistage spinal fusion related to multiple osteopenia/degeneration related pathological fractures of thoracolumbar spine.

- *Patient 2*: A 57-year-old male, post–L2-ilium posterior spinal instrumentation and fusion (PSIF), increasing wound discharge, history of multiple surgeries on the spine consequent to L3 burst fracture, likely resulting from radiotherapy for his testicular cancer. Prior history of cerebrospinal fluid (CSF) leak.

- *Patient 3*: A 70-year-old woman, post-left acoustic neuroma resection presenting with watery discharge from nose (CSF rhinorrhea).

FINDINGS

Delayed images show radiotracer activity in the region of nasopharynx. Pledgets positive for CSF leak with pledget to plasma count ratio of more than 1.5 bilaterally.

COMMENTS

CSF leak may occur from the nose (rhinorrhea), from the external auditory canal (otorrhea), or from a traumatic or operative defect in the skull or spine. Head trauma accounts for 50% to 80% of all cases of CSF leak, and up to 16% are iatrogenic.

Blunt trauma is the most common cause (30% of patients with a skull-base fracture). Postoperative CSF leak has been noted in 0.5% to 15% of patients with transsphenoidal surgery. Other causes include excessive weight lifting. Meningitis occurs in 25% to 50% of untreated traumatic CSF fistulas and in 10% of patients in the first week after trauma with head injury. Most CSF leaks resolve spontaneously within 7 days, and almost all leaks cease within 6 months. CSF fistula of spontaneous origin is often intermittent, persisting in at least 60% of cases if untreated. The risk of meningitis is higher with spontaneous CSF fistula than with traumatic CSF fistula. A number of investigations have been suggested in the algorithm for the diagnosis of a CSF fistula and include immunoelectrophoretic study of the discharge for the presence of beta-2 transferrin, high-resolution, thin-section axial and coronal cranial and facial CT including all the paranasal sinuses and petrous temporal bones in the scans; magnetic resonance (MR) cisternography. Radionuclide cisternography is performed by administering a lumbar or cervical subarachnoid intrathecal injection of In-111-DTPA in a 500-μCi dose. In-111 has minimal background activity and does not accumulate in the brain.

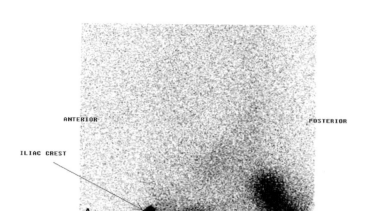

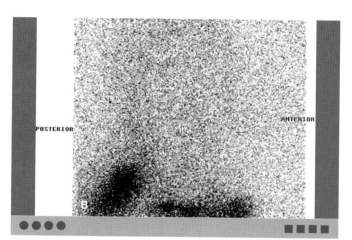

A. and **B.** Delayed 24-hour anterior and posterior images show focal collection of CSF in the region of lower lumbar spine. Also, there is increased tracer activity noted in the pelvic cavity in front of the bladder. Findings are highly suspicious for CSF leak. (*Images courtesy of Bhasker R. Koppula, MD.*)

PEARLS

- Trauma is the commonest cause for CSF leaks. Postoperative leak can be a complication of cranial surgery, particularly transsphenoidal surgical resection.

- Injection site is typically in the lumbar region but can be in different locations depending on the site of the leak.

- Sensitivity for the nuclear medicine CSF leak study is 50% to 100% and the specificity is 100%.

- SPECT helps in localizing small leaks in the head.

Images are acquired 2, 6, 12, and 24 hours after injection of the isotope. Follow-up 48- or 72-hour scans are possible with In-111 and useful in the detection of intermittent CSF leaks. The entire spine is scanned up to 24 hours in cases of spontaneous intracranial hypotension, spinal trauma, or postoperative CSF leaks. Cotton pledgets are placed in the nose before the intrathecal space injection of the isotope for rhinorrhea. These are placed closest to the cribriform plate, in the middle meatus, and in the sphenoethmoidal recess of the right and left nasal cavities with blood samples obtained and counted at the same time points. Higher ratio of pledget/serum counts confirms the diagnosis with confidence. For otorrhea, one cotton pledget is placed in each external auditory canal. The sensitivity is in the range of 50% to 100% and the specificity is almost 100% for contemporary radionuclide cisternography.

ADDITIONAL IMAGES (C-F)

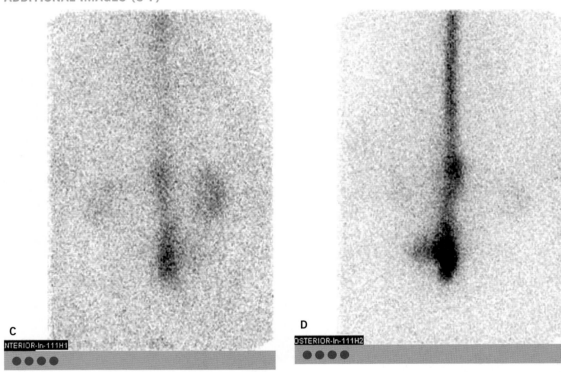

C., D., E., and **F.** Delayed 24-hour images show pooling of the radiotracer in the extrathecal space below the left kidney, lateral to midline on the anterior/posterior images. On the left lateral image, the tracer is seen posterior to the spinal canal. Findings are highly suspicious for CSF leak from the lumbar spinal canal. (*Images courtesy of Bhasker R. Koppula, MD.*)

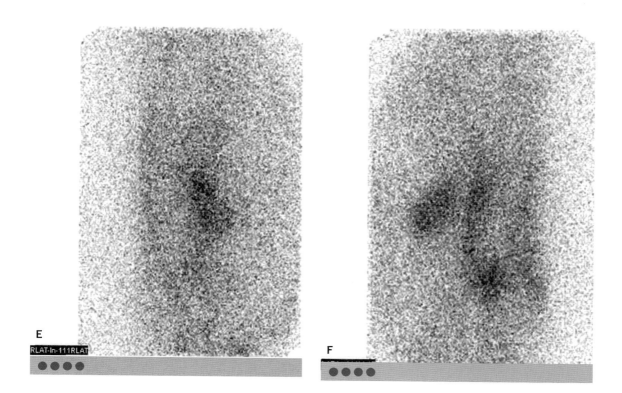

E

RLAT-In-111RLAT

F

Bhasker R. Koppula, MD

PRESENTATION

A patient presents with headache, vomiting, or confusion either alone or in combination. There is a history of CSF shunt in place and, depending on the onset the length of shunt, presence can vary.

DIFFERENTIAL DIAGNOSES

- *Proximal limb obstruction*: Low or negative opening pressure; no retrograde flow of tracer into the ventricular system if complete obstruction; positive flow retrogradely if incomplete obstruction and with maneuvering

- *Distal limb obstruction*: High opening pressure; drainage of the tracer distally, if incomplete or partial obstruction, with different maneuvers; no flow of CSF, if complete and high-grade obstruction

- *Gravity-/position-dependent flow*: Normal or high opening pressure; no drainage in the supine position; however, in sitting position or with walking, there would be flow of CSF distally

- *Overdrainage syndrome*: Low opening pressure; rapid draining of the CSF distally

- *Defective valve mechanisms*

COMMENTS

A ventriculoperitoneal (VP) shunt is the most commonly used CSF diversionary procedure in the presence of an obstructed ventricular system or normal pressure hydrocephalus. Modern VP shunts contain several components, usually including a proximal ventriculostomy catheter (shunt tubing), a pressure-sensitive valve and reservoir, and a distal peritoneal catheter. CSF shunt malfunction is a common complication that is difficult to diagnose and manage. The rate of shunt failure after 1 year can be up to 30%, and up to 50% of shunts require some form of revision within 6 years of placement. The leading cause of shunt malfunction is mechanical failure and could be due to ventricular catheter obstruction, valve malfunction, distal catheter obstruction, pressure mismatch, or component disconnection as well as infection. Shunt malfunction manifests clinically, with nonspecific symptoms and signs, including headache, nausea, abdominal pain, vomiting, lethargy, irritability, fever, increasing head size, persistent bulging of the anterior fontanel in children, and seizures. The following investigations are performed to evaluate shunts:

Plain radiographs (shunt series): The entire course of the shunt can be evaluated for disconnections, kinks, breaks, or migration of the shunt tubing which can be confirmed by other imaging methods. CT scan of the head is performed to check for changes in ventricular size or other evidence of increased intracranial pressure.

Radionuclide shuntogram: Following injection of 0.2 mCi of Tc-99m pertechnetate of In-111 DTPA into the shunt reservoir under aseptic conditions, static sequential images are obtained in supine position. Images can also be obtained in sitting position or after ambulating the patient as clinically permitted to facilitate the flow of CSF in cases of gravity-/position-dependent flow conditions. Other commonly used maneuver, if patient cannot be ambulated due to neurologic status, is pumping of the reservoir and repeating the imaging. Static images of the abdomen are obtained as needed to demonstrate radionuclide presence in the peritoneal cavity. Radionuclide scintigraphy is performed to evaluate the patency of the shunt. Sonography and MRI are performed to evaluate the peritoneal end of the shunt and central nervous system (CNS) infection and/or hemorrhage, respectively. Ventriculoatrial shunts and lumboperitoneal shunts can also be used for CSF diversions, though done rarely. Lumboperitoneal shunts have a high prevalence of tonsillar herniation, brain stem compression, and syringomyelia and may result in scoliosis and nerve root deficits. If tracer appears trapped within the reservoir on the supine images, obtain images in sitting position or after making the patient walk as neurologically and clinically allowed. If patient is unable to walk due to neurologic status, pumping of the reservoir should be done. Make sure to compare the plateaus of the activity on the images obtained after the maneuvers with the initial set of images.

PEARLS

- Always check for the number of shunts and location of the reservoir before the procedure, from shunt series of radiographs or from CT or MRI if obtained.

- Check for any obvious breaks or kinks in the distal catheter tubing which would obviate the need for the shuntogram procedure.

- Specifically look for the distal tip of the distal catheter tip—keeping in mind that the tip can be normally placed in the right atrium, pleural spaces, gallbladder, urinary bladder apart from the most usual location that is the peritoneal space.

- Asepsis is of paramount importance during the entire procedure. A small sample of CSF is obtained for microbiological testing.

Case A

Bhasker R. Koppula, MD

PRESENTATION

A 36-year-old females, status post right occipital arteriovenous malformation (AVM) resection with VP shunt presenting with enlarging ventricles on CT.

FINDINGS

- Shunt series show single reservoir in the left frontal region and did not show any breaks or kinks in the shunt tubing.

- Shuntogram:
  - Negative opening pressure.
  - Supine images obtained immediately after tracer injection show very mild tracer activity in the distal-most portion of the proximal catheter with no flow into the distal limb.
  - Upright images show trapping of tracer in the reservoir with no proximal or distal flow of tracer. Abdominal image obtained in upright position shows no tracer activity in the peritoneal cavity.
  - Images obtained after pumping of the reservoir show no retrograde flow into the ventricular system. The abdominal images obtained after pumping the reservoir show tracer activity in the lower abdomen.

DIFFERENTIAL DIAGNOSIS

Proximal limb obstruction, probably involving the proximal ventricular catheter at its origin.

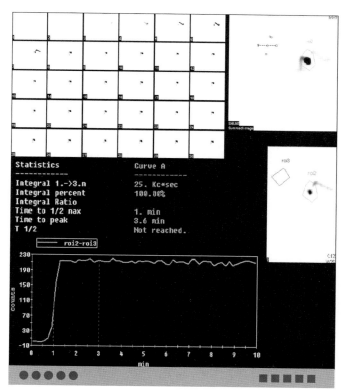

A. Early images after the tracer injection showing minimal tracer activity in the distal-most portion of the proximal limb in supine position. (*Image courtesy of Bhasker R. Koppula, MD.*)

ADDITIONAL IMAGES (B-D)

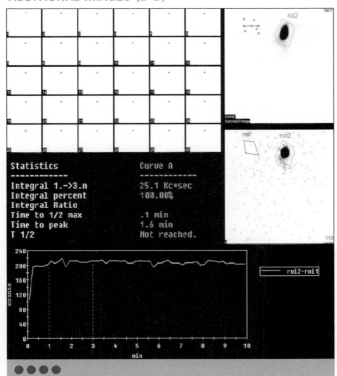

B. Sequential images of the head obtained in sitting position showing tracer trapped within the reservoir. (*Image courtesy of Bhasker R. Koppula, MD.*)

C. Abdominal anterior image in sitting position, prior to reservoir pumping, with no sign of tracer activity in the abdomen. (*Image courtesy of Bhasker R. Koppula, MD.*)

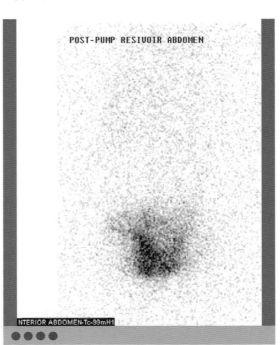

D. Abdominal anterior image in sitting position, after reservoir pumping, showing tracer activity dispersed in the peritoneal cavity. (*Image courtesy of Bhasker R. Koppula, MD.*)

Case B

Bhasker R. Koppula, MD

PRESENTATION

A 48-year-old male with a long-standing history of hydro-cephalus and multiple shunt revisions. Presented with balance disturbance and worsening headache. Enlarging ventricles on the CT.

FINDINGS

- Plain radiographs show a loop in the distal catheter, on the right side of the neck.

- Shuntogram:
  - Opening pressure 24 cm of water.
  - No flow of tracer into the distal limb on supine images.
  - No distal flow of CSF on upright images and on reservoir pumping.
  - Retrograde flow of CSF into the ventricular system on both upright imaging and on post-reservoir pumping images.
  - No tracer activity is found in the abdomen.

DIFFERENTIAL DIAGNOSIS

Distal catheter limb obstruction.

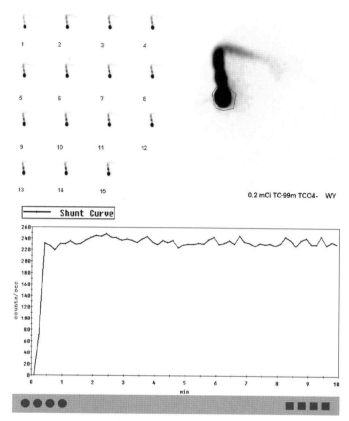

A. Immediate supine images with tracer in the reservoir. (*Image courtesy of Bhasker R. Koppula, MD.*)

ADDITIONAL IMAGES (B-F)

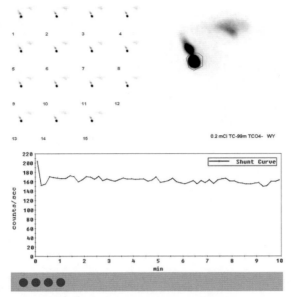

0.2 mCI TC-99m TCO4- WY

B. Images in upright position with retrograde flow of tracer into the ventricles. (*Image courtesy of Bhasker R. Koppula, MD.*)

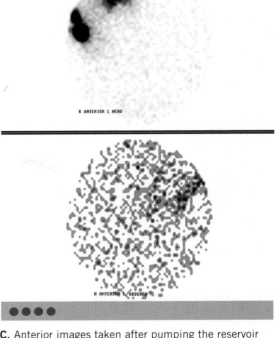

R ANTERIOR L HEAD

R ANTERIOR L ABDOMEN

C. Anterior images taken after pumping the reservoir with retrograde flow of tracer. (*Image courtesy of Bhasker R. Koppula, MD.*)

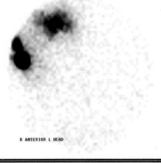

R ANTERIOR L HEAD

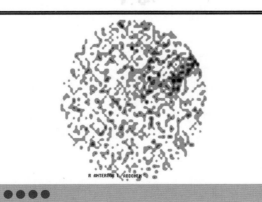

R ANTERIOR L ABDOMEN

D. Abdominal images show no tracer activity in the peritoneal cavity. (*Image courtesy of Bhasker R. Koppula, MD.*)

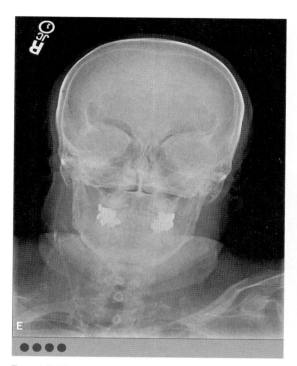

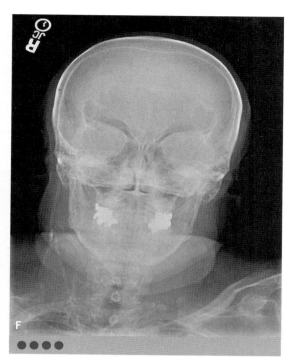

E. and **F.** These images show a loop in the distal catheter limb on the right side of the neck. (*Images courtesy of Bhasker R. Koppula, MD.*)

Bhasker R. Koppula, MD

PRESENTATION

A 72-year-old female with a history of hydrocephalus and VP shunt presenting with 1 day history of nausea, vomiting, and ataxia.

FINDINGS

- Shunt series radiographs: Reservoir in right occipital region; otherwise, normal.
- Shuntogram:
  - Opening CSF pressure of 17 cm of water.
  - Initial images show tracer in the reservoir with mild reflux into the ventricles.
  - The radiotracer is cleared when the patient is imaged in the upright position with the estimated T1/2 of 5 to 6 minutes.
  - The abdominal images show radiotracer in the peritoneal cavity, localized near the shunt tip with minimal dispersion in the peritoneal cavity.
- Ultrasonography: It shows localized collection of fluid at the tip of the distal catheter limb in the right lower quadrant.

DIFFERENTIAL DIAGNOSIS

Distal limb malfunction with position-dependent CSF drainage into the CSF pseudocyst in the abdomen.

A. Initial images showing tracer in the reservoir with some reflux into the ventricles. (*Image courtesy of Bhasker R. Koppula, MD.*)

ADDITIONAL IMAGES (B-D)

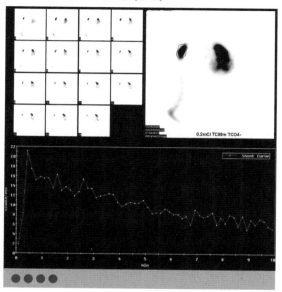

B. Images in upright position show CSF flowing through the distal catheter limb. (*Image courtesy of Bhasker R. Koppula, MD.*)

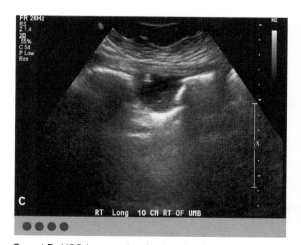
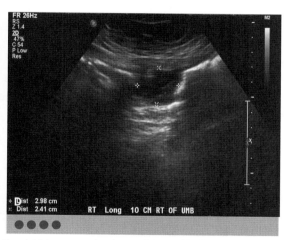

C. and **D.** USG images showing localized collection of CSF in the right lower quadrant, consistent with CSF pseudocyst. (*Images courtesy of Bhasker R. Koppula, MD.*)

Joseph Rajendran, MD

PRESENTATION

Patient with a known history of occipital meningioma, status postsurgical resection now with recurrent symptoms being considered for radiosurgery.

FINDINGS

Planar and SPECT images of the head obtained at 4 and 24 hours following injection of 5 mCi of In-111 octreotide show a focus of increased uptake in the region corresponding to MR abnormality. SPECT images help in localization and correlation with other cross-sectional images and can also be helpful in radiation therapy planning.

DIFFERENTIAL DIAGNOSES

- *Metastases from a somatostatin receptor-positive tumor*: Unlikely because of the absence of any other foci in the body

- *Meningioma*: Most likely because of the location of the focus

- *Well-differentiated astrocytoma*: Typically not somato-statin avid

- *Other somatostatin-expressing tumors*: Pituitary adenoma; unlikely because of the more lateral location of octreotide-avid disease in the current patient

- *Primary brain tumor*: Location of the abnormality and changes on radiologic examination

COMMENTS

Meningioma affects approximately 2 cases per 100,000 individuals in the United States and accounts for about 20% of all primary intracranial neoplasms. Meningiomas are slow-growing tumors and in some cases are incidentally discovered. However, meningiomas can cause serious symptoms as a result of functional effect on adjacent brain structures. Somatostatin is a neuropeptide taken up in the somatostatin receptors (SSTRs) that are expressed on the surface of several target cell types. The subtypes of human SSTRs that are commonly associated with meningioma are 2, 3, and 5. The expression of SSTR decreases with increasing degree of malignant changes in the tumor at which point FDG-PET will show increased uptake compared to Octreoscan. Sensitivity, specificity, and positive and negative predictor values for octreotide imaging for evaluating brain tumors were 100, 50, 75, and 100, respectively. False-positive data were found in three patients (metastases, chronic inflammation, and lymphoma). Octreotide imaging along with brain MRI

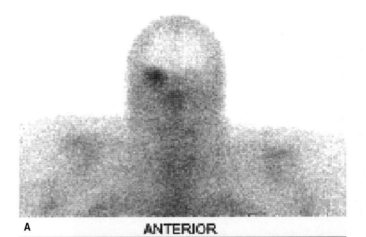

A

ANTERIOR

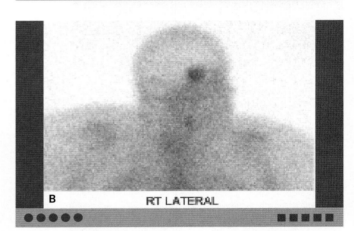

B

RT LATERAL

A. and **B.** Planar In-111 pentetreotide anterior images show a focus of increased tracer uptake in the right orbit.

PEARLS

- Octreotide is an octapeptide analogue of somatostatin that can bind to somatostatin receptors with a longer half-life than natural somatostatin.

- Octreotide has been labeled with either I-123 or In-111 for scintigraphic localization.

- Octreotide imaging is rarely used in the primary diagnosis of meningioma.

- Octreotide imaging is useful for planning radiotherapy (typically stereotactic radiosurgery) of meningioma, which can result in reduction in size and uptake over several months and in the follow-up of these patients.

is useful in differentiating meningiomas from other lesions. It may also increase the diagnostic specificity of conventional MRI when differentiating meningioma from other dural-based pathologies, while the addition of FDG-PET differentiates benign from malignant lesions. Octreotide imaging is helpful in radiation therapy planning and field placement, particularly in cases recurrent after surgical excision.

ADDITIONAL IMAGES (C-E)

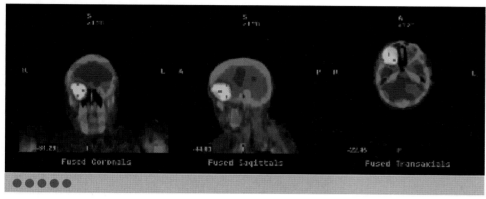

C. In-111 pentetreotide fused SPECT/CT images clearly show the uptake in the right orbit in coronal, sagittal, and axial planes.

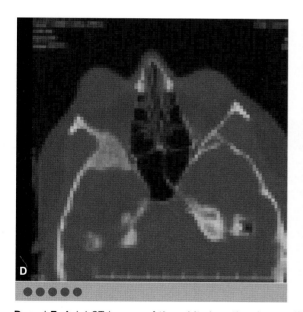

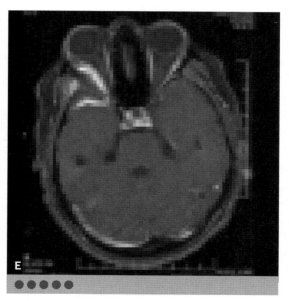

D. and **E.** Axial CT images of the orbit show the abnormality in the posterior right orbit corresponding to the focus of abnormal uptake seen on Octreoscan.

Joseph Rajendran, MD

PRESENTATION

Patient is status postclipping of aneurysm. Patient underwent Tc-99m ECD SPECT cerebral blood flow images prior to surgery and periodically as needed postoperation.

FINDINGS

Cerebral perfusion images were obtained 35 minutes after the intravenous injection of 30 mCi of Tc-99m ECD. SPECT images show surgical site and infarct in the right anterior frontal region and show areas of reduced perfusion in bilateral parietal regions suggestive of vasospasm.

DIFFERENTIAL DIAGNOSIS

• *Infarct*: Usually shows decreased perfusion to the region along with abnormalities in other images as well. On serial imaging, the pattern of perfusion does not show changes.

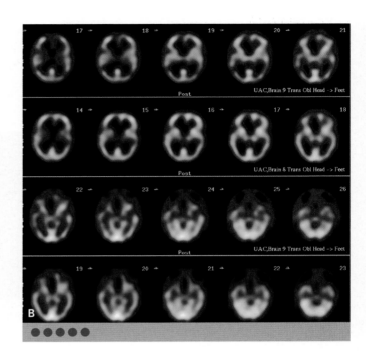

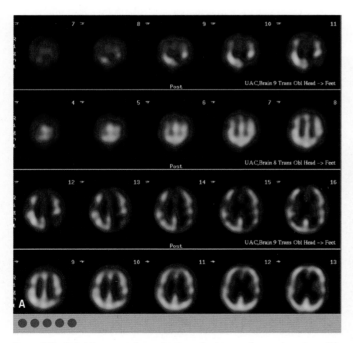

A. and **B.** Axial images of cerebral perfusion performed on two different days show an area of severely decreased perfusion in the right frontal region consistent with infarct and surgical site and areas of moderately reduced perfusion in bilateral parietal regions indicating vasospasm (rows 1 and 3 in image A). There is significant improvement in perfusion to bilateral parietal regions on perfusion images performed on Day 9 of hospitalization (rows 2 and 4 in image B).

COMMENTS

The incidence of intracranial aneurysms is approximately 1% to 6% of the general population. It can be multiple in up to one-third of cases and is seen in people from 40 to 60 years of age. Majority of the aneurysms are found in the anterior circulation and remain without symptoms for several years. Subarachnoid hemorrhage (SAH) is the most

PEARLS

• **Early identification of vasospasm is critical for intervention to correct the problem and to avoid serious and permanent sequelae.**

• **Baseline brain SPECT scan is helpful to follow postsurgery changes. Simultaneously displaying the last two image sets help evaluate subtle changes.**

• **Serial brain SPECT helps track changes in the postoperative period. Comparison is made to the most recent brain SPECT.**

• **Intensity of uptake is referenced to that of cerebellum and images are examined for symmetry and for both spatial and temporal changes. Particular attention should be paid to the basal ganglia, thalami, and brain stem (seen best on sagittal images).**

common presentation and might be the first presentation. Vasospasm is a serious complication that can result in severe ischemia and can occur in regional blood vessels as surgery or in a remote part of the cerebral vasculature away from the bleeding/surgical site. Transcranial Doppler (TCD) is frequently used to identify changes in the large- and medium-caliber blood vessels. However, brain SPECT is very sensitive in evaluating distal cerebral blood vessels. All the imaging modalities are complementary rather than exclusive of one over the other.

Tc-99m ECD, a neutral lipophilic compound, is currently the most commonly used radiotracer for imaging cerebral perfusion and after reconstitution is stable for 6 hours and has a rapid clearance from the blood. Tc-99m HMPAO, also a lipophilic compound, has a greater extraction fraction and is stable for 2 hours after reconstitution. Baseline images prior to any intervention would be very helpful in assessing changes on serial images done during the course of illness.

Vivek Manchanda, MD

PRESENTATION

Man in his seventh decade of life with maxillary sinus mass.

FINDINGS

Mildly increased FDG activity in the left maxillary sinus soft tissue mass with erosion of medial wall.

DIFFERENTIAL DIAGNOSES

- *Carcinoma*
- *Metastasis*
- *Sarcoma (ie, rhabdomyosarcoma)*
- *Esthesioneuroblastoma*
- *Plasmacytoma*
- *Lymphoma*
- *Inverting papilloma*
- *Wegener granulomatosis*
- *Infection such as fungal*

COMMENTS

Adenoid cystic carcinoma is seen most commonly in the fifth decade of life. There is no sex predilection, and it is seen in salivary glands and other glandular tissue such as lacrimal glands, ceruminous glands of external auditory canal,

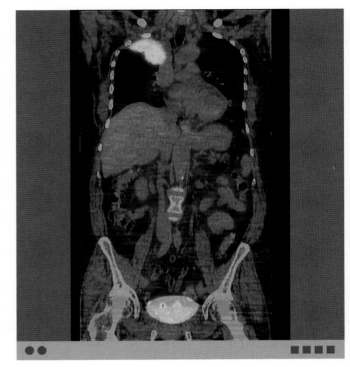

B. Different patient with adenoid cystic metastasis to right upper lobe, coronal fused PET/CT.

esophagus, breast, Bartholin glands of vulva, uterine cervix, and prostate.

Adenoid cystic carcinoma is characterized by prolonged history of slow growth, multiple recurrences, and late metastases. Another feature of these cancers is the perineural spread of the disease. Studies have shown that there is no correlation with survival based on perineural spread alone.

Adenoid cystic carcinoma has variable FDG activity and many tumors are mildly FDG avid. The perineural spread of disease may be missed on FDG-PET.

Distant metastases are most commonly seen in the lungs, which tend to be multiple. Classically, these patients are followed for a long time as distant metastases can be seen after 10 years.

Surgery is the mainstay of therapy and best survival results are with surgery and radiation therapy.

FDG-PET may be used for radiation therapy planning and for follow-up of treatment.

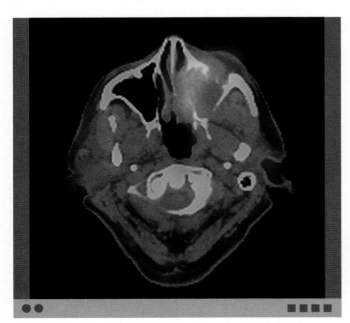

A. Adenoid cystic cancer of left maxillary sinus with erosion of medial wall of the sinus. Axial fused PET/CT.

PEARLS

- Adenoid cystic carcinoma has variable FDG activity and many tumors are mildly FDG avid.
- The perineural spread of disease may be missed on FDG-PET.

Vivek Manchanda, MD

PRESENTATION

Female in early seventies with swollen tongue and difficulty swallowing.

FINDINGS

Hypermetabolic floor of mouth lesion with hypermetabolic left level 2 lymph node.

DIFFERENTIAL DIAGNOSES

- *Floor of mouth squamous cell cancer*

- *Inflammation*

- *Infection/abscess*

It is less likely to be inflammation given the level of activity and intensely hypermetabolic node. Biopsy showed invasive squamous cell cancer.

COMMENTS

Majority of the oropharyngeal cancers are squamous cell and include soft palate, tonsils, tonsillar pillars, lateral and posterior pharyngeal walls, and posterior one-third of tongue.

Base of tongue tumors are very likely to spread to nodes. Tumors of tonsillar pillar tend to be superficial and spread over a broad region, whereas tonsillar fossa tumors are bulky at presentation. Adenoid cystic cancer of the soft palate is less aggressive and has a typical perineural spread. Pharyngeal wall tumors are often advanced at presentation and spread bilaterally in the neck.

FDG-PET is useful in initial staging and restaging of advanced locoregional disease. It is also important in evaluation of recurrence and assessment of response to therapy. FDG-PET is also important in radiation therapy planning.

FDG-PET can delineate a previously unidentified primary tumor in about 20% to 50% of cases. However, false-positive findings can be seen in benign inflammatory lesions, lesions less than 5 mm, and in small lesions in areas with high background activity such as the base of the tongue or palatine tonsils. In isodense lesions, distorted anatomy, or obliterated fat planes, FDG-PET may help.

Criteria for separating reactive from metastatic lymph nodes on CT and MR are necrosis, extracapsular spread, and size.

PET may detect occult distant metastases and synchronous malignancies. It has been suggested that PET/CT is more accurate when performed 2 to 3 months after completion of radiation therapy than earlier, eliminating false positives from inflammation.

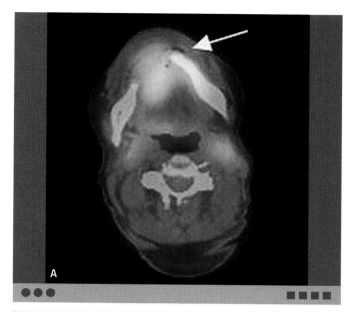

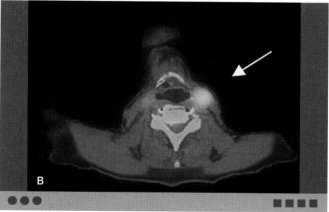

A. and **B.** Floor of mouth cancer with nodal metastases. No distant metastases. Axial FDG fused PET/CT.

PEARLS

- **Squamous cell cancers of the floor of mouth are extremely FDG avid.**

- **FDG-PET can delineate a previously unidentified primary tumor in about 20% to 50% of cases.**

- **FDG-PET is useful in initial staging and restaging of advanced locoregional disease. It is also important in evaluation of recurrence and assessment of response to therapy. FDG-PET is also important in radiation therapy planning.**

- **Radiation (without chemo) is treatment of choice for most oropharyngeal cancers.**

ADDITIONAL IMAGES (C-F)

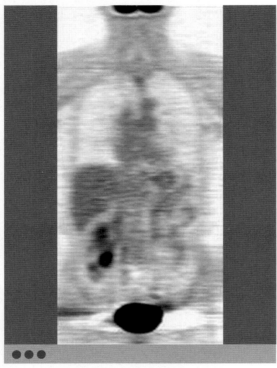

C. Corresponding coronal FDG-PET with no distant metastases.

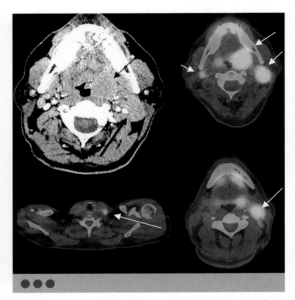

D. Left tonsillar cancer with bilateral level 2 and left supraclavicular metastases. Axial CT (*black arrow*), fused axial PET/CT images (*white arrows*).

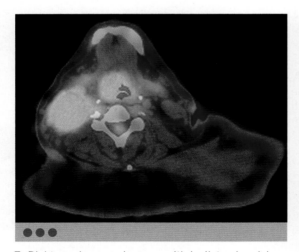

E. Right oropharyngeal cancer with ipsilateral nodal disease. Axial fused PET/CT.

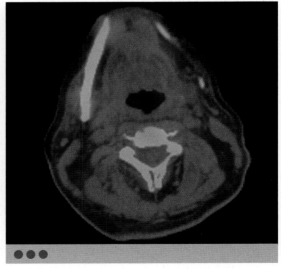

F. Good response after treatment for right oropharyngeal cancer with nodal metastases. No metabolically active disease. Fused PET/CT.

Vivek Manchanda, MD

PRESENTATION

Ataxia, nystagmus weakness, multiple cerebellar/motor cortex lesions on MRI, in 35-year-old female.

FINDINGS

Multiple foci of increased FDG uptake in the brain including left occipital lobe and bilateral cerebellum, corresponding to enhancing lesions on MR. No systemic disease.

DIFFERENTIAL DIAGNOSES

- *Infection such as cysticercosis, histoplasmosis, tuberculosis*

- *Noninfectious inflammatory processes such as sarcoidosis and multiple sclerosis*

- *Primary CNS lymphoma*

- *Metastases such as from melanoma and lung*

It is difficult to distinguish the etiologies on the basis of FDG-PET and, majority of times biopsy is needed to make a final diagnosis. Meningiomas are typically non–FDG avid.

COMMENTS

Sarcoidosis is a multisystemic idiopathic granulomatous disease of unknown cause (with noncaseating granulomas). Lymph nodes, lungs, skin, eyes, and bones are frequently involved. Neurologic manifestations of sarcoidosis include meningoencephalopathy, cranial neuropathy, hypothalamic dysfunction, hydrocephalus, myelopathy, and peripheral neuropathy. Radiologically, it can present in many different ways, including dural mass or thickening, leptomeningeal granulomas, brain parenchymal lesions, and nerve involvement.

CNS sarcoidosis has been reported in approximately 5% of patients with systemic sarcoidosis.

The diagnosis of neurosarcoidosis is based on the documentation of systemic sarcoidosis and exclusion of other neurologic diseases.

Dural-based lesions tend to be isointense with gray matter on T1, hypointense on T2, and enhance uniformly with intravenous gadolinium on MR. Differential diagnoses include meningioma (typically FDG negative), lymphoma, adenocarcinoma, chronic meningitis, and granulomatous infection.

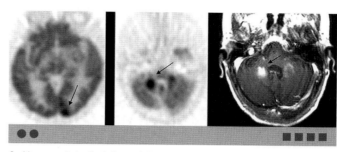

A. Hypermetabolic left occipital and bilateral cerebellar (*black arrows*) and corresponding enhancing lesions on MR (*black arrow*). Axial FDG-PET right and center. Post gad axial T1W MR, left.

Meningeal sarcoidosis is associated with enhancing brain parenchymal lesions (80%) and cranial nerves (60%). Leptomeningeal infiltration typically involves the suprasellar and frontal basal meninges. The granulomatous lesions may coalesce to form mass-like lesions, mainly in the region of the optic chiasm, floor of the third ventricle, and pituitary stalk. Differential diagnoses include tuberculosis (TB), Wegener granulomatosis, fungal/pyogenic meningitis, lymphoma, demyelination (which can be FDG avid), meningioangiomatosis, acute lymphoblastic leukemia (ALL), and leptomeningeal carcinomatosis.

Diffusely enhancing intraparenchymal granulomas (isointense on T1 and iso- to hyperintense on T2 MR) can be found in the hypothalamus, brain stem, and cerebral and cerebellar hemispheres.

Nonenhancing parenchymal lesions are commonly seen in periventricular white matter, brain stem, and basal ganglia.

The facial nerve is the most frequently involved cranial nerve in sarcoidosis, usually presenting as Bell palsy.

Spinal cord lesions tend to be extramedullary. The cervical spine is frequently involved.

PEARLS

- **Radiologically, sarcoidosis can present in many ways, including dural mass or thickening, leptomeningeal granulomas, brain parenchymal lesions, and nerve involvement.**

- **Brain sarcoidosis can be extremely FDG avid and difficult to distinguish from CNS lymphoma and infection.**

DIFFERENTIAL DIAGNOSIS IMAGES (B-F)

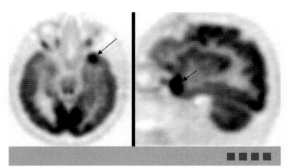

B. High-grade anterior temporal glioma, axial and sagittal FDG-PET (*black arrows*).

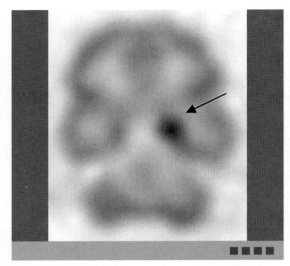

C. Axial FDG-PET, left temporal encephalitis (*black arrow*).

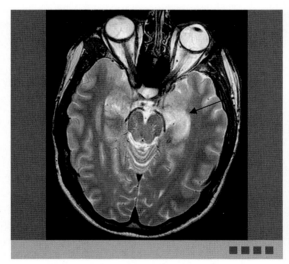

D. Corresponding T2W axial MR image with left temporal encephalitis.

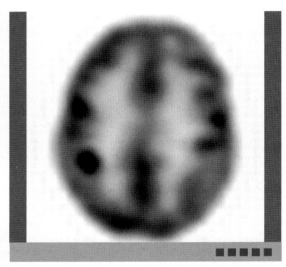

E. Melanoma metastasis in right parietal lobe, axial FDG-PET.

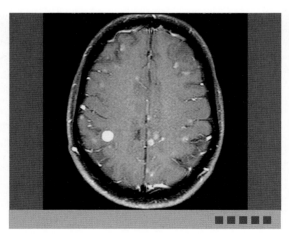

F. Post gad T1W axial MR with numerous metastases from melanoma, many of which are below PET resolution.

Vivek Manchanda, MD

PRESENTATION

Man in midseventies with memory loss.

FINDINGS

Mildly decreased FDG metabolism in biparietal (left worse than right) and moderately decreased metabolism in bitemporal regions, posterior cingulate gyrus, and sensorimotor preservation.

DIFFERENTIAL DIAGNOSES

- *Alzheimer dementia*

- *Frontotemporal dementia (FTD)*

- *Vascular dementia*

The findings are typical for Alzheimer dementia given biparietal, bitemporal, posterior cingulate hypometabolism, and preservation of sensorimotor cortex metabolism.

COMMENTS

Bilateral temporoparietal hypometabolism is the classic metabolic abnormality associated with Alzheimer disease (AD). In earlier stages, the pattern can be asymmetric. Posterior cingulate gyrus hypometabolism, preservation of sensorimotor, and visual cortex metabolism are some of the other features of AD. Moderate AD involves decreased metabolism of midfrontal lobes, bilateral parietal lobes, and the superior temporal regions. In patients with severe AD, the same regions are more severely affected. Differential diagnoses include bilateral parietal subdural hematomas, strokes, and bilateral parietal radiation therapy ports. CT and MR comparison is important. PET findings may correspond to atrophy of parietotemporal lobes.

FTDs show hypometabolism in frontal and anterior temporal areas and anterior cingulate gyrus. The temporoparietal, occipital, and subcortical areas are relatively preserved. The left hemisphere is more commonly involved and the asymmetric hypometabolism is commoner in FTD than AD. Pick disease, a neurodegenerative dementia, has histopathologic findings of Pick bodies. The patients have cognitive and language dysfunction and behavioral changes. Bilateral hypometabolism of frontal and anterior temporal lobes may correspond to frontal and temporal lobe atrophy on CT and MR images. Differential diagnoses include other frontal lobe dementias, schizophrenia, and alcoholism.

Diffuse glucose hypometabolism in the entire cortex including the occipital region is a typical feature of dementia of Lewy body (DLB) and distinct from AD. Clinically, DLB patients show progressive and fluctuating cognitive decline with recurrent visual hallucinations, systematized delusions, and spontaneous parkinsonian symptoms.

The multi-infarct dementias and dementia due to AIDS are

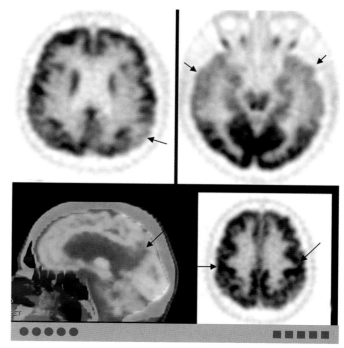

A. (*Top left*) Left parietal hypometabolism. (*Top right*) Moderately decreased FDG metabolism in bitemporal regions. (*Bottom right*) Decreased posterior cingulate metabolism. (*Bottom left*) Sensorimotor preservation; Alzheimer dementia pattern.

characterized by multiple asymmetric areas of hypometabolism. Crossed cerebellar diaschisis may be seen in vascular and Alzheimer dementia. Vascular dementia combined with AD is the commonest form of dementia recognized in the outpatient setting.

Dementia due to Parkinson disease (PD) and AD can show bilateral temporal hypometabolism on the FDG-PET scan. Dementia due to PD occurs late, whereas, progressive decline of memory is prominent in AD and the neuropsychiatric features occur later.

PEARLS

- Bilateral symmetric or asymmetric parietal and superior temporal lobe hypometabolism is characteristic of AD. Frontal lobe is involved in severe AD.

- Sensorimotor and visual cortex preservation and posterior cingulate hypometabolism are also features of AD.

- FTD is characterized by bilateral frontal and anterior temporal lobe hypometabolism.

- DLB dementia typically involves diffuse cortical hypometabolism including the visual cortex. The patients may clinically have visual hallucinations.

ADDITIONAL IMAGE

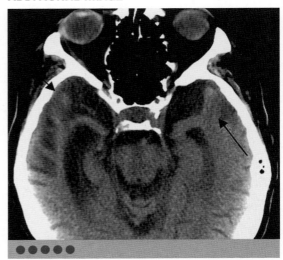

B. Corresponding noncontrast CT with bilateral temporal lobe atrophy.

DIFFERENTIAL DIAGNOSES IMAGE

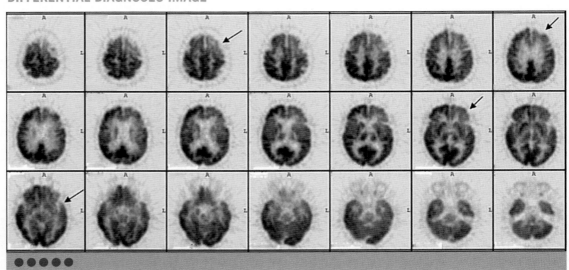

C. Moderate to severe decrease in metabolism in left frontal and inferior frontal, and mild decrease in metabolism in left anterior temporal lobe. (*Image courtesy of David H. Lewis, MD.*)

Vivek Manchanda, MD

PRESENTATION

Female in midseventies with rapidly progressing neurological deficit.

FINDINGS

Diffuse hypometabolism in left superficial and deep grey matter, involving left thalamus and basal ganglia with midline shift. There is crossed cerebellar diaschisis.

DIFFERENTIAL DIAGNOSES

- *Stroke*
- Low-grade tumor.
- *Gliomatosis cerebri*

Although severe AD cannot be excluded, the combination of diffuse hypometabolism and midline shift and rapid deterioration in signs and symptoms suggest a more aggressive process such as tumor.

COMMENTS

Gliomatosis cerebri involves diffuse growth of neoplastic glia (large areas, usually more than one hemisphere, brain stem, and cerebellum).

Clinical signs and symptoms are nonspecific (eg, headache). Signs and symptoms may be mild or severe (in contrast to brain involved at presentation).

Peak age for gliomatosis cerebri is between second and fourth decades. Progression is variable (depends on well-differentiated astrocytes to increased mitosis).

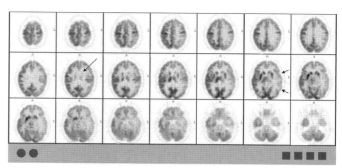

A. Diffusely decreased metabolism in both grey and white matter in left thalamus with evidence of midline shift.

CT is nonspecific and there is minimum density change. (May be read normal!)

MR is nonspecific. T2 may show subtle increased signal in large areas of brain.

FDG-PET shows diffuse hypometabolism in superficial and deep grey matter, consistent with diffuse infiltration. There is poor contrast between normally hypometabolic white matter and hypometabolic low-grade tumors.

PEARLS

- Diffuse hypometabolism in the brain involving one or more large areas, usually corresponding to increased signal on T2 is characteristic of gliomatosis cerebri.

- CT may be read normal. Signs and symptoms may be minimal or severe (in contrast to the imaging findings).

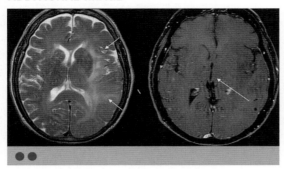

B. Left, axial T2 flair with diffuse left cerebral hyperintensity (*white arrows*) and left T1W post gad image with midline shift and no enhancement (*white arrow*).

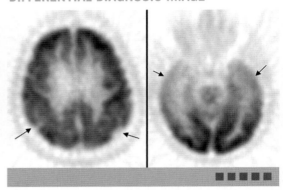

C. Axial FDG-PET with Alzheimer dementia, mild bilateral parietal and bilateral temporal hypometabolism (*black arrows*).

Vivek Manchanda, MD

PRESENTATION

Man in early eighties with a lump in the neck.

FINDINGS

Hypermetabolic right glottic mass.

DIFFERENTIAL DIAGNOSES

- *Primary squamous cell cancer*
- *Metastasis*
- *Lymphoma*
- *Infection*

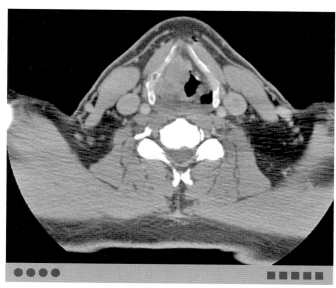

B. Corresponding axial CT with right glottic squamous cell cancer.

COMMENTS

Majority of the laryngeal cancers are squamous cell cancers.

The supraglottic larynx (above the level of true vocal cords) is composed of false vocal cords, laryngeal side of aryepiglottic folds, upper arytenoids and the epiglottis, and paraglottic and preepiglottic fat/spaces.

The glottis includes anterior and posterior commissures in addition to true vocal cords.

The subglottic larynx extends from inferior to true vocal cords to the inferior margin of the cricoid cartilage.

Metastatic adenopathy is most commonly seen with supraglottic cancer due to rich lymphatic network.

FDG-PET is useful in initial staging and restaging, evaluation of recurrence, assessment of response to therapy,

and radiation treatment planning. FDG-PET/CT is also helpful in detecting distant metastases.

In the assessment of regional nodes, N1 is defined as metastasis in a single ipsilateral node less than or equal to 3 cm. N2a is defined as metastasis in a single ipsilateral node 3 to 6 cm in greatest dimension, N2b as multiple ipsilateral nodes less than or equal to 6 cm in greatest dimension, and N2c as metastases in bilateral or contralateral nodes less than or equal to 6 cm in greatest dimension. N3 is defined as metastases in a lymph node greater than 6 cm in greatest dimension.

MR is important in distinguishing cartilage invasion, which might be equivocal on CT.

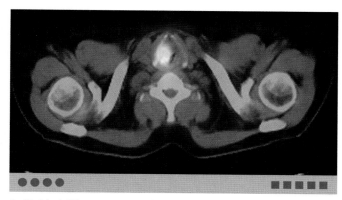

A. Right glottic squamous cell cancer, fused PET/CT.

PEARLS

- **FDG-PET is useful in detecting distant metastases and initial staging and restaging along with assessing response to therapy and radiation treatment planning.**

- **Among laryngeal cancers, metastatic adenopathy is most commonly seen with supraglottic cancer because of rich lymphatic network.**

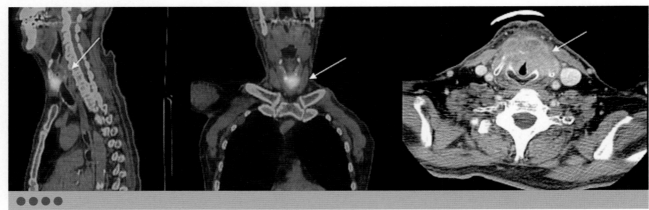

C. Fused PET/CT of left hypermetabolic nonmoving vocal cord. Biopsy was negative, but the follow-up CT showed large mass. Rebiopsy showed invasive squamous cell cancer.

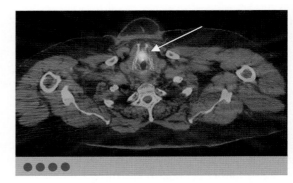

D. Different patient with recurrent laryngeal cancer. Axial fused PET/CT.

Vivek Manchanda, MD

PRESENTATION

Man in midsixties with left lung cancer, for staging.

FINDINGS

Intensely hypermetabolic right tongue lesion and hypermetabolic left lung cancer.

DIFFERENTIAL DIAGNOSES

• *Primary tongue cancer with primary lung cancer*

• *Inflammatory lesion in tongue*

Given that the patient has a history of smoking, synchronous oral cancer is most likely, which was proven by biopsy.

COMMENTS

Majority of the oral cancers are squamous cell and extremely FDG avid.

Synchronous cancers of the lungs, larynx, or esophagus may be present in 10% to 15% of patients, related to smoking.

Oral cavity cancers include area of suprahyoid neck anterior to oropharynx, below sinonasal region.

Initial staging is done by CT and MR. CT is better in detecting cortical bone invasion and MR is better in defining tumor-muscle interface. Distant metastases are rare at presentation, hence initial screening with FDG-PET may not be cost effective. In selected patients, however, FDG-PET can be useful in staging spread to the neck nodes. Patients with advanced locoregional disease are at risk for distant metastases, especially lungs.

FDG-PET is also useful in evaluation of recurrence and response to the treatment.

The nonbreath-held, noncontrast CT of the chest obtained with PET may not detect small nodules at the lung bases.

FDG-PET can complement contrast-enhanced CT (especially in cases of artifacts) in characterizing the T stage, including extension across midline, into muscles, and invasion of maxillary bone.

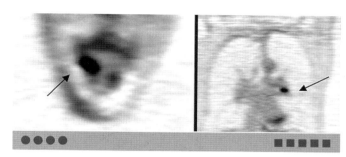

A. Coronal FDG-PET with incidental right tongue cancer in a patient with left lung cancer.

The risk of nodal metastasis is site dependent; higher with oral tongue, floor of mouth, and buccal mucosa in comparison to hard palate and upper gum.

Level 4 or 5 metastases is rare in absence of lymphadenopathy at levels 1 to 3. FDG-PET may detect disease in up to 4- to 5-mm nodes in an untreated patient. On CT, round morphology and lack of fatty hilum in lymph nodes is more likely to be metastatic.

PEARLS

• **FDG-PET is extremely useful in evaluation of recurrence and response to therapy.**

• **Since distant metastases is rare in initial presentation of oral cancers, initial staging with FDG may not be cost-effective.**

• **In selected cases (dental/metal artifacts), however, disease in small (4-5 mm) neck nodes (including contralateral nodes) may be detected by FDG-PET.**

• **Patients with advanced locoregional nodal disease are at higher risk for distant metastases, especially lungs. A breath-hold CT obtained with FDG-PET may be more useful.**

ADDITIONAL IMAGE

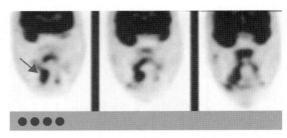

B. Right tongue cancer in different patient (*arrow*).

Vivek Manchanda, MD

PRESENTATION

Man in late twenties with nasopharyngeal mass.

FINDINGS

Intensely hypermetabolic nasopharyngeal mass with involvement of base of skull.

DIFFERENTIAL DIAGNOSES

- *Nasopharyngeal carcinoma*
- *Juvenile Angiofibroma*
- *Lymphoma*
- *Plasmacytoma (older)*
- *Infection*

COMMENTS

The commonest nasopharyngeal carcinoma is squamous cell type. These cancers tend to be very FDG avid.

FDG-PET is useful in identifying primary tumor site in cervical metastases and also in detecting unsuspected distal metastases.

There is synchronous lung cancer in about 8% to 10% patients with primary head and neck cancers.

Most of the nasopharyngeal cancers arise in the fossa of Rosenmüller. It is common for these cancers to spread into the surrounding structures including the base of skull. About 5% to 10% of the tumors may have intracranial extension. The incidence of distant metastases is higher in nasopharyngeal cancer as compared to other head and neck cancers.

Nasopharyngeal tumors spread to nodes bilaterally and to the posterior triangle nodes.

Follow-up of treatment with FDG-PET scanning is very accurate. Resolution of FDG activity after one cycle of chemo radiation predicts complete remission and longer survival. Radiation has minimal effect on the FDG uptake in normal structures, but there may be mild early postradiation uptake from inflammation.

High standardized uptake value (SUV) in the primary tumor correlates with poor prognosis; however, nodal SUV does not predict prognosis. Postoperatively, there may be increased FDG activity related to surgery. High SUV after treatment is a reliable predictor of local recurrence.

It is difficult for FDG-PET/CT to distinguish between benign and malignant salivary gland tumors. Carcinomas, tumors, and pleomorphic adenomas can all be metabolically active.

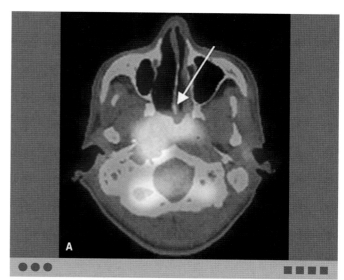

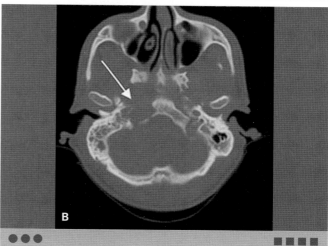

A. and **B.** Hypermetabolic nasopharyngeal mass with base of skull involvement, and crosses midline. Axial fused PET/CT (*top*) and axial CT (*bottom*).

PEARLS

- Majority of nasopharyngeal cancers are squamous cell and hence very FDG avid.

- Nasopharyngeal cancers may spread to base of the skull or intracranially and are most likely to metastasize distantly in comparison to other head and neck cancers.

- Level of FDG activity cannot distinguish nasopharyngeal cancer from NHL involving Waldeyer ring.

- Malignant and benign salivary gland tumors cannot be differentiated on basis of PET.

ADDITIONAL IMAGES (C-G)

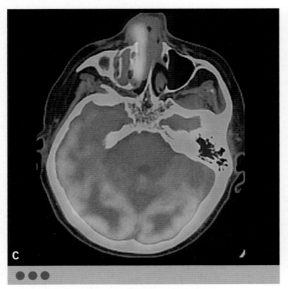

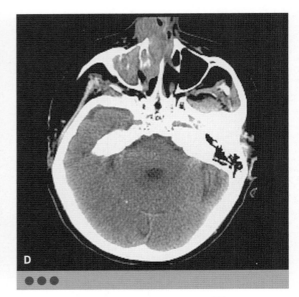

C. and **D.** Another patient with right nasopharyngeal cancer. Axial fused PET/CT and corresponding CT.

DIFFERENTIAL DIAGNOSES IMAGES (F-G)

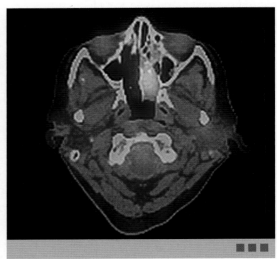

F. Esthesioneuroblastoma. Axial fused PET/CT.

E. Metastatic mediastinal and right femoral poorly differentiated nasopharyngeal cancer in 44-year-old male. Coronal fused FDG-PET.

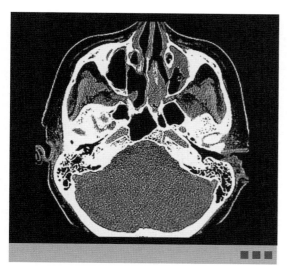

G. Corresponding CT.

Vivek Manchanda, MD

PRESENTATION

New right parietal lesion in a patient with a history of previous glioblastoma multiforme in the right temporal lobe.

FINDINGS

Photopenia corresponding to postsurgical changes and radiation necrosis, right temporal lobe. FDG uptake corresponding to new lesion with central photopenia with increased heterogenous peripheral FDG activity in the right parietal lobe, with maximum SUVs from 7.6 to 9.4, concerning for recurrent tumor. Central photopenia suggests necrosis. SUV of contralateral white matter is 4.8 and contralateral grey matter is 11.0.

DIFFERENTIAL DIAGNOSES

- Radiation necrosis in the right parietal lobe is unlikely given the new hypermetabolic lesion is away from the radiation field. Also the metabolic activity is higher than contralateral white matter, also suggestive of disease involvement.

- Abscess is unlikely given no clinical features associated with an infectious process.

- Metastasis, tumefactive multiple sclerosis.

COMMENTS

FDG can be used to differentiate recurrent glioblastoma multiforme from postradiation changes. The clinical and imaging characteristics of recurrent glioblastoma and postradiation changes can be similar. Late delayed radiation injury can occur from 4 months to years and is due to vascular endothelial injury or direct damage to oligodendroglia. This stage of injury can be confused with recurrent tumor. Both tumor and late delayed radiation injury can present on CT or MRI as a contrast-enhancing mass with edema and mass effect. Areas of radiation injury have lower glucose metabolism than tumor or normal brain tissue

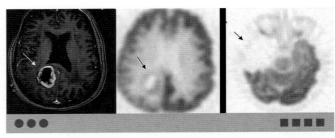

A. Photopenia corresponding to right temporal lesion, postsurgical. Right parietal peripherally hypermetabolic lesion, corresponding to peripherally enhancing MR lesion, concerning for recurrence. Central photopenia suggests necrosis.

as they are less cellular. (Usually, they show photopenia or lower metabolism than contralateral white matter.)

Recurrent tumors usually have an increased metabolism (more than contralateral white matter, equal to contralateral grey matter, or greater than contralateral grey matter in the region of enhancement on post-Gd MR images).

However, increased uptake can sometimes also be seen during normal healing processes during the first several months following radiation or surgery.

Other potential causes of false-positive studies are abscess and seizure foci. If the patient has a history of seizures, it is prudent to coordinate the PET examination with the neurology team for concurrent EEG.

Many physicians are using MR perfusion, FDG-PET, and MR spectroscopy to increase the specificity to distinguish radiation necrosis from tumor recurrence.

PEARLS

- Areas of radiation injury show decreased metabolism and areas of tumor recurrence show increased metabolism in a broad sense. However, false positives and false negatives have been reported.

- Comparison of FDG activity with contralateral white matter and contralateral grey matter is advisable.

ADDITIONAL IMAGE

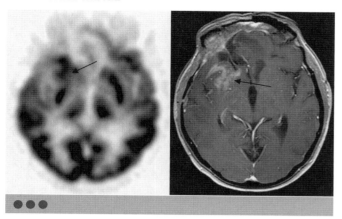

B. Axial FDG-PET (*right*) with right inferior frontal hypermetabolic focus and axial contrast-enhanced MR (*left*) with recurrence of tumor.

Vivek Manchanda, MD

PRESENTATION

Child with complex partial seizures. PET for localization.

FINDINGS

Interictal PET shows left medial temporal hypometabolism, corresponding to mesial temporal sclerosis in MR, consistent with lateralization of the seizure activity to the left.

COMMENTS

Functional brain imaging is most helpful in localizing partial seizures and less helpful in isolating the focus in generalized seizure disorders.

In general, during an epileptic seizure, cerebral metabolism and cerebral blood flow are markedly increased. On contrary, during the interictal period, both cerebral metabolism and cerebral blood flow are decreased.

In terms of specific brain structures, the temporal lobe is the most common focus of partial epilepsy. Most of the patients with nonlesional temporal lobe epilepsy have findings of hippocampal sclerosis on high-resolution MRI scan. Many patients with nonlesional temporal lobe epilepsy and electroclinically well-lateralized temporal lobe seizures have no evidence of MRI abnormality, but have concordant hypometabolism on FDG-PET.

Most of the data has suggested that in patients with temporal lobe epilepsy, the presence of temporal lobe hypometabolism is associated with a positive outcome after ipsilateral temporal lobectomy. The degree of hypometabolism, however, may not be that important according to some studies, whereas some studies have suggested that hypometabolism of at least 15% is considered significant.

There has been at least one study comparing the sensitivity of interictal PET with ictal SPECT, where ictal SPECT was considered more sensitive than interictal PET.

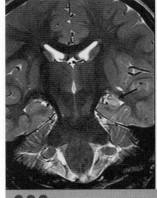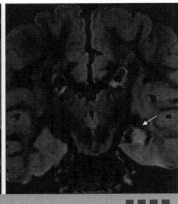

B. Corresponding coronal T2W MR with abnormal left mesial temporal signal. Axial flair with abnormal left mesial temporal signal.

It has been suggested that the metabolic dysfunction of thalamus, ipsilateral to the seizure focus, may become more severe with long-standing temporal and frontal lobe epilepsy, and also with secondary generalization of seizures.

In comparison to patients with unilateral temporal lobe hypometabolism, patients with bilateral temporal lobe hypometabolism have a higher percentage of generalized seizures and are more likely to have bilateral, diffuse, or extratemporal seizure onsets. Some studies have stressed the importance of mesial temporal lobe hypometabolism; others have predicted lateral temporal hypometabolism as a good predictor of surgical outcome.

Performing ictal PET is logistically difficult given the short half-life of FDG. Carbon-11 flumazenil (11C-FMZ) has shown promise in being more specific and sensitive than FDG-PET.

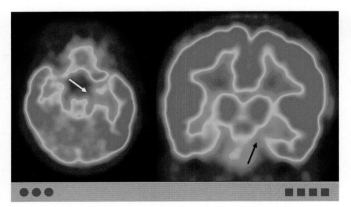

A. Left mesial temporal hypometabolism, axial and coronal views. Axial and coronal color-coded FDG-PET images.

PEARLS

- Mesial temporal hypometabolism and lateral temporal hypometabolism have been described as good predictors of surgical outcome in different studies.

- Patients with contralateral thalamic hypometabolism may be associated with more postoperative seizures.

- Functional brain imaging is most helpful in localizing partial seizures.

ADDITIONAL IMAGES (C-F)

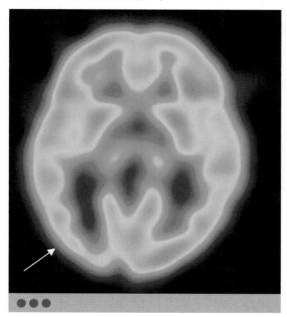

C. Right occipital hypometabolism in an infant with infantile spasms.

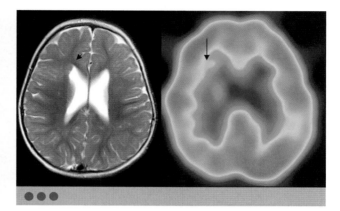

D. Heterotopia in an infant with infantile spasms, MR and FDG-PET (*arrows*).

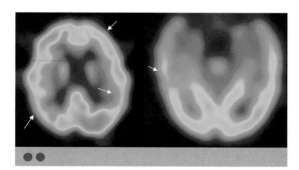

E. Patchy areas of hypometabolism in bilateral cortices with arrows in infantile spasm. Axial color coded FDG-PET.

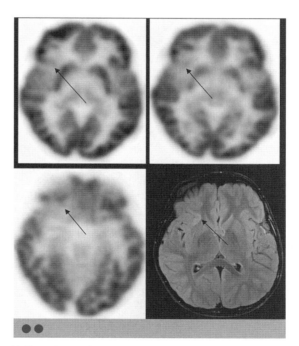

F. Frontal-type focal seizures in 8-year-old boy. (*Top left and top right*) Right inferior frontal and operculum hypometabolism as compared to left. (*Bottom left*) Right orbitofrontal hypometabolism. (*Bottom right*) Right inferior frontal subtle signal abnormality. Axial flair MR (*black arrow*). Right inferior frontal lobectomy showed focal cortical dysplasia, type II with areas of gliosis.

Vivek Manchanda, MD

PRESENTATION

Man in his midseventies, FDG-PET.

FINDINGS

Asymmetrically hypermetabolic left vocal cord, no mass.

DIFFERENTIAL DIAGNOSES

- *Physiologic*
- *Metastasis*
- *Cancer*
- *Teflon injection/granuloma*
- *Papilloma*

COMMENTS

Vocal cord paralysis from direct compression of the recurrent laryngeal nerve would result in superphysiologic FDG uptake in the contralateral normal vocal cord.

Similarly vocal cord paralysis from stroke/other neurologic conditions may result in increased FDG uptake in non-paralysed vocal cord, as in the index case.

Some benign lesions in the vocal cords can accumulate FDG and can be misinterpreted as malignancies. One such issue involves increased FDG uptake at the site of Teflon (Polytetrafluoroethylene) injection, which was a preferred method of treatment for symptomatic vocal cord paralysis

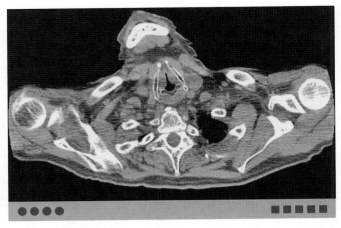

B. Corresponding CT, no mass in left vocal cord.

until recent past and was used to instigate a local inflammatory response. On CT, Teflon typically manifests as high-density material in the vocal cord that can extend into the soft tissues.

Laryngeal papillomas are more commonly seen in children and less common in persons older than 30 years. It is due to laryngeal infection with the HPV (human papillomavirus). Patients may present with hoarseness, respiratory difficulty, and stridor.

Papilloma recurrences in affected pediatric patients necessitate regular follow-ups. The patients may develop lung papillomatosis, which can be extremely FDG avid. These lesions may cavitate. It is difficult to ascertain a sarcomatous conversion in a lung papilloma on the basis of FDG-PET. However, serial CTs or follow-up PET may be helpful as these lesions in the lungs mostly wax and wane.

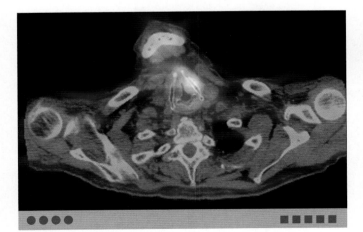

A. Axial fused PET/CT, hypermetabolic left vocal cord without mass, due to right vocal cord paralysis.

PEARLS

- Vocal cord paralysis from direct compression of the recurrent laryngeal nerve or stroke results in superphysiologic FDG uptake in the contralateral normal vocal cord.

- Teflon injection and papillomas may be associated with increased FDG activity.

DIFFERENTIAL DIAGNOSES IMAGES (C-D)

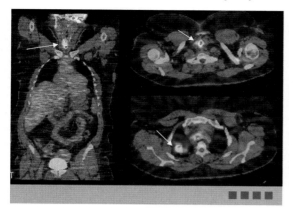

C. Laryngeal and lung papilloma with tracheostomy.

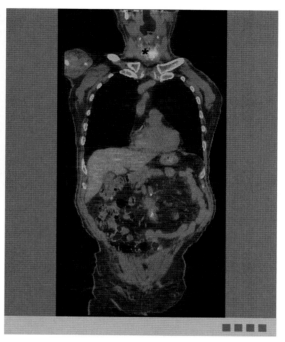

D. Left vocal cord carcinoma (*black star*). Coronal fused FDG-PET

Chapter 8

RENAL

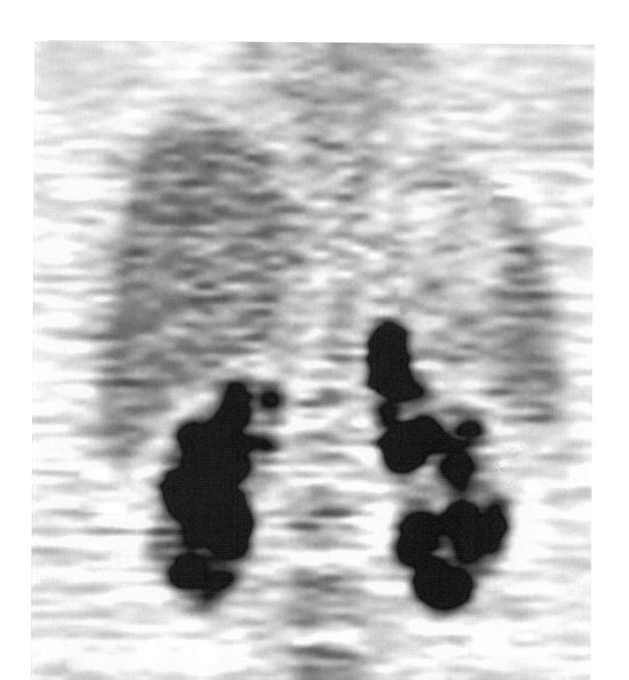

Case 8–1 Bilateral Kidneys and B-Cell Lymphoma and FDG-PET

Vivek Manchanda, MD

PRESENTATION

Man in early forties with bilateral kidney masses, known non-Hodgkin lymphoma (NHL).

FINDINGS

Increased FDG activity in both kidneys, corresponding to multiple hypodense kidney masses.

DIFFERENTIAL DIAGNOSES

- *Bilateral renal involvement in NHL*
- *Leukemia*
- *Metastases*
- *Multiple abcesses/infected cysts*

Lymphoma may present as nonenhancing masses of soft tissue attenuation. Focal fungal infections are usually small lesions in an immunocompromised patient with hepatic and splenic lesions. Bilateral and diffuse renal enlargement with preservation of reniform shape is the most common presentation of leukemia.

COMMENTS

Primary renal lymphoma is rare as kidneys do not have lymphoid tissue. Renal lymphoma is usually a B-cell lymphoma or Burkitts lymphoma.

Mostly, renal lymphoma is clinically asymptomatic and radiologic detection seldom influences staging and treatment. Follow-up data in patients with renal lymphoma suggests that recurrence in the kidneys is associated with bad prognosis.

Although it is difficult to assess kidney metabolism with Fluorodeoxyglucose-positron emission tomography (FDG-PET) given the FDG excretion, FDG-PET shows intensely hypermetabolic foci corresponding to hypodense masses in or around the kidneys, which enhance poorly with contrast on CT in renal lymphomas. Venous phase images may help detect small lesions in the medullary portion. Hilar region or obstruction of collecting system is best seen on the excretory phase.

Majority of patients have multiple lymphomatous masses (hematogenous dissemination). Bilateral kidney involvement is common. Solitary mass is seen in 10% to 25% of patients. Contiguous extension to the kidneys or perinephric space or diffuse renal enlargement (especially in Burkitt lymphoma) can also be seen.

Aggressive rhabdoid tumors of the kidneys can arise centrally and resemble lymphoma.

In a newborn, bilateral nephroblastoma and in myelofibrosis/thalassemia; extramedullary hematopoiesis (EMH) can be a differential. FDG uptake in nephroblastoma has been

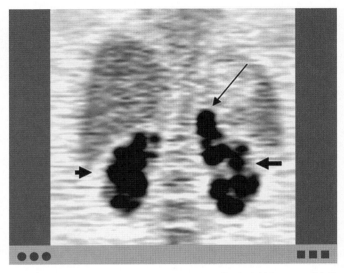

A. Multiple hypermetabolic masses in the bilateral kidneys and left adrenal (*long arrow*) in a patient with known DLBC lymphoma.

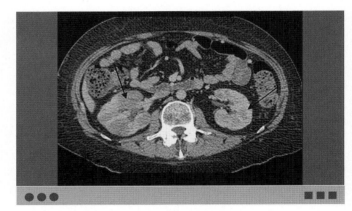

B. Corresponding contrast-enhanced CT with nonenhancing masses (*black arrows*).

described as variable, related to pathologic heterogeneity. FDG uptake in EMH is typically mild.

On MR, renal lymphoma is of low intermediate signal on both T1 and T2 images, similar to that of spleen and lymph nodes. It enhances weakly after contrast administration. On ultrasound (US), lymphomatous masses are typically hypoechoic and homogeneous.

PEARLS

- Most lymphomas involving kidneys are either diffuse large B-cell (DLBC) or high-grade Burkitts lymphoma, which are intensely hypermetabolic on FDG-PET.

- Corresponding CT usually shows multiple hypodense masses which do not enhance with contrast administration.

ADDITIONAL IMAGE

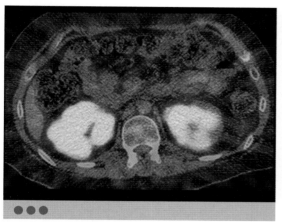

C. Axial fused PET/CT. DLBC.

DIFFERENTIAL DIAGNOSIS IMAGES (D-E)

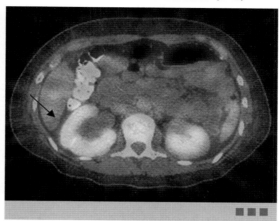

D. Axial fused PET/CT with right difffuse cortical activity without masses, from hydronephrosis (*black arrow*).

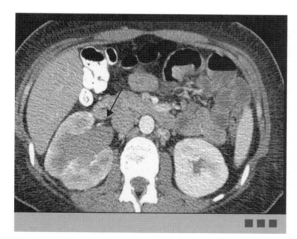

E. Corresponding contrast-enhanced CT (*black arrow*).

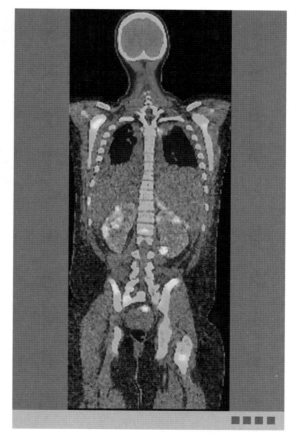

F. Coronal fused PET/CT. Bilateral renal disease, Burkitt lymphoma. Note diffuse bony and peritoneal disease.

Vivek Manchanda, MD

PRESENTATION

Intense focal FDG activity adjacent to bladder.

DIFFERENTIAL DIAGNOSES

- *Bladder diverticulum*
- *Artifact*
- *Adjacent node/metastasis*

Adjacent node/disease focus/artifact is unlikely given the clearly seen outpouching from the bladder wall, contiguous with bladder.

COMMENTS

Bladder diverticula are herniations of the bladder mucosa through the bladder wall musculature which can be identified on the FDG-PET/CT scan and localized easily. Some narrow-mouthed diverticula may not show any FDG accumulation.

They most commonly occur lateral and superior to the ureteral orifices. They may also occur at the dome of the bladder, in orders of bladder outlet obstruction such as posterior urethral valves or prune belly syndrome.

Congenital bladder diverticula are the commonest, mainly solitary, and located at the junction of the bladder trigone and detrusor.

Acquired diverticula are usually multiple and a result of obstruction, infections, or iatrogenic causes. Examples of obstruction include urethral valves, strictures, and neuropathic bladder. Many of these diverticula resolve spontaneously after correction of the obstruction.

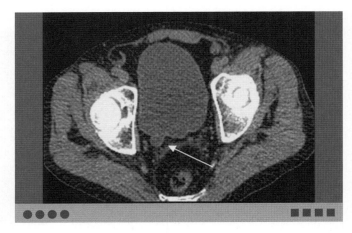

B. Corresponding axial CT (*arrow*).

Urachal sinus derives from a persistently patent urachus and may be seen as an outpouching with FDG activity on PET. Intense radiotracer activity will be seen tracking to umbilicus, if there is persistent patent urachus. Vesicourachal diverticulum, an outpouching at the apex of the bladder, results from an incomplete closure of the proximal urachus.

Bladder ears are lateral protrusions of the bladder through the internal inguinal ring and into the inguinal canal. The bladder positioning improves with growth. Bladder agenesis is rare and generally incompatible with life.

Megacystitis, an enlarged bladder, is associated with high-grade vesicoureteral reflux and can be seen in posterior urethral valves, Ehlers-Danlos syndrome, urethral diverticulum, microcolon hypoperistalsis syndrome, sacral meningomyelocele, sacrococcygeal teratoma, and pelvic neuroblastoma.

Bladder duplication is rare. Complete duplication (two urethras) is more common than incomplete duplication. Associated anomalies include duplicated penis, vagina, uterus, lumbar vertebrae, and hindgut. Bladder septation anomalies are rare and may be complete or incomplete.

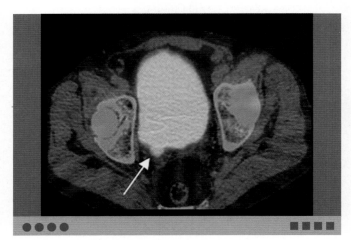

A. Axial fused PET/CT, bladder diverticulum (*white arrow*).

PEARLS

- Bladder diverticula, urachal sinus, and vesicourachal diverticulum are some of the bladder anomalies, which can cause false-positive findings on a PET/CT scan.

- Prostatic hypertrophy and pelvic masses can distort the shape of the bladder and should be kept in mind while reading PET/CTs.

ADDITIONAL IMAGES (C-D)

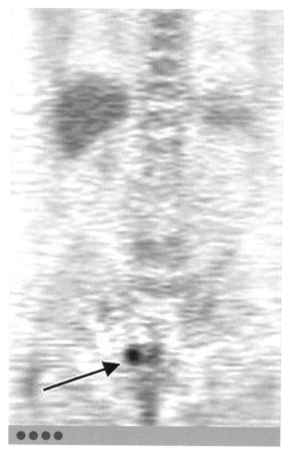

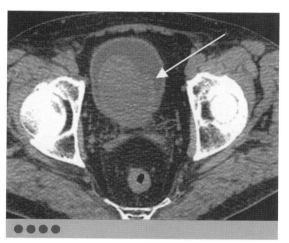

D. Prostatic hypertrophy, axial noncontrast CT (*white arrow*).

C. Coronal FDG-PET, with focal FDG activity in the pelvis, representing bladder diverticulum.

DIFFERENTIAL DIAGNOSIS IMAGES (E-H)

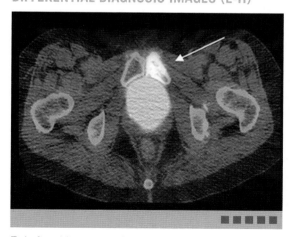

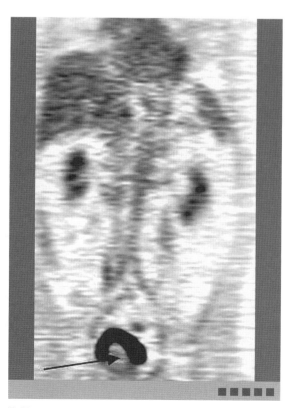

E. Left pubic metastasis and bladder (*white arrow*). Axial fused PET/CT.

F. Photopenic artifact from prostatic hypertrophy. Coronal FDG-PET.

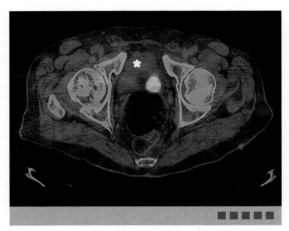

G. Axial fused PET/CT with focal hypermetabolic left transitional cell cancer and catheterized bladder (*white star*).

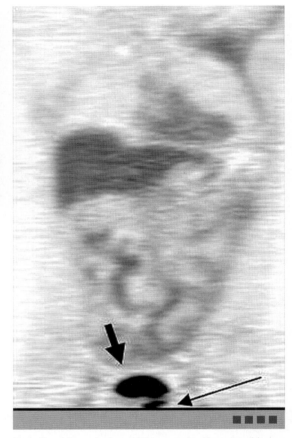

H. Left pubic metastases (*thin arrow*) adjacent to bladder (*thick arrow*). Coronal FDG-PET.

Vivek Manchanda, MD

PRESENTATION

Nonvisualization of one kidney on the PET scan.

FINDINGS

Absence of left kidney with hypermetabolic myometrium of bicornuate uterus.

DIFFERENTIAL DIAGNOSES

• *Surgical removal of left kidney*

• *Congenital absence of left kidney*

Congenital absence of one kidney is associated with Müllerian anomalies and is the most likely cause in this case. Surgical absence of a kidney should be suspicious for previous cancers such as renal cell carcinoma (RCC).

COMMENTS

If the kidney has not been removed surgically, it is important to evaluate PET scan for the clues of other congenital anomalies.

The most common anomalies associated with the unilateral renal agenesis are Müllerian ductal anomalies in females and seminal vesicle anomalies in males.

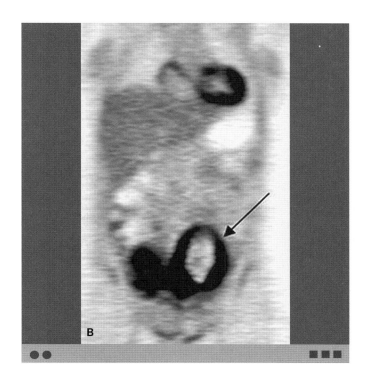

One-half of Mayer-Rokitansky-Küster-Hauser syndrome patients have vaginal atresia with other variable Müllerian duct abnormalities such as bicornuate or septated uterus and unilateral renal anomalies.

One of the commonest renal anomalies is horseshoe kidney in which the inferior poles of both the kidneys are fused. On the PET/CT, the fusion of the lower poles can be visualized easily on both PET and CT. The incidence of Wilms' tumor in horseshoe kidney is higher than that for the general population.

One or both kidneys may be displaced with or without other renal malformations. Duplication of ureter and renal pelvis may be seen.

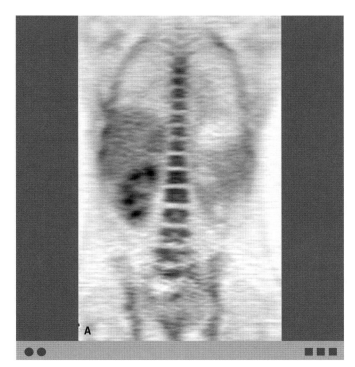

A. and **B.** Congenital absence of left kidney (Image A) and bicornuate uterus (*arrow*), postpartum (Image B). Coronal FDG-PET.

PEARLS

• **It is important to comment on congenital renal anomalies on the PET/CT and recognize other anomalies associated with them.**

• **The most common anomaly associated with unilateral renal agenesis is Müllerian ductal anomaly in females and seminal vesicle cysts in males.**

• **Viability of renal transplant can be commented upon the PET/CT scan.**

Of the two types of polycystic renal disease, autosomal dominant usually presents in adulthood and autosomal recessive in infancy. It is twice as frequent in males as in females. Classic multicystic dysplastic kidney appears as a mass of noncommunicating cysts resembling a bunch of grapes with no discernible parenchyma and no function on Tc MAG3 scan.

Prune belly syndrome in males has dilated urinary bladder and ureters with flabby abdominal wall. It may be associated with renal dysplasia.

Viability of renal transplant can be commented upon the PET scan.

ADDITIONAL IMAGES (C-F)

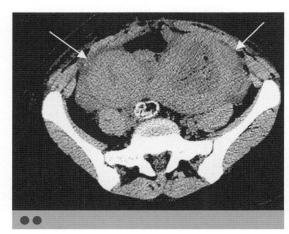

C. Corresponding CT for the images A and B.

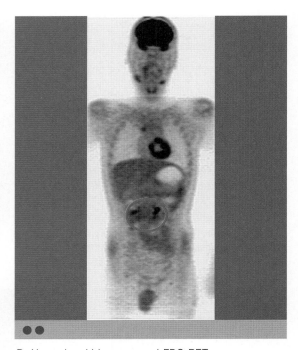

D. Horseshoe kidney, coronal FDG-PET.

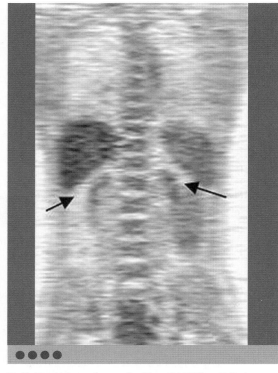

E. Native kidneys (*arrows*) with mild FDG activity in a patient with transplanted kidney (Image H). Coronal FDG-PET.

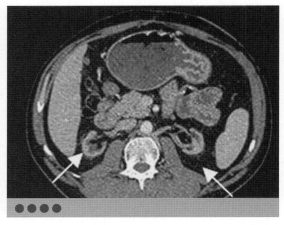

F. Corresponding CT.

DIFFERENTIAL DIAGNOSIS IMAGES (H-I)

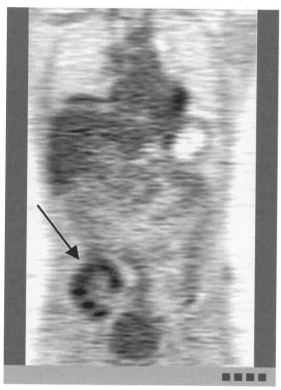

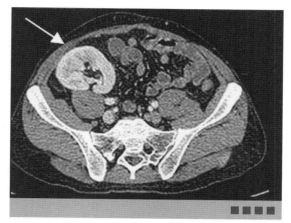

I. Corresponding CT.

H. Right pelvic transplanted kidney (*arrow*). Coronal FDG-PET.

Vivek Manchanda, MD

PRESENTATION

Right kidney mass in patient in midsixties with hematuria.

FINDINGS

Isometabolic right kidney mass.

DIFFERENTIAL DIAGNOSES

- *Primary renal cell cancer*
- *Lymphoma*
- *Metastasis*

Given the history of hematuria and no known primary, isometabolic kidney mass is most consistent with primary renal cell carcinoma (RCC). Metastases to kidneys can have variable FDG activity, based on primary tumor histology. Lymphoma is unlikely as most renal lymphomas are DLBC, which are intensely metabolically active.

COMMENTS

The increased background activity of healthy renal tissue and normal FDG excretion in urine can make visualization of primary renal cancers by PET difficult. They can be isometabolic or hypermetabolic (more likely) or FDG negative (less likely). In multiple studies, the range of sensitivity

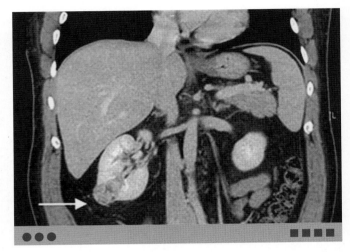

B. Corresponding contrast CT (*arrow*).

spans from 30% to 70% for detection of primary RCC with ^{18}F-FDG-PET.

Inconsistent FDG uptake in RCC remains unexplained. Correlation between glucose transporter 1 (GLUT-1) and PET hypermetabolism has been suggested but not proven. It has also been hypothesized that the isometabolic nature of primary renal cancers may be due to a lack of accessibility of FDG. Some researchers have suggested that PET-positive patients had higher tumor grade and increased GLUT-1. Per some studies, FDG-PET has proven to be more sensitive for metastatic lesions from primary RCC than primary tumors themselves.

FDG-PET has very high specificity in characterizing indeterminate renal cysts and results have been consistent in multiple studies. It is important to compare both contrast-enhanced CT and PET to characterize a cystic renal lesion. Ultrasound/ MR can be used for further characterization.

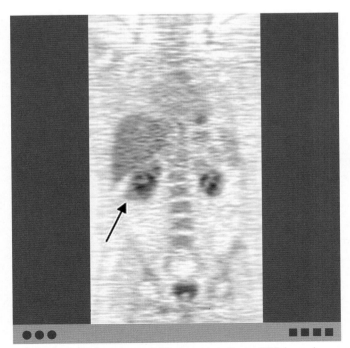

A. Patient A: Right primary RCC, isometabolic on PET (*arrow*).

PEARLS

- Up to one-third of primary RCC may not be FDG avid. Most lesions are iso- or hypermetabolic to the renal parenchyma.

- Differential FDG uptake in RCC is unexplained. FDG activity in metastases to kidneys and primary RCC may be similar.

- FDG-PET is more sensitive for detection of RCC metastases (typically lytic on CT) than primary RCC.

- FDG-PET is highly specific in characterizing indeterminate renal cysts.

FDG-PET can be used as a complementary tool when conventional scans are suspicious but equivocal for metastatic RCC or solid renal mass.

FDG-PET is highly sensitive and specific for detection of metastases to bone. Classically, metastatic renal cancer is osteolytic and sclerotic lesions are rare.

Angiomyolipoma is typically hypometabolic, but along with oncocytoma, can be falsely FDG avid. Absolute radiologic differentiation of oncocytoma from RCC is difficult.

FDG-PET would not be useful in differentiating hypertrophied columns of Bertin/pseudotumor from RCC.

ADDITIONAL IMAGES (C–H)

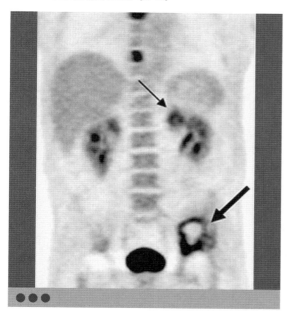

C. Patient B: Left renal hypermetabolic RCC (*thin arrow*) in a patient with left hip (*thick arrow*) and vertebral metastases from head and neck squamous cell cancer.

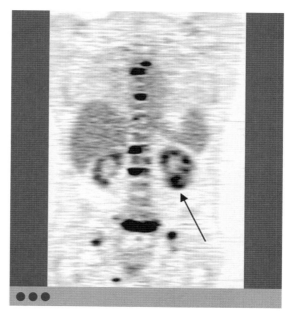

D. Patient C: Left kidney primary RCC (*arrow*) with multiple metastases.

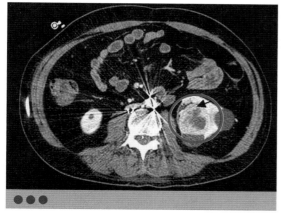

E. Corresponding CT.

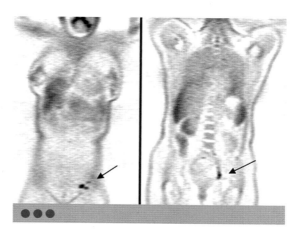

F. Patient D: Left inguinal and internal iliac nodal metastases from RCC (*arrows*), non–attenuation corrected (NAC) image.

DIFFERENTIAL DIAGNOSIS IMAGES (G-I)

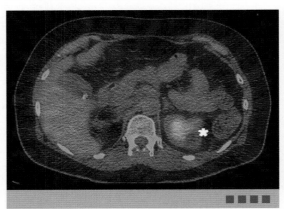

G. Hypometabolic left renal angiomyolipoma. Axial fused PET/CT (*white star*).

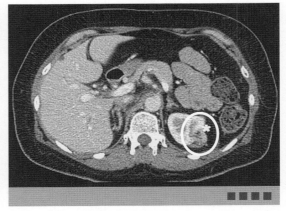

H. Corresponding CT (*white star*).

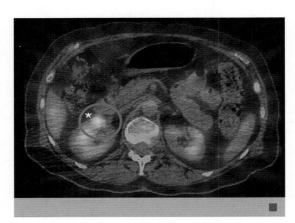

I. Right renal metastasis from papillary thyroid cancer.

Vivek Manchanda, MD

PRESENTATION

A 34-year-old with cervical cancer.

FINDINGS

Retention of radiotracer in the left collecting system with dilated pelvicalyceal system on the corresponding CT scan.

DIFFERENTIAL DIAGNOSES

- *Left ureteral obstruction from cervical cancer causing hydronephrosis*

- *Diffuse metastasis involving kidney*

The hydronephrosis seen on the CT scan and cervical mass are most consistent with left ureteral obstruction from cervical cancer.

COMMENTS

Fluorine 18 FDG can be considered an expensive functional renal imaging agent as it is not reabsorbed in the proximal tubules, unlike glucose.

The high excretion of FDG makes it difficult to assess metabolism for renal disease, but it can still provide important

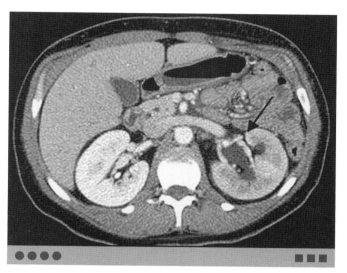

B. Corresponding CT.

physiological information. In the dynamic data, the parenchymal and pelvic curves can be differentiated with separate peaks.

In the index case, unilateral hydronephrosis from ureteral compression has resulted in backpressure, stalling the egress of FDG tracer from renal parenchyma into the pelvis.

Similarly, a blockage from stone in the ureterovesical junction can result in FDG accumulation in the ureter and in the renal pelvis, causing hydronephrosis.

Functionality of a stent can be assessed as a blocked stent would retain the FDG activity in the pelvis.

Urinary leak from renal trauma, kidney transplantation, and nephrostomy tube removal can be visualized. The nephrostomy tubes will show FDG activity, corresponding to the tube and the FDG activity may appear to track outside the renal contour.

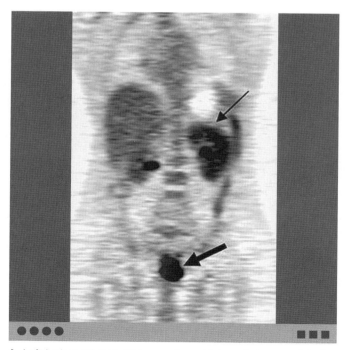

A. Left hydronephrosis (*thin arrow*), and intensely hypermetabolic cervical cancer (*thick arrow*), coronal FDG-PET.

PEARLS

- **FDG, unlike glucose, is not resorbed in the proximal tubules and as such can give important physiological information.**

- **Hydronephrosis, ureterovesical junction (UVJ) obstruction, urinary leak, acute tubular necrosis (ATN), and stent function are some of the physiological parameters that can be characterized on the PET scan.**

- **Unilateral hydronephrosis in a patient with cervical cancer is an independent factor for stage III cervical cancer.**

As an aftereffect of radiation, radiation therapy can cause transient or permanent functional defect in the irradiated kidneys. Radiofrequency ablation of a renal mass would result in a corresponding photopenic defect on an FDG-PET scan.

ADDITIONAL IMAGES (C–I)

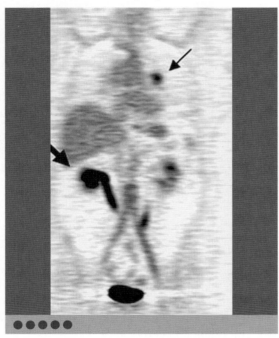

C. Right ureteral obstruction, caused by stone in the ureter (*thick arrow*), coronal FDG-PET. Left lung cancer (*thin arrow*).

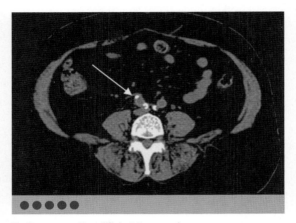

D. Corresponding CT (*white arrow*).

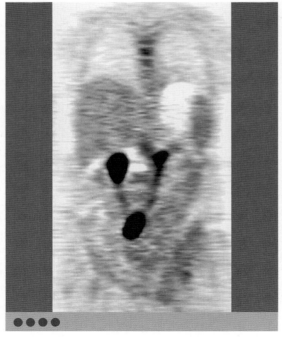

E. Urinary diversion and neobladder, coronal FDG-PET.

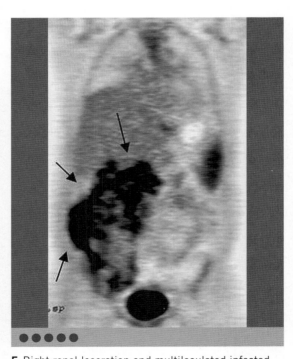

F. Right renal laceration and multiloculated infected hematoma in the right abdomen (*arrows*). Coronal FDG-PET.

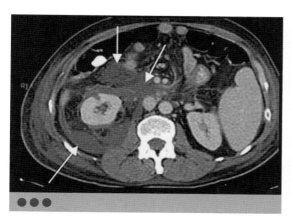

G. Corresponding CT.

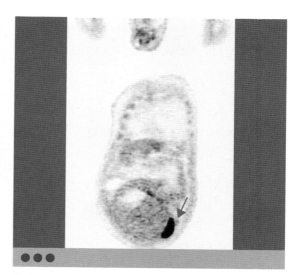

H. Pelvic mass displacing bladder (*arrow*). Coronal FDG-PET.

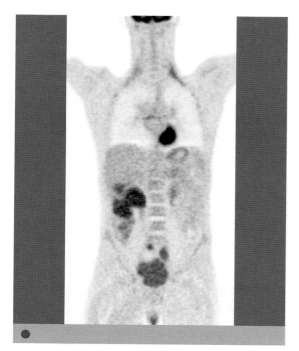

I. Right hydroureteronephrosis and insertion of right ureter to left side of bladder. Coronal FDG-PET.

Vivek Manchanda, MD

PRESENTATION

Man in early sixties with sigmoid colon cancer.

FINDINGS

Focal FDG uptake in the right lateral wall of the bladder which is catheterized with retrograde filling of the bladder. Intense FDG uptake in the known sigmoid colon cancer.

DIFFERENTIAL DIAGNOSES

- *Bladder diverticulum*
- *Residual urine*
- *Image artifact*
- *Transitional cell cancer (TCC)*

Residual urine in a retrogradely filled bladder is possible in the dependent portion of the bladder, but unlikely in the lateral wall. Image artifact can be produced if clamped

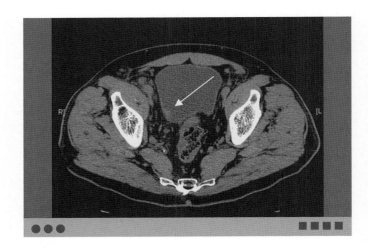

catheter is released between acquisition of PET emission images. Bladder diverticulum is seen as an outpouching.

COMMENTS

Bladder epithelial cancer is the commonest genitourinary tract cancer, with TCC accounting for 90%. Chemical agents such as aniline dye and nicotine are associated with bladder carcinogenesis.

Gross or microscopic hematuria is the commonest presentation of TCC. Patients are usually older than 50 years (peak seventh decade). Men: women ratio is 3:1 with white predominance.

Squamous cell carcinoma (5%) is associated with chronic inflammation, especially from bilharziasis. Adenocarcinoma (2% of all) is associated with urachal remnant.

About 60% of bladder tumors are detected on urograms as intravesical filling defects. CT is limited to evaluate depth

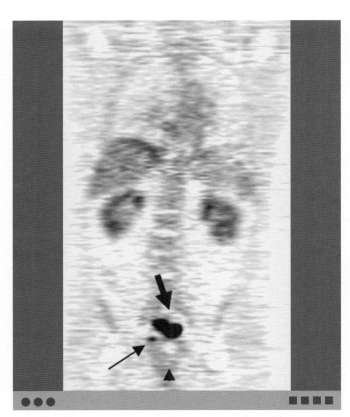

A. and **B.** Right posterolateral hypermetabolic focus (TCC, *thin black arrow*) and sigmoid cancer (*thick black arrow*). Retrogradely filled bladder (*arrowhead*). Coronal FDG-PET.

PEARLS

- **Since FDG is excreted in urine, evaluation of TCC is difficult. But it can be eliminated by retrograde filling of the bladder.**

- **Focal FDG uptake in the nondependent portion of bladder should be worked up for primary bladder cancer with cystoscopy and biopsy.**

- **FDG-PET has excellent sensitivity in detecting distant metastases.**

of disease. It can evaluate perivesical and local pelvic extension. MRI is superior to CT for local tumor growth and detection of bone marrow infiltration.

Few studies have addressed the role of FDG-PET in bladder cancer because of renal excretion of FDG. PET is useful for identifying sites of disease not found by conventional imaging, in particular, PET may identify unsuspected pelvic, para-aortic, mediastinal, or supraclavicular nodal metastases, sometimes sparing the patient's inappropriate surgery. FDG-PET has very high sensitivity for distant metastases, but sensitivity for detection of disease in the local nodes is moderate.

In urothelial cancer, the role of PET is still being defined, but it has a high positive predictive value and can be used for problem solving in patients with indeterminate findings on conventional imaging.

ADDITIONAL IMAGE

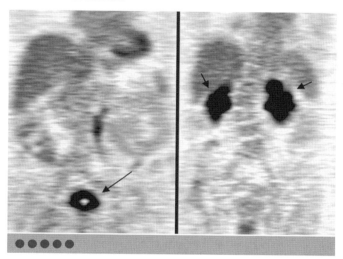

C. Intensely hypermetabolic circumferentially thickened bladder wall (*long arrow*) from TCC with bilateral hydronephrosis (*small arrows*).

DIFFERENTIAL DIAGNOSIS IMAGES (D-G)

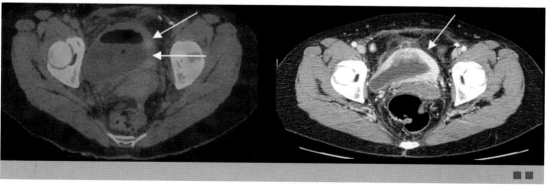

D. Mildly hypermetabolic bladder wall metastases from invasive lobular breast cancer. Axial fused PET/CT (*white arrows*) and corresponding-contrast-enhanced CT (*white arrow*).

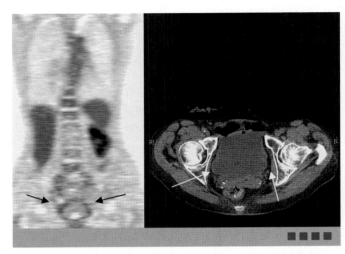

E. Mildly hypermetabolic bladder wall (chronic inflammation) in a catheterized and retrogradely filled bladder, corresponding to chronically thickened bladder wall. Coronal FDG-PET with corresponding CT.

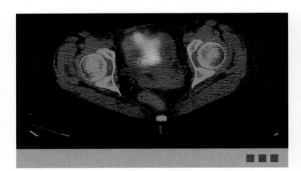

F. Leiomyosarcoma of bladder in a 29-year-old female.

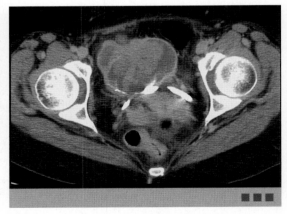

G. Leiomyosarcoma of bladder, corresponding CT.

Bhasker R. Koppula, MD

PRESENTATION

A 42-year-old female, status post–multiple abdominal surgeries and retroperitoneal and intraperitoneal abscess, presenting with right hydronephrosis with J-stent in place in the collecting system.

FINDINGS

Posterior abdominal images of Tc-99m MAG3 (mercapto acetyl triglycine) renogram show progressive accumulation of tracer in the collecting system in the right kidney and show no drainage even after Lasix (furosemide) administration. Delayed images obtained show slow tracer accumulation in the perinephric space and thence into the bag outside the body which drains the perinephric space. Features are consistent with obstructed right collecting system and obstructed J-stent within the collecting system and urine extravasation into the perinephric space.

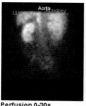
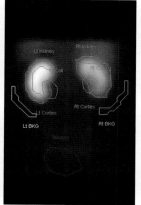
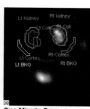

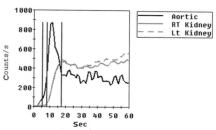

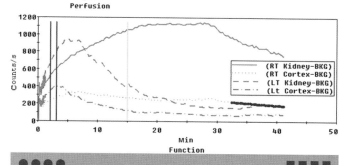

B. Tc-99m MAG3 renogram curves show prompt uptake and concentration in both kidneys with delayed excretion in the right kidney even after Lasix administration at 15 minutes. However, there is slow clearance of tracer from the collecting system best seen after 30 minutes which resulted from slow urine leak into the retroperitoneal space. (*Image courtesy of Bhasker R. Koppula, MD.*)

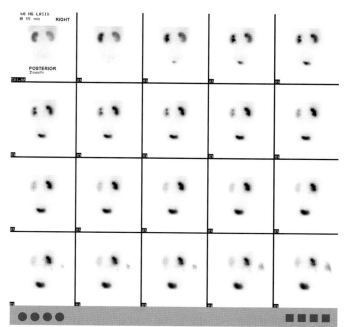

A. Sequential dynamic posterior images from MAG3 renogram show progressive accumulation of the tracer within the right collecting system. No significant clearance of tracer is noted even after the administration of Lasix. Features are consistent with obstruction of the right collecting system. However, the images obtained after the administration of Lasix show subtle accumulation of the radiotracer in the perinephric space inferior to the right kidney. Also, there is progressive accumulation of the tracer outside the body into the drainage bag which is in turn drained by a perinephric space drainage catheter. (*Image courtesy of Bhasker R. Koppula, MD.*)

PEARLS

- Tc-99m MAG3 renal imaging is helpful in identifying urine extravasation as a cause of localized or diffuse fluid collections in the retroperitoneal or intraperitoneal compartments.

- Delayed images may have to be obtained to document slow and delayed leaks.

- Caution needs to be exercised in interpreting extrarenal activity because of normal physiological excretion of Tc-99m MAG3 in the gastrointestinal tract. Correlation with CT or ultrasound will be helpful.

DIFFERENTIAL DIAGNOSES

- External trauma to the kidneys, ureters, or bladder resulting from either blunt or penetrating injuries.

- Iatrogenic injury to the renal collecting system, ureters, or bladder during surgical procedures. For example, necrosis of the ureters caused by ligation of ureters or injury resulting from gynecologic surgeries. Invasion by adjacent malignant process or inflammatory processes.

- Differential diagnoses for focal perinephric/periureteral collections include lymphoceles particularly after surgical procedures like lymph node dissections and resolving hematomas.

COMMENTS

Extravasation of urine refers to leak of urine from the renal collecting systems, ureters, or the bladder into the perinephric space, periureteral space, or into perivesical spaces. If the urine leaks into the peritoneal space, it can result in urinary ascites. Most common causes of urinary extravasation include iatrogenic trauma or external trauma, resulting from blunt or penetrating injuries to the kidneys, ureters, or the urinary bladder.

Clinical presentation of patients with urinary extravasation depends on the etiology and location of urine collection. However, in the presence of diffuse peritoneal extravasation resulting in urinary ascites it might be difficult to establish the etiology of the source of fluid collection by clinical and/or standard radiographic methods. Also, anatomic imaging can provide information about the presence or absence of a focal fluid collection without necessarily giving information about the etiology causing the collection. Noninvasive scintigraphic imaging with radiopharmaceuticals is helpful in such situations confirming urinary leak as the etiology as well as the most probable site of urinary extravasation. Renal radionuclide imaging is usually performed with dynamic imaging of the blood flow, uptake, and clearance of tracer over a period of time with or without Lasix administration. Tc-99m MAG3 is the most commonly used tracer for renal scintigraphic evaluation. In addition to various semiquantitative functional analyses that are possible by generating time activity curves, static and delayed (2-4 hours) imaging of the abdomen and pelvis is very helpful in identifying the cause of fluid accumulation. However, normal excretion of Tc-99m MAG3 by the hepatobiliary system might complicate interpretation. High sensitivity and lack of local tissue toxicities make radioisotope renogram the most attractive test for this purpose.

ADDITIONAL IMAGES (C-E)

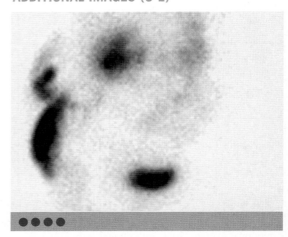

C. Static image after 30 minutes in anterior projection shows radiotracer outside the body in the drainage bag draining the perinephric space. (*Image courtesy of Bhasker R. Koppula, MD.*)

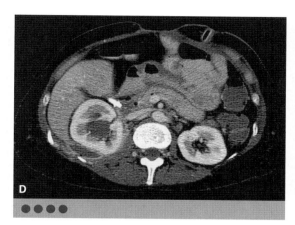
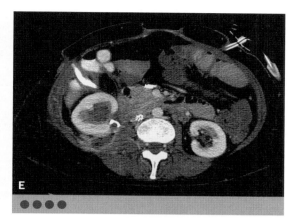

D. and **E.** Representative axial CT images at the level of kidneys show fluid collection in the right retroperitoneal space which is drained by perinephric drainage catheter. Also, note the J-stent in the right pelvis. (*Images courtesy of Bhasker R. Koppula, MD.*)

Joseph Rajendran, MD

PRESENTATION

A 68-year-old male suffers ruptured AAA (abdominal aortic aneurysm). Emergency surgical repair is successful. Patient goes into acute renal failure (ARF). Six weeks later, with a presumptive diagnosis of ATN, creatine levels and urine output are discordant. Question of vascular disruption or acute tubular necrosis (ATN).

FINDINGS

Flow phase demonstrates prompt, normal perfusion of both kidneys. Time activity curves (TAC) and parenchymal phase demonstrate accumulation of MAG3 in the renal parenchyma but none in the collecting system. No tracer is seen in the bladder. Sixty milligrams of Lasix (furosemide) was administered at 10 minutes.

DIFFERENTIAL DIAGNOSIS

The differential diagnosis would include severe, long-standing bilateral renal obstruction; however this is unlikely because at least some tracer usually escapes into the collecting system.

The other possibility is renal failure due to prerenal causes, for example acute hypovolemia but the history usually directs to that diagnosis.

COMMENT

ATN is typically caused by varying degrees of tubule cell damage as a result of tissue death prolonged renal ischemia,

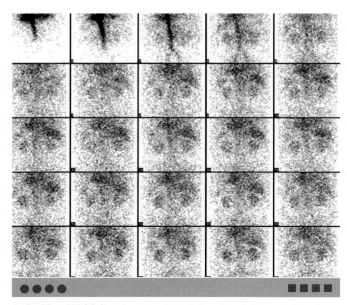

A. Tc-99m MAG3 flow images show delayed and decreased perfusion to the both kidneys.

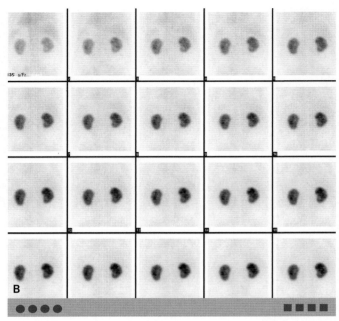

B. Sequential renal function images show uptake in the parenchyma with significantly prolonged retention. There is minimal accumulation in the collecting systems.

nephrotoxins, and sepsis. ATN presents with ARF that leads to a rise in products such as BUN and creatinine. The most common etiologies of ARF belong to the following groups: prerenal, intrinsic renal (parenchymal), and postrenal. Thus history is important in clinching the diagnosis. ATN is typically caused by an acute ischemic or toxic effect. In the case of transplant ATN, acute episodes of severe reduction in renal perfusion are the most common etiologic causes. Nephrogenic

---

PEARLS

- In ATB perfusion to the kidneys can be normal until very late in the disease process.

- Absence of activity in the collecting system excludes high-grade outflow obstruction as the primary cause.

- Tc-99m MAG3 is the agent of choice as it has the highest renal extraction and is very useful under impaired renal function.

- Postischemic ATN is the common cause for renal transplant dysfunction; increased with longer cold ischemia time.

- Cyclosporine toxicity can produce the same abnormalities. Perfusion will be retained.

- Acute rejection has significantly decreased perfusion to the transplanted kidney as compared to well-preserved perfusion in ATN (differentiating point).

toxicity can be caused by a variety of drugs including amino-glycosides and radiographic contrast media. Early phases of ATN manifest with oliguria but late phases present with polyuria; however, ATN manifests for a prolonged period. The specific gravity of the urine is a constant at 1010 as the kidneys lose their ability to concentrate. Tc-99m MAG3 is a tubular excretion agent, that is, it is not filtered at the level of the glomerulus but instead is taken up by the parenchyma and actively excreted by the tubules making it an excellent agent for testing tubular function. Failure to remove MAG3 from the parenchyma indicates failure of the tubules to function. Renogram in ATN shows an obstructive pattern of curves with no or very little activity in the collecting system. When transplanted kidney is evaluated, the perfusion phase shows essentially normal perfusion (depending on the status of the vascular supply) but no excretion with flat curves. This differentiates it from acute rejection where the perfusion is grossly diminished but the pattern of curves remains the same.

ADDITIONAL IMAGES (C-F)

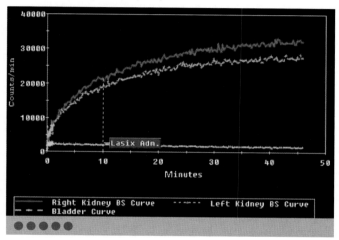

C. Renogram curves show delayed concentration and excretion in both kidneys. Activity in both kidneys continues to rise indicating an "obstructive pattern."

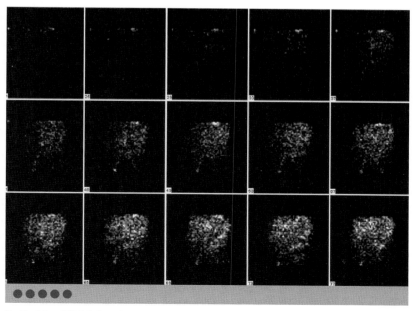

D. Tc-99m MAG3 flow images show delayed and decreased perfusion to the transplanted kidney in the pelvis.

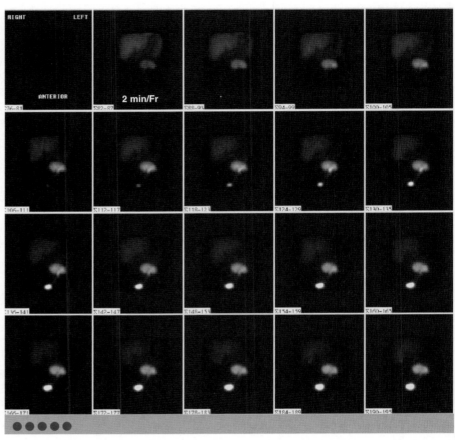

E. Sequential renogram images show persistent parenchymal activity in the transplanted kidney consistent with ATN. Note absence of prominet uptake in the collecting system.

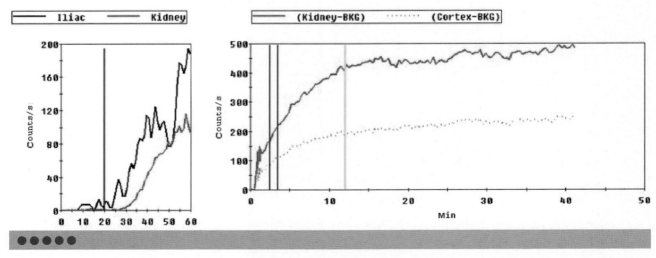

F. Renogram curves show decreased perfusion to the transplanted kidney compared to iliac vessel (*left image*) and significantly decreased excretion in the transplanted kidney.

Chapter 9

VASCULAR

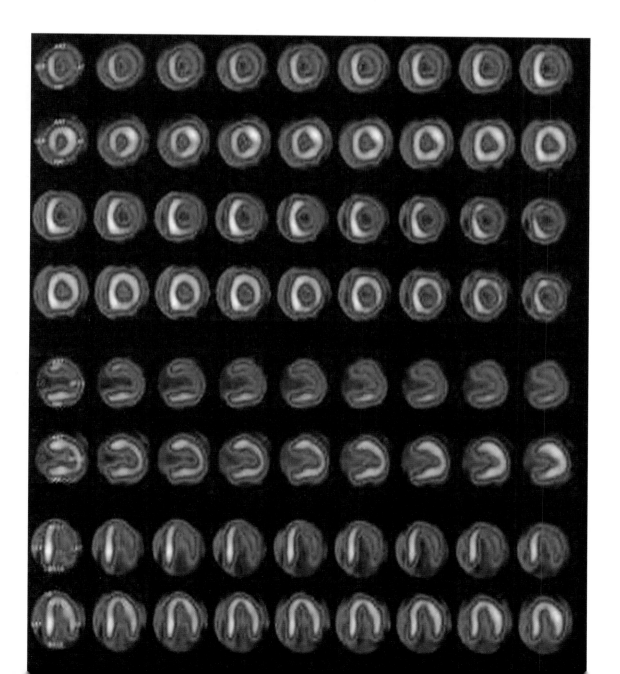

Case 9–1 Cardiac PET Perfusion

Vivek Manchanda, MD

PRESENTATION

Man in midfifties with hypercholesterolemia, hypertension, and diabetes with chest pain.

FINDINGS

Scintigraphic evidence of a large-sized region of moderate, reversible myocardial perfusion involving the entire antero-lateral, true lateral, apical, and distal one-third of the inferoapi-cal wall of the left ventricle. Dilatation of left ventricle cavity size with stress.

DIFFERENTIAL DIAGNOSES

• *Artifact*

• *Ischemia*

The findings are most consistent with true ischemia, provided there is no misregistration of attenuation (CT) and emission images, which can create an artifact.

COMMENTS

Rubidium-82 (Rb-82) and nitrogen 13 ammonia (N 13-NH$_3$) are the myocardial perfusion agents. Fluorodeoxyglucose (FDG) is used for viability assessment.

The advantages of positron emission tomography (PET) CT over single photon emission computed tomography (SPECT) are in patients with a body mass index (BMI) greater than 30 kg/m^2. In such patients, abnormal results on PET are more reliable. Also, cardiac PET has better spatial resolution and has the ability to provide quantitative measurement of physiologic parameters. In addition to lower radiation exposure than other forms of nuclear stress testing, patients benefit from reduced examination time. Cardiac PET is equally sensitive and slightly more specific in comparison to SPECT for detection of coronary artery disease (CAD), when compared with cardiac catheterization results. It has better predictive accuracy than SPECT for CAD diagnosis. It also reduces diagnostic uncertainty in patients with equivocal SPECT scans.

Myocardial perfusion imaging (MPI) with PET can be accomplished with the flow tracers Rb-82 or N 13-NH$_3$, at rest and during pharmacologic (usually dipyridamole) or exercise stress. Normal myocardial perfusion with adequate stress is indicative of absence of significant CAD.

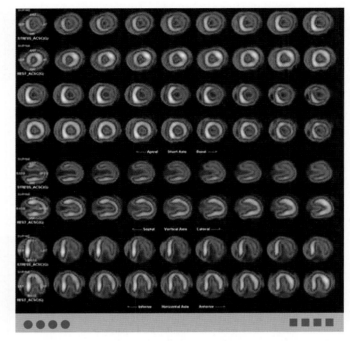

A. Moderate myocardial ischemia involving the entire anterolateral, true lateral, apical, and distal one-third of the infero-apical wall of the left ventricle. Dilatation of left ventricular cavity size with stress. N13-ammonia PET. (*Image courtesy of James Caldwell, MD, UWMC.*)

Stress-induced regional myocardial perfusion abnormalities are indicative of hemodynamically significant CAD. Impaired regional myocardial perfusion in both stress and rest suggests the presence of an irreversible myocardial injury.

Quantitative measurement of regional flow reserve assessed by PET can help monitor the progression or regression of CAD.

PEARLS

• **Perfusion imaging with cardiac PET has equal sensitivity and higher specificity in comparison to SPECT perfusion.**

• **Regional flow reserve can be assessed by PET perfusion study.**

• **Multi-attenuation imaging series and visual coregistration of attenuation and emission images can significantly reduce artifacts.**

Vivek Manchanda, MD

PRESENTATION

Man in late fifties, for evaluation of CAD.

FINDINGS

Mild to moderately decreased radiotracer activity in the lateral wall in both stress and rest images.

DIFFERENTIAL DIAGNOSES

- *Artifact*

- *Scar*

- *Stunned/hibernating myocardium*

In a patient with no prior evidence of myocardial damage, and given that the lateral wall artifacts are commonest in PET/CT, findings are most consistent with artifact.

COMMENTS

In a nuclear medicine clinic, after informed consent, N 13-NH_3 is injected, with the patient at rest. After the injection of N 13-NH_3, dynamic PET images are acquired for about 4 minutes followed by gated images for 15 minutes. After that, as N 13-NH_3 is decaying, a multislice cine CT attenuation scan is acquired (typically for 3.2 seconds, 0.8 rotations/s). A stress test is then performed by infusion of dipyridamole over 4 minutes. During minutes following the dipyridamole infusion, a second attenuation scan is performed. One minute later, beginning with the higher dose of N 13-NH_3, dynamic-mode PET images are acquired over 4 minutes. After dynamic image acquisition is complete, gated images are acquired for 15 minutes followed by a final cine CT attenuation scan. Beta-blockers are held for the stress test.

Misregistration of attenuation CT and emission images is common in PET rest-dipyridamole perfusion imaging and is associated with artifactual defects. This misregistration is directly predicted by the BMI and displacement of the diaphragm downward after stress with dipyridamole. It is also inversely related to heart size.

The artifactual defects in the cardiac perfusion PET/CT due to misregistration between CT and emission images are typically anterolateral or lateral. These, however, do not

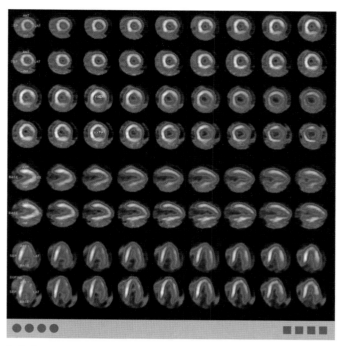

A. Left ventricular lateral wall artifact on PET. (*Image courtesy of Bhasker R. Koppula, MD.*)

correspond to the coronary distribution territories. Manual registration of emission and CT images or automatic emission-driven correction can resolve the artifact. There is quantitative relationship of artifacts to the extent of misregistration between CT and PET emission images.

PEARLS

- PET marker for hibernating myocardium is the mismatch between hypoperfusion of the region of interest and normal or increased uptake of FDG in that region.

- Lateral and anterolateral wall artifacts are the commonest in cardiac PET/CTs and are most commonly due to misregistration of PET and CT.

DIFFERENTIAL DIAGNOSIS IMAGE

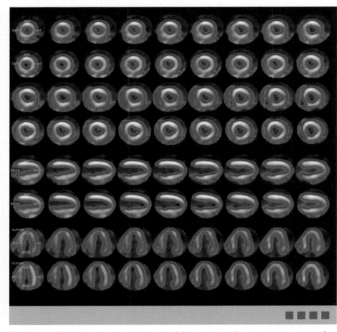

B. Mild left ventricular lateral wall ischemia. (*Image courtesy of Bhasker R. Koppula, MD.*)

Vivek Manchanda, MD

PRESENTATION

A woman in her late twenties; with incidental left posterior mediastinal masses.

FINDINGS

Mild diffuse FDG activity corresponding to left posterior mediastinal mass.

DIFFERENTIAL DIAGNOSES

- *Neurogenic tumor*
- *Lymphoma*
- *Well-differentiated sarcoma*
- *Lymphangioma*
- *Extramedullary hematopoiesis*
- *Other vascular tumors*

Lymphomas are usually very FDG avid. Neurogenic tumors vary in FDG activity. Lymphangiomas, benign tumors derived from blood vessels usually have none to minimal FDG activity. Biopsy showed PEComa (perivascular epithelioid cell derived).

COMMENTS

PEComas are benign tumors with perivascular epithelioid cell differentiation and include angiomyolipoma,

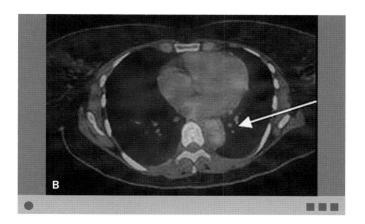

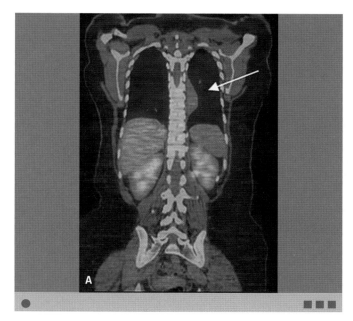

A. and **B.** Mild linear FDG activity in the left posterior mediastinum (fused PET/CT).

lymphangiomyomatosis, and clear cell "sugar" tumor of the lungs.

These tumors share a distinctive cell type (perivascular epithelioid cell, which does not have a known normal tissue counterpart).

These are seen mainly in females and are composed of epithelioid and occasionally spindle cell with clear to granular eosinophilic cytoplasm, prominent nucleoli, and a focal association with blood vessels. Prominent vascular/lymphatic spaces can be identified.

There is a subset of PEComas which behave in a malignant fashion and metastasize with marked hypercellularity, high mitotic activity, cytologic atypia, and coagulative necrosis and may show increased FDG activity. Case report of intensely FDG-avid PEComa of lung has been described.

PEComas may potentially arise from any anatomic location, but the most common sites of involvement are visceral (gastrointestinal and uterine), retroperitoneal, and abdominopelvic sites. Some of these tumors arise in somatic soft tissue and skin. Immunohistochemistry is almost always positive for melanocytic and smooth muscle markers.

PEARLS

- PEComas are benign tumors with perivascular epithelioid cell differentiation and are a group of neoplasms that include angiomyolipoma, lymphangiomyomatosis, and clear cell "sugar" tumor of the lungs.

- Per literature review so far, PEComas have not shown FDG activity greater than the mediastinal blood pool. FDG-PET may have a role in identifying metastases in aggressive subset of PEComas.

- Although some hemangiopericytomas behave in a benign fashion, many are locally invasive, metastasize and cause death, and are moderately FDG avid.

MR usually shows heterogeneous enhancement with gadolinium. On CT, some of these lesions may enlarge. They have variable FDG activity, mostly similar to that of mediastinal blood pool.

Hemangiopericytomas are slow-growing vascular tumors derived from the pericytes of Zimmerman, which surround the capillary wall. They are usually located in the soft tissues of the upper and lower extremities, pelvis, and the retroperitoneal space. Many hemangiopericytomas are locally invasive at the time of diagnosis or recur following removal, then metastasize, and cause death. Occasionally, hemangiopericytomas may exhibit calcification and bone erosion. FDG activity associated with hemangiopericytomas is variable and high FDG activity has been associated with poor prognosis.

ADDITIONAL IMAGES (C–G)

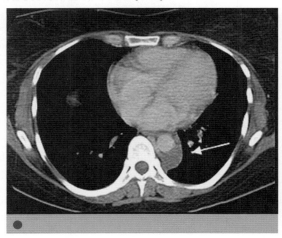

C. Contrast CT.

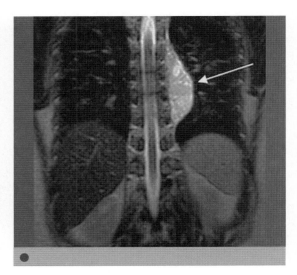

D. T2 MR with high signal.

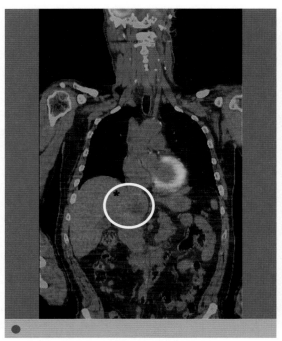

E. Hemangiopericytoma metastasis to liver (*black star*), mild circumferential FDG activity; coronal fused FDG-PET.

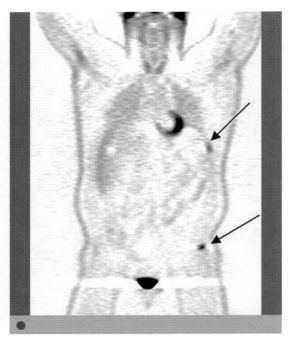

F. Left iliac and left rib metastasis from hemangiopericytoma. Coronal nonattenuation-corrected image, FDG-PET. Different patient.

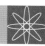

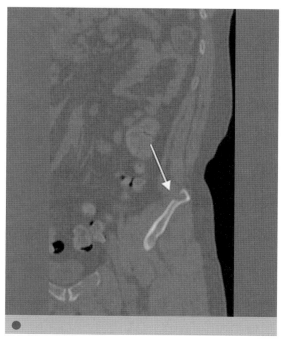

G. Corresponding CT.

Vivek Manchanda, MD

PRESENTATION

Man in midfifties with right upper quadrant (RUQ) pain and vomiting.

FINDINGS

Intense FDG uptake in right hepatic vein corresponding to the thrombus seen on the CT scan.

DIFFERENTIAL DIAGNOSES

- *Infectious thrombus/thrombophlebitis*

- *Tumor thrombus from hepatocellular cancer, cholangio-carcinoma, melanoma, etc*

- *Phlebothrombosis (bland thrombus)*

Without underlying interventional procedure, thrombophlebitis is unlikely. Bland thrombi are usually FDG negative.

COMMENTS

Tumor thrombus is a rare complication of many solid cancers such as renal cell carcinoma (RCC), Wilms tumor, testicular tumor, adrenal cortical carcinoma, lymphoma, pancreatic

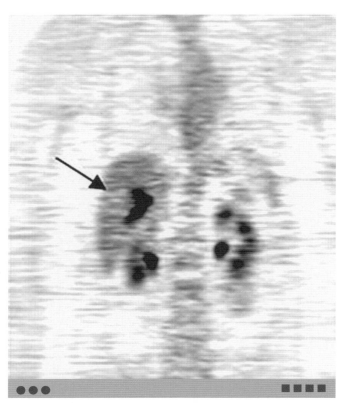

A. Right hepatic vein tumor thrombus from melanoma, attenuation corrected, coronal filtered back projection image. (AC, FBP image).

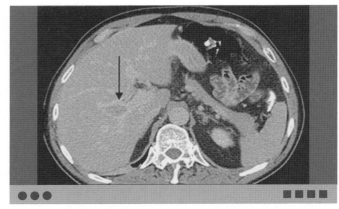

B. Corresponding axial contrast-enhanced CT.

cancer, osteosarcoma, Ewing sarcoma, and melanoma. Recognition of this complication by PET/CT can change the management plan and prevent unnecessary long-term anticoagulation treatment because of a diagnosis of cancer-related venous thrombus. The index case represents a patient who presented with RUQ pain and was found to have melanoma in the gallbladder. He also had tumor thrombus in the right hepatic vein seen in the images. Enhancement of the tumor thrombus may be seen on CT with contrast.

There have been a few reports describing acute venous thrombosis with FDG accumulation, likely from glucose uptake in the presence of platelet-aggregating factors and cytokines, including growth factors. It appears that there is a spectrum of FDG activity related to thrombi and throm-bophlebitis, with the phlebothrombi which do not cause any inflammation of the veins at one end of the spectrum and septic thrombophlebitis on the other.

Septic thrombophlebitis causes increased FDG uptake by increased glycolysis and may be difficult to distinguish from tumor thrombus. There is usually a history of recent

PEARLS

- It may be difficult to distinguish tumor thrombus from septic thrombophlebitis by FDG-PET alone. However, bland thrombi are usually FDG negative.

- Increased glycolysis is responsible for increased FDG uptake in both septic thrombophlebitis and tumor thrombus.

- Tumor thrombus may be seen in cancers such as RCC, testicular tumor, adrenal cortical carcinoma, lymphoma, and others.

- FDG accumulation can be seen physiologically in the central line.

intervention, such as a central line. Diffuse soft tissue inflammation may be seen on the CT scan. The patient may show clinical signs and symptoms of infection. Evaluation of tumor thrombus, including extension can be done with MR and ultrasound, but in cancers which are FDG avid with multiple thrombi, FDG-PET can discriminate between the benign and tumor thrombi.

Pulmonary emboli are typically not FDG avid and the infarcts caused by pulmonary emboli are typically photopenic.

DIFFERENTIAL DIAGNOSIS IMAGES (C-H)

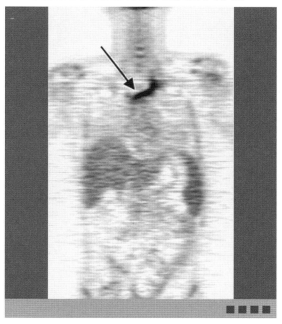

C. Thrombophlebitis in the left brachiocephalic vein, coronal FDG-PET.

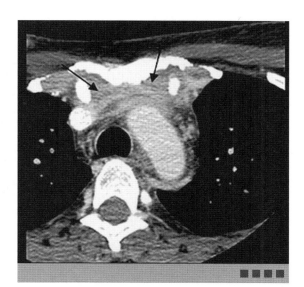

D. Corresponding CT.

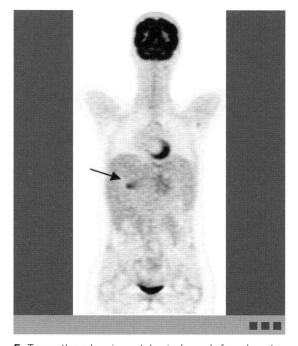

E. Tumor thrombus in portal vein (*arrow*), from hepatocellular carcinoma (HCC). Coronal FDG-PET.

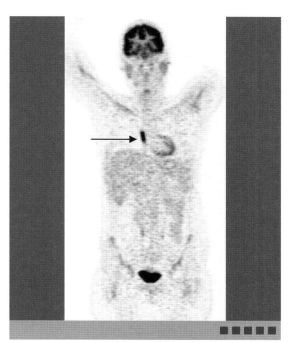

F. FDG activity in central line. Coronal FDG-PET.

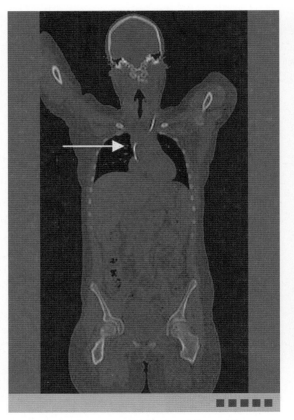

G. Corresponding coronal CT (*central line, white arrow*).

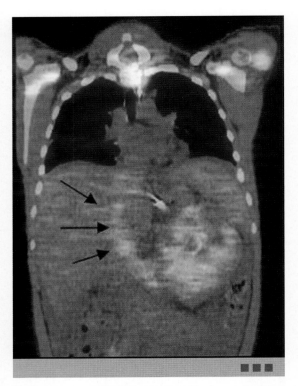

H. Fused coronal PET/CT, adrenocortical cancer with invasion of IVC.

Vivek Manchanda, MD

PRESENTATION

A man in his late thirties with shortness of breath.

FINDINGS

Intense FDG activity in right pulmonary artery with extravascular extension.

DIFFERENTIAL DIAGNOSES

- *Pulmonary embolism*
- *Infected embolus*
- *Metastatic thrombus*: Melanoma
- *Pulmonary artery sarcoma*

Bland pulmonary emboli usually have none to mild FDG activity.

COMMENTS

The level of FDG activity is unlikely to be due to bland pulmonary embolism and is more likely due to metastatic tumor thrombus or primary tumor, such as angiosarcoma.

Angiosarcoma is a rare malignant neoplasm of vascular endothelium, characterized by rapidly proliferating anaplastic cells derived from blood vessels and lining irregular, blood-filled spaces. They are aggressive with high local recurrence, spread widely, and have a high rate of lymph node and systemic metastases. Angiosarcomas may not produce symptoms

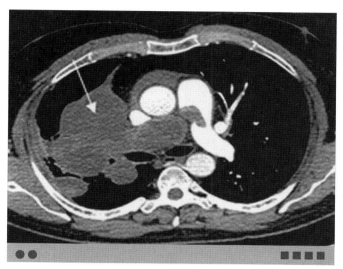

B. Corresponding CT.

until late. They tend to have very nonspecific appearance on imaging.

Angiosarcomas can arise in soft tissues (extremities, retroperitoneum), organs (such as liver, lungs, and heart), breasts, skin, head and neck, and bones.

Depending on the grade of angiosarcomas, there may be variability in FDG uptake.

It is important in patient preparation to include prolonged fasting (sometimes > 6 hours) to assess for lesions close to heart. Myocardial uptake can be reduced by switching metabolism of myocardium from glucose to free fatty acids. MR or FDG-PET can both be helpful in detecting recurrence of disease. A breath-hold chest CT in a patient with sarcomas, including angiosarcomas is important.

It can be difficult to differentiate radiologically between pulmonary artery sarcoma and thromboembolism, although chest CT findings in patients with advanced disease are more specific and show contrast enhancement on MR.

CT findings suggestive of pulmonary artery sarcoma include hypodense filling defect in the proximal or main pulmonary artery with expansion and extraluminal extension.

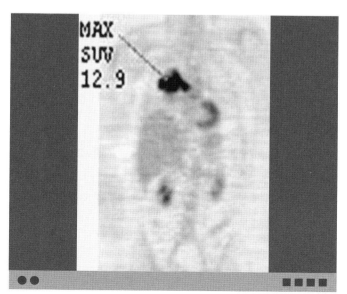

A. Pulmonary artery sarcoma, coronal FDG-PET.

PEARLS

- **Bland thrombi usually have none to mild FDG activity, whereas pulmonary artery sarcomas are usually intensely FDG avid.**

- **Prolonged fasting is important to characterize lesions close to heart.**

ADDITIONAL IMAGES (C-D)

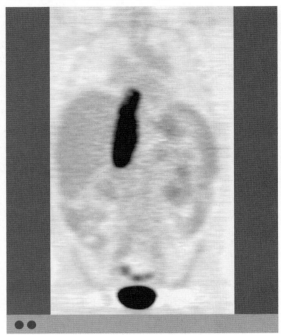

C. Intensely metabolically active inferior vene cava (IVC) sarcoma, FDG-PET.

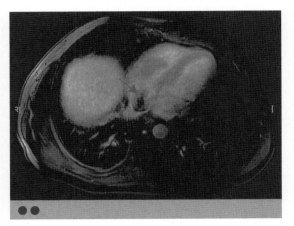

D. Axial gradient echo MR sequence with evidence of extension of tumor in the right atrium (*arrow*).

DIFFERENTIAL DIAGNOSIS IMAGES (E-G)

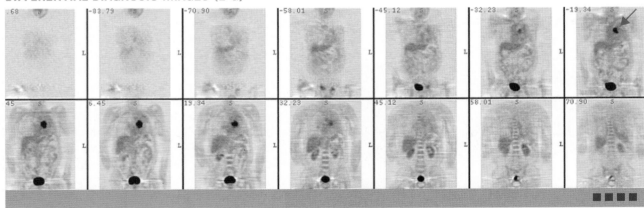

E. Left hilar non–small-cell cancer, mimicking normal myocardial uptake. Coronal FDG-PET.

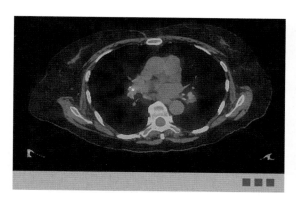

F. Bilateral pulmonary artery emboli, mild FDG activity. Fused PET/CT.

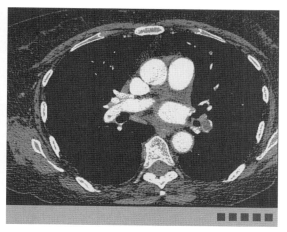

G. Corresponding bilateral pulmonary artery emboli, with filling defects.

Vivek Manchanda, MD

PRESENTATION

Man in midsixties evaluated for myocardial viability.

FINDINGS

Severe perfusion defect in distal anterior, apical, and inferior wall. FDG activity in the same region, indicating viability.

DIFFERENTIAL DIAGNOSIS

Viable myocardium: Since glucose is the normal substrate for heart, increased FDG activity in the non-/less perfused myocardium is most consistent with viable myocardium. Scar would show decreased/nonperfusion and no corresponding FDG activity.

COMMENTS

Viable myocardium may be characterized by integrity of cell membrane, intact mitochondria, preserved glucose and fatty acid metabolism, and intact resting perfusion, etc.

Integrity of cell membrane viability can be assessed with delayed thallium redistribution or absence of delayed hyperenhancement on MRI.

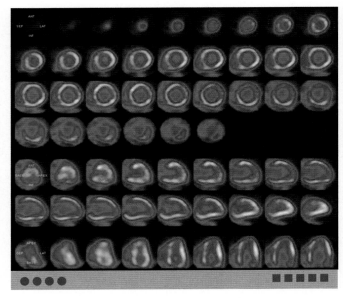

B. FDG uptake in the same region, indicating viability. FDG-PET viability scan.

Technetium sestamibi (Tc-MIBI) and Tc-tetrofosmin uptake is related to intact mitochondria.

Flourine-18 (^{18}F)-FDG-PET detects glucose metabolism in viable myocardium. Resting perfusion can be assessed by Tc-sestamibi and Tc-tetrofosmin uptake, and immediate thallium uptake. Inotropic reserve can be assessed by dobutamine stress echocardiogram.

In a nondiabetic patient, preparation for the FDG viability study includes fasting for 6 to 12 hours and then administering a glucose load, which results in rising plasma glucose and insulin levels, resulting in glucose as the preferred substrate for myocardial metabolism. In a diabetic patient, more elaborate glucose loading protocol with insulin is followed.

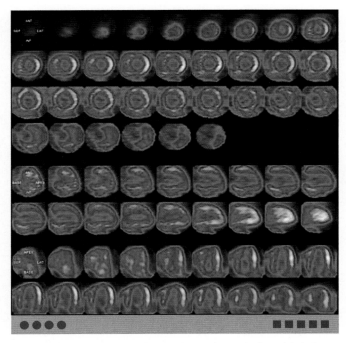

A. Severe perfusion defect in distal anterior, apical, and inferior wall. N13-Ammonia PET.

PEARLS

- Increase in FDG uptake relative to regional myocardial blood flow (perfusion-metabolism mismatch) indicates myocardial viability.

- Regional reductions in FDG uptake proportional to myocardial perfusion (perfusion-metabolism match) indicate scar.

- MR is more sensitive in detecting subendocardial scars than FDG-PET, due to latter's limited spatial resolution.

Impaired regional myocardial perfusion in both stress and rest suggests the presence of an irreversible myocardial injury. Increase in FDG uptake relative to regional myocardial blood flow (perfusion-metabolism mismatch) indicates myocardial viability. On contrary, regional reductions in FDG uptake proportional to myocardial perfusion (perfusion-metabolism match) indicate scar.

Stunned myocardium shows contractile dysfunction despite perfusion normalization. The etiology involves successive ischemic episodes. Stunning is difficult to differentiate from hibernation, which may coexist, but both hibernating and stunned myocardium are examples of reversible ischemia-induced myocardial mechanical dysfunction, and will be FDG avid on a viability FDG-PET study.

Contrast-enhanced MR is more sensitive for subendocardial scar than FDG-PET.

Naoya Hattori, MD, PhD

PRESENTATION

A 65-year-old male with a history of chest pain and dyspnea on exertion for 3 months.

FINDINGS

Stress MPI with Tc-99m tetrofosmin shows moderate-sized severe hypoperfusion in the proximal part of anteroseptal wall. Resting perfusion scan on the previous day shows complete normalization of the anteroseptal wall.

DIFFERENTIAL DIAGNOSIS

- *Inducible ischemia*: Careful review of raw images will show the normal location of arm during stress and rest imaging. Similarly, inspection of gated and attenuation-corrected images will show normal perfusion and wall motion in the affected segment.

COMMENTS

SPECT has high-contrast resolution and allows three-dimensional display of myocardial perfusion, therefore is a standard method of myocardial perfusion imaging. However, reconstructed three-dimensional images sometimes show artifact because of patient movement or attenuation due to chest wall, breasts, and diaphragm. The source of artifact often locates outside of reconstructed area, thus examination of raw images helps to identify the artifact. The present case shows soft tissue attenuation due to inability to raise the arm during imaging because of arthritis which became worse due to the resting scan done on a previous day. Planar images (left anterior oblique [LAO] and right anterior oblique [RAO]) were added to confirm the preserved perfusion in anteroseptal wall. Two-dimensional planar imaging requires shorter time than SPECT and is free from reconstruction artifact, thus it is considered to be useful when SPECT images are not properly acquired. Another method to correct for the problem of attenuation is to use attenuation correction using a moving rod source of gadolinium-153 (Gd-153) or X-ray source (eg, SPECT/CT) to generate attenuation maps for raw myocardial perfusion images and reconstruct attenuation-corrected images.

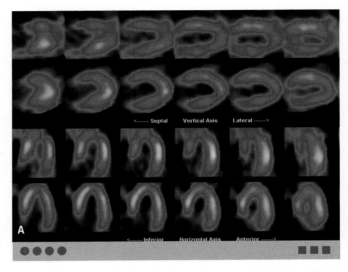

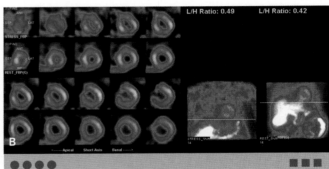

A. and **B.** Tc-99m tetrofosmin stress and rest myocardial perfusion SPECT images show an apparent perfusion defect (moderate sized and mild) in the anterior wall that improves on rest images suggestive of ischemia. Note lateral position of the left arm on raw images. (*Images courtesy of Naoya Hattori, MD, PhD and Sharon McRae, ARNP.*)

PEARLS

- **Myocardial perfusion SPECT images may contain artifact from soft tissue attenuation.**

- **Examination of raw projection images may help identify the source of artifact.**

- **On gated imaging, an area of attenuation shows reduced perfusion but that segment shows normal wall motion and thickens and brightens indicating normal perfusion.**

- **Planar images may help interpretation when SPECT shows severe artifacts.**

- **Applying attenuation correction will help identify this problem and correct for apparent "perfusion defects."**

ADDITIONAL IMAGE

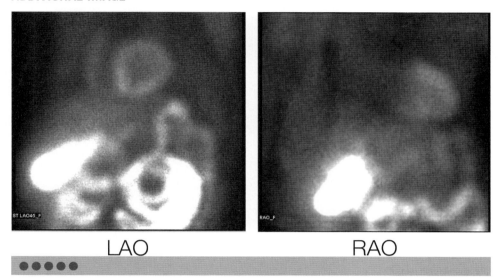

LAO   RAO

● ● ● ● ●

C. Tc-99m tetrofosmin stress planar perfusion images in LAO and RAO views show normal perfusion to the anterior wall after placing the left arm above the shoulder. (*Image courtesy of Sharon McRae, ARNP.*)

Naoya Hattori, MD, PhD

PRESENTATION

A 58-year-old male with atypical chest pain and dyspnea on exertion.

FINDINGS

Pharmacologic stress perfusion scan using Tc-99m tetrofosmin shows small-sized mild hypoperfusion in basal lateral wall. Resting perfusion scan using ^{201}Tl (thallium 201) shows completely normalized perfusion in the area, suggesting inducible ischemia. The size of left ventricle looks larger in stress image. Transient ischemic dilatation (TID) score is 1.49.

DIFFERENTIAL DIAGNOSIS

Perfusion abnormality is seen in the small area of lateral wall, suggesting single vessel disease in left circumflex artery. However, apparently enlarged size of left ventricle may indicate global ischemia due to known multivessel disease.

COMMENTS

TID is reported to be a sign of severe multivessel CAD. Either poststress dilatation of left ventricle or steal effect of subendocardial blood flow may explain the phenomenon. TID score greater than 1.35 has been reported to be a marker of dilation secondary to ischemic heart disease. When applying the score, however, one should be careful

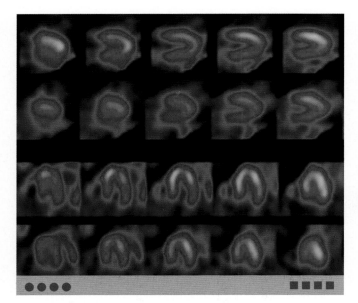

A. Stress (Tc-99m tetrofosmin) and resting (^{201}Tl) perfusion images in multiple projections show "dilated" left ventricular chamber. TID score was 1.49 (automatic) and 1.26 (after manual adjustment). (*Image courtesy of Naoya Hattori, MD, PhD and Sharon McRae, ARNP.*)

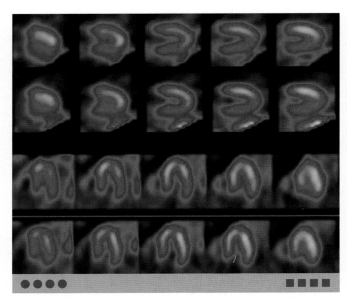

B. Resting scan was repeated on the next day using Tc-99m tetrofosmin, showing no TID effect. TID score was 0.97. (*Image courtesy of Naoya Hattori, MD, PhD and Sharon McRae, ARNP.*)

to check the result of edge detection of the left ventricle to be more accurate. It is also important to pay attention to the image quality of stress and resting scans. In particular, dual isotope protocol using resting ^{201}Tl and stress Tc-99m agents may be overestimating TID score because of apparently smaller left ventricular cavity with ^{201}Tl images caused by scatter and lower count statistics. When there is true stress-induced cavity dilatation, the images show an extra slice or two in the respective rows of stress images. In the case example presented here, the resting myocardial perfusion study was repeated using Tc-99m tetrofosmin the next day. Although the reversible ischemia was confirmed in the lateral wall, the size of left ventricle on the resting images did not differ significantly from the stress images. With the current trend in performing MPI with low-/high-dose Tc-99m agent, it will not be a significant issue because of similar physical characteristics for the two tracers.

PEARLS

- **TID may indicate multivessel CAD.**

- **Dual isotope protocol using resting ^{201}Tl and stress Tc-99m agents may overestimate TID score and this fact should be taken into account when interpreting.**

- **With the current trend in performing MPI with low-dose/ high-dose ^{99m}Tc agent, it will not be a significant issue.**

Chapter 10

PEDIATRIC CASES

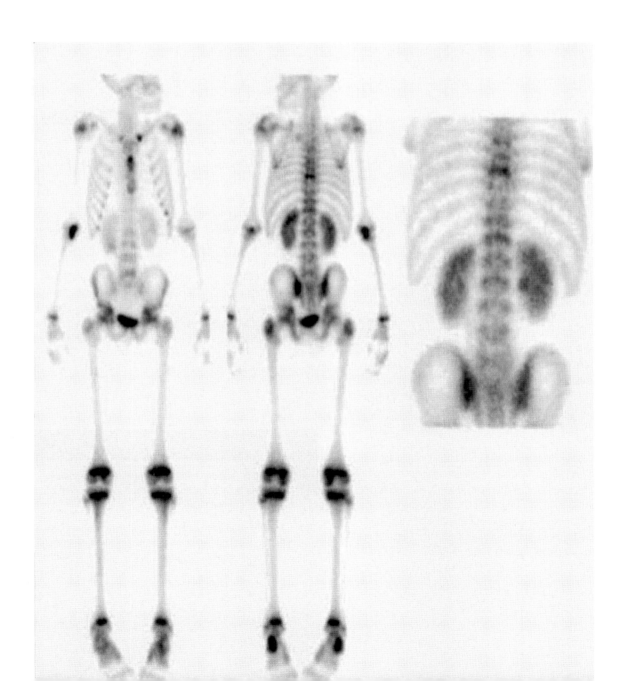

Marguerite T. Parisi, MD, MS Ed

PRESENTATION

A 14-year-old adolescent male with a 4-month history of back pain and weight loss.

FINDINGS

Bone scan (image A) demonstrates bilateral nephromegaly with delayed cortical retention of radiotracer. There are multiple vertebral compression fractures. The constellation of findings suggests leukemia.

DIFFERENTIAL DIAGNOSES

- Bilateral nephromegaly (without hydronephrosis):
  - *Neoplastic infiltrative processes*: Leukemia/lymphoma
  - Sickle nephropathy
  - Acute urate nephropathy/spontaneous tumor lysis syndrome
  - Post-chemotherapy renal toxicity
  - Infection
- Multiple vertebral body compression fractures:
  - *Infiltrative neoplastic processes*: Leukemia, lymphoma, Langerhans cell histiocytosis (LCH)
  - *Metastases*
  - *Trauma*
  - *Diskitis*

COMMENTS

Leukemia, representing 25% to 35% of all pediatric malignancies, is the most common form of childhood cancer. Characterized by multisystemic organ involvement, the bone marrow is the site of origin of this disease. Patient symptomatology at initial presentation is a reflection of diminished production of normal blood elements. For example, pallor, fatigue, and shortness of breath are the results of anemia; thrombocytopenia causes bruising, bleeding, or purpura. Granulocytopenia predisposes these patients to infection while bone marrow expansion results in arthralgia, arthritis, and bone pain.

Acute lymphocytic leukemia (ALL) is the most common form of pediatric leukemia; chronic leukemias represent only 2.6% of pediatric leukemias. While the death rate from pediatric leukemia has declined 60% over the last three decades, leukemia remains the leading cause of cancer deaths in children and young adults. Overall survival rate for children with leukemia who are younger than 5 years is 88%; it is 65% for all other ages.

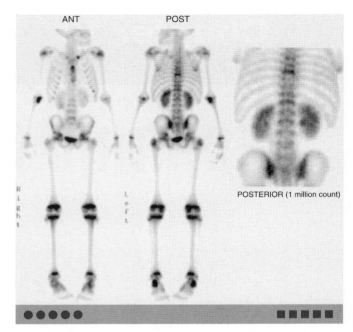

A. Anterior and posterior whole-body and a 1 million count posterior spot scintiphoto of spine from a Tc-99m MDP (methylene diphosphonate) bone scan.

Greater than 25% of patients with leukemia will have symptoms referable to the musculoskeletal system. Radiologic findings can include osteopenia, metaphyseal lucent lines, periostitis, diffuse and focal lytic lesions, pathologic fractures including vertebral collapse (as seen in this case), sclerotic lesions, and avascular necrosis. Scintigraphy does not play a role in the staging of this disease. However, nuclear medicine imaging may aid in establishing the diagnosis and can be vital in the evaluation of both early and late complications of therapy in those with leukemia.

PEARLS

- **Consider leukemia in the differential diagnosis of patients with bone and joint pain, particularly when disease course is protracted.**

- **Alteration in normal tracer biodistribution can be a vital distinguishing factor in establishing the diagnosis.**

ADDITIONAL IMAGES (B-I)

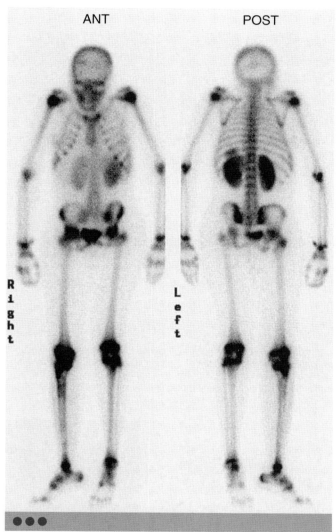

B. Sickle cell nephropathy: Anterior and posterior whole-body images from a Tc-99m MDP bone scan in a 16-year-old with knee pain reveal bilateral nephromegaly with prolonged cortical retention of tracer, findings consistent with sickle nephropathy. Note uptake in the small, atrophied, autoinfarcted spleen superior to the left kidney. Abnormal uptake in the right tibia is either infarct or osteomyelitis.

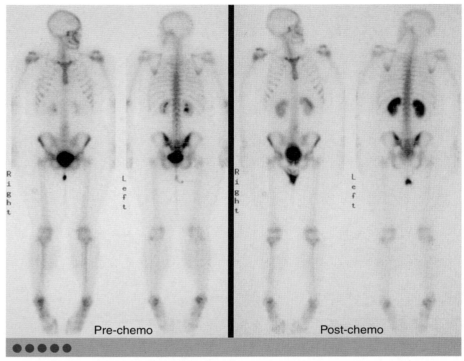

C. Post-chemotherapeutic nephrotoxicity: A 15-year-old with pelvic Ewing sarcoma. Pre-chemotherapy bone scan (*pre-chemo image*) is normal. Following chemotherapy (*post-chemo image*), there is prolonged cortical retention of tracer in mildly enlarged kidneys consistent with post-chemotherapy nephrotoxicity. Chemotherapy-induced nephrotoxicity, typically a transient phenomenon, is thought to occur secondary to direct toxicity to renal tubules.

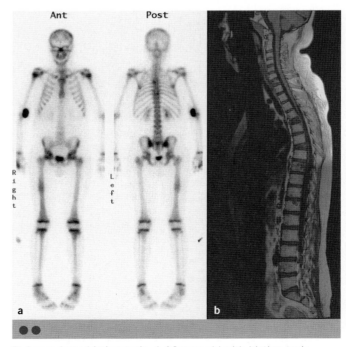

D. Langerhans histiocytosis: A 19-year-old with histiocytosis. Anterior and posterior whole-body images (*a*) from a bone scan reveal lesions in the skull and right femur as well as multiple mid-thoracic vertebral compression fractures, the latter better shown on corresponding view from sagittal T1 MRI (*b*).

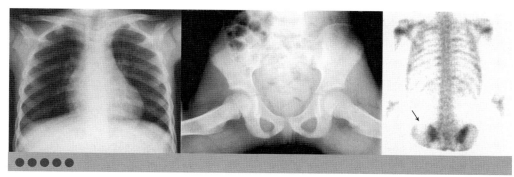

E. Leukemia: Plain films of the chest and pelvis; posterior spot view from a Tc-99m MDP bone scan. A 5-year-old with low back and rib pain. Plain film radiographs of the chest (*left*) and pelvis (*middle*) are normal. Bone scan (*right*) abnormalities including multiple bilateral rib lesions and lytic lesion in left iliac wing (*arrow*) led to diagnosis of leukemia.

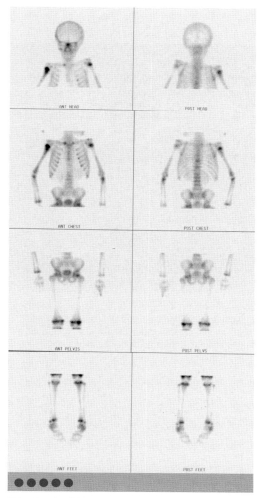

F. Leukemia: A 5-year-old with diffuse lymphadenopathy, fever, and bilateral leg pain. Anterior and posterior spot views of the skeleton from a bone scan reveal heterogeneous uptake in lower thoracic and lumbar spine, as well as diffuse tracer uptake following bone marrow distribution, findings of leukemia with marrow expansion and multiple vertebral compression fractures. Pathologic right humeral fracture also noted.

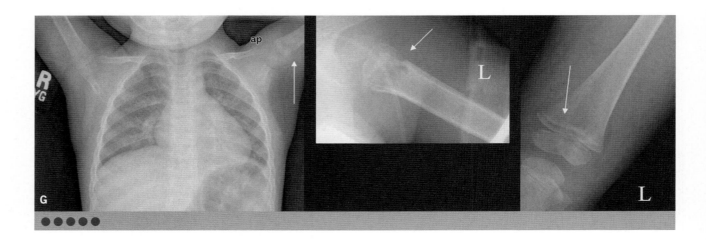

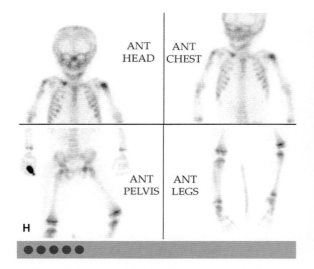

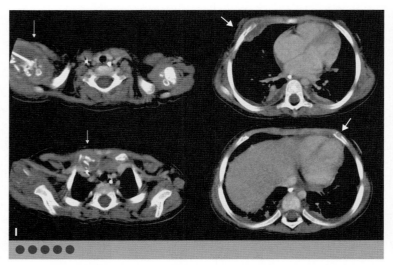

G., H., and **I. Leukemia:** Infectious complications. A 2-year-old previously healthy female presents with 4 days of fever, lethargy, hemodynamic instability, profound anemia, and pancytopenia. Plain films (image G) of the chest (*left*) and proximal humerus (*middle*) reveal bony demineralization with focal lytic lesions (*arrows*). AP view of the distal left femur (*right*) shows classic metaphyseal lucent lines of leukemia. Bone scan performed 2 weeks later (image H) reveals multiple areas of abnormal uptake due to multifocal *Staphlococcus aureus* osteomyelitis with abscess formation well demonstrated on corresponding CT (image I; *arrows*).

Marguerite T. Parisi, MD, MS Ed

PRESENTATION

Abnormal neonatal thyroid screening laboratory results.

FINDINGS

No radiotracer uptake in expected position of thyroid gland. Rather, there is tracer uptake in an ectopic, sublingual thyroid gland (image A).

DIFFERENTIAL DIAGNOSES

Differential diagnoses for neonatal hypothyroidism are as follows:

- *Thyroid dysgenesis*: Lingual thyroid, thyroid agenesis

- *Maternal thyroid-blocking antibodies*

- *Organification defects*

COMMENTS

Congenital hypothyroidism occurring outside endemic regions is termed sporadic and occurs in approximately 1 in 4000 live births. Women are affected about twice as often as men. Sporadic congenital hypothyroidism can be categorized as either transient or permanent. Transient hypothyroidism is due to transplacental maternal thyrotropin receptor-blocking antibodies or maternal ingestion of drugs such as propylthiouracil. Permanent hypothyroidism is caused by thyroid dysgenesis (abnormal thyroid formation during embryogenesis) or less commonly by abnormal thyroid hormonogenesis (abnormal hormone production).

Thyroid hormone is essential for normal central nervous system development, bone growth, and maturation. Newborn screening programs for congenital hypothyroidism are essential in identification of "at-risk" neonates. Prompt institution of treatment with thyroid replacement in the first 2 weeks of life prevents or ameliorates permanent neurologic and physical defects. If results of screening tests are abnormal and confirmed by findings from serum thyroid function tests, thyroid scintigraphy with Tc-99m pertechnetate or I-123 is recommended to diagnose thyroid dysgenesis or a congenital error of thyroxine production, respectively. Ultrasound has also been used to identify ectopic thyroid glands but is less accurate than scintigraphic methods.

In the last 30 years, industrialized nations have systematically implemented neonatal thyroid screening programs. These programs have been extremely successful in eradicating the severe mental deficiency that formerly resulted from congenital hypothyroidism. While newborn screening remains the

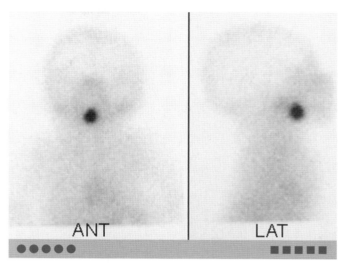

A. Anterior and right lateral images of the head and neck from a Tc-99m pertechnetate scan in a 7-day-old with congenital hypothyroidism.

most important tool for early detection of congenital hypothyroidism, nuclear scintigraphy is vital in confirming screening findings and in identifying the etiology of this condition in individual patients. Recognition of the radiographic manifestations of congenital hypothyroidism also plays a role in arousing suspicion and in diagnosis of those patients missed clinically or with screening.

PEARLS

- Tc-99m pertechnetate is the preferred radiotracer in the assessment of congenital hypothyroidism in the neonate or young child. As compared to I-123, Tc-99m pertechnetate delivers less radiation dose to the patient and is less expensive. It is readily available and does not require any patient preparation. Its imaging is easier to perform and can be completed within 30 minutes.

- Tc-99m pertechnetate is trapped by the thyroid gland as are the radioactive iodides but does not undergo organification. Thus, it can help in distinguishing agenesis from dyshormonogenesis.

- In the older child presenting with midline neck mass, scintigraphy with either Tc-99m pertechnetate or I-123 should be obtained to distinguish a thyroglossal duct cyst from an ectopic thyroid gland.

ADDITIONAL IMAGES (B-G)

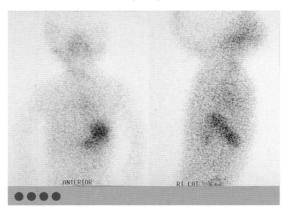

B. Thyroid agenesis: Anterior and lateral views of the head, neck, and chest from a Tc-99m-pertechnetate scan in a neonate with congenital hypothyroidism reveal thyroid agenesis.

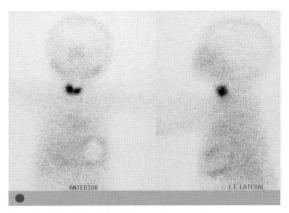

C. Dyshormonogenesis: Tc-99m pertechnetate scan (anterior and lateral views of head, neck, and chest) in another neonate with congenital hypothyroidism. There is increased uptake in an enlarged bilobed thyroid gland in normal/expected position. This may be either due to dyshormonogenesis or, less likely, maternal blocking antibodies.

ANT   LAT

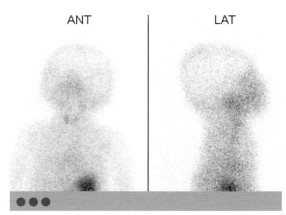

D. Anterior and lateral views from a Tc-99m pertech-netate scan reveal a poorly functioning bilobed gland in expected location in a 1-week-old with congenital hypothyroidism.

ANT   LAT

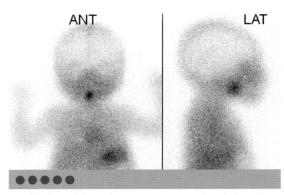

E. Another example of lingual thyroid in a neonate with congenital hypothyroidism, demonstrated on anterior and lateral views from a Tc-99m pertechnetate scan.

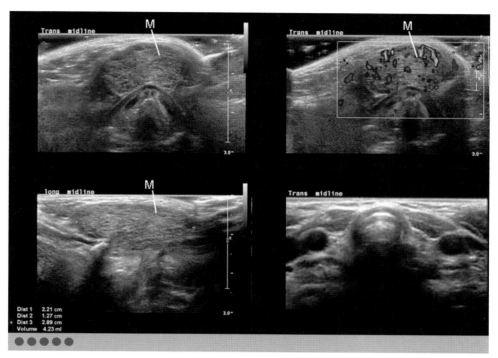

F. Lingual thyroid: Views from a neck ultrasound in a 4-year-old with enlarging solid-appearing midline neck mass (M) just superior to the hyoid bone. No thyroid gland is identified in expected location (lower right image).

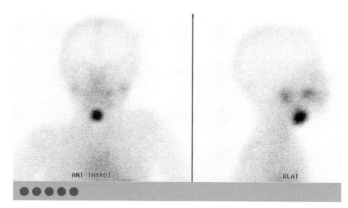

G. Lingual thyroid: Anterior and lateral views of the head from a Tc-99m pertechnetate scan performed immediately after the above ultrasound (image F) shows that the neck "mass" is an ectopic, lingual thyroid gland.

Case 10–3 Unanticipated or "Corner Findings" Identified Scintigraphically

Marguerite T. Parisi, MD, MS Ed

PRESENTATION

A 3-year-old with fever of unknown origin (FUO).

FINDINGS

Bone scan (image A) demonstrates bilaterally enlarged kidneys. There is heterogeneous radiotracer uptake in the left kidney with areas of cortical photopenia; there is prolonged cortical retention of tracer on the right. No osseous abnormalities are identified. CT (image B) confirms low-density pyogenic areas and enlarged kidneys, consistent with pyelonephritis.

DIFFERENTIAL DIAGNOSES

Bilaterally enlarged, nonhydronephrotic kidneys:
• *Infection*: Glomerulitis, hemolytic uremic syndrome, pyelonephritis (unilateral or bilateral)

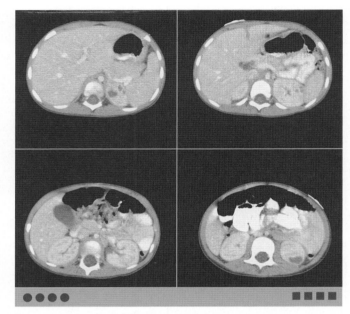

B. Axial images from contrast-enhanced CT confirm bilateral nephromegaly with focal abscesses.

• *Leukemia/lymphoma*

• *Sickle cell nephropathy*

• *Other infiltrative processes*: Protein deposition

COMMENTS

FUO is conventionally defined as fever of greater than 102°F persisting for more than 4 weeks. FUO has many etiologies; the most common are infection, neoplasia, autoimmune diseases, and idiopathic pathology. If the etiology of patient's

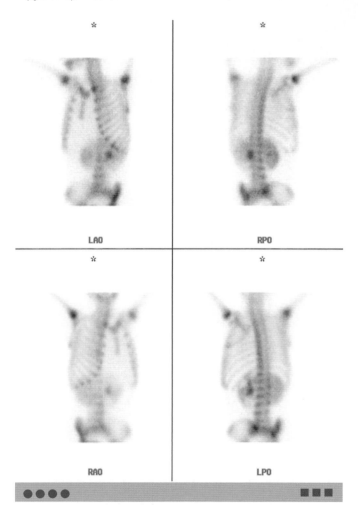

A. Delayed spot scintiphotos from a Tc-99m bone scan show enlarged kidneys with focal areas of decreased tracer uptake. No osseous abnormalities are present.

PEARLS

• The astute observer can identify unexpected pathology on nuclear imaging studies which may alter patient diagnosis or treatment.

• To detect critical but unanticipated findings, utilize a systematic approach to image interpretation which includes assessment of expected normal radiotracer biodistribution.

• Avoid "tunnel vision." Look beyond the specific clinical question asked and review all information available, including patient history and correlative imaging. Consider a broad differential diagnosis when analyzing cases.

fever is not established with conventional radiologic imaging, nuclear medicine is employed. Gallium scanning with 24- and 48-hour imaging is the most useful scintigraphic study for determining the etiology of FUO. However, because of the imaging characteristics of gallium, including higher kiloelectron volt (keV) energies, prolonged half-life of the tracer, longer time to study completion and higher radiation dose to patient, bone scan is typically the first scintigraphic technique employed.

Awareness of the normal biodistribution of each radiotracer is of crucial importance when assessing any nuclear medicine study. Unexpected pathology which may alter diagnosis or treatment can be identified by utilizing a systematic approach to study interpretation which includes deliberate evaluation of expected tracer biodistribution. In the above example, nephromegaly with heterogeneous renal cortical tracer uptake leads to the unanticipated diagnosis of pyelonephritis. As was seen in Case 10–1, the patient with leukemia, alteration in normal renal uptake of the bone agent helped to pinpoint the diagnosis. Additional examples of alteration of expected tracer biodistribution leading to unanticipated diagnoses are presented below.

ADDITIONAL IMAGES (C-H)

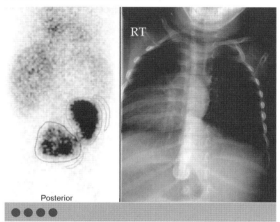

C. Cross-fused renal ectopia with unanticipated situs inversus totalis. Summed posterior flow images (*left*) from a Tc-99m MAG3 (mercapto acetyl triglycine) renogram reveal a cross-fused ectopic kidney on the right (*circles*) and unanticipated situs inversus totalis with left-sided liver and dextrocardia confirmed on chest radiograph (*right*).

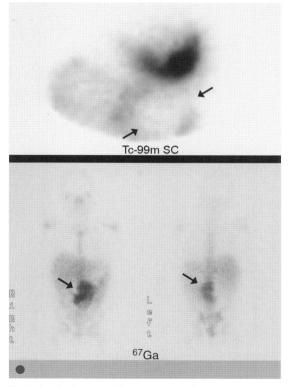

D. Abdominal mass, (biopsy-proven *Mycobacterium avium-intracellulare*) incidentally identified on gastric emptying study and confirmed on gallium study. A 14-year-old with AIDS and complaints of early satiety. Small bowel displacement by photopenic mass (*arrows, top*) is incidentally identified on anterior image from sulfur-colloid gastric emptying study. Gallium scan (*bottom*) shows intense abnormal abdominal uptake at site of "cold lesion" on gastric emptying study, due to biopsy-proven *M. avium-intracellulare* (*arrows*).

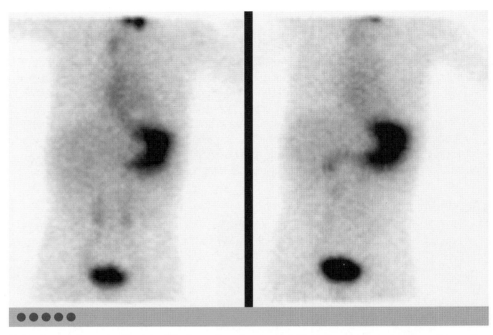

E. Gastroesophageal reflux identified on otherwise normal Meckel scan. Anterior views from a Tc-99m pertechnetate Meckel scan reveal transient gastroesophageal reflux (*left*) which clears promptly (*right*).

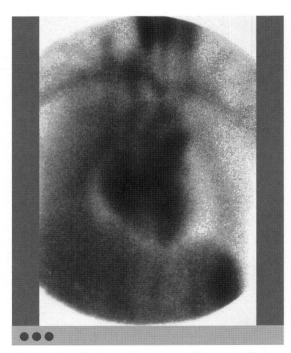

F. Pericardial effusion incidentally identified on multigated acquisition (MUGA) scan. MUGA scan to assess for cardiac toxicity following adriamycin therapy in a 15-year-old with ALL shows an unexpected pericardial effusion. Ejection fraction was normal.

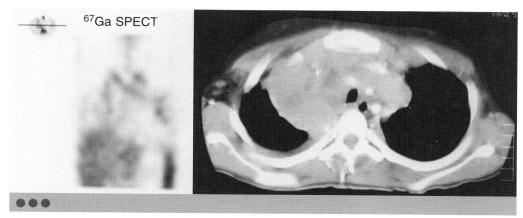

G. Superior vena cava (SVC) syndrome: 16-year-old adolescent female with malignant thymoma. Coronal SPECT image from staging gallium scan (*left*) shows tracer retention in the SVC as well as the branciocephalic and subclavian veins due to SVC syndrome caused by a large, heterogenous anterior mediastinal mass (contrast-enhanced CT, *right*).

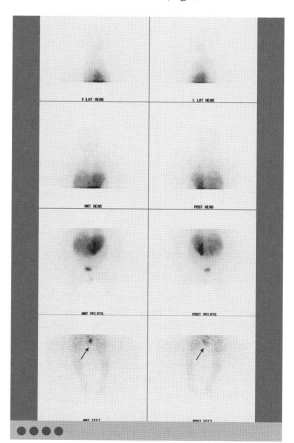

H. Unexpected scrotal metastases from neuroblastoma identified on I-123 MIBG (metaiodobenzylguanidine) scan. Anterior and posterior spot images from an I-123 MIBG scan in an infant with neuroblastoma. In addition to uptake in the large, bilobed MIBG-avid abdominal mass, there is an unexpected left scrotal metastases (*arrows*), a finding which changes tumor stage, treatment protocol, and overall prognosis.

Marguerite T. Parisi, MD, MS Ed and Helen Nadel, MD

PRESENTATION

A 9-month-old infant presenting with irritability and decreased lower extremity movement.

FINDINGS

Bone scan (image A) reveals abnormal uptake in multiple ribs, in distal right femur, and proximal left tibia, consistent with fractures. Chest and bilateral knee radiographs (images B and C) confirm the fractures and demonstrate that the fractures are in various stages of healing, classic findings in nonaccidental trauma.

DIFFERENTIAL DIAGNOSES

Multiple fractures:

- *Nonaccidental trauma*

- *Trauma*

- *Fragility fractures*: Prematurity, birth trauma, vitamin deficiencies, scurvy
  - *Rickets*
  - *Osteogenesis imperfecta*

- *Pathologic fractures secondary to malignancy*

COMMENTS

Child abuse, a problem that transverses all socioeconomic groups, affects approximately 1.5 million children per year in the United States and results in 5000 deaths annually. Most incidents occur in children younger than 1 year; boys and girls are equally affected. Skeletal trauma is identified in 11% to 55% of patients and is more commonly seen in younger age groups (1–3 years). Characteristic imaging findings include multiple fractures, fractures in various stages of healing, fractures that result from unusual mechanisms of injury or occur in unusual locations (metaphyseal corner fractures, posterior rib fractures, metacarpal, metatarsal, spinous process, sternum, and scapular fractures), and spiral long bone fractures occurring in infants and toddlers younger than 1 year. Periosteal new bone formation may be indicative of remote trauma but, as an isolated finding, is nonspecific. The metaphyseal corner or bucket handle fracture, also typically seen in patients younger than 1 year, is pathognomonic of nonaccidental trauma.

Bone scintigraphy is complementary to radiographic skeletal survey in the identification and documentation of skeletal injuries from nonaccidental trauma. It is extremely helpful in the first week post-injury as it may detect fractures before plain films are positive.

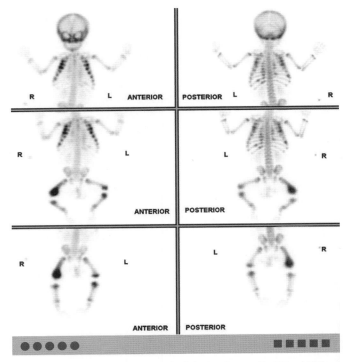

A. Anterior and posterior spot scintiphotos from a Tc-99m MDP bone scan of the entire axial and appendicular skeleton demonstrates multiple rib, distal right femoral, and proximal left tibial fractures, consistent with child abuse.

Nonskeletal manifestations of child abuse include but are not limited to bruising, burns, solid organ injuries involving the liver, spleen, pancreas, or kidneys; lung injury; duodenal hematoma or bowel perforation, subdural hematoma, intracranial and retinal hemorrhage, brain ischemia, or brain death.

PEARLS

- **Knowledge of child development, mechanics of childhood skeletal injuries, locations of injury, and sequential findings of skeletal healing are crucial to diagnosing child abuse.**

- **Recognition and appropriate reporting of child abuse is a cornerstone of treatment—removing the child from a hostile environment.**

- **Scintigraphy is less sensitive than plain films in the identification of metaphyseal corner fractures, which are located adjacent to the normally radio-avid physes.**

- **Correlate scintigraphic findings with radiographs to determine fracture age.**

- **Having a bone disease or fragile bones does not preclude the possibility of nonaccidental injury.**

ADDITIONAL IMAGES (B-J)

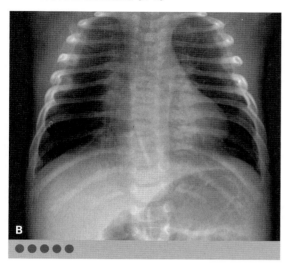

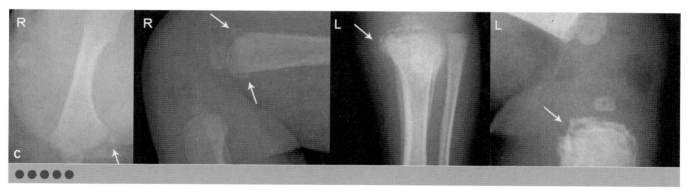

B. and **C.** AP chest (image B) and bilateral two-view radiographs of the knees (image C) confirm the presence of multiple fractures in various stages of healing, including bilateral anterior and posterior rib fractures (image B) and classic metaphyseal corner/bucket handle fractures (image C)—an acute fracture involving the distal right femur and a healing fracture in the proximal left tibia.

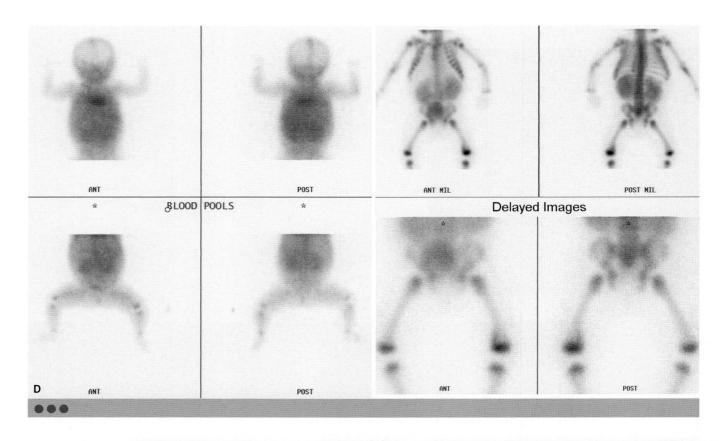

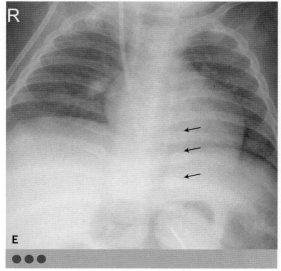

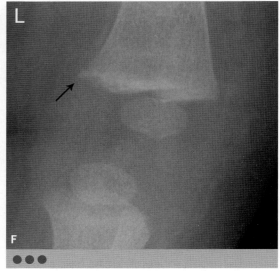

D.,E., and F. Fragility fractures due to renal insufficiency. A 6-month-old patient hospitalized for renal insufficiency was evaluated for persistent fevers despite antibiotics. Anterior and posterior blood pool and delayed spot scintiphotos from a Tc-99m bone scan (image D) reveal poor renal function (*blood pool images*) with prolonged cortical retention in bilaterally enlarged kidneys (*delayed images*). Abnormal osseous uptake shown in distal left femoral metaphysis as well as in several contiguous left posterior ribs raised suspicion of nonaccidental trauma. Plain film radiographs of the chest (image E) and distal left femur (image F) confirm healing posterior rib fractures (*arrows*) and a subacute left distal femoral metaphyseal corner fracture (*arrow*). In this case, despite extensive investigation, no evidence of child abuse was identified.

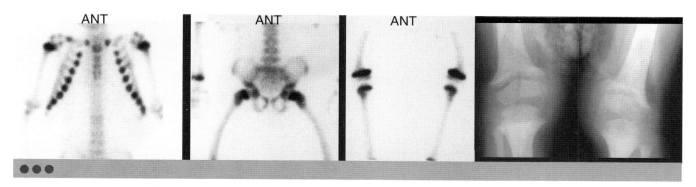

G. Rickets: A 2-year-old with complaint of left leg pain. Anterior spot scintiphotos from a Tc-99m bone scan (*left*) show marked increased uptake in anterior ribs (rachitic rosary), lower extremity bowing, widening and increased uptake in metaphyses of long bones, findings consistent with rickets and corroborated on plain films of the knees (*right*). Although no lower extremity fracture was identified, bone scan showed a right clavicular fracture.

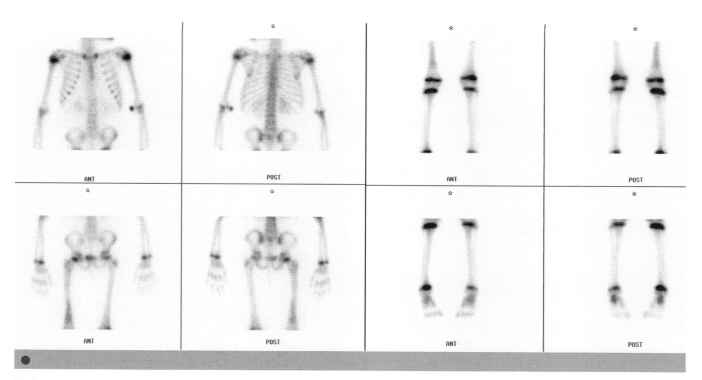

H. Osteogenesis imperfecta: Bone scan (anterior and posterior images) in a 7-year-old patient with osteogenesis imperfecta reveals normal uptake but flattening of multiple vertebral bodies as well as heterogeneous uptake in the right femoral shaft, site of known remote healing diaphyseal fracture.

431

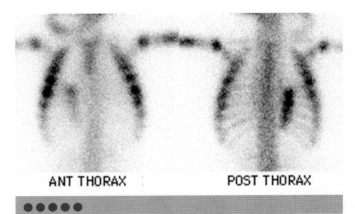

ANT THORAX   POST THORAX

●●●●●

I. Child abuse: Rib fractures. Anterior and posterior spot images of the thorax from a Tc-99m MDP bone scan show bilateral anterior and posterior rib fractures secondary to child abuse in a 6-month-old child with subdural and parenchymal hemorrhages on head CT (*not shown*). (*Image courtesy of Helen Nadel, MD.*)

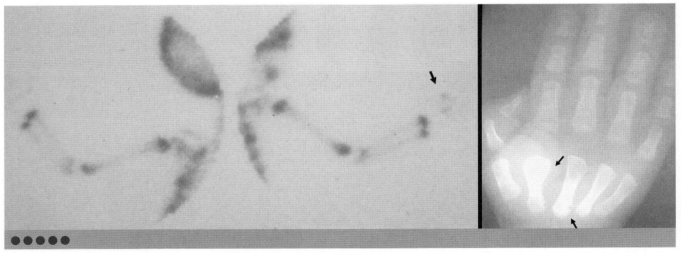

●●●●●

J. Child abuse: Small bone fractures. A 6-week-old infant with healing fractures in the small bones of the hands, shown on spot views from Tc-99m bone scan (*left, arrows*) and corroborating plain film radiograph (*right, arrows*), are due to being stepped on. (*Image courtesy of Helen Nadel, MD.*)

Marguerite T. Parisi, MD, MS Ed

PRESENTATION

An afebrile 2-year-old presents with refusal to bear weight.

FINDINGS

Initial plain films and hip ultrasound were interpreted as normal. Bone scan (image A) with blood pool imaging (*top, left*) revealed left femoral shaft hyperemia and, on delayed imaging (*bottom, left*), persistent abnormal oblique linear uptake. Review of plain films (image A, *right*), using magnification, confirmed a toddler fracture.

DIFFERENTIAL DIAGNOSIS

Refusal to bear weight/causes of leg pain: Toddler's fracture, osteomyelitis, nonaccidental trauma, shin splint, hip joint effusion, diskitis, osteoid osteoma, primary or secondary malignancy (leukemia, neuroblastoma).

COMMENTS

A toddler's fracture is a clinically subtle, nondisplaced lower extremity fracture, occurring in a child who is starting to walk, typically between the ages of 1 and 2 years, although these may present in older children up to age 5 years. The most common sites of toddler's fractures include the tibial shaft, proximal tibia, cuboid, and calcaneus. These injuries tend to heal without residual deformity.

Radiographs may initially be normal or demonstrate soft tissue swelling. Callus formation or, in the small bones of the feet, sclerotic bands, seen between 10 and 14 days later with repeat imaging, confirm the diagnosis. The radionuclide bone scan is highly sensitive in detection of toddler's fractures as it becomes positive as early as 1 to 2 days following initial injury. The bone scan, with its ability to image the whole body, may demonstrate additional abnormalities that lead to an alternative diagnosis.

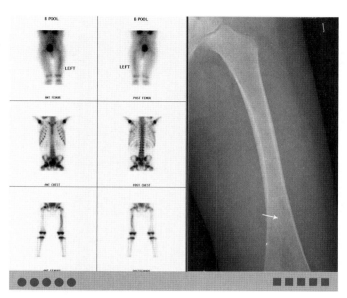

A. Tc-99m MDP bone scan (*left*) including anterior and posterior blood pool images (*left, top*) shows a femoral shaft toddler's fracture, subtly noted on plain film (*right, arrow*).

PEARLS

- If initial radiographs and hip ultrasound are normal, obtain bone scan.

- Blood pool imaging is a mandatory component of the bone scan in this clinical scenario. The presence of marked, focal hyperemia on blood pool imaging helps to distinguish osteomyelitis from toddler's fracture (less hyperemia).

- The whole body should be imaged in children of all ages when performing a bone scan.

ADDITIONAL IMAGES (B-F)

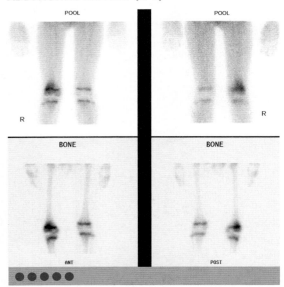

B. Distal femoral osteomyelitis: Bone scan; anterior and posterior blood pool (*top*) and delayed spot views of the femurs from a bone scan show marked metaphyseal hyperemia and persistent delayed uptake consistent with distal right femoral osteomyelitis.

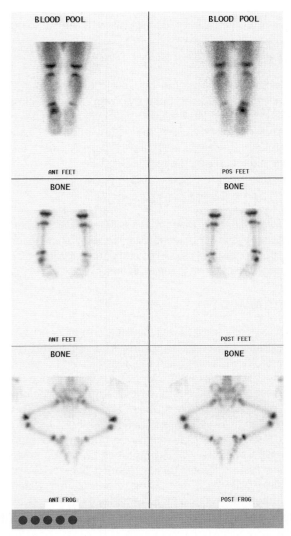

C. Calcaneal osteomyelitis: Bone scan; anterior and posterior blood pool (*top*) and delayed spot scintiphotos of the lower extremities from a whole-body bone scan in a 1-year-old with calcaneal tenderness, fever, and elevated inflammatory markers show hyperemia and persistently delayed calcaneal uptake consistent with osteomyelitis.

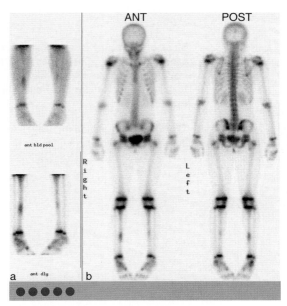

D. Shin splints: Bone scan; anterior blood pool and delayed spots of the lower extremities (*a; top, bottom*) and anterior and posterior delayed whole-body images from a bone scan in an athletic teen with leg pain. There is focal bilateral midshaft tibial uptake present consistent with shin splints. Patient age, history, and bilateral involvement distinguish these from toddler's fractures.

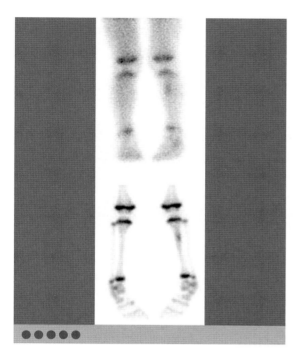

E. Toddler's fracture: Anterior blood pool (*top*) and delayed (*bottom*) spot scintiphotos from a whole-body bone scan in an 18-month-old afebrile patient refusing to bear weight. Toddler's fracture is present in the proximal left tibial shaft.

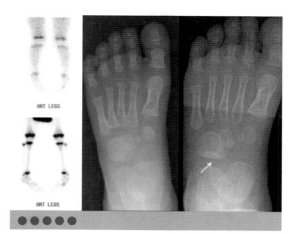

F. Toddler's fracture, left cuboid bone: Bone scan; initial and follow-up radiographs. Anterior blood pool (*top left*) and delayed (*bottom left*) spot images of the lower extremities from a whole-body bone scan in an afebrile 2-year-old reveal focal uptake in the left cuboid bone consistent with toddler's fracture. Initial radiographs (*middle*) were normal. Two weeks later, repeat radiographs (*right, arrow*) reveal sclerosis consistent with healing fracture, confirming diagnosis.

Marguerite T. Parisi, MD, MS Ed

PRESENTATION

An afebrile 6-year-old complains of right hip and back pain which is worse at night.

FINDINGS

Spot images from a bone scan (image A) demonstrate intensely increased uptake in the posterior elements on the right at the L4 level, confirmed with single photon emission computed tomographic (SPECT) imaging (image B, *top*). Corresponding CT images (image B, *bottom*) identify a lucent lesion with central nidus consistent with osteoid osteoma as the etiology of the scintigraphic abnormality.

DIFFERENTIAL DIAGNOSES

Focal increased uptake in posterior elements on bone scan:

• *Osteoid osteoma/osteoblastoma*

• *Spondylolysis*

• *Osteomyelitis secondary to spinal epidural abscess*

• *Mimicker*: Ectopic kidney

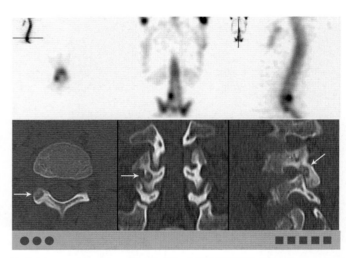

B. Axial, coronal, and sagittal Tc-99m MDP SPECT images (*top*) and corresponding CT images (*bottom*) in identical planes show abnormal radiotracer uptake in right pedicle at L4 level is due to an osteoid osteoma.

COMMENTS

Osteoid osteoma is a benign bone-forming lesion. Commonly presenting between the ages of 10 and 20 years, males are affected twice as often as females. The classic symptoms of osteoid osteoma are pain at night relieved by aspirin. The femoral neck, the tibia, and the posterior elements of the spine are the most frequently involved sites of osteoid osteoma. Classically, radiographs and/or CT demonstrate a lucent nidus surrounded by an exuberant zone of sclerosis. On bone scan, there is focal intense radiotracer uptake corresponding to the exuberant sclerosis surrounding the lesion.

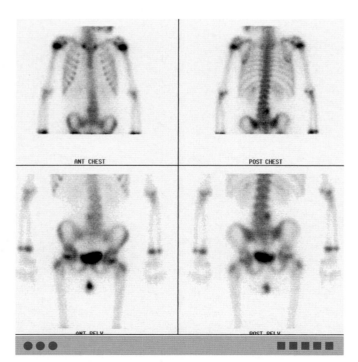

A. Anterior (*left*) and posterior (*right*) spot scintiphotos of the spine and pelvis from a Tc-99m MDP bone scan demonstrate abnormal uptake on the right at the L4 Level.

PEARLS

• **Bone scintigraphy is highly sensitive but nonspecific.**

• **Performing SPECT during bone scintigraphy improves disease detection.**

• **Routinely image the whole body in children of all ages when performing bone scans.**

• **Do not underestimate the importance of blood pool imaging.**

ADDITIONAL IMAGES (C-H)

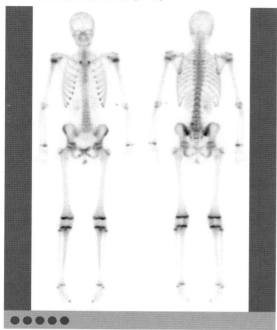

C. Spondylolysis: Tc-99m MDP bone scan in a 13-year-old with low back pain. Anterior and posterior whole-body views show abnormal uptake in the posterior elements at L5 level consistent with spondylolysis.

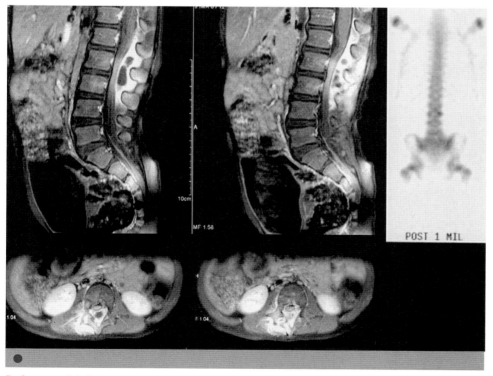

D. Osteomyelitis from spinal epidural abscess: A 17-month-old with fever and refusal to bear weight. Sagittal (*top left*) and axial (*bottom left*) T2 MRI images of the lower spine show a spinal epidural abscess with osteomyelitis at the L3 level, seen as a solitary focus of increased uptake on posterior spot spine image from bone scan (*right*). Spinal epidural abscess is a rare, nonmalignant cause of spinal cord compression.

437

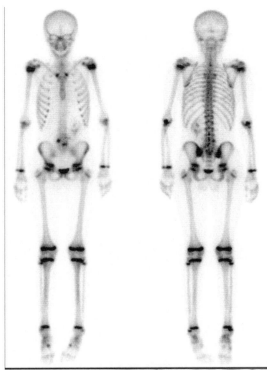

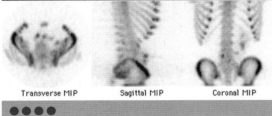

Transverse MIP   Sagittal MIP   Coronal MIP

E. Ectopic pelvic kidney mimicking abnormal posterior element uptake: Anterior and posterior whole-body bone scan (*top*) shows two foci of abnormal uptake best seen in the anterior view, mimicking a lower lumbar vertebral abnormality. This uptake is due to the presence of an ectopic, right pelvic kidney, seen on SPECT images (*bottom*) and suspected on whole-body scintigraphy. (*Image courtesy of Helen Nadel, MD.*)

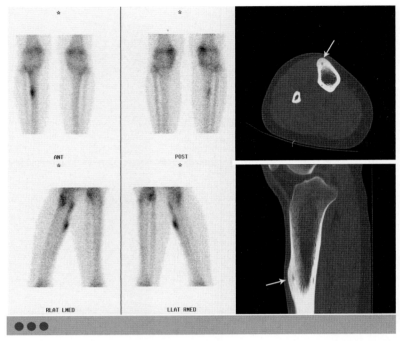

ANT   POST

RLAT LMED   LLAT RMED

F. Osteoid osteoma: Anterior and posterior spot scintiphotos of the tibias (*left*) from a whole-body bone scan in a 17-year-old patient with leg pain at night reveal intense uptake in the proximal tibia anteriorly due to an osteoid osteoma (*arrows*) confirmed on axial (*top right*) and sagittal (*bottom right*) CT images in bone algorithm.

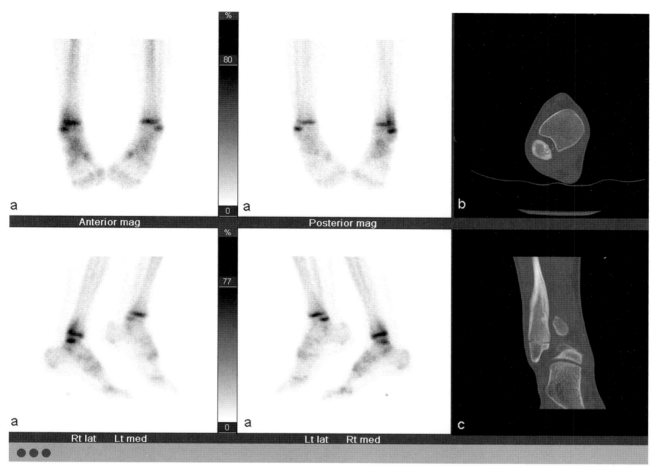

G. Osteoid osteoma: Anterior and posterior spot views of the ankles from bone scan (*left* and *middle*) and corroborating axial (*top right*) and coronal (*bottom right*) CT images in bone window of a distal right fibular osteoid osteoma.

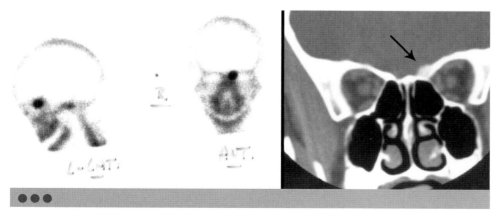

H. AP and left lateral skull views from bone scan (*left*) of a 15-year-old with headache reveal intense uptake in a left superior orbital osteoid osteoma confirmed on coronal CT bone windows (*arrow, right*).

Marguerite T. Parisi, MD, MS Ed

PRESENTATION

Low back pain.

FINDINGS

Bone scan (image A) reveals abnormal uptake at the L4 vertebral level. Subsequent SPECT imaging in coronal, sagittal, and axial planes (image B, *top*) demonstrates decreased uptake pertaining to the left aspect of the L4 vertebral body (rather than increased uptake on the right as was suspected at first glance). Corresponding CT imaging (image B, *bottom*) in the same planes confirms vertebra plana, a classic finding in Langerhans cell histiocytosis (LCH).

DIFFERENTIAL DIAGNOSES

Vertebral destruction/vertebra plana:
- *LCH*

- *Leukemia and metastatic tumors*

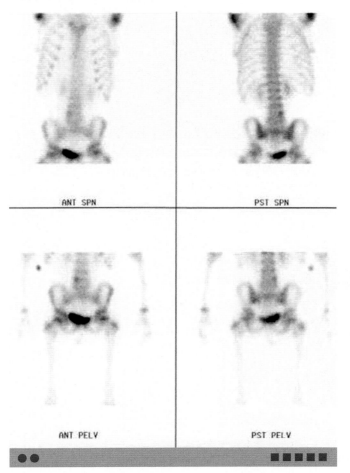

ANT SPN   PST SPN

ANT PELV   PST PELV

A. LCH presenting with vertebra plana: Tc-99m bone scan; anterior and posterior spot scintiphotos of the spine and pelvis with abnormal L4 uptake.

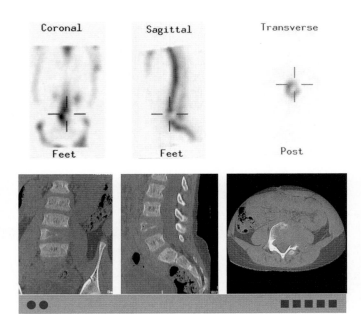

Coronal   Sagittal   Transverse

Feet   Feet   Post

B. Subsequent SPECT imaging of the spine (*top row*) confirms decreased uptake on the left at L4. Correlative CT imaging in similar planes (*bottom row*) reveals vertebra plana (vertebral destruction with preserved disc space).

- *Fracture*
- *Infection:* "cold" osteomyelitis; diskitis (disk space narrowed), fungal (disc space preserved)

COMMENTS

LCH encompasses several different entities characterized by a proliferation of abnormal histiocytes that contain Birbeck granules. Although various hypotheses have been

PEARLS

- **Bone scintigraphy is highly sensitive but nonspecific.**

- **Performing SPECT during bone scintigraphy improves disease evaluation.**

- **Plain film and scintigraphic skeletal surveys are complementary in the evaluation of osseous involvement in LCH as both modalities may miss lesions.**

- **Organ dysfunction rather than organ involvement is the crucial factor in predicting outcome in LCH. Rather than defining the extent of organ involvement, the role of the radiologist is to recognize the protean manifestations of LCH thereby leading to prompt diagnosis.**

proposed, the cause remains unknown. Occurring at any age, the peak age for LCH occurs between 1 and 4 years. In children, incidence is approximately 2 to 5 cases per million per year with a slight male predominance.

Three general forms of LCH were initially described: Letterer-Siwe disease, Hand-Schüller-Christian disease, and eosinophilic granuloma. As many as 50% of cases of LCH cannot be easily placed into one of these categories.

Patients with Letterer-Siwe LCH present during the first year of life with a fulminant course and disseminated disease due to diffuse bone marrow infiltration and resultant hematopoietic dysfunction. Hepatosplenomegaly, lymphadenopathy, and pulmonary involvement are noted; bone involvement is rare. Despite aggressive therapy with systemic chemotherapeutic agents, death may ensue within 1 to 2 years.

Hand-Schüller-Christian disease, a more chronic disseminated form of LCH, usually occurs in patients between the ages of 3 and 6 years. Bone involvement ("geographic skull"), diabetes insipidus, and exophthalmos are the triad of features most often seen.

The eosinophilic granuloma form of LCH involves localized disease in bone (75%) and/or lungs, with onset often in late childhood or in early adulthood. The clinical course is generally benign, and spontaneous remissions are common.

Imaging of LCH patients usually begins with plain films including chest x-ray and radiographic skeletal survey. The bones most frequently involved in LCH are the skull followed by the proximal femur, ribs, and pelvis. Osseous skull lesions of LCH are typically sharply marginated lytic lesions; in long bones, lesions may be accompanied by periostitis that may mimic more malignant lesions. In the spine, the disease manifests with vertebra plana or vertebral body collapse. At nuclear bone scintigraphy, osseous lesions of LCH can have either increased or decreased radiotracer uptake.

ADDITIONAL IMAGES (C-G)

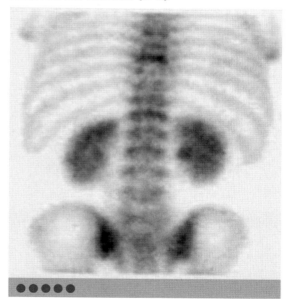

C. Multiple vertebral compression fractures due to leukemia (see Case 10–2). Posterior spot view from bone scan shows multiple compression fractures in thoracic and lumbar spine. Enlarged kidneys with delayed cortical retention suggest acute tumor lysis syndrome and help differentiate leukemia from LCH.

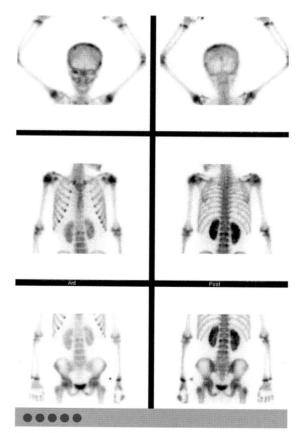

D. Another case of leukemia. Spot anterior (*left*) and posterior (*right*) scintiphotos from a bone scan reveal mildly enlarged kidneys with marked, prolonged cortical retention, skull lesions, multiple lumbar vertebral compressions, and prominent diffuse osseous uptake in marrow distribution caused by leukemia and mimicking LCH.

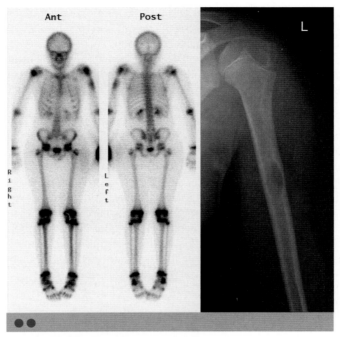

E. Eosinophilic granuloma: Whole body bone scan (*left*) in the anterior and posterior projections in a 12-year-old reveals focal uptake in a left humeral shaft lesion. Plain film X-ray (*right*) shows a sharply marginated lytic lesion, classic for eosinophilic granuloma.

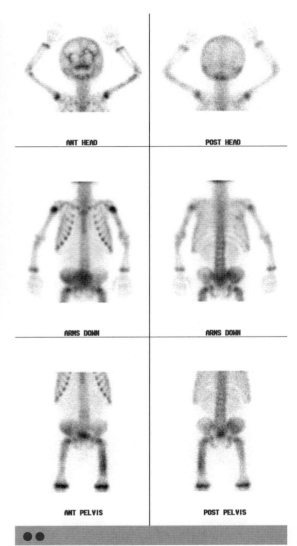

ANT HEAD   POST HEAD

ARMS DOWN   ARMS DOWN

ANT PELVIS   POST PELVIS

F. Langerhans cell histiocytosis: Spot images from a bone scan demonstrate a lytic left supraorbital skull lesion, as well as increased uptake in the right iliac wing, left humerus, and both femoral shafts consistent with LCH.

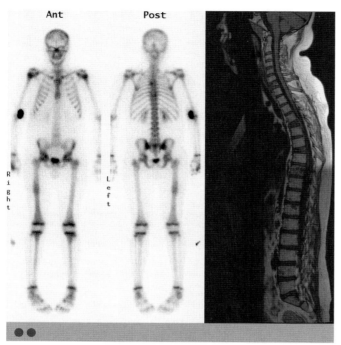

G. LCH: Anterior and posterior views from a whole body bone scan (*left*) demonstrate skull lesions, a right midshaft femoral lesion, and multiple midthoracic vertebral compressions from LCH. Correlative sagittal T1 spine MRI (*right*) confirms vertebra plana at these levels but demonstrates additional lesions in the cervical and lumbar spine.

Shawn E. Parnell, MD

PRESENTATION

An 11-year-old male with remote history of trauma now presents with left knee effusion, severe pain, and inability to bear weight for 1 week.

FINDINGS

Increased uptake on blood pool images (image A) in soft tissues and physes of the left knee and the lateral aspect of the distal femoral epiphysis; focal increased uptake in lateral distal femoral epiphysis on delayed images (image B).

DIFFERENTIAL DIAGNOSES

- *Osteomyelitis*
- *Fracture*
- *Eosinophilic granuloma*
- *Chondroblastoma*

COMMENTS

Acute epiphyseal osteomyelitis is rare in children, and can occur with or without involvement of the adjacent metaphysis or joint space. Its scintigraphic appearance parallels that of osteomyelitis in other locations.

The most common organism implicated in pediatric osteomyelitis is *Staphylococcus aureus*, which accounts for 80% to 90% of cases. Other less common etiologies include group B streptococcus, *Neisseria meningitidis*, mycobacteria, brucellosis (which may cause spondylodiscitis), *Salmonella* in those with sickle cell disease, *Aspergillosis* in immunocompromised children, and congenital syphilis.

The differential considerations for hot epiphyseal lesions on bone scan in children include acute fracture, which may have similar increased radiotracer uptake on early and delayed images. Correlative plain films and/or MRI can help differentiate these processes. Chondroblastoma, the most common primary epiphyseal tumor in children, is another consideration. It can occur in epiphyseal/apophyseal locations throughout the skeleton, most commonly in the proximal humerus and proximal tibia. Finally, eosinophilic granuloma can be single or multifocal hot lesions, with predilection for the calvarium, ribs, spine, and long bones particularly the femur and the humerus.

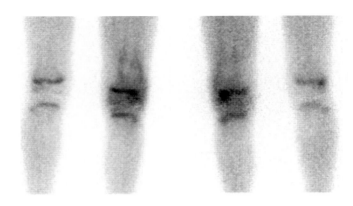

A. Osteomyelitis: Anterior and posterior blood pool images from Tc-99m MDP bone scan show increased soft tissue, physeal, and distal lateral femoral epiphyseal uptake.

In considering a differential diagnosis for multifocal warm osteomyelitis, one should include CRMO (chronic recurrent multifocal osteomyelitis). This is a self-limiting relapsing disorder of unknown etiology which affects predominantly the metaphyses. Biopsy in these cases rarely identifies a causative organism.

PEARLS

- Metaphysis is the most common location for hematogenous osteomyelitis, but epiphysis can be involved either with or without metaphyseal involvement.

- Patterns of spread of hematogenous osteomyelitis vary by age group, depending on presence or absence of the physeal barrier.

- To differentiate between cellulitis, septic arthritis, and osteomyelitis, both early-phase imaging to detect hyperemia (blood flow and/or blood pool) and delayed-phase imaging to detect osseous involvement is necessary.

- Imaging with indium In-111 Oxine (In-111 oxyquinoline)-labeled white blood cells is not recommended in children because of its high radiation burden.

ADDITIONAL IMAGES (B-O)

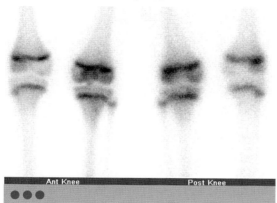

B. Osteomyelitis: Delayed scintiphotos of the knees from the bone scan (anterior and posterior projections) show focal uptake in the distal lateral femoral epiphysis.

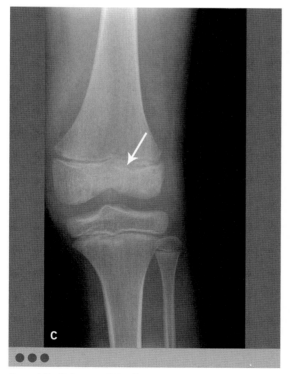

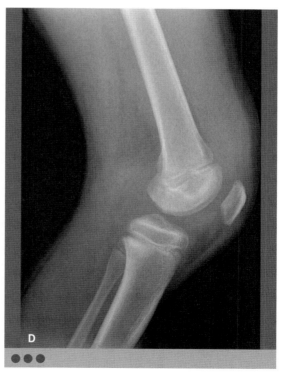

C. and **D. Osteomyelitis:** Correlative frontal (image C) and lateral (image D) knee radiographs show sclerosis and mild irregularity of the lateral femoral condyle (*arrow*) and large knee joint effusion. No fracture is seen.

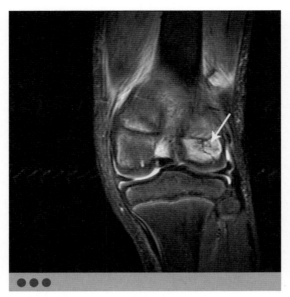

E. Osteomyelitis: Correlative coronal STIR image shows increased signal throughout the lateral femoral condyle (*arrow*), with internal linear low signal representing fracture, presumably a predisposing factor.

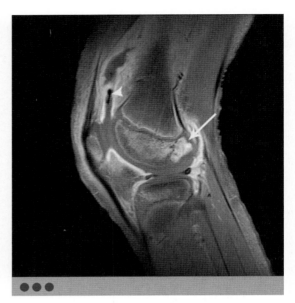

F. Osteomyelitis: Correlative sagittal T1 post-gadolinium (post-Gd) image shows focal enhancement in the fractured lateral femoral condyle (*arrow*), small joint effusion, and synovial enhancement. Note that focal low signal within effusion represents air from joint aspiration (*arrowhead*).

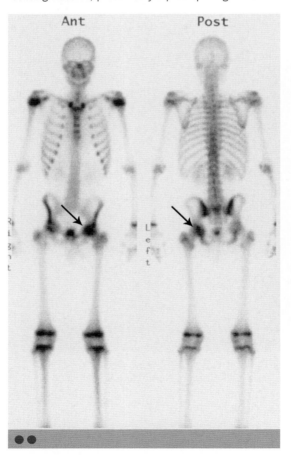

G. Chondroblastoma: Anterior and posterior whole-body delayed images from bone scan show focal increased radiotracer uptake in the left femoral head (*arrows*).

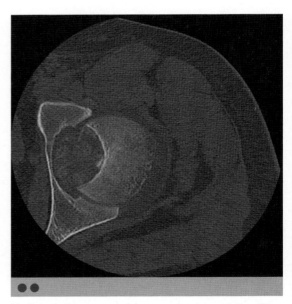

H. Chondroblastoma axial noncontrast correlative CT through left hip shows a well-circumscribed lytic lesion of the capital femoral epiphysis with cortical breakthrough.

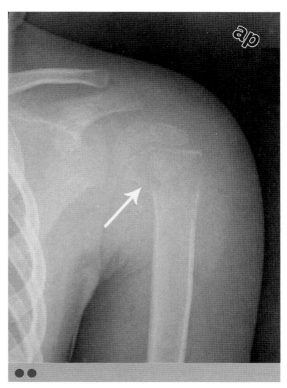

I. Eosinophilic granuloma: AP left shoulder film shows lytic destruction of the proximal metaphysis (*arrow*) with pathologic fracture.

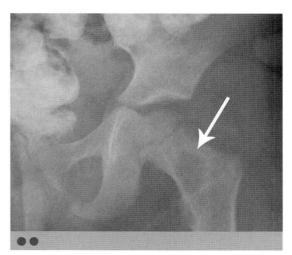

J. Eosinophilic granuloma: AP pelvis film shows well-circumscribed lytic lesion in the left femoral neck (*arrow*).

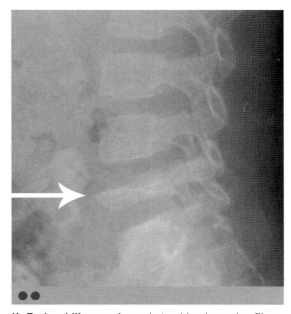

K. Eosinophilic granuloma: Lateral lumbar spine film shows characteristic vertebral plana of EG at L5 (*arrow*). No corresponding scintigraphic abnormality was seen.

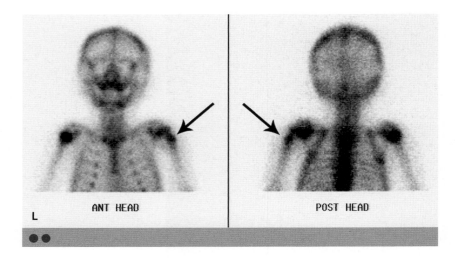

ANT HEAD   POST HEAD

L

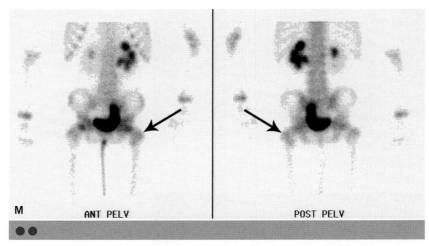

ANT PELV   POST PELV

M

L. and **M. Eosinophilic granuloma:** Anterior and posterior delayed images from bone scan show corresponding asymmetric uptake in the right proximal humerus and left femoral neck (*arrows*). Incidental note of left hydronephrosis.

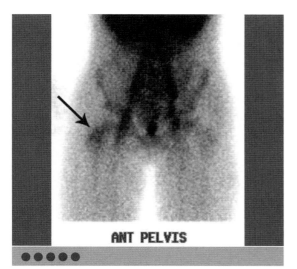

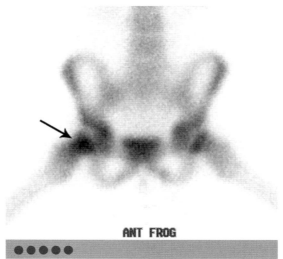

N. Right proximal femoral osteomyelitis in its more common metaphyseal location. Increased uptake of right hip (*arrow*) on blood pool image.

O. Corresponding increased uptake in the proximal right femoral metaphysis (*arrow*) on delayed images.

Shawn E. Parnell, MD

PRESENTATION

A 6-year-old boy with streptococcal toxic shock following 5 days of fever, neck pain, and abdominal pain. Hip effusions were seen on CT obtained at outside institution.

FINDINGS

Photopenia of right hip with surrounding hyperemia on blood pool images (image A). Corresponding proximal femoral photopenia on delayed images and lack of enhancement on MR (image B).

DIFFERENTIAL DIAGNOSES

- *Cold osteomyelitis*
- *Avascular necrosis*
- *Bone cyst*
- *Geode*

COMMENTS

Pediatric osteomyelitis most commonly develops from hematogenous spread, from either asymptomatic or symptomatic bacteremia. Typically, it originates in the metaphysis, where there is relatively slow blood flow. Spread of infection is related to the vascular anatomy of the epiphysis, physis, and metaphysis and varies according to age. Prior to age 18 months and after physeal closure, transphyseal vessels supply the epiphysis. From age 18 months until physeal closure, capillaries in the metaphysis do not cross the physis, and instead terminate as slow flow venous lakes.

Osteomyelitis classically demonstrates focal hyperemia on blood pool and focal increased bone uptake on delayed images. Some children can, however, early in the course of their disease, demonstrate focal photopenia on delayed images, particularly when associated with rapid onset of symptoms, severe bone pain, and high fever. Increased joint pressure can also cause a transiently photopenic joint.

The differential for cold lesions in the proximal femur would include avascular necrosis of the femoral head, most commonly occurring in the elementary school age group. Unicameral bone cyst could create focal photopenic lesion, although this lesion is more commonly evaluated by plain film, which is virtually diagnostic. Unicameral bone cyst (UBC) is most common in the 5- to 15-year-old age group, and is commonly located in the proximal humerus, followed by the proximal femur, with these two sites accounting for nearly 90% of cases. Geodes would be an unlikely consideration in children without underlying abnormal

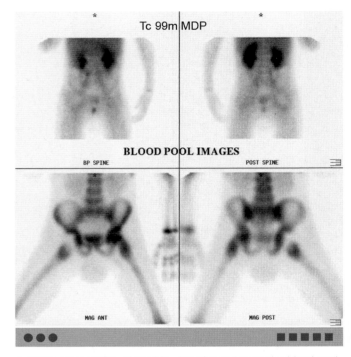

A. Cold osteomyelitis of the hip: Anterior and posterior blood pool images (*top*) and delayed magnified views of the pelvis (*bottom*) from bone scan show early photopenia with surrounding rim of increased uptake and late focal photopenia and mild lateral displacement of the right hip.

mechanics from hip dysplasia or other congenital hip malformation.

PEARLS

- Osteomyelitis may appear very early as photopenic area due to thrombosis and vascular compression from bone marrow edema.

- Correlation between blood pool and delayed scans can be helpful to differentiate between avascular necrosis and cold osteomyelitis, with the latter demonstrating adjacent hyperemia on blood pool phase.

- Bone scan may also be negative for osteomyelitis in the first 24 hours before increased bone turnover has occurred.

- MR is useful in evaluating for pediatric pelvic osteomyelitis, providing early detection and treatment of otherwise occult pyomyositis. Also MR is beneficial for long bone osteomyelitis in which patient is not improving on standard therapy and to detect complications such as subperiosteal abscess.

ADDITIONAL IMAGES (B-H)

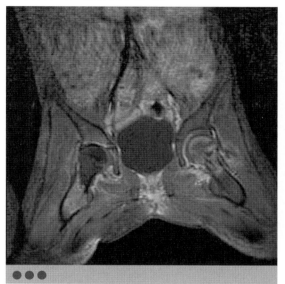

B. Cold osteomyelitis of the hip: Correlative Coronal T1 fat saturation post-Gd of the pelvis shows abnormal low signal in the right femoral head and proximal femoral metaphysis indicating avascular necrosis, with enhancing more distal femoral metaphysis compatible with osteomyelitis.

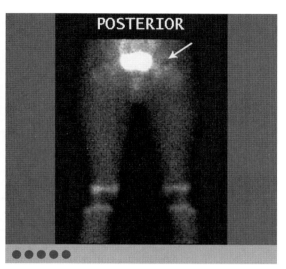

C. Avascular necrosis of the right hip: Posterior blood pool images of the pelvis from bone scan show subtle decreased uptake over the right hip (*arrow*).

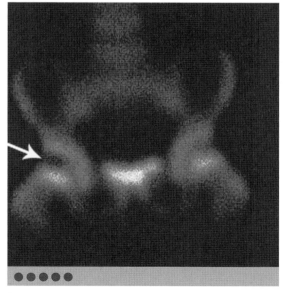

D. Avascular necrosis of the right hip: Delayed anterior images show focal photopenia of the right femoral head (*arrow*).

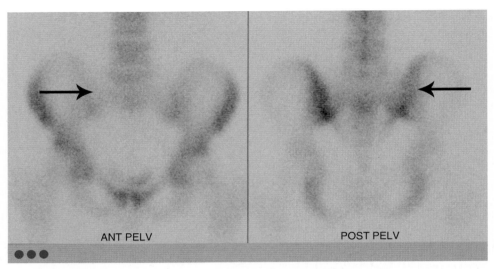

ANT PELV POST PELV

E. Aneurysmal bone cyst: Anterior and posterior delayed images from bone scan show asymmetric decreased uptake at the right sacroiliac joint (*arrows*).

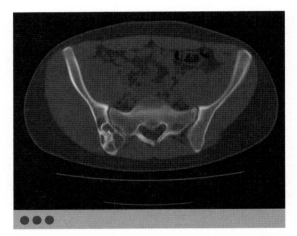

F. Aneurysmal bone cyst: Correlative noncontrast CT of the pelvis shows multiloculated, slightly expansile lytic lesion of the right ilium.

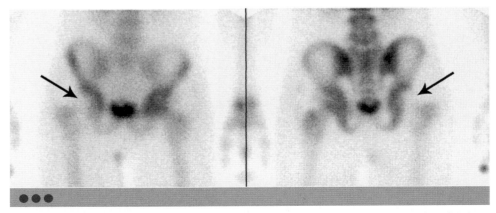

G. Cold osteomyelitis of the hip: Anterior and posterior delayed pelvic spot images show focal photopenia (*arrows*), involving right proximal femoral epiphysis and metaphysis and mild lateral displacement of the femoral head.

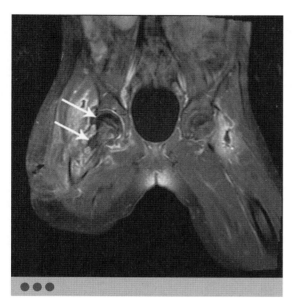

H. Cold osteomyelitis of the hip: Follow-up coronal T1 fat saturation post-Gd MR image after incision and drainage shows focal abnormal low signal consistent with avascular necrosis involving portions of the right femoral head and neck (*arrows*), as well as abnormal increased enhancement of the metaphysis indicating osteomyelitis.

Marguerite T. Parisi, MD, MS Ed

PRESENTATION

A 2-year-old with palpable abdominal mass.

FINDINGS

Axial images from a contrast-enhanced CT (Figure A) scan reveal a large mass arising from or invading the left kidney, either Wilms tumor or neuroblastoma. There is adjacent retroperitoneal adenopathy present which encases the aorta. Anterior images from whole-body Tc-99m MDP bone and corresponding I-131 metaiodobenzylguanidine (MIBG) scans (Figure B) both demonstrate uptake in the left upper quadrant (LUQ) mass. MIBG avidity confirms a diagnosis of neuroblastoma and excludes Wilms tumor as the etiology of the tumor. Retroperitoneal lymphadenopathy and diffuse osseous metastatic disease are more easily identified on MIBG than on corresponding bone scan.

DIFFERENTIAL DIAGNOSES

- *Retroperitoneal malignancies* of childhood
  - *Neuroblastoma*
  - *Wilms Tumor*
  - *Renal cell carcinoma* (RCC)

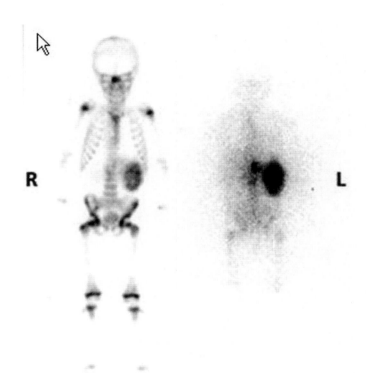

Tc-99m MDP   I-131 MIBG

B. Anterior views from whole-body bone scan (*left*) and corresponding I-131 MIBG scan (*right*). (*Reprinted with permission from: Parisi MT. Cases of the day (pediatrics): Neuroblastoma Masquerading as Wilms Tumor—Figure 3c. Presented at the Radiological Society of North America Scientific Assembly and Annual Meeting, Chicago, IL; November 26-December 1, 2000.*)

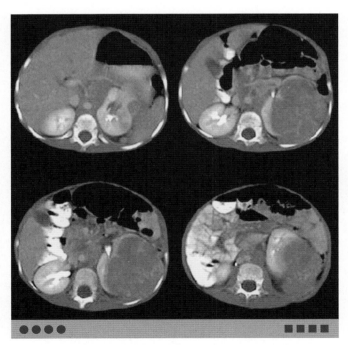

A. Four contiguous axial views from the CT scan. (*Reprinted with permission from: Parisi MT. Cases of the day (pediatrics): Neuroblastoma Masquerading as Wilms Tumor—Figure 3a. Presented at the Radiological Society of North America Scientific Assembly and Annual Meeting, Chicago, IL; November 26-December 1, 2000.*)

PEARLS

- MIBG is highly sensitive and specific for neuroblastoma.

- I-123 MIBG is preferred to I-131 MIBG as it has a shorter half-life, better imaging characteristics allowing for performance of SPECT imaging, and delivers a lower radiation dose to the patient.

- SPECT imaging (I-123) improves disease detection.

- Administer appropriate oral doses of supersaturated potassium iodide (SSKI) to block thyroid uptake of tracer.

- Routinely perform whole body imaging in children of all ages; include lateral views of calvarium.

- *Other renal tumors*: Clear cell sarcoma and rhabdoid tumor
- *Pheochromocytoma*: Rare
- *Adrenocortical carcinoma*: Very rare

- *MIBG-avid tumors*
  - *Neuroblastoma*
  - *Pheochromocytoma*
  - *Carcinoid tumors*

COMMENTS

Neuroblastoma is the third most common childhood malignancy, accounting for 10% of all pediatric tumors and 15% of cancer-related deaths in children. Originating in neural crest cells, 70% of neuroblastomas are located within the adrenal glands, 15% in the posterior mediastinum, 10% in the pelvis, and 5% in the neck. Fifty percent of patients are diagnosed within the first year of life, 75% by age 2 years, and 90% by age 4 years. These children are typically ill-appearing at diagnosis, presenting with vague systemic manifestations, including fever and malaise. Unusual paraneoplastic presentations occur in 10% of patients and include opsoclonus-myoclonus syndrome (1%-3%) or refractory diarrhea from tumor secretion of vasoactive intestinal peptide (7%). Elevated urinary catecholamine levels are detected in up to 80% of the cases.

Up to 50% of infants and 70% of older children with neuroblastoma will have metastases at the time of diagnosis. The most common sites of metastatic disease are cortical bone and bone marrow, liver, lymph nodes, and skin.

Wilms tumor is the most common renal neoplasm of childhood. Up to 15% of the patients with Wilms tumor have associated anomalies (horseshoe kidney) or predisposing conditions (hemihypertrophy or Beckwith-Wiedemann syndrome; sporadic aniridia). Unlike patients with neuroblastoma, those with Wilms tumor tend to be healthy and present with an asymptomatic abdominal mass. The mean age at time of diagnosis of Wilms tumor is $3^1/_2$ years. At diagnosis, only 12% of those with Wilms tumor will have metastatic disease, manifested either as local tumoral or vascular extension into the renal vein or inferior vena cava (IVC) or as hematogenous spread to the lungs or liver. Bone metastases are extremely rare.

The classic CT findings distinguishing neuroblastoma from Wilms tumor are presented in Figure C.

The preoperative diagnosis of neuroblastoma is typically established on the basis of patient age, clinical and laboratory features, the site of the primary tumor, its imaging appearance, and the patterns of metastatic spread. In confusing cases in which intrarenal invasion by neuroblastoma masquerades as a Wilms tumor, nuclear scintigraphy is crucial to diagnosis and to disease staging.

ADDITIONAL IMAGES (C-H)

Distinguishing CT Features

Neuroblastoma	Wilms Tumor
• Calcification >80%	• Calcification = 10%
• Encases vessels	• Displaces vessels
• Crosses midline	• Doesn't cross midline
• Spinal canal extension	• No spinal canal extension
• Metastases:	• Metastases:
– bones common	– lungs common
– lungs rare	– bones rare

C. Classic CT features distinguishing neuroblastoma from Wilms tumor.

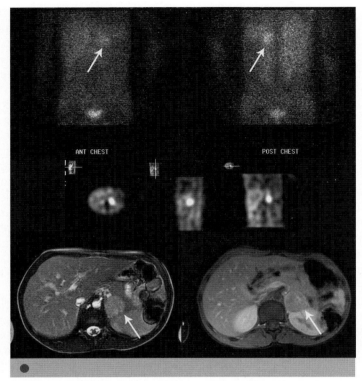

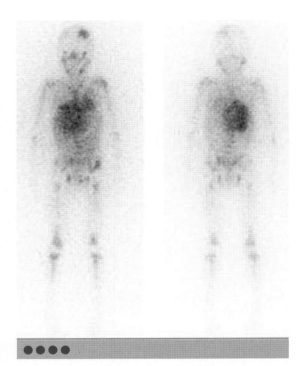

D. Pheochromocytoma: Anterior and posterior spot (*top*) and SPECT (*middle*) views from an I-123 MIBG scan in a 9-year-old with hypertension show increased uptake in a left adrenal pheochromocytoma, corresponding to mass seen on (*arrows*) axial T2 (*left*) and postcontrast T1 (*right*) MRI images (*bottom*).

E. Stage IV neuroblastoma: Anterior (*left*) and posterior (*right*) images from an I-123 MIBG scan in a patient with stage IV neuroblastoma. There is uptake in the large primary mass in the right upper quadrant (RUQ), in a cortical skull metastases, and diffusely throughout the bone marrow of the axial and appendicular skeleton.

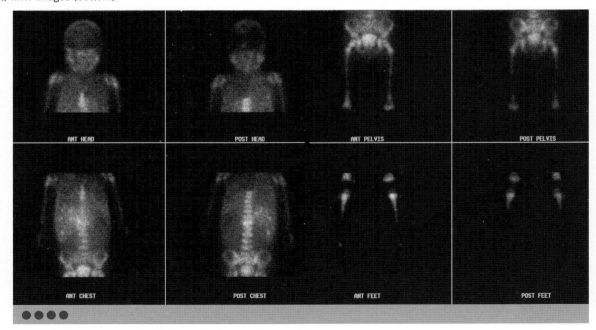

F. Stage IV neuroblastoma with diffuse bone marrow metastases: Anterior and posterior images from an I-123 MIBG scan in a 3-year-old patient with relapsed stage IV neuroblastoma. Osseous metastatic disease (with focal cortical T12 lesion and diffuse bone marrow involvement) is so extensive that the study resembles a bone scan. The presence of diffuse hepatic uptake with numerous metastases distinguishes this study from a Tc-99m bone scan. Photopenic area in the left upper chest, including portions of the thoracic spine, is due to recent radiation therapy.

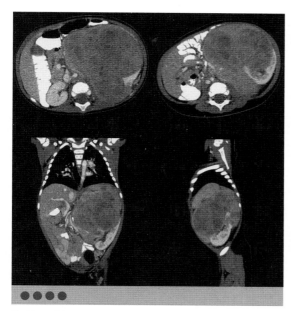

G. Neuroblastoma mimicking Wilms tumor: Axial (*top left* and *right*), coronal (*bottom left*), and sagittal (*bottom right*) views from a contrast-enhanced CT scan in a 2-year-old with a large, heterogeneous LUQ mass either arising from or invading the left kidney.

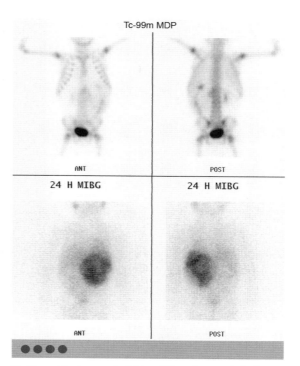

H. Neuroblastoma mimicking Wilms tumor: Anterior and posterior views of the torso from a Tc-99m MDP bone scan (*top*) show subtle tracer uptake in the mass which displaces and stretches the left kidney. Corresponding views from an I-123 MIBG scan (*bottom*) show massive uptake in the large mass, confirming it is a neuroblastoma, not a Wilms tumor as was suggested by the CT.

Marguerite T. Parisi, MD, MS Ed

PRESENTATION

A 3-year-old with abdominal mass diagnosed as neuroblastoma.

FINDINGS

Staging evaluation included bone scan (Figure A, *left*) and corresponding I-123 MIBG scan (*right*). I-123 MIBG scan delineates not only the primary tumor, but thoracic soft tissue metastatic disease not seen on Tc-99m MDP bone scan. Diffuse osseous metastatic disease is also more easily appreciated on the MIBG scan.

COMMENTS

Overall prognosis in neuroblastoma is dependent on patient age, tumor stage, and other factors, including N-myc oncogene amplification. The spectrum of treatment for those with neuroblastoma ranges from supportive care in stage IV disease, to definitive excision (stage I), and ultimately to extensive chemotherapy with autologous bone marrow transplant for those with stage IV disease. This makes precise definition of disease extent crucial in those with neuroblastoma.

Nuclear medicine, with its ability to provide whole-body assessment of disease extent, plays a pivotal role in the evaluation of those with neuroblastoma. There are five radiotracer agents that have been used in the diagnosis, staging, and therapeutic response monitoring of those with neuroblastoma: technetium 99m methylene diphosphonate (Tc-99m MDP), metaiodobenzylguanidine (MIBG), somatostatin receptors (indium-111 octreotide), monoclonal antibodies, and fluorine 18 fluorodeoxyglucose positron emission tomography (^{18}F-FDG-PET). The two most commonly used are Tc-99m MDP and MIBG radiolabeled with either iodine-131 or, preferably, iodine-123 (I-131 MIBG or I-123 MIBG).

When compared with conventional radiographic skeletal surveys in those with neuroblastoma, the Tc-99m MDP bone scan identifies more patients with unsuspected osseous metastatic disease and demonstrates additional sites of disease in 80% of those with known metastases. Uptake of Tc-99m MDP is seen in 35% to 65% of the primary soft tissue tumors as well. On bone scan, osseous metastases typically appear as areas of abnormally increased or decreased radiotracer uptake involving both the appendicular and axial skeleton. Lesions are primarily metaphyseal, often symmetric and located close to the normally radiotracer-avid epiphyses, findings which can increase the difficulty in correctly identifying extent of disease. As bone scans are sensitive but not specific, entities such as infection, fracture, and benign and healed metastases can mimic active osseous metastatic lesions of neuroblastoma.

Developed in 1980 by D.M. Wieland, MIBG is a structural analogue of norepinephrine and guanethidine which is 92% sensitive and 100% specific for neuroblastoma in the

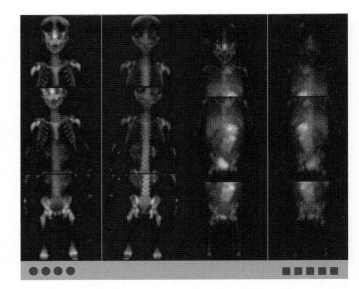

A. Staging Tc-99m bone scan (*left*) and corresponding spot images from an I-123 MIBG scan (*right*) in a 3-year-old with newly diagnosed neuroblastoma. Uptake in the primary abdominal soft tissue mass is present on both studies. The extent of the primary mass is better delineated with MIBG which additionally shows a soft tissue metastases in the left upper thorax. Cortical bone metastases in the right orbit, left skull as well as symmetric lesions in the proximal humeri, proximal and distal femurs, and left skull are better seen on the MIBG scan which also shows diffuse bone marrow involvement not seen on the bone scan.

PEARLS

- Normal MIBG biodistribution includes uptake in the salivary glands, heart, liver, and urinary bladder. Occasionally there can be uptake in normal adrenal glands and in bowel.

- Lack of MIBG uptake in normal bones improves detection of the osseous metastatic lesions of neuroblastoma when compared to bone scans. Epiphyseal uptake of MIBG, in the absence of antecedent bone scan, is abnormal.

- Bone scans demonstrate cortical bone abnormalities. MIBG can demonstrate both cortical bone and bone marrow involvement by neuroblastoma.

- Fluorine-18 FDG is particularly useful in staging and therapeutic response monitoring in those 10% of patients whose neuroblastomas are not MIBG avid.

- In-111 octreotide localizes in a variety of neuroendocrine and non-neuroendocrine tumors as well as in inflammatory lesions, making it sensitive in but not specific for the detection of neuroblastoma. Additionally, physiologic uptake of octreotide in liver, spleen, kidneys, and bowel may obscure tumor visualization in neuroblastoma.

- Radiolabeled (I-123 or I-131) monoclonal antibodies (3F8, G$_{D2}$, among others) are highly sensitive and specific for neuroblastoma. Limited trials, limited availability, and high cost have precluded widespread usage.

pediatric population. The uncomplicated normal biodistribution, the lack of MIBG uptake in normal bone, and the ability of MIBG to image both cortical and bone marrow sites of neuroblastoma, combined with improved rates of disease detection compared with Tc-99m MDP scintigraphy, make MIBG the single best radiotracer for imaging neuroblastoma. I-131 MIBG has also been used as a systemic radiotherapeutic agent in advanced stage neuroblastoma.

ADDITIONAL IMAGES (B-H)

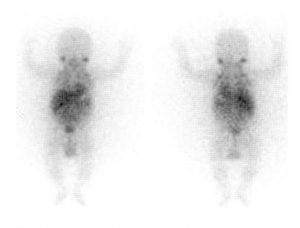

B. Normal I-123 MIBG scan: Normal surveillance I-123 MIBG scan in an infant with neuroblastoma. Anterior and posterior images show expected uptake in salivary glands, heart, liver, urinary bladder, and bowel.

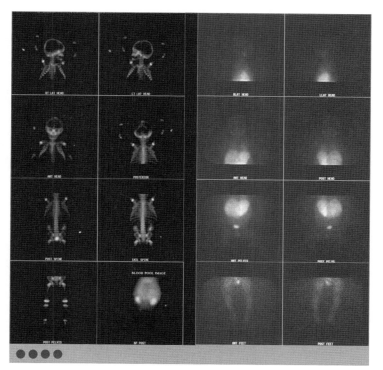

C. Neuroblastoma: Paired Tc-99m MDP and I-123 MIBG scans. Anterior and posterior spot scintiphotos from a Tc-99m MDP (*left*) show mass effect upon the kidneys from a large neuroblastoma. Extent of the large, bilobed mass which crosses midline is easily appreciated on the accompanying I-123 MIBG scan (*right*). Additionally identified only on the MIBG scan is a hematogenous metastases in the left scrotum. No evidence of osseous metastatic disease.

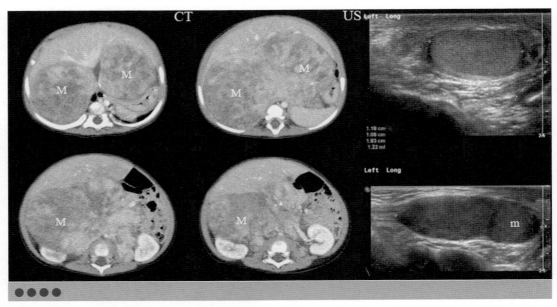

D. Correlative imaging; CT and US of neuroblastoma: Correlative axial images from contrast-enhanced CT (*left*) delineate the huge bilobed neuroblastoma (M) which crosses midline and displaces the liver and kidneys, demonstrated in Figure C. US (*right*) confirms the left scrotal metastases (m) adjacent to the normal left testes.

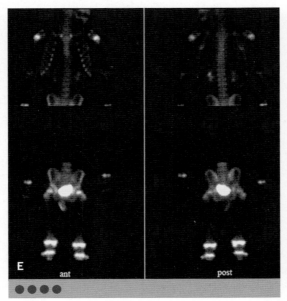

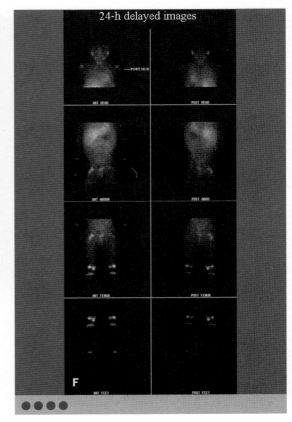

E., F., G., and **H. Neuroblastoma:** Paired Tc-99m MDP and I-123 MIBG scan. Anterior and posterior spot scintiphotos from a Tc-99m bone scan (Figure E, *left*) and I-123 MIBG scan (Figure F, *right*) in a neuroblastoma patient. MIBG better shows known proximal and distal right femoral metastases as well as a new left knee lesion. Initially, symmetric physeal uptake (image F) was presumed to represent residual "shine-through" from antecedent bone scan. Pesistence of symmetric physeal uptake of tracer on 48 hour imaging (image G) was the first indication of progressive disease, better seen 1 month later with repeat I-123 MIBG imaging (image H). Epiphyseal uptake of MIBG, in the absence of antecedent bone scan, is always abnormal.

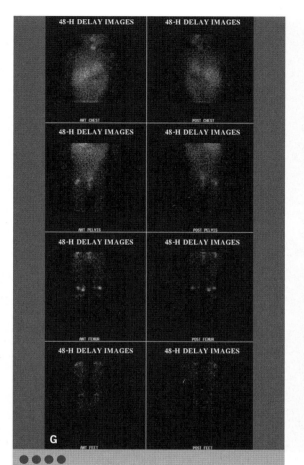

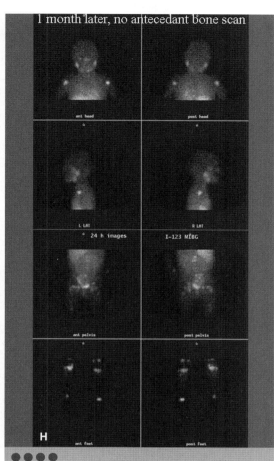

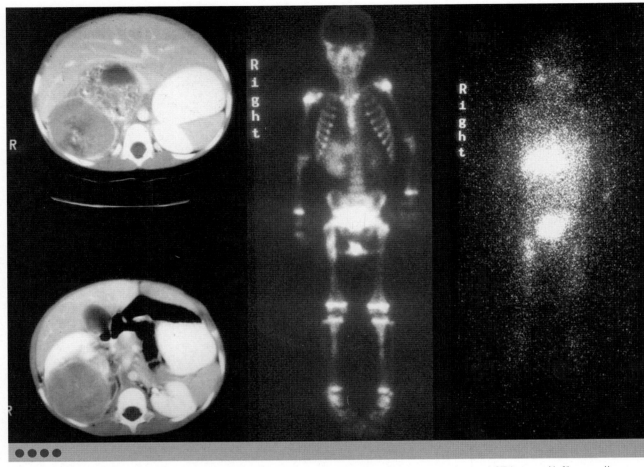

I. Neuroblastoma: CT; paired Tc-99m MDP and I-131 MIBG scan. Selected axial contrast-enhanced CT images (*left*), as well as anterior whole-body images from corresponding bone (*center*), and I-131 MIBG (*right*) scans in a patient with RUQ neuroblastoma. Uptake in the primary abdominal tumor is seen on both scintigraphic studies. Despite poor resolution of the I-131 MIBG scan, more osseous lesions are detected than on bone scan, including right orbit, skull base, left arm, left sacrum, bilateral femurs, and tibias.

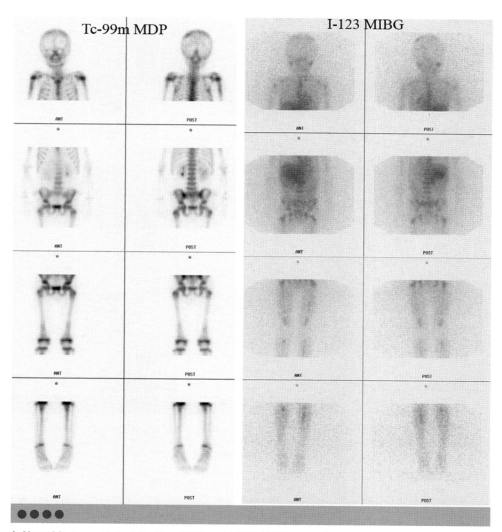

J. Neuroblastoma: Paired Tc-99m MDP and I-123 MIBG scan. Anterior and posterior views from a Tc-99m MDP bone scan (*left*) and paired I-123 MIBG scan (*right*) in a 4-year-old with neuroblastoma. I-123 MIBG scan better delineates the primary tumor in the right upper abdomen. Identification of cortical bone metastases are easier to identify on MIBG than on bone scan. Additionally, unlike bone scans, MIBG can identify diffuse bone marrow disease which is present in this patient.

Marguerite T. Parisi, MD, MS Ed

PRESENTATION

Surveillance I-123 MIBG scan in a 4-year-old with previous history of neuroblastoma.

FINDINGS

There is absence of the normal MIBG biodistribution as evidenced by lack of expected radiotracer uptake in salivary glands, heart, and liver. Rather, tracer uptake in the stomach, kidneys, urinary bladder, and, subtly, in the thyroid gland, is a biodistribution most compatible with that of radioactive iodine (image A).

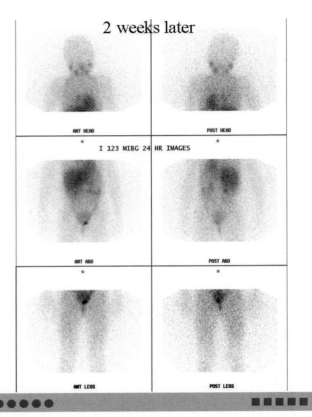

B. Repeat I-123 MIBG scan (anterior and posterior) performed 2 weeks later shows normal study with no evidence of residual or recurrent neuroblastoma.

DIFFERENTIAL DIAGNOSIS

- Altered biodistribution of MIBG:
  - *Interfering medications*
  - *Hyperavid neoplasm*
  - Quality control problem with poor MIBG labeling (as in this case)

PEARLS

- **Awareness of the normal biodistribution of MIBG is crucial for accurate disease detection and staging.**

- **Prior to administering either I-123 or I-131MIBG, one should always check for the presence of interfering medications. In children these most commonly include cold preparations containing pseudoephedrine or phenylpropanolamine.**

- **Always administer appropriate amounts of SSKI for thyroid blockade prior to MIBG administration.**

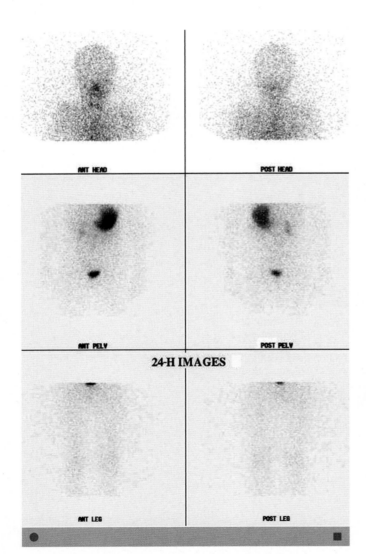

A. Altered MIBG biodistribution resulting in non-diagnostic study. Anterior and posterior spot scintiphotos from an I-123 MIBG scan in which a poor radiotracer labeling process resulted in an iodine, *not* MIBG, biodistribution.

COMMENTS

In nuclear medicine, a radiotracer (the combination of a nonradioactive pharmaceutical and a radioactive atom) is administered which allows functional imaging of organs in which that radiotracer preferentially accumulates. The unique chemistry, anticipated biodistribution, and target organ for each radiotracer is used to evaluate and diagnose specific pathologic processes.

When evaluating any nuclear medicine study, one must always be cognizant of the normal biodistribution of the radiotracer used. When labeled with either I-131 or, preferably, I-123, MIBG uptake should normally be seen in the salivary glands, heart, liver, normal adrenal glands, urinary bladder, and, occasionally, in gut (image B). In this case (image A), the normal MIBG distribution is absent, replaced by that of radioactive iodine. This is secondary to a quality control issue in which there is poor labeling either because of an insufficient quantity of MIBG or dissociation of MIBG from its I-123 label. This results in a nondiagnostic study. Awareness of this appearance will avoid misdiagnosis of left upper quadrant neuroblastoma.

ADDITIONAL IMAGES (C-H)

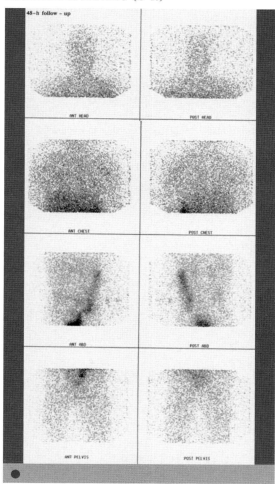

C. Altered MIBG biodistribution due to interfering medications: Anterior and posterior spot scintiphotos from an I-131 MIBG scan in a 16-year-old patient with biopsy-proven pheochromocytoma. The presence of interfering medications—in this case antihypertensive drugs—resulted in altered MIBG distribution with absence of uptake in known left posterior thoracic mass as well as in expected normal sites.

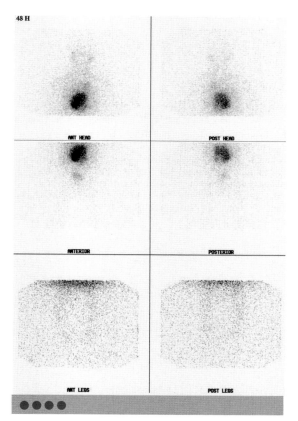

D. Altered MIBG biodistribution due to hyperavid neoplasm: Anterior and posterior scintiphotos from an I-131 MIBG scan in a 2-year-old with hyperavid abdominal neuroblastoma. The marked radiotracer accumulation in the midabdominal mass results in an altered MIBG biodistribution with decreased tracer uptake in salivary glands, heart, liver, and urinary bladder.

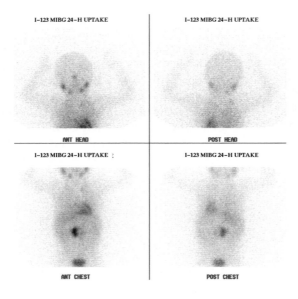

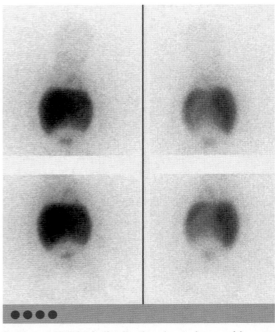

E. Neuroblastoma: I-123 MIBG scan following four cycles of chemotherapy in the 2-year-old with neuroblastoma whose staging images are shown in image D. There is now, decrease in size and tracer uptake in residual midabdominal neuroblastoma. In addition, expected physiologic MIBG uptake is present in salivary glands, heart, liver, and bladder.

F. Altered MIBG biodistribution due to hyperavid neoplasm: An 18-month-old with malaise, weight loss, and abdominal mass. Anterior and posterior scintiphotos from an I-123 MIBG scan reveal altered biodistribution with decreased uptake in expected sites of radiotracer uptake due to the presence of a hyperavid neuroblastoma.

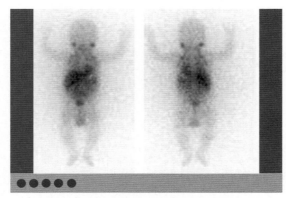

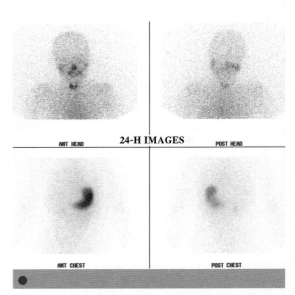

24-H IMAGES

G. Normal I-123 MIBG scan. Anterior and posterior images from a normal I-123 MIBG scan with expected physiologic uptake in salivary glands, heart, liver, and urinary bladder.

H. Additional example of altered MIBG biodistribution due to quality control issues. This occurred on the same day as the index case (image A). Again, note anterior and posterior scan shows a normal iodine rather than an MIBG radiotracer distribution.

Marguerite T. Parisi, MD, MS Ed

PRESENTATION

A 12-year-old female child diagnosed at age 6 with stage IIB neuroblastoma of right neck. She underwent tumor resection, chemotherapy, and radiation therapy. Subsequently, surveillance CT scan at age 12 suggested disease recurrence in right neck (image A, *circle*).

FINDINGS

Anterior scintiphotos from I-123 MIBG (image A, *center*) and corresponding ¹⁸F-FDG-PET scans (*right*) demonstrate that the recurrent mass (*arrows*) is only minimally MIBG but markedly FDG avid.

DIFFERENTIAL DIAGNOSES

- Recurrent non-MIBG but FDG-avid neuroblastoma
- *Adrenocortical carcinoma*
- *Ganglioneuroma*
- *Development of secondary tumor*
- *Soft tissue inflammatory lesion*

COMMENTS

Fluorine-18 FDG-PET uptake is nonspecific and can be seen in variety of tumors as well as in inflammatory processes. FDG uptake in malignancies is related to the enhanced glycolytic metabolism of tumor cells as compared to normal cells. FDG uptake is proportional to tumor cell burden and tumor cell proliferation.

Sites of physiologic FDG uptake include brain, tonsils, lymphoid tissue at Waldeyers ring in the throat, parotid, salivary glands, vocal cords, thymus, myocardium, liver, spleen, gastrointestinal (GI) tract, kidneys, and bladder. Avid FDG uptake is seen in most neuroblastomas prior to chemo or radiation therapy. As FDG uptake is independent of the type 1 catecholamine uptake mechanism of MIBG, FDG is a useful radiotracer for those 10% of neuroblastomas that fail to accumulate or have poor accumulation of MIBG.

The respective roles of MIBG and ¹⁸F-FDG-PET in neuroblastoma remain in evolution. Contrary to intuition, tumor-to-background ratios are higher for MIBG than for FDG-PET.

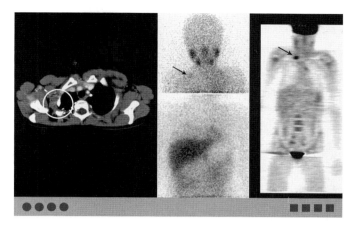

A. Axial image from contrast-enhanced CT scan (*left*) with soft tissue mass in right neck (*circle*). Anterior scintiphotos from I-123 MIBG scan (*center*) and corresponding ¹⁸F-FDG-PET scan (*right*) reveal minimal MIBG uptake but marked FDG avidity in the right neck mass (*arrows*). Excisional biopsy confirmed recurrent neuroblastoma.

MIBG is rated superior to FDG-PET in assessment of bone and marrow disease, detecting more sites of osseous metastases. MIBG is often superior to FDG-PET during and after chemotherapy. FDG is better than MIBG in early-stage disease and sometimes better than MIBG for assessment of primary/residual mass lesions and nonosseous metastases.

PEARLS

- Fluorine-18 FDG-PET cannot replace standard imaging modalities in newly diagnosed neuroblastoma patients. Tc-99m MDP and I-123 MIBG are mandatory in initial staging evaluation.

- Fluorine-18 FDG-PET is useful in those 10% of neuroblastoma patients who are non-MIBG avid.

- FDG-PET may assist in assessment of the proliferative and malignant potential of neuroblastoma.

- In conjunction with bone marrow aspirate, FDG may, in the absence of or after resolution of cranial vault lesions, supplant standard imaging modalities including MIBG in routine follow-up, simplifying restaging.

ADDITIONAL IMAGES (B-D)

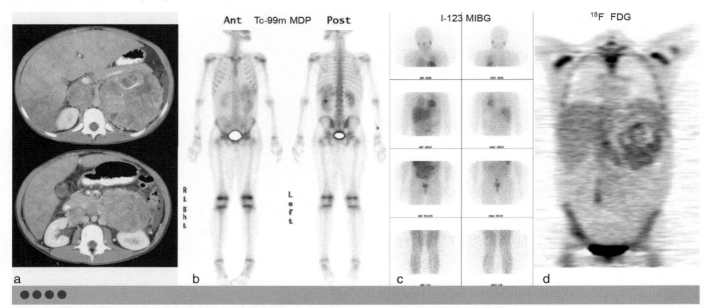

B. Adrenocortical carcinoma: A 12-year-old girl with weight loss and palpable heterogeneous left abdominal mass (axial CT, *a*). Anterior and posterior images from whole-body bone scan (*b*) reveal uptake in the mass which inferiorly displaces the left kidney. I-123 MIBG scan (*c*) is negative. Single coronal FDG-PET image (*d*) shows PET avidity in this biopsy-proven adrenocortical carcinoma, a rare pediatric malignancy.

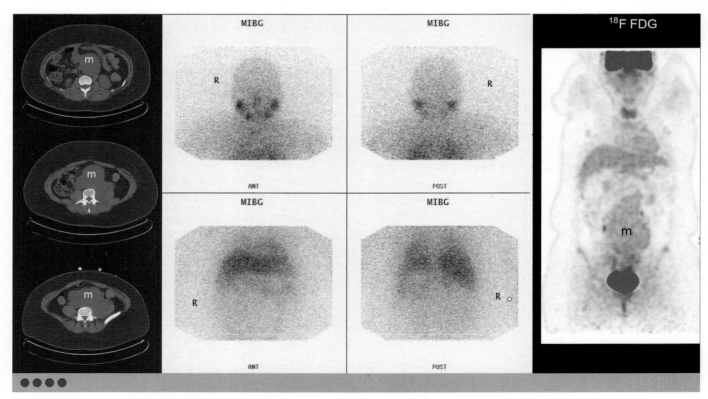

C. Ganglioneuroma: Noncontrast axial CT images (*left*) show a midline retroperitoneal mass (m) which is non-MIBG avid (*center*). The biopsy-proven ganglioneuroma (m) is FDG avid (*right*). Only 30% of ganglioneuromas are MIBG avid.

468

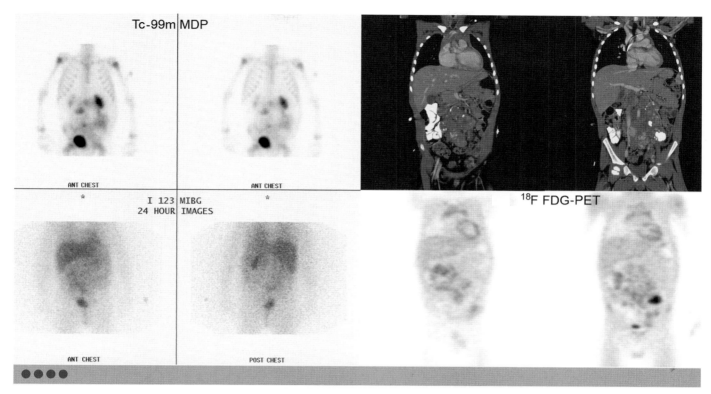

D. Additional example of poorly MIBG-avid neuroblastoma which is better evaluated with FDG-PET; a 3-year-old child with large abdominal neuroblastoma. There is extensive Tc-99m MDP uptake (*top left*) in the large, heterogeneous, and calcified mass. Minimal I-123 MIBG uptake (*bottom left*) is present. Coronal contrast-enhanced CT (*top right*) and corresponding images from FDG-PET show the mass to be FDG avid. As in this case, ^{18}F-FDG-PET is useful in those 10% of neuroblastoma patients whose tumors are poorly or non-MIBG avid.

Nghia Jack Vo, MD, and Marguerite T. Parisi, MD, MS Ed

PRESENTATION

A 4-month-old male infant with persistent jaundice, abnormal liver enzymes, and light-colored stools presents for evaluation of suspected biliary atresia (BA).

FINDINGS

Initial (image A) as well as 7- and 24-hour delayed (image B) images from a Tc-99m hepatobiliary scan demonstrate lack of excretion of radiotracer into bowel, a finding which given patient age, is highly suspicious for BA. Poor hepatic function as demonstrated by delayed hepatic uptake and prolongation of the blood pool activity in conjunction with splenomegaly on initial images suggest cirrhosis with portal hypertension. Limited views from abdominal CT scan (image C, *left*) and ultrasound with color flow Doppler (image C, *centre* and *right*) demonstrate absence of gallbladder, cavernous transformation of the portal vein (*arrow*), splenomegaly, a spontaneous splenorenal shunt, and recanalization of the umbilical vein (*arrowhead*), findings consistent with surgical diagnosis of BA, and portal hypertension.

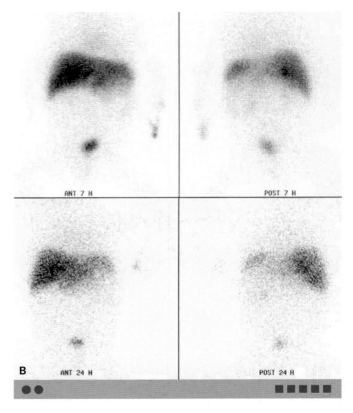

B

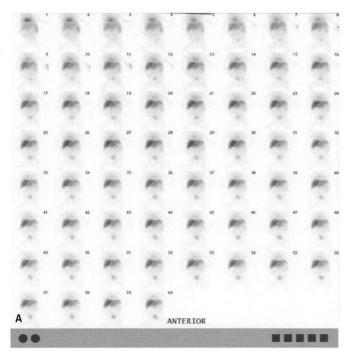

A

A. and **B.** Initial sequential anterior 1-minute (image A) as well as 7- and 24-hour anterior and posterior delayed images (image B) from a Tc-99m hepatobiliary scan in a 4-month-old infant with persistent jaundice, abnormal liver enzymes. There is poor hepatic function and splenomegaly consistent with cirrhosis as well as absence of bowel excretion of radiotracer, findings consistent with BA.

DIFFERENTIAL DIAGNOSES

- *Neonatal hepatitis*
- *Alagille syndrome* (arteriohepatic dysplasia)
- *Bile-plug syndrome*
- *Choledochal malformations*

PEARLS

- Early diagnosis of BA and surgical intervention (before 3 months) is essential for patients with BA before the onset of cirrhosis which portends a poor prognosis.

- Pretreatment with oral phenobarbital increases the diagnostic accuracy of hepatobiliary scintigraphy.

- Delayed imaging of up to 24 hours may be necessary to identify GI tract activity.

- A small gallbladder may be present on ultrasound in as many as 25% of patients with BA. The common bile duct, however, is never seen.

- Mebrofenin and disofenin, both labeled with Tc-99m, are the preferred radiotracer agents because of their greater hepatic extraction and less renal excretion.

COMMENTS

Jaundice is common in the newborn, occurring in up to 80% of preterm and 50% of term infants. In the vast majority of instances, jaundice is transient. Physiologic jaundice is caused by the combination of increased bilirubin production resulting from increased breakdown of fetal erythrocytes, decreased excretory capacity related to low levels of ligandin in hepatocytes, and low activity of the bilirubin-conjugating enzyme glucuronyl transferase. Physiologic jaundice typically presents on days 2 to 3 of life.

Nonphysiologic jaundice is defined as jaundice occurring in the first 24 hours of life or lasting more than 1 week; bilirubin rising faster than 5 mg/dL/d; a total bilirubin of greater than 15 mg/dL (in term infants); or direct bilirubin of greater than 2 mg/dL. Hyperbilirubinemia is classified as either conjugated (direct) or unconjugated (indirect). Etiologies of nonphysiologic unconjugated hyperbilirubinemia include increased lysis of red blood cells (RBCs) as can be seen with Rh, ABO incompatibility, RBC enzyme defects (glucose-6 [G-6] phosphatase dehydrogenase deficiency) or structural abnormalities (hereditary spherocytosis), and decreased hepatic uptake of conjugation of bilirubin (Crigler-Najjar and Gilbert syndromes, hypothyroidism, breast milk jaundice). Jaundice presenting in the first 24 hours of life is typically due to unconjugated hyperbilirubinemia and requires immediate evaluation and treatment, typically phototherapy; occasionally exchange transfusion is recommended to prevent bilirubin encephalopathy.

Causes of nonphysiologic conjugated (direct) hyperbilirubinemia can be divided into hepatocellular diseases, including neonatal hepatitis (idiopathic, bacterial, viral, eg, hepatitides B and C, and TORCH infections), hepatic ischemia, metabolic disorders, and biliary tree disorders such as bile-plug syndrome (due to dehydration, sepsis, hemolytic disorders, cystic fibrosis, or parenteral alimentation), choledochal malformations, Alagille

syndrome, and BA. Jaundice persisting beyond 2 weeks of age is usually due to conjugated hyperbilirubinemia and is the clinical scenario most typically encountered by the radiologist or nuclear medicine specialist. These children need immediate evaluation to distinguish between BA, which requires prompt surgical intervention, and those including neonatal hepatitis and bile-plug syndrome which can be managed medically.

BA, an anomaly in which there is absence, obliteration, or severe deficiency in the extrahepatic biliary tree, affects between 1/10,000 to 1/15,000 newborns. The pathogenesis of this disorder is poorly understood with congenital disorders of hepatobiliary ontogenesis and acquired etiologies (infectious or toxic agents) implicated. Often confused with neonatal hepatitis, early diagnosis and palliative treatment of BA with the Kasai portoenterostomy procedure prior to 8 weeks of age is effective in relieving biliary obstruction in 80% to 90% of patients. When performed after 3 months of age or in the setting of biliary cirrhosis, success rate of the Kasai procedure drops to less than 50%. Complications of the Kasai procedure include the failure to achieve adequate bile drainage, cholangitis (up to 50%), and, even in those with initial surgical success, progressive liver disease with cirrhosis and portal hypertension (in up to 60%) necessitating liver transplantation.

The key imaging study for patients suspected of BA is hepatobiliary scintigraphy. The excretion of radiotracer into the GI tract essentially excludes BA. Patients with severe hepatic dysfunction can have delayed identification and excretion of radiotracer into the GI tract. Often delayed imaging up to 24 hours is needed before radiotracer activity in the GI tract can be identified. The use of phenobarbital significantly increases bile flow in the liver and its pretreatment use several days prior to the imaging study significantly increases the accuracy of hepatobiliary scintigraphy (5 mg/kg/d administered orally in two divided doses in the 5 days prior to imaging). When no gut excretion is seen, liver biopsy is used to distinguish BA from severe neonatal hepatitis.

ADDITIONAL IMAGES (C-L)

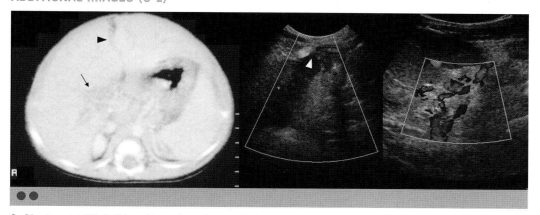

C. Single axial CT (*left*) and two views from color Doppler ultrasound (*right*) of patient shown in images A and B confirm absent gallbladder, cavernous transformation of the portal vein (*arrow*), splenomegaly, a spontaneous splenorenal shunt, and recanalization of the umbilical vein (*arrowhead*), findings consistent with surgical diagnosis of BA and portal hypertension.

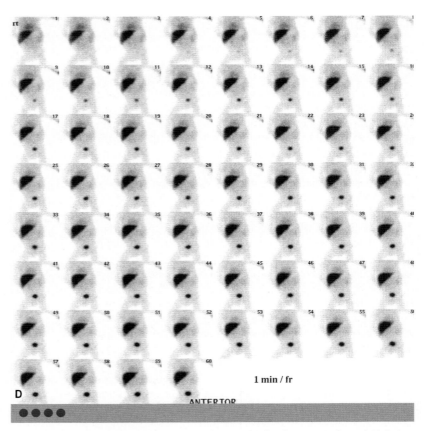

D. and **E. Idiopathic neonatal hepatitis:** Sequential 1-minute anterior scintiphotos from a Tc-99m hepatobiliary scan in a 1-month-old former premature infant with persistent hyperbilirubinemia reveal prompt hepatic uptake. Prolongation of blood pool activity and persistent tracer retention within the liver is consistent with hepatocellular dysfunction. Excretion of tracer into the gut at 4 (image D, *top*) and 9 (*bottom*) hours excludes BA and is consistent with ultimate diagnosis of idiopathic neonatal hepatitis.

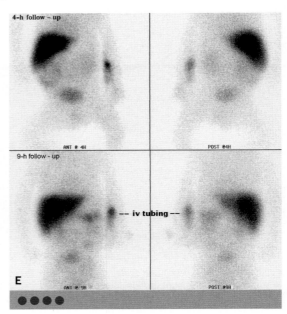

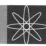

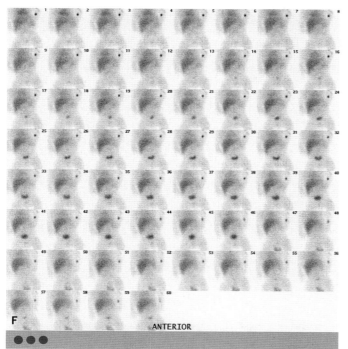

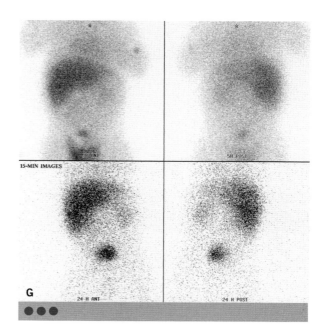

F. and G. Hepatic dysfunction secondary to total parenteral nutrition (TPN) cholestasis. A 1-month-old infant on TPN for short gut syndrome secondary to malrotation with midgut volvulus has persistent direct hyperbilirubinemia. Initial sequential 1-minute anterior images from a Tc-99m choletec hepatobiliary scan (Figure F) show poor hepatic uptake of the radiotracer, marked prolongation of blood pool, and significant soft tissue activity, findings consistent with severe hepatic dysfunction. Absence of excretion into the biliary tree and gut on delayed imaging at 5 (Figure G, *top*) and 24 (*bottom*) hours could represent BA or severe hepatic dysfunction. Liver biopsy, mandatory in this situation, excluded BA. Patients with severe hepatic injury or dysfunction—in this case the result of severe TPN cholestasis—may not have sufficient hepatocyte function to excrete isotope into the GI tract.

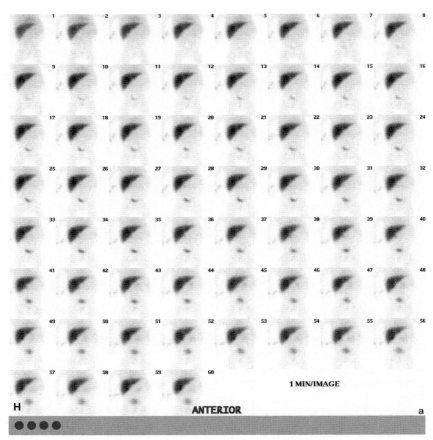

H. and **I. Idiopathic neonatal hepatitis:** A 2-month-old with elevated bilirubin and concern for BA. Sequential initial anterior 1-minute images from a hepatobiliary scan show prompt hepatic uptake. There is faint excretion of tracer in the region of the porta hepatis by 30 minutes, and possibly into a small gallbladder by 48 minutes. Delayed imaging (image I, *right*) at 5 hours confirms tracer excretion into bowel, thereby excluding BA. Significant retention of tracer in the liver on delayed imaging reflects hepatocyte dysfunction and is consistent with neonatal hepatitis.

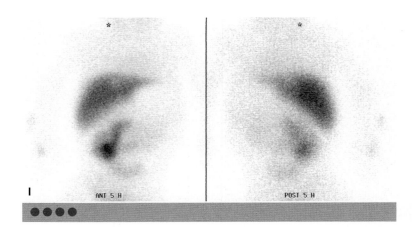

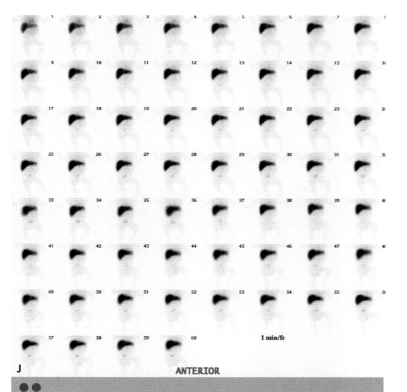

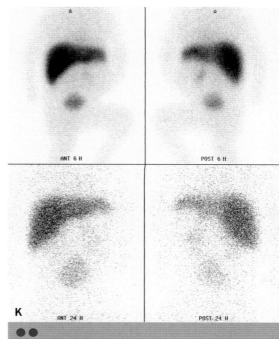

J., K., and L. BA: A 7-week-old with elevated direct hyperbilirubinemia worrisome for BA. Initial anterior images from a Tc-99m choletec hepatobiliary scan (image J) reveal prompt, homogeneous hepatic uptake but no excretion into biliary tree or bowel. Delayed anterior and posterior imaging at 6 (image K, *top*) and 24 (*bottom*) hours shows prolonged hepatic retention of tracer and absent bowel excretion concerning for BA. (Do not confuse renal excretion of radiotracer as seen in image K with gut.) View from intraoperative cholangiogram (image L) obtained at time of Kasai procedure shows absence of the extrahepatic bile ducts consistent with BA.

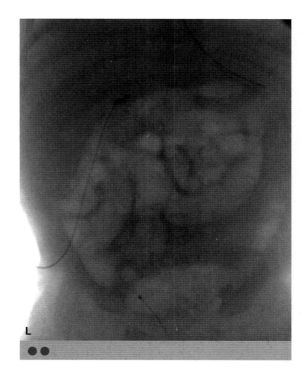

Nghia Jack Vo, MD and Marguerite T. Parisi, MD, MS Ed

PRESENTATION

A 1-year-old, status post–liver transplant, with fever, abdominal pain, and an intra-abdominal fluid collection adjacent to the transplant.

FINDINGS

Views from an ultrasound (image A) in a 1-year-old status post–liver transplant demonstrate a fluid collection in the porta hepatis, adjacent to the liver. The gallbladder is surgically absent. Hepatobiliary iminodiacetic acid (HIDA) scan (images B and C) demonstrates prompt and homogeneous uptake in the transplant liver. There is progressive accumulation of radiotracer in a focal fluid collection within the porta hepatis, corresponding to that seen on ultrasound and consistent with a bile leak, confirmed surgically. This is obstructing biliary drainage into bowel.

- Etiologies of bile leaks:
  - *Abdominal trauma*
  - *Iatrogenic biliary duct injury*: Status post–laparoscopic cholecystectomy or liver transplant

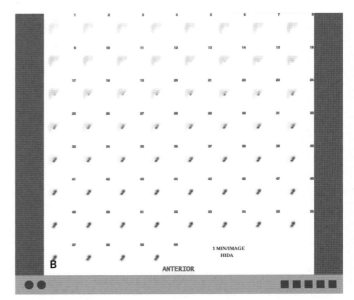

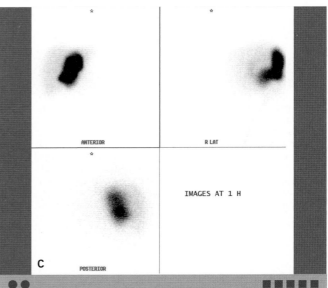

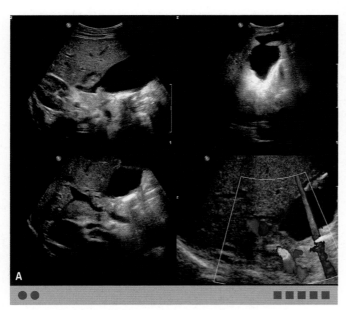

A., B., and **C.** Views from an abdominal ultrasound (image A) showing an RUQ fluid collection adjacent to the transplant liver in the porta hepatis. As expected, the gallbladder is surgically absent. Initial 1-minute anterior (image B) and 1-hour delayed (image C) scintiphotos from a hepatobiliary scan show prompt and homogeneous uptake by a normally functioning transplant liver. There is progressive accumulation of radiotracer in a focal fluid collection within the porta hepatis, corresponding to that seen on ultrasound and consistent with a bile leak, confirmed surgically. This is obstructing biliary drainage into bowel.

PEARLS

- Blunt abdominal trauma is a common etiology for biliary injury and bile leak in children.

- Beyond its utility in diagnosing bile leaks in liver transplant patients, hepatobiliary scintigraphy can also assess vascularity, hepatic parenchymal function, and biliary drainage.

- The "blind end sign," related to the Roux-en-Y anastomosis in liver transplant patients, is a potential pitfall which be confused with a bile leak on hepatobiliary scintigraphy. Delayed imaging is useful in distinguishing this normal postoperative appearance from a true bile leak.

DIFFERENTIAL DIAGNOSIS

Liver transplant: Radiotracer retention in the blind end of the Roux-en-Y hepaticojejunostomy limb ("blind end sign").

COMMENTS

Bile leaks in children are commonly associated with blunt abdominal trauma or are complications of surgical procedures such as liver transplants. Additionally, in adults, bile duct injury associated with laparoscopic cholecystectomy is a well-recognized potential complication due to the limited field of view available during the procedure.

Although bile leaks are relatively uncommon, prompt diagnosis and treatment are essential. The patient's clinical condition can rapidly deteriorate due to sepsis or bile peritonitis. CT and US have high sensitivity in detecting the presence of a fluid collection but have limited utility in differentiating a bile leak from other fluid collections such as ascites, hematoma, or a seroma.

Hepatobiliary scintigraphy is an effective technique for the evaluation of a suspected bile leak. It has the benefit of being noninvasive, physiologic, highly specific, and sensitive. The presence of a gradually increasing radiotracer collection that does not migrate like bowel contents or clear from around the liver is typical of a bile leak. A less common manifestation of a bile leak is gradually increasing accumulation of radiotracer diffusely throughout the peritoneum.

As the frequency of liver transplantation in the pediatric population increases, biliary complications can be a significant source of morbidity. The Roux-en-Y hepaticojejunostomy is a reconstruction performed during liver transplantation or as part of repair of BA. In this procedure, there is a blind ending Roux limb into which biliary drainage occurs. Radiotracer can focally accumulate and persist in the blind loop of the Roux limb, mimicking a bile leak. However, this "blind end sign" appearance of radiotracer will typically fluctuate with time and eventually migrate with bowel, excluding bile leak as the etiology of the collection.

ADDITIONAL IMAGES (D-G)

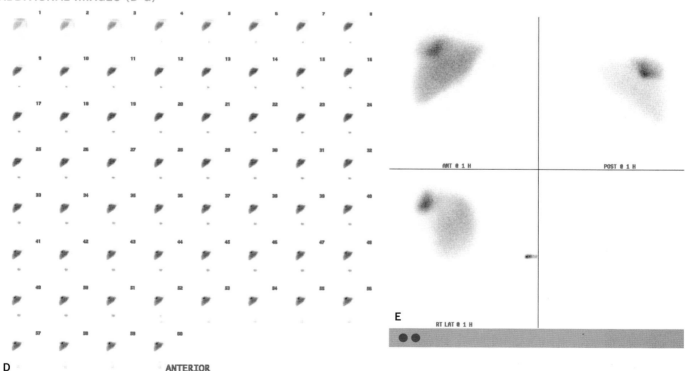
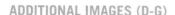

D. and **E. Another example of bile leak.** Sequential 1-minute anterior scintiphotos from a Tc-99m HIDA scan (Figure D) in a 4-year-old status post–liver transplant reveal mild delay in but homogeneous tracer uptake by the liver. There is a focal collection of radiotracer, which accumulates along the right posterior dome of the liver, consistent with bile leak. This persists on delayed anterior, posterior, and right lateral images obtained at 1 hour (Figure E). Mild delay in hepatic uptake of tracer in conjunction with prolonged retention within the liver and absent excretion into bowel is consistent with a component of hepatic dysfunction.

477

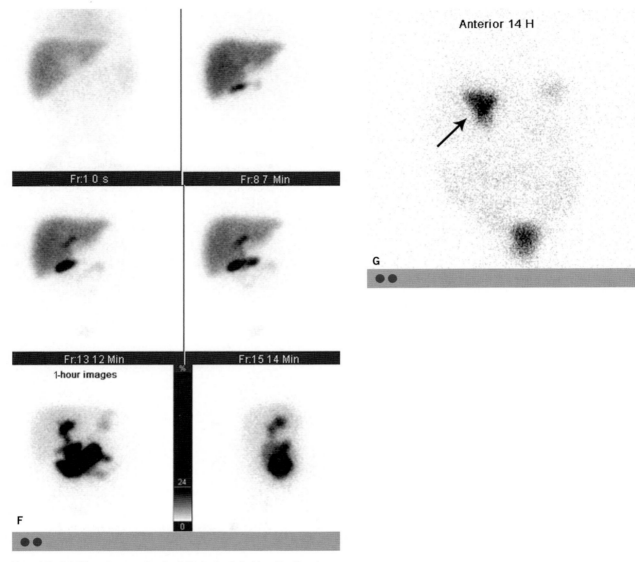

F. and **G. Additional example of a bile leak.** A fluid collection is identified on CT (*not shown*) in a 1-year-old with fever, status post–liver transplant. Selected early and 1-hour anterior images from a Tc-99m choletec study (image F) reveal prompt hepatic tracer uptake and excretion into bowel. Additionally, corresponding to site of CT abnormality, there is a photopenic defect in the subhepatic space. Progressive accumulation of tracer within this site which persists at 14 hours (image G, *arrow*) confirms the presence of a bile leak and differentiates it from residual tracer in the Roux-en-Y loop.

Marguerite T. Parisi, MD, MS Ed

PRESENTATION

An 8-year-old with acute on chronic pancreatitis and abnormal ultrasound.

FINDINGS

Ultrasound (image A) reveals a cystic lesion containing debris in the porta hepatis located between the gallbladder and the pancreatic head. Subsequent DISIDA (diisopropyl iminodiacetic acid) scan (images B and C) demonstrates radiotracer accumulation in the abnormality, which is separate from the gallbladder, consistent with a choledochal cyst and confirmed on intraoperative cholangiogram (image D).

DIFFERENTIAL DIAGNOSES

- Cystic abnormalities in close proximity to the biliary tree
  - *Choledochal cyst*
  - *Gut duplication* (duodenal and/or gastric duplications)
  - *Pancreatic pseudocyst*
  - *Hepatic cysts, including hydatid cysts*

COMMENTS

Choledochal cysts, a spectrum of malformations of the extra- and intrahepatic bile ducts, are congenital anomalies of unknown etiology. There are two distinct clinical groups. The infantile type occurs in newborns or infants younger than 1 year of age whose presentation with obstructive jaundice and acholic stools mimics biliary atresia (BA). The adult form occurs in those older than 1 year of age who present with the classic triad of pain, jaundice, and palpable mass. Complete excision is the treatment of choledochal cysts. Malignancies (cholangiocarcinoma) can arise in choledochal cysts with an incidence up to 20 times that of the normal population. The incidence of cholangiocarcinoma developing in those with choledochal cysts is related to patient age at time of resection and ranges from 0.7% if patient is younger than 10 years at time of resection to 6.8% if resection occurs between ages of 10 and 20 years and up to 14.3% if resection occurs between 20 and 30 years. Thus prompt diagnosis and treatment is essential to overall prognosis.

The Todani system is utilized to classify choledochal cysts. Type I choledochal cyst in which there is cystic or fusiform dilatation of the common bile duct (CBD) is the most common type, occurring in more than 90% of cases. In type II, there is a diverticulum of the normal-sized CBD; in type III or choledochocele there is a cystic dilatation of the distal CBD which protrudes into the duodenum. Type IV is characterized by a dilated CBD with intrahepatic

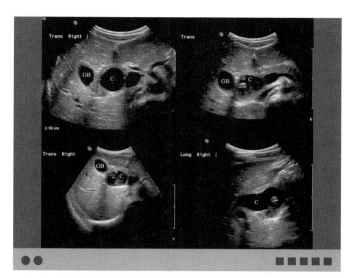

A. Views from an abdominal ultrasound in an 8-year-old patient with acute on chronic pancreatitis reveal a cystic structure (C) with internal debris located in the porta hepatis between the gallbladder (GB) and the pancreatic head, suspicious for choledochal cyst.

biliary dilatation whereas in type V (Caroli disease), there is intrahepatic biliary dilatation with a normal-sized CBD.

Ultrasound is typically the best initial imaging study for those with suspected choledochal cysts. Magnetic resonance cholangiopancreatography (MRCP) with its high spatial resolution, ability to demonstrate detailed anatomy, and noninvasive nature is then employed in further assessment. MRCP is 90% to 100% sensitive and 73% to 100% specific for the diagnosis of choledochal cyst. Combining this with its lack of ionizing radiation and absence of postprocedural complications, MRCP is replacing endoscopic retrograde cholangiopancreatography (ERCP), the previous gold standard, as the diagnostic test of choice. ERCP is reserved for those with difficult or complex cases. Hepatobiliary scintigraphy can both make the diagnosis of choledochal cyst and provide important functional information regarding biliary obstruction.

PEARLS

- **Nuclear medicine hepatobiliary scan (using Tc-99m iminodiacetic [IDA] compounds) can not only diagnose choledochal cysts but provide functional information regarding biliary tree obstruction.**

- **Delayed imaging up to 24 hours and/or the use of cholecystokinin (CCK) may be helpful in full evaluation of those with choledochal cysts.**

ADDITIONAL IMAGES (B–L)

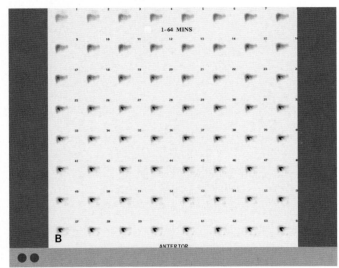

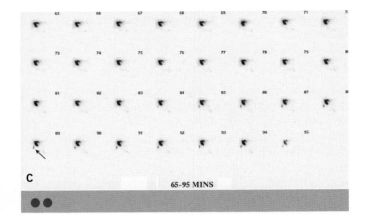

B. and C. Sequential 1-minute anterior images from a Tc-99m DISIDA scan reveal progressive accumulation of radiotracer within the cystic mass in the porta hepatis initially seen on ultrasound, (image A) confirming a diagnosis of choledochal cyst. Tracer excretion into the gallbladder (image C, *arrow*) is also present.

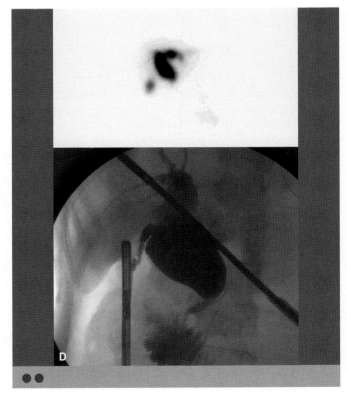

D. Single representative image from the DISIDA scan (*top*) is compared to the intraoperative cholangiogram (*bottom*). Both studies confirm the diagnosis of type I choledochal cyst.

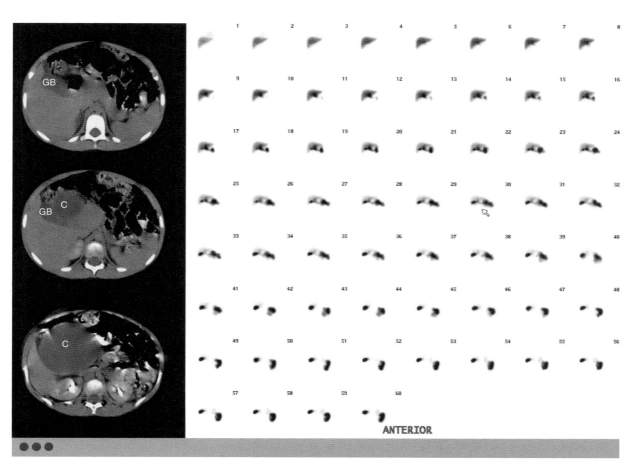

E. Duodenal duplication cyst: Three axial views from a contrast-enhanced CT (*left*) in a 5-year-old girl with a palpable RUQ cystic mass (C) in close proximity to the gallbladder (GB), suspicious for choledochal cyst. Sequential 1-minute anterior views from a Tc-99m choletec scan (*right*) show prompt hepatic uptake and excretion into the bowel (10 minutes) and into gallbladder (14 minutes), which are displaced by the photopenic mass. The absence of radiotracer excretion into the mass excludes a diagnosis of choledochal cyst. A duodenal duplication cyst was confirmed by surgical pathology.

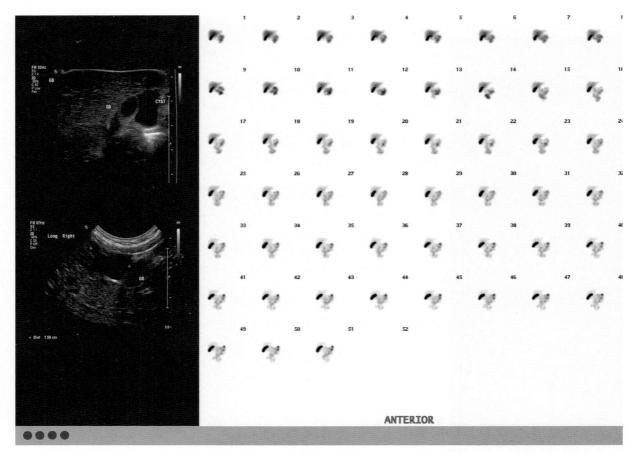

F. Hepatic cyst: Limited views from an ultrasound (*left*) in a 14-month-old male child confirms cystic liver lesion initially diagnosed antenatally, adjacent to but not definitely connected to the gallbladder or biliary tree. An anterior Tc-99m hepatobiliary scan (*right*) obtained to exclude a choledochal cyst showed prompt hepatic uptake and excretion into the bowel and gallbladder (with protracted retention of tracer within). Delayed imaging at 6 and 24 hours (*not shown*) failed to show excretion into the cystic lesion, likely a simple hepatic cyst.

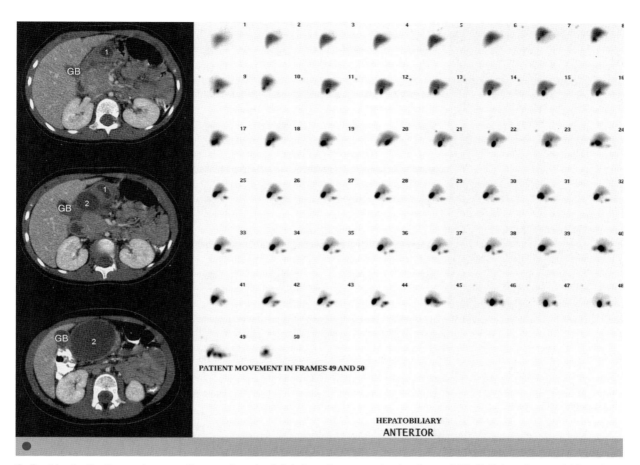

PATIENT MOVEMENT IN FRAMES 49 AND 50

HEPATOBILIARY
ANTERIOR

G. Gastric duplication and pancreatic pseudocysts: Axial views from a contrast-enhanced CT (*left*) in a 2-year-old female child with pancreatitis and two RUQ cystic lesions (1, 2) in close proximity to the gallbladder (GB). Sequential anterior 1-minute images from a Tc-99m choletec scan (*right*), obtained to ascertain if either cystic lesion represented a choledochal cyst, show normal hepatic uptake and excretion into gallbladder and bowel. No tracer excretion into either of the cystic masses could be shown, excluding a diagnosis of choledochal cyst. Surgical excision confirmed two cystic mass lesions: one a gastric duplication cyst and the second a pancreatic pseudocyst.

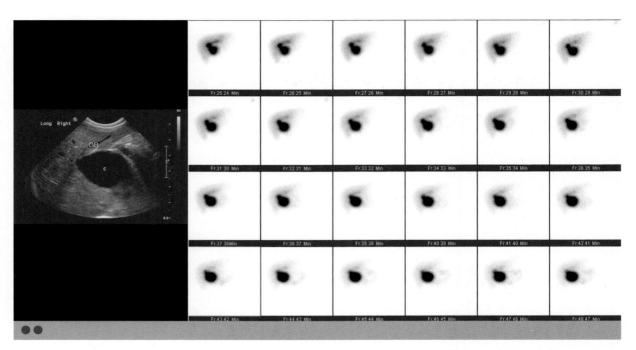

H. Choledochal cyst: Single view from an ultrasound (*left*) in a 9-month-old female infant presenting with failure to thrive, gastroesophageal reflux, and elevated liver function tests reveals a large cystic mass (C) in the porta hepatis in close proximity to the gallbladder (GB) and without a separately identifiable CBD. Select images from a Tc-99m hepatobiliary scan (*right*) show excretion into a bilobed structure in the porta hepatis, representing the gallbladder superiorly and the type I choledochal cyst inferiorly.

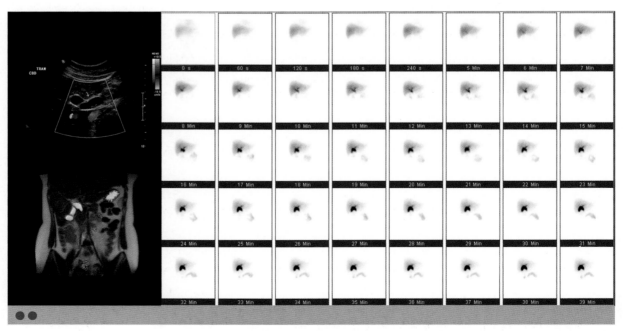

I. Ultrasound (*left, top*) and single coronal HASTE (half-fourier acquisition single shot turbo spin echo) image from an MRI (*left, bottom*) in a 5-year-old with type I choledochal cyst reveals dilatation of the CBD. Sequential anterior 1-minute images from a hepatobiliary scan (*right*) confirm tracer accumulation in the choledochal cyst, confirming diagnosis.

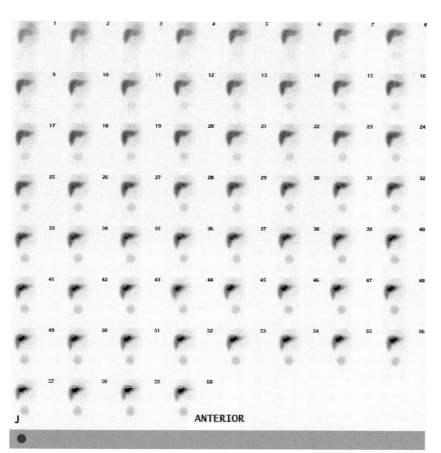

ANTERIOR

J., K., and **L.** Sequential anterior 1-minute scintiphotos from a hepatobiliary scan (image J) in a child with recurrent abdominal pain and jaundice reveal tracer excretion into markedly dilated intrahepatic and common bile ducts. This is confirmed on 5-hour delayed images (image K, *top*); 24-hour delayed images (*bottom*) exclude biliary obstruction by confirming excretion of tracer into gut. Findings are consistent with type IV choledochal cyst and are also well shown on coronal HASTE sequences from MRI (image L).

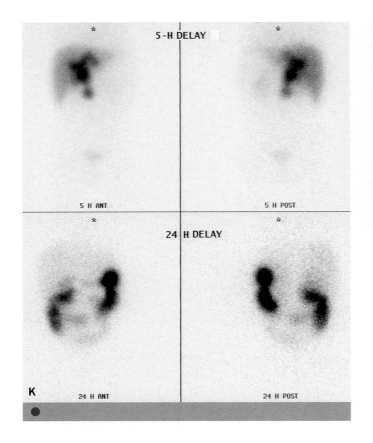

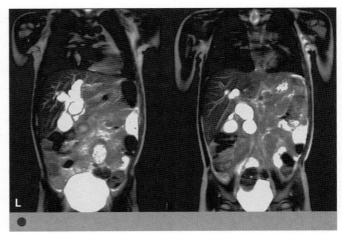

Nghia Jack Vo, MD and Marguerite T. Parisi, MD, MS Ed

PRESENTATION

A 12-year-old with severe liver disease, clubbing of the digits, dyspnea, hypoxemia, and concern for pulmonary embolism.

FINDINGS

Anterior and posterior whole-body views from a Tc-99m macroaggregated albumin (MAA) perfusion study (image A) reveal extensive abnormal uptake in the brain, kidneys, and throughout the soft tissues of the axial and appendicular skeleton, consistent with hepatopulmonary syndrome. No perfusion defect is found in the lungs to suggest pulmonary embolus.

DIFFERENTIAL DIAGNOSES

- *Intracardiac right-to-left shunt*

- *Free or unbound pertechnetate*

- *Pulmonary arteriovenous fistula* (AVF)/*arteriovenous malformation* (AVM)

COMMENTS

In patients with liver disease (typically cirrhosis but also occurring in those with acute liver failure), pulmonary symptoms of hypoxemia are commonly present, related to dilated pulmonary vessels and resultant shunting. This is termed hepatopulmonary syndrome (HPS). HPS is not rare, occurring in 47% of patients with end-stage liver disease and 38% of those with less severe liver disease. The presenting symptoms of HPS are nonspecific (hypoxia, shortness of breath, digital clubbing, and dyspnea on exertion) and must be distinguished from multiple other potential etiologies, including pulmonary embolus.

Patients with nonspecific pulmonary symptoms and liver disease are often imaged with Tc-99m MAA due to the concern for potential pulmonary embolus as the source of their symptoms. In the absence of a ventilation/perfusion (V/Q) mismatch, additional scintigraphic information should be sought. Whole-body imaging can be used to detect the presence of extrapulmonary activity which is indicative of a right-to-left shunt. Normally, MAA particles do not traverse the normal capillary bed (8-15 µm). In HPS, the MAA particles (20-100 µm) will bypass the normal pulmonary capillaries through the abnormally dilated pulmonary vascular structures and become trapped in systemic capillary beds in proportion to the shunt flow. The presence of a right-to-left shunt has been reported to occur in up to 40% of patients with cirrhosis and hypoxemia, confirming the diagnosis of HPS.

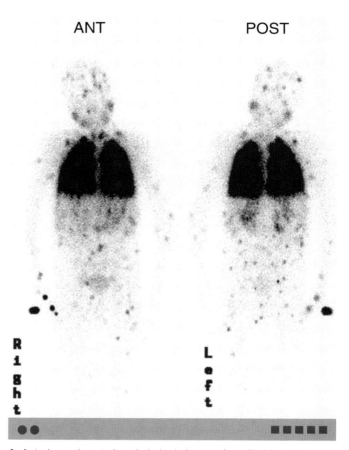

ANT   POST

Right   Left

A. Anterior and posterior whole-body images from Tc-99m MAA perfusion scan in a 12-year-old with severe liver disease reveal extensive abnormal uptake in the brain, kidneys, and throughout the soft tissues of the axial and appendicular skeleton, consistent with HPS. No perfusion defect in the lungs to suggest pulmonary embolism.

PEARLS

- Always include images of the cranium and kidneys when performing Tc-99m MAA perfusion imaging in children, especially in those with documented cardiac and/or liver disease.

- The presence of extrapulmonary MAA (shunting) in the setting of liver disease is virtually diagnostic of HPS.

- The association between pulmonary vascular dilation with resultant hypoxemia and liver disease are well documented. The factors leading to HPS have not been established.

- Normal shunt fraction of MAA is less than 5%.

Progressive decline in oxygenation in those with HPS can occur despite stable hepatic function. In patients with HPS, mortality can be as high as 41% by 2.5 years after onset of dyspnea. Definitive treatment for those with chronic liver disease and HPS is transplantation, but with the development and progression of HPS, the intra- and postoperative risk is increased. Therefore early prompt diagnosis of HPS may lead to earlier transplantation.

ADDITIONAL IMAGE

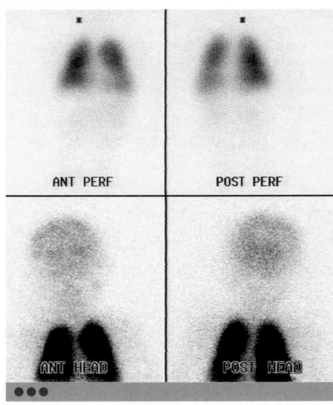

B. Intracardiac right-to-left shunt: 2-month-old infant with history of transposition of the great arteries (TGA) status post–atrial septostomy and Blalock-Taussig shunt; new desaturations. Perfusion images from a Tc-99m MAA perfusion study reveal relatively symmetric and homogeneous radiotracer uptake in the lungs. Uptake in the brain is consistent with an intracardiac right-to-left shunt. Intracardiac right-to-left shunt can be distinguished from HPS on the basis of patient history.

Marguerite T. Parisi, MD, MS Ed and Nghia Jack Vo, MD

PRESENTATION

A 5-year old presents with painless gastrointestinal bleeding. Other clinical presentations in those with Meckel diverticulum include abdominal pain or bowel obstruction. Meckel diverticulum may also be identified incidentally when abdominal imaging (CT, US, or MRI) or surgery is performed for other indications.

FINDINGS

Sequential 1-minute anterior scintiphotos from a Tc-99m pertechnetate Meckel scan (image A) reveal a focus of abnormal uptake in the right lower quadrant (RLQ) appearing coincidentally with uptake in the stomach and persisting throughout the entirety of the study. Delayed scintiphotos at 40 minutes demonstrate that the abnormal focus is located anteriorly (image B, *arrows*) distinguishing this from ureteral activity. Findings are consistent with a Meckel diverticulum containing ectopic gastric mucosa.

DIFFERENTIAL DIAGNOSES

- *False-positive scan:*
  - Urinary tract activity
  - Intestinal duplication cysts (containing ectopic gastric mucosa)
  - Intussusception with associated hyperemia; inflammatory bowel disease; other hyperemic inflammatory or neoplastic processes
  - Vascular malformation

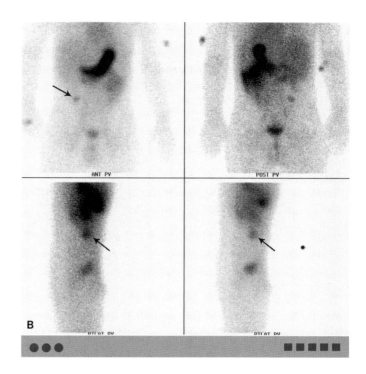

B

- *False-negative scan:*
  - Poor patient positioning
  - Meckel diverticulum with impaired blood supply or containing only small amounts of ectopic gastric mucosa
  - Rapid transit of pertechnetate due to gut irritation

PEARLS

- The normal biodistribution of Tc-99m pertechnetate includes the thyroid gland, salivary glands, choroid plexus, and gastric mucosa. The primary route of excretion is through renal clearance.

- Nuclear scintigraphic identification of a Meckel diverticulum using Tc-99m pertechnetate requires the presence of ectopic gastric mucosa. The most common presentation in children is painless rectal bleeding.

- Lateral views are mandatory to differentiate ectopic gastric mucosa anteriorly from normal urinary tract activity.

- Pharmacologic interventions such as the use of cimetadine may increase sensitivity in detecting Meckel diverticulum on pertechnetate scans.

- Meckel diverticulum can serve as a lead point for intussusception presenting primarily as a bowel obstruction, typically in those diverticulum that do not contain ectopic gastric mucosa.

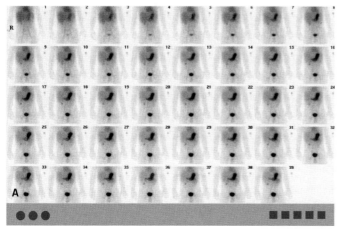

A

A. and B. Sequential 1-minute anterior images (image A) and delayed post void (PV) images in anterior, posterior right, and left lateral projections (image B) from Tc-99m pertechnetate scan reveal abnormal uptake in a Meckel diverticulum containing ectopic mucosa.

COMMENTS

Meckel diverticulum, an omphalomesenteric duct remnant, is the most common GI tract congenital anomaly. The omphalomesenteric duct is a fetal structure that connects the umbilical cord to a segment of GI tract that generally develops into the ileum. Thus, the most common location of a Meckel diverticulum is in the RLQ. Incomplete regression of the duct adjacent to the ileal end results in an outpouching along the antimesenteric side of the bowel that contains all four intestinal wall layers.

The vast majority of Meckel diverticula (96%) are asymptomatic. When symptomatic, various presentations can occur, including bleeding, RLQ abdominal pain, or bowel obstruction. Most Meckel diverticula do not contain gastric mucosa. Those Meckel diverticula that are associated with bleeding invariably will have ulcerated ectopic gastric or pancreatic mucosa within.

The presence of ectopic gastric mucosa in patients with symptomatic Meckel diverticula permits physiologic radionuclide imaging with the use of a Tc-99m pertechnetate. Pertechnetate is gradually secreted by gastric mucosa and classic findings in those with Meckel diverticula containing ectopic mucosa will demonstrate focal increased radiotracer activity accumulating in the RLQ or midabdomen over a period of 30 to 60 minutes. Lateral views are helpful to differentiate accumulation of activity anteriorly within the Meckel diverticulum from unrelated physiologic renal or ureteral activity. Technetium pertechnetate imaging is reported to be 95% accurate in the detection of ectopic gastric mucosa.

False-positive studies have been reported as a result of urinary tract activity, inflammatory bowel disease, and intestinal duplication cysts that also contain gastric mucosa. False-negative radionuclide studies can occur in the presence of a Meckel diverticulum which lacks or contains only small amounts of ectopic gastric mucosa or which has an impaired blood supply. Other sources of false-negative studies include local bowel irritability with rapid transit or clearance of the pertechnetate.

The use of cimetidine or glucagon may increase the sensitivity of pertechnetate imaging in detection of Meckel diverticulum by inhibiting the release of the pertechnetate from the ectopic gastric mucosa or by decreasing bowel motility, respectively.

ADDITIONAL IMAGES (C-G)

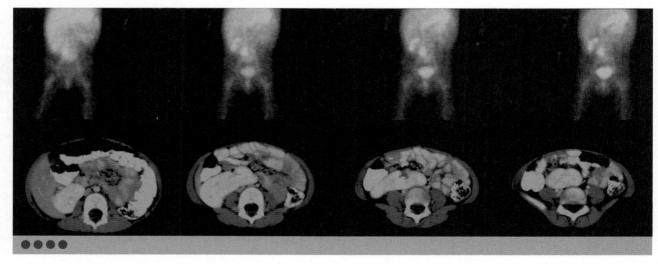

C. Cross-fused renal ectopia mimicking Meckel diverticulum: A 4-year-old with painless GI bleeding. Selected sequential anterior images from a Tc-99m pertechnetate scan (*upper row*) show tracer uptake in stomach and urinary bladder and in two adjacent foci in the RLQ of the abdomen. Corresponding axial views from contrast-enhanced CT (*bottom row*) confirm the presence of a cross-fused ectopic kidney, accounting for the unexpected radiotracer uptake in the RLQ of the abdomen. No evidence of a Meckel diverticulum containing ectopic gastric mucosa was found. Urinary tract activity is the most common cause of a false-positive Meckel scan.

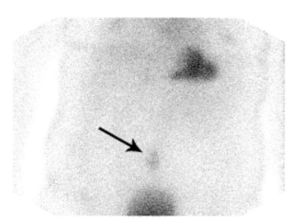

ANT

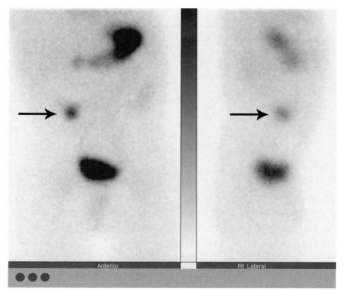

D. Appendicitis mimicking Meckel diverticulum: A 13-year-old adolescent female with GI bleed, history of positive Meckel scan at outside facility, and negative laparoscopy. Anterior view from repeat Tc-99m pertechnetate scan shows abnormal tracer uptake at midline, superior to the bladder (*arrow*). Surgical exploration showed an inflamed, edematous appendix located above the bladder and corresponding to the site of abnormal uptake on Meckel scan. No evidence of Meckel diverticulum was found. Hyperemic inflammatory lesions such as an inflamed appendix may be a cause of a false-positive pertechnetate scan.

E. Additional example of Meckel diverticulum; a 1-year-old with rectal bleeding. Anterior and lateral images obtained at 45 minutes following IV administration of Tc-99m pertechnetate show abnormal uptake in the RLQ of the abdomen (*arrows*), consistent with a Meckel diverticulum containing ectopic gastric mucosa. Anterior location of tracer uptake distinguishes a Meckel diverticulum from physiologic activity in the ureter.

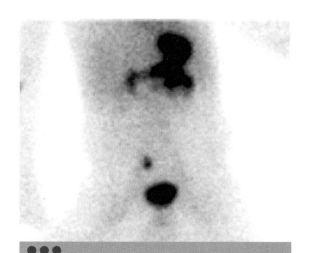

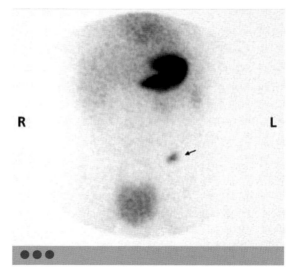

F. Additional example of Meckel diverticulum; a 9-year-old with bloody stools and low hematocrit. Anterior view from Tc-99m pertechnetate scan shows abnormal radiotracer uptake in the lower abdomen, confirmed to represent a Meckel diverticulum.

G. Atypical location of Meckel diverticulum: Anterior scintigraphic image from a Tc-99m pertechnetate scan shows abnormal uptake (*arrow*) in the left lower quadrant (LLQ) in a 2-year-old boy presenting with GI bleeding who was suspected of having an ileal duplication. Pathologic examination revealed a Meckel diverticulum in atypical location. (*Reprinted with permission from: Parisi MT. Cases of the day (pediatrics): gastric duplication—Figure 1c. Presented at the Radiological Society of North America Scientific Assembly and Annual Meeting, Chicago, IL; November 26-December 1, 2000.*)

Marguerite T. Parisi, MD, MS Ed and Nghia Jack Vo, MD

PRESENTATION

- Latent or subclinical (asymptomatic)
- Asymmetric limb circumference
- Extremity swelling (soft pitting edema to fibrosis)
- Hyperkeratosis
- Cellulitis

FINDINGS

Absent or delayed radiotracer migration in the involved limb and poorly visualized or absent lymph nodes are diagnostic of lymphedema (image A). Dermal diffusion or backflow can result from the absence of normal lymphatic channels.

DIFFERENTIAL DIAGNOSES

- *Deep venous thrombosis (DVT)*
- *Myxedema*
- *Venous insufficiency*
- *Congestive heart failure* (CHF)/*fluid overload*
- *Iatrogenic lymph* flow obstruction (postsurgical) or radiotherapy
- *Lymphatic infiltration* (malignancy)

COMMENTS

Lymphedema is the abnormal accumulation of protein-rich fluid into the interstitium. This most commonly involves the lower extremity (80%) but can also involve the upper extremity, genitalia, or trunk. The underlying cause is the result of lymphatic transport dysfunction. Lymphedema is typically divided into primary (idiopathic) and secondary causes (infection, trauma, surgery, radiation, neoplasm, venous obstruction). Primary or congenital lymphedema is the most common type in the children, with incidence of 1.5/100,000 persons younger than 20 years.

Swelling of the involved extremity is the most common presenting symptom in children with congenital lymphedema. Many other disease processes—including congestive heart or renal failure, hypoproteinemic states, DVT, or venous insufficiency—may present with extremity swelling and may be difficult to distinguish from lymphedema.

The diagnosis of lymphedema can typically be made clinically. In various circumstances, imaging is useful for a more definitive diagnosis. Lymphoscintigraphy, first introduced in 1953, is a relatively noninvasive, repeatable, and easily performed test that provides physiologic and anatomic

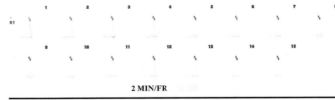

2 MIN/FR

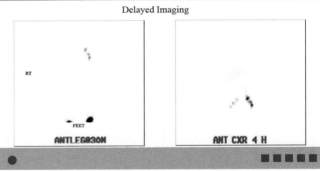

Delayed Imaging

A. A 1-year-old child with right leg swelling. Sequential anterior scintiphotos (2 min/frame) of the lower extremities from a Tc-99m sulfur colloid lymphoscintigram (*top*) show prompt ascent of tracer in normal-appearing lymphatic channels on the left. No lymphatic channels are visualized in the right leg. Delayed imaging at 30 minutes (*bottom left*) shows tracer uptake in normal-sized inguinal nodes on the left. Dermal diffusion or backflow into right inguinal nodes on 4-hour images (*bottom right*) is due to the absence of normal lymphatic channels and confirms a diagnosis of primary (congenital) lymphedema on the right.

information of lymphatic transport and depiction of regional nodes that can be used to diagnose lymphedema. Intradermal introduction of small aliquots of triple filtered Tc-99m sulfur colloid into the web spaces of each foot followed by timed imaging of the lower limb and pelvis from 60 to 120 minutes allows for the observation of normal lymphatic activity in the regional lymph nodes of

PEARLS

- **Congenital lymphedema can occasionally be difficult to distinguish clinically from various other causes of limb swelling. Lymphoscintigraphy is a noninvasive test that can be used to confirm the diagnosis.**

- **Triple filtered Tc-99m sulfur colloid is placed intradermally into the web spaces between the toes bilaterally and imaging is performed for at least 60 to 120 minutes.**

- **Cross-sectional imaging with US, CT, or MRI can be helpful for congenital lymphedema, but are more useful for identifying alternative diagnosis in patients with limb swelling**

the groin (inguinal and iliac lymph nodes). A normal study will demonstrate symmetric inguinal nodal activity typically within 30 minutes. Absent or delayed radiotracer transport failing to demonstrate normal inguinal or pelvic nodes along with secondary findings such as dermal diffusion or backflow (due to accumulation of radiotracer in the dilated channels of the dermis) are consistent with and can confirm the clinical diagnosis of congenital lymphedema.

Lymphoscintigraphy may also be used to confirm a diagnosis of either congenital or acquired chylothorax (image C) or chyloperitoneum. The same technique is employed with delayed imaging up to 24 hours or until tracer activity is demonstrated within the liver. Radiotracer accumulation in nonphysiologic locations within the chest or abdomen confirms the diagnosis.

Another use of lymphoscintigraphy in children is to aide in localizing sentinel nodes (images E and F) for biopsy in those with melanomas and soft tissue sarcomas.

ADDITIONAL IMAGES (B-E)

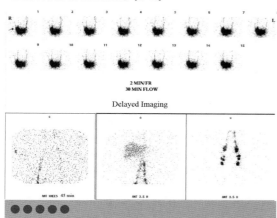

B. Normal lymphoscintigraphy study in a 14-year-old adolescent female with right lower extremity swelling. Early anterior sequential images (*top*) show a nonspecific 6-minute delay in ascent of tracer into lymphatic channels on the right. Delayed imaging at 45 minutes (*bottom left*) and at 3.5 hours (*bottom right*) confirm symmetric time of appearance and uptake into inguinal nodes bilaterally. No abnormal sites of tracer uptake are identified. The study is concluded when tracer is shown within the liver (*bottom middle*).

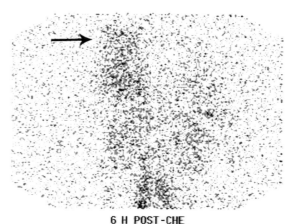

6 H POST-CHE

C. Lymphoscintigraphy confirming a left chylothorax. A 16-year-old status post–motor vehicle accident presents with persistent pleural fluid following chest tube drainage, pleurodesis, and thoracic duct ligation. Single posterior view of the chest and upper abdomen from a lymphoscintigram obtained 6 hours following radiotracer injection shows accumulation of radiotracer in the left thorax (*arrow*), consistent with recurrent chylothorax.

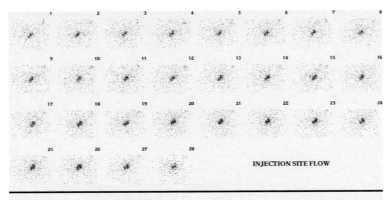

INJECTION SITE FLOW

Delayed Imaging

Tc-99m MDP

BLOOD POOLS

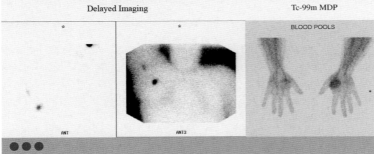

ANT

ANT3

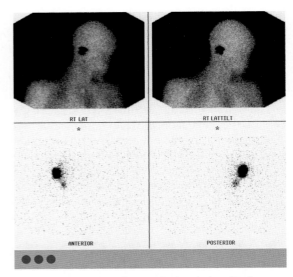

RT LAT

RT LATTILT

ANTERIOR

POSTERIOR

E. Another example of a sentinel node localization procedure in a 5-year-old with a malignant soft tissue neoplasm adjacent to the right ear (injection site top images). Tracer uptake is seen in a sentinel node located inferior to the injection site and along the angle of the jaw on the right on delayed images (*bottom row*).

D. Lymphoscintigraphy for sentinel node localization in a 14-year-old with hyperemic soft tissue sarcoma in the right hand, shown on blood pool images from a Tc-99m bone scan (*bottom right*). Early sequential dynamic images (*top*) following four intradermal injections of small amounts of triple filtered Tc-99m sulfur colloid (each consisting of approximately 0.125 mCi in 0.1 mL of saline placed circumferentially around the lesion) show progressive decrease in the amount of radiotracer remaining around the injection site. Delayed static imaging at 15 and 30 minutes (*bottom left* and *center*, respectively) shows intense uptake of tracer in a sentinel node in the central axilla as well as one in a more peripheral node.

Marguerite T. Parisi, MD, MS Ed and Christopher J. Hurt, MD

PRESENTATION

A 4-year-old with ventriculoperitoneal (VP) shunt, headache, and nausea and vomiting.

FINDINGS

Initial "flow" images (20 s/image for 5 minutes) and time activity curves from a Tc-99m cerebrospinal fluid (CSF) shunt study (image A) reveal prompt egress of tracer from the VP shunt reservoir with normal T1/2 time of 60 seconds. Delayed anterior images over the chest and abdomen obtained at 5 and 15 minutes following tracer administration show tracer within the distal limb of the shunt (image B, *left*) and free dispersal into the peritoneum (image B, *right*) indicative of a normally functioning, nonobstructed shunt.

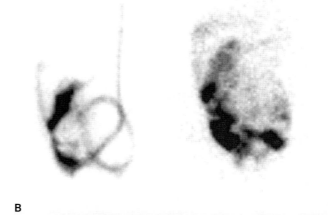

B

ANTERIOR CHEST 5 MIN   ANTERIOR ABD 15 MIN

DIFFERENTIAL DIAGNOSIS

Shunt malfunction:
- *Proximal limb obstruction*

- *Distal limb obstruction*
  - Kink or disruption
  - Pseudocyst formation
  - Erosion of distal shunt tube into viscus organ

- Inconclusive study due to radiotracer extravasation or suboptimal injection

PEARLS

- Determination of the type of CSF shunt present, knowledge of the mechanics of its operation, combined with review of correlative imaging when available, will enable tailoring of the radionuclide procedure, thereby increasing sensitivity and specificity.

- Determination of CSF opening pressure (upon accessing the shunt reservoir and immediately prior to radiotracer injection) is a crucial piece of information in distinguishing proximal from distal limb obstructions in those with CSF shunts. In proximal limb obstructions, opening pressures are low (0-2 cm of water) or have negative values; in distal limb obstructions, opening pressures are typically high (>15 cm of water).

- In those with VP shunts, patency is determined by rapid egress of tracer from the reservoir into the distal tubing and free dispersal in the peritoneum.

- In those with VA shunts, patency is determined by rapid egress of tracer from the reservoir into distal tubing, followed by uptake in thyroid gland, stomach, and urinary bladder indicating dispersal in the blood pool.

- Maneuvers such as pumping of the reservoir, having the patient sit or stand upright or even walk around may distinguish a true shunt obstruction from a gravity-dependent or "sluggish" system. Failure to obtain reflux of tracer into the ventricular system after pumping the reservoir is indicative of a proximal limb obstruction.

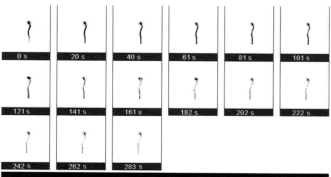

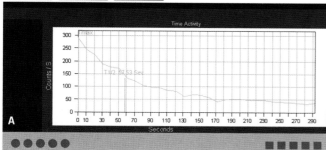

A. and **B.** Initial (image A) and delayed (image B) anterior images from a normal Tc-99m CSF shunt study.

COMMENTS

Hydrocephalus, a condition in which there is an increased volume of intracranial CSF, can be congenital (eg, aqueductal stenosis, Chiari II malformation, Dandy-Walker malformation) or acquired (eg, meningitis, prior intracranial hemorrhage, brain tumors). Hydrocephalus may be due to either obstruction of CSF flow within the ventricular system (obstructive or intraventricular obstructive hydrocephalus), decreased CSF reabsorption (communicating or extraventricular obstructive hydrocephalus), or increased CSF production as can occur with choroid plexus papillomas.

Function of the diversionary CSF shunts—either ventriculoatrial (VA) or, more commonly, VP—used to treat hydrocephalus can be evaluated scintigraphically using Tc-99m agents, including Tc-99m or Tc-99m DTPA. The procedure involves antiseptic injection of the radiotracer into the shunt reservoir with subsequent anterior early/"flow" images (10 s/frame for 5 minutes) over the head with generation of time activity curve and determination of clearance half-time. Delayed anterior images (5 min/frame) at 10 and 15 minutes are obtained of the chest and abdomen, respectively. Normal clearance half-time of the tracer in a patent shunt should be less than 10 minutes. Opening CSF pressure determination upon accessing the shunt reservoir should be a routine component of the procedure. Normal CSF opening pressure should be between 0 and 15 cm of water. A sample of CSF should be obtained and sent to pathology for culture and Gram stain.

Shunt malfunctions may result from a faulty or incorrectly set valve. Proximal limb obstructions are more common in former premature infants. Distal limb obstruction can be due to kinking or disruption of the shunt tubing, pseudocyst formation, or erosion of the tubing into a viscous organ like bowel or bladder which can result in meningitis.

ADDITIONAL IMAGES (C-K)

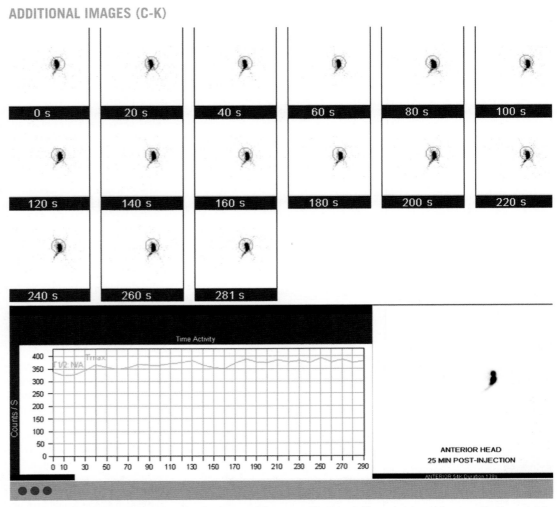

C. Proximal limb obstruction: Early (*top*), time activity curve (*bottom left*), and delayed images (*bottom right*) from a VP shunt study in a 5-year-old with headache and anorexia. Lack of egress of tracer from the shunt reservoir, absence of retrograde tracer flow into the ventricles, in conjunction with an opening CSF pressure of −27 cm of water is consistent with a proximal shunt obstruction.

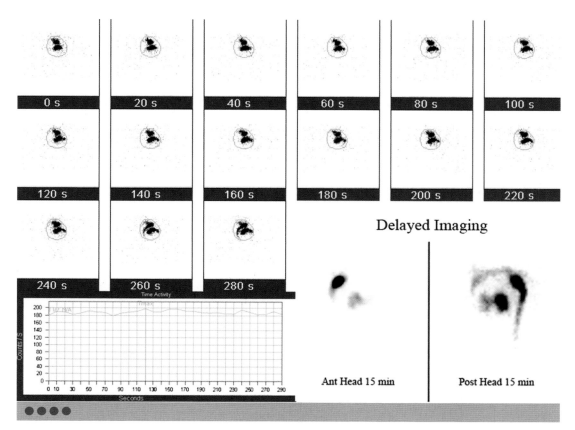

D. Distal limb obstruction with reflux into ventricles: VP shunt study in an 18-year-old with headache, dizziness, and increasing ventricular size on the CT. Early images (*top*) show prompt retrograde tracer flow into ventricles and flat time-activity curve (*bottom left*). Delayed images (*bottom right*) confirm above findings with tracer persisting in shunt tubing overlying the head and neck. In conjunction with elevated opening pressures, findings are consistent with obstruction of the distal limb of the shunt.

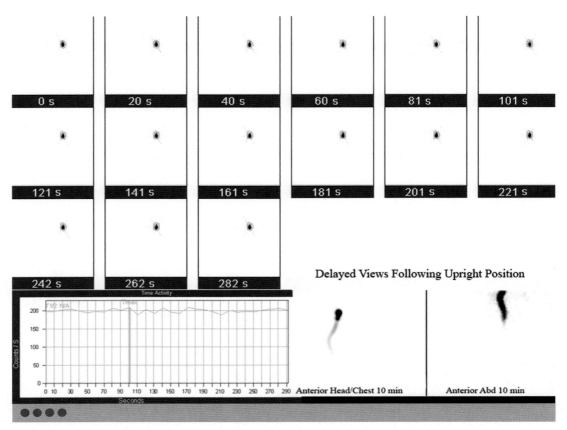

E. Distal limb obstruction: Another example of distal shunt obstruction in a 7-year-old with headache, vomiting, but stable CT. With patient supine, early images (*top*) and time-activity curve (*bottom left*) show no egress of tracer from the shunt reservoir. Following upright positioning, there was gravity-dependent drainage of tracer into shunt tubing extending to the level of the upper abdomen but no peritoneal spill.

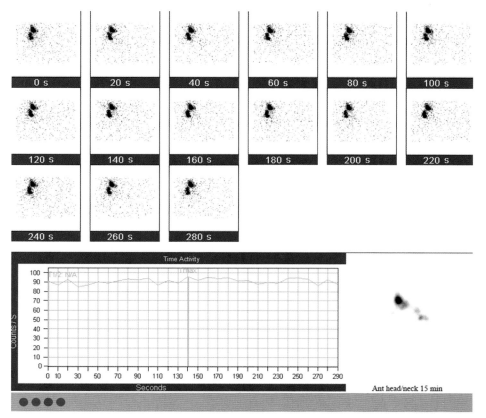

F. Distal limb obstruction due to tube disruption: Early (*top*) and delayed (*bottom right*) images from a VP shunt in a 17-year-old with headache show a distal limb obstruction with tracer accumulating in focal collections at the level of the neck.

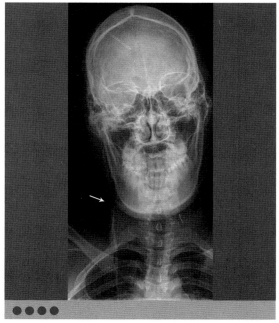

G. Plain film imaging (*arrow*) confirms disruption of shunt tubing in the neck at site of focal tracer collections seen on scintigraphy.

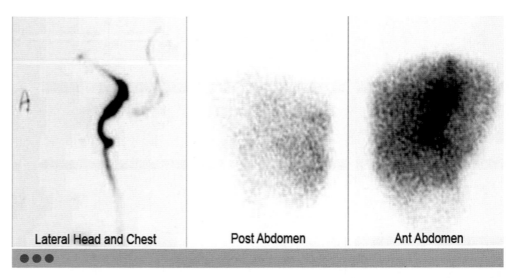

| Lateral Head and Chest | Post Abdomen | Ant Abdomen |

● ● ●

H. VP shunt pseudocyst: Views from a VP shunt series show egress of tracer into a massive pseudocyst in the abdomen. The lack of visualization of the kidneys and shape of collection distinguishes this from free peritoneal spill.

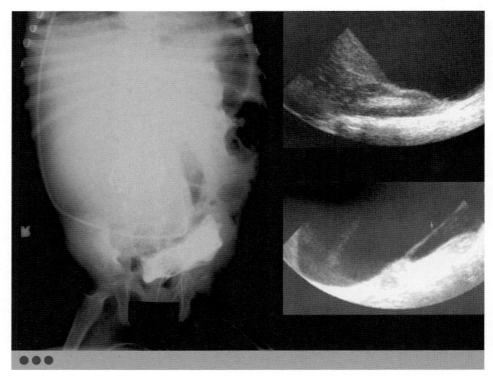

● ● ●

I. Single film of the abdomen (*left*) (with contrast in the bladder from antecedent CT) and two views from US (*right*) confirm the large pseudocyst, causing mass effect upon bowel and bladder.

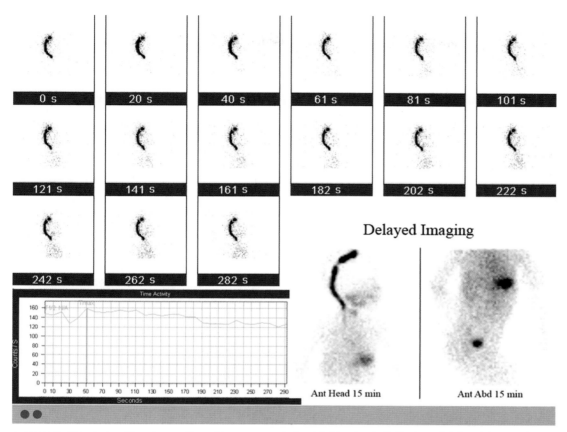

J. Inconclusive study with extravasation of tracer around shunt tubing in skull. Early and delayed images from a VP shunt study demonstrate extravasation of tracer into a pseudocollection tracking around the proximal shunt tubing in the calvarium. Extravasation is confirmed by the presence of tracer in the thyroid gland, stomach, and bladder.

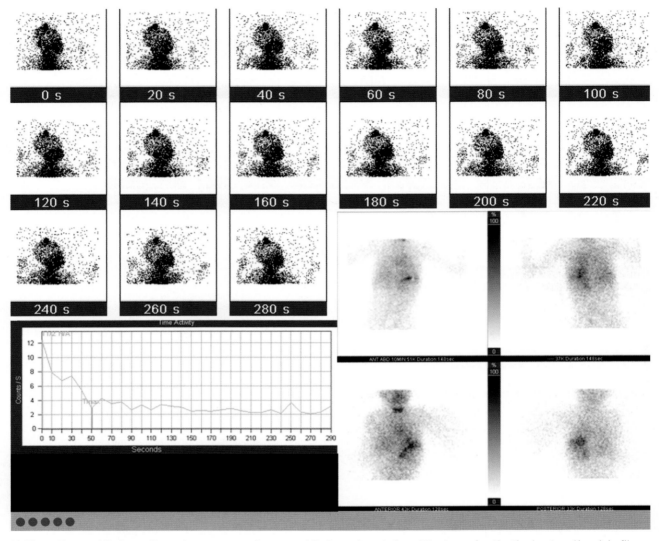

K. Normal/patent VA shunt: Normal appearance of a patent VA shunt; knowledge of the type of patient's shunt and/or plain films will distinguish this appearance from tracer extravasation as was seen in image J.

Grace S. Phillips, MD and Marguerite T. Parisi, MD, MS Ed

PRESENTATION

A 4-year-old female child with a history of febrile urinary tract infections.

FINDINGS

Posterior views from a radionuclide cystogram (RNC) (image A) in a 4-year-old being reevaluated for vesicoureteral reflux (VUR) demonstrates radioactivity within the bilateral upper renal collecting systems consistent with reflux.

DIFFERENTIAL DIAGNOSIS

The scintigraphic finding of retrograde extension of radiotracer activity into the collecting systems on RNC is fairly specific for VUR. Occasionally, activity external to the patient (urine contamination) may simulate reflux. Vesicoureteral reflux may also be indirectly identified on MAG3 renography. This is evidenced by either a visual increase in the amount of tracer seen in the collecting system following initial excretion into the ureter or a "spike" in the time activity curve. The main differential diagnoses for intermittent increase in the MAG3 time activity curve following initial ureteral excretion

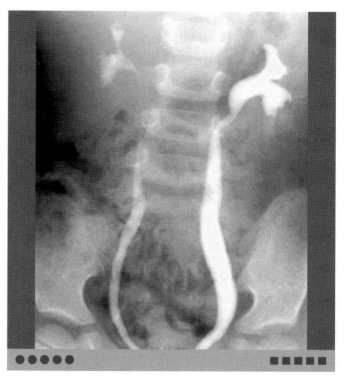

B. Voiding cystourethrogram (VCUG) confirms left grade III and right grade II VUR seen on antecedent radionuclide cystogram (image A).

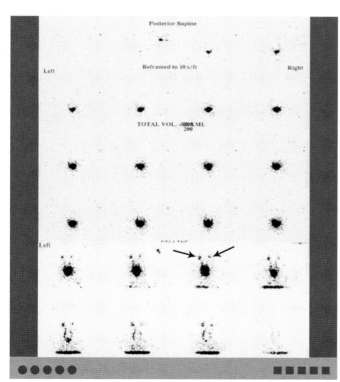

A. Posterior views from a radionuclide cystogram in a 4-year-old being reevaluated for VUR show radioactivity within both upper renal collecting systems consistent with vesicoureteral reflux.

PEARLS

- Fluoroscopic voiding cystourethrogram (VCUG) yields better anatomical detail compared to radionuclide cystogram (RNC).

- VCUG is preferred for the initial evaluation for VUR in males.

- RNC results in decreased radiation exposure compared to VCUG, even with the advent of pulsed flouroscopy. RNC can be used as the first examination in girls and for follow-up examinations in boys.

- Radionuclide cystogram is more sensitive than conventional VCUG for VUR because imaging is continuous.

- Controversy exists in the literature regarding the efficacy of prophylactic antibiotics in preventing renal damage in those with VUR. In the future, therefore, the imaging algorithm for children with a UTI may change.

- A rough guideline for urinary bladder filling capacity is (patient age + 2) multiplied by 30 cc.

is patient motion or augmentation of excretory response due to diuretic augmentation.

COMMENTS

VUR is defined as the abnormal retrograde flow of urine from the urinary bladder into the ureter and/or renal collecting system. VUR most commonly presents in children who are younger than 2 years, and is typically diagnosed during the workup of a urinary tract infection (UTI). Higher grades of VUR may be suspected prenatally in patients with a dilated collecting system. There is an increased incidence of VUR in patients with duplex collecting system, multicystic dysplastic kidney (MCDK), horseshoe kidney, and contralateral ureteropelvic junction (UPJ) obstruction. Regarding the natural history of VUR, 80% of patients with VUR outgrow it by puberty. The prognosis of VUR depends on several factors, including the degree of reflux, duration, frequency of UTIs, and presence of renal scarring. There has been recent controversy in the literature regarding the efficacy of antibiotic prophylaxis in preventing renal scarring or reflux nephropathy in patients with VUR.

The typical radiographic workup for suspected VUR includes renal ultrasound and voiding cystourethrogram (VCUG). If VCUG shows VUR, radionuclide cystogram (RNC) may be utilized in follow-up studies as it generally involves less radiation exposure than VCUG, though at the expense of diminished anatomic detail.

Nuclear medicine renal cortical imaging using dimercaptosuccinic acid (DMSA) is the gold standard for evaluating renal scarring, one of the sequelae of VUR. When assessing for renal scarring, DMSA scintigraphy should be performed at least 6 months following the resolution of a UTI. Focal defects seen on DMSA scan performed earlier than 6 months after a UTI may relate to either scarring (nonreversible defect) or to pyelonephritis (potentially reversible defect).

The degree of VUR is graded on a scale of I through V. Grade I VUR involves reflux into the ureter. With grade II VUR, contrast or radiotracer extends into nondilated ureter and collecting system. Grade III extends into the collecting system with mild dilatation of ureter and calyces. Grade IV shows increasing tortuosity and ectasia of the ureter and increasing dilatation of the upper collecting system. Grade V implies massive dilatation and tortuosity of the ureter, and profound dilatation of the upper collecting system with loss of papillary impressions. Intrarenal reflux may also be seen with grade V VUR.

ADDITIONAL IMAGES (C-G)

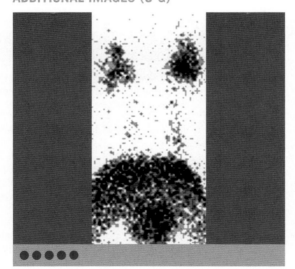

C. Posterior views from a radionuclide cystogram in a 6-year-old show radioactivity within dilated bilateral upper collecting systems, corresponding to radiographic grade IV VUR.

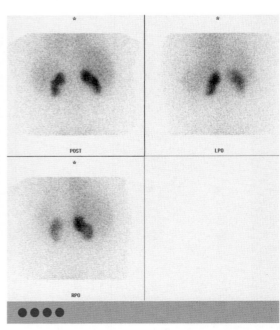

D. Focal defects as well as small size of the left kidney on posterior renal cortical imaging (DMSA scan) are consistent with scarring from reflux nephropathy.

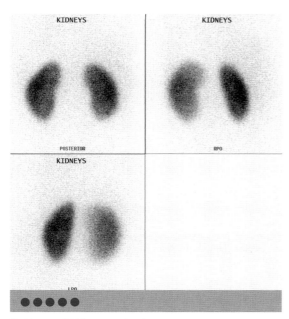

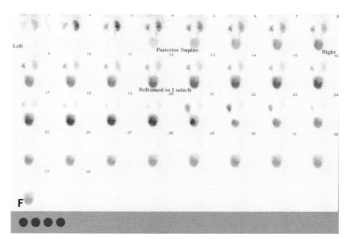

E. Normal DMSA examination.

F. and **G.** Posterior images from a radionuclide renogram MAG3 study (image F) in a 5-year-old with a history of pyelonephritis and left grade V VUR show a poorly functioning, scarred left kidney. At 21 to 24 minutes there is increased activity within a massively dilated left collecting system, which is also reflected in the time-activity curve (image G), consistent with grade V VUR.

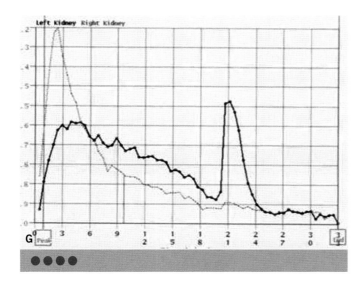

Grace S. Phillips, MD and Marguerite T. Parisi, MD, MS Ed

PRESENTATION

A 4-month-old with a history of severe left-sided hydronephrosis, diagnosed antenatally.

FINDINGS

Ultrasound image (image A) demonstrates moderate hydronephrosis. Posterior images from MAG3 radionuclide renogram (image B) demonstrate mild delay in perfusion to and uptake by an enlarged left kidney. Central photopenic defect is compatible with moderate hydronephrosis. There is progressive accumulation of radioactivity within a dilated renal collecting system with minimal, if any, response to Lasix (furosemide) administration. These findings are consistent with high-grade ureteropelvic junction (UPJ) obstruction.

DIFFERENTIAL DIAGNOSES

- *Congenital megacalycosis*

- *Hydronephrotic form of multicystic dysplastic kidney (MCDK)*

- *Infundibular stenosis*

- *Ureterovesical junction obstruction*

- *Nonobstructive pelviectasis*

COMMENTS

UPJ obstruction is the most common cause of hydronephrosis and also of a palpable abdominal mass in the newborn. Etiology of UPJ obstruction is multifactorial, with contributing factors that include anatomical abnormalities, abnormal peristalsis, and delayed recanalization of the fetal ureter. The

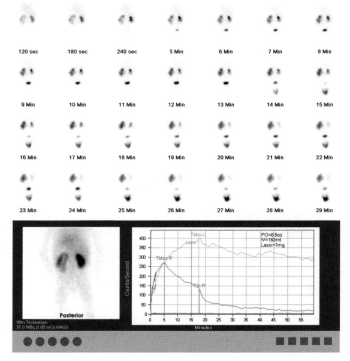

B. Posterior images from MAG3 radionuclide renogram show mild delay in perfusion to and uptake by an enlarged left kidney. Central photopenic defect is compatible with moderate hydronephrosis. There is progressive accumulation of radioactivity within a dilated renal collecting system with minimal, if any, response to Lasix administration. These findings are consistent with high-grade left UPJ obstruction. Normal right renal function is present.

PEARLS

- Adequate patient hydration is crucial in children.

- Attention to technical detail is important. Technique and time of Lasix administration should be identical in follow-up assessment.

- Lasix challenge will distinguish true obstruction from nonobstructive pelviectasis.

- Image for at least 30 minutes after Lasix administration.

- MAG3 radionuclide examination is useful to assess renal function, whereas DMSA may be used to assess for renal ectopia or agenesis.

- Attention to the normal biodistribution in nonrenal imaging studies can result in diagnosis of unanticipated but crucial findings, as demonstrated in Figure E.

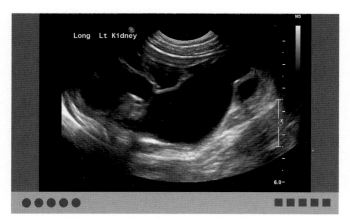

A. Longitudinal ultrasound image demonstrates moderate pelvicaliectasis with disproportionate dilatation of the renal pelvis and absence of ureteral dilatation, classic for UPJ obstruction.

classic ultrasound features of UPJ obstruction include hydronephrosis with disproportionate dilatation of the renal pelvis as compared to the degree of calyceal dilatation. There is typically a normal-sized, nondilated ureter.

Magnetic resonance urography (MRU) and renal scintigraphy may assess renal function of the affected kidney and help determine the need for surgery. Although MRU avoids the use of ionizing radiation, it is more expensive than renal scintigraphy and frequently requires sedation in the pediatric population. VCUG may be indicated to assess for VUR, which may coexist with UPJ obstruction in 10% to 14% of cases.

Congenital megacalycosis should be considered in the differential diagnosis of UPJ obstruction. Congenital megacalycosis is characterized by nephromegaly with greater than 20 calyces present. Calyces are abnormally shaped, typically polygonal in morphology. A dilated pelvis is present, but without obstruction. Of note, patients with congenital megacalycosis are predisposed to stone formation.

ADDITIONAL IMAGES (C-J)

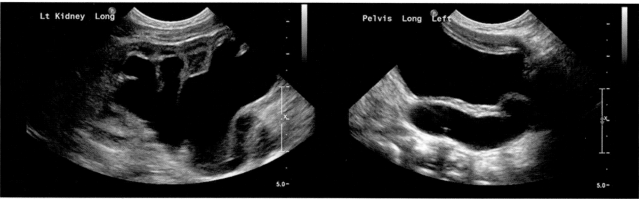

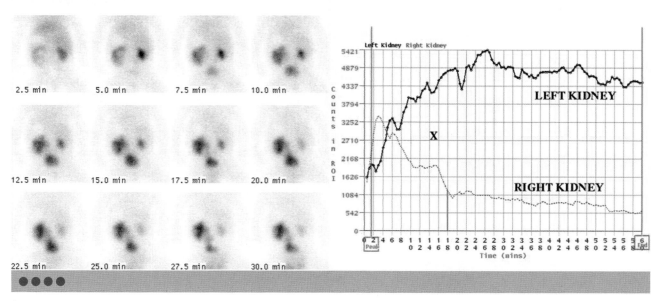

C. Ultrasound images (*top*) show severe left hydroureteronephrosis due to an obstructing ureterocele at the left UVJ. Obstructive hydroureteronephrosis is confirmed on diuretic renogram (*bottom*) and is distinguished from UPJ obstruction by the presence of activity within the dilated left ureter.

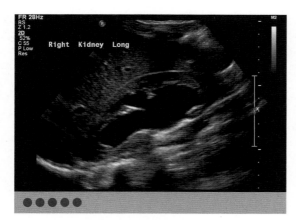

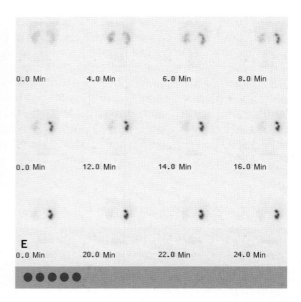

0.0 Min   4.0 Min   6.0 Min   8.0 Min

0.0 Min   12.0 Min   14.0 Min   16.0 Min

E
0.0 Min   20.0 Min   22.0 Min   24.0 Min

D., E. and **F. Partial UPJ Obstruction:** Ultrasound (image D) shows moderate right hydronephrosis with a UPJ configuration. Posterior views from an MAG3 renogram (image E) and corresponding time-activity histogram (image F) show moderate right hydronephrosis with incomplete washout of residual radiotracer from the dilated renal collecting system (image F) consistent with a partial right UPJ obstruction. Left kidney is normal.

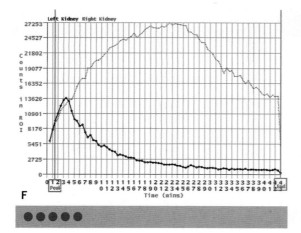

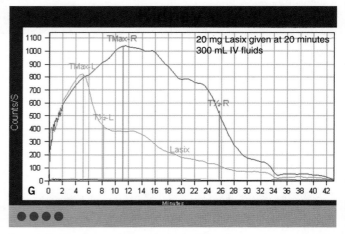

G. and **H. Nonobstructive pelviectasis:** There is complete washout of residual radioactivity from a dilated right renal collecting system, with activity approaching baseline on the time-activity curve by the end of the study.

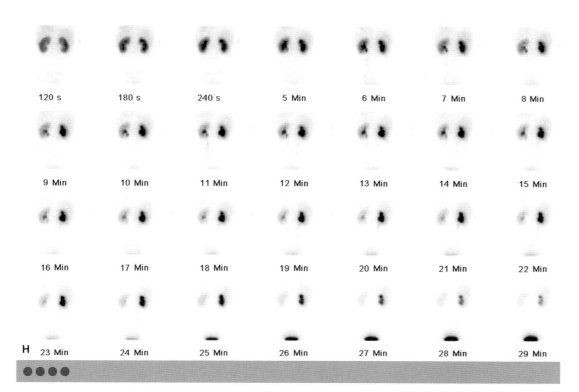

120 s	180 s	240 s	5 Min	6 Min	7 Min	8 Min
9 Min	10 Min	11 Min	12 Min	13 Min	14 Min	15 Min
16 Min	17 Min	18 Min	19 Min	20 Min	21 Min	22 Min
23 Min	24 Min	25 Min	26 Min	27 Min	28 Min	29 Min

H

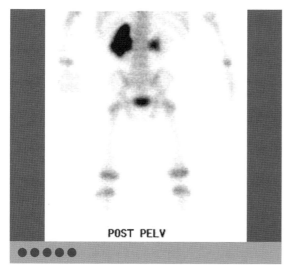

POST PELV

I. Incidentally noted accumulation of activity within a dilated left collecting system on bone scan in a 1-year-old patient who presented with a swollen left wrist. Subsequent diuretic renogram (*not shown*) confirmed high-grade UPJ obstruction.

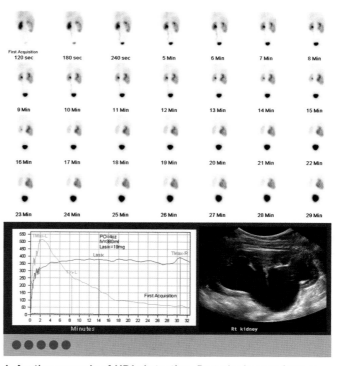

J. Another example of UPJ obstuction: Posterior images from an MAG3 renogram (*top*) with corresponding time-activity curve (*bottom left*) demonstrate marked right hydronephrosis with progressive accumulation of tracer in the dilated collecting system and lack of excretion, findings of a high-grade right UPJ obstruction with classic ultrasound appearance (*bottom right*).

Grace S. Phillips, MD and Marguerite T. Parisi, MD, MS Ed

PRESENTATION

A 3-month-old with a history of a renal anomaly diagnosed in utero.

FINDINGS

Longitudinal ultrasound image (image A) of the left kidney shows numerous cysts of varying sizes, without clear communication with the renal pelvis, and no definite renal parenchyma. Right kidney was normal (*not shown*). Posterior summed flow views from a nuclear medicine (MAG3) renogram (image B) show prompt radiotracer uptake by the right kidney. There is a large photopenic defect and absent uptake corresponding to the enlarged, nonfunctioning left kidney which exerts significant mass effect upon the spleen. The presence of mass effect suggests that this is multicystic dysplastic kidney (MCDK) or severe hydronephrosis as opposed to renal agenesis.

DIFFERENTIAL DIAGNOSES

Differential diagnoses for scintigraphic mimickers of MCDK are
- *Solitary kidney*
- *Cross-fused renal ectopia*
- *Severe hydronephrosis/UPJ obstruction*
- *Severe reflux nephropathy*

COMMENTS

MCDK is the most common cystic renal lesion. It is the second most common cause of a palpable abdominal mass in

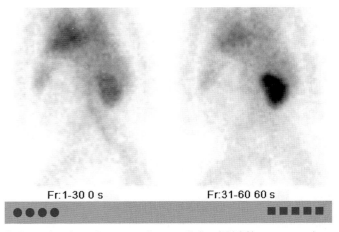

B. Posterior views from a nuclear medicine (MAG3) renogram show normal function in the right kidney and absence of uptake in the enlarged, nonfunctioning left kidney, with significant mass effect upon the spleen. The presence of mass effect suggests that this is MCDK or severe hydronephrosis as opposed to renal agenesis.

the newborn (after UPJ obstruction). MCDK occurs sporadically in 1 in 4000 births. MCDK results during embryology from upper ureteral atresia occurring in the metanephric phase during the seventh through the tenth week of nephrogenesis. With MCDK, the ipsilateral renal vessels are typically atretic or absent. The ipsilateral ureter is also absent, or hypoplastic and blind-ending. Absent flow to the ipsilateral kidney helps distinguish MCDK from severe hydronephrosis on scintigraphy. Associated genitourinary anomalies involving the contralateral kidney occur in approximately one-third of patients and include VUR in 20% to 25% and UPJ obstruction in 12%.

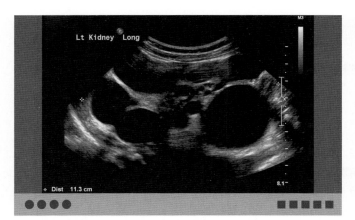

A. Longitudinal ultrasound image of the left kidney shows numerous cysts of varying sizes, without clear communication with the renal pelvis, and no definite renal parenchyma. Right kidney was normal (*not shown*).

PEARLS

- **Nuclear scintigraphy documents lack renal function, confirming diagnosis of MCDK.**

- **Flow imaging may be helpful. Documentation of absence of flow in MCDK helps distinguish MCDK from severe hydronephrosis or other causes of a poorly functioning kidney.**

- **Approximately one-third of those with MCDK have a contralateral renal abnormality, including UPJ obstruction or VUR, both of which may be diagnosed scintigraphically.**

- **Renal ectopia may be difficult to differentiate from renal agenesis with a contralateral duplex system, as seen in image K.**

MCDK is typically diagnosed either pre- or postnatally by ultrasound. Classic ultrasound features are an aggregate of cysts of varying sizes that do not communicate with the collecting system, with little or no surrounding renal parenchyma. Over time, the cystic mass typically involutes. At renal scintigraphy, no renal uptake is demonstrated. Bilateral MCDK, as depicted in images C and D, is incompatible with life.

The differential diagnosis for absence of radiotracer uptake within a kidney on renogram also includes unilateral renal agenesis. Unilateral renal agenesis occurs in approximately 1 in 1000 births, and may result from aplasia of the wolffian duct or absence of the ureteric bud with lack of metanephric tissue induction. There may be associated absence of ipsilateral ureter, vessels, and hemitrigone. Anomalies of the spine, GI tract, or genital tract may also be present. When unilateral renal agenesis is secondary to involution of an MCDK, the urinary bladder is normally developed and the ipsilateral distal ureter is hypoplastic.

Ultrasound is the cornerstone of evaluation and diagnosis of both MCDK and renal agenesis. Nuclear cortical scintigraphy may be used to distinguish agenesis from renal ectopia. CT or MRI may be used to further evaluate associated genital anomalies. VCUG is recommended as patients with a solitary kidney have a higher incidence of VUR.

ADDITIONAL IMAGES (C-L)

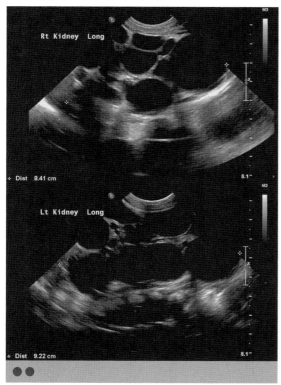

C. A 1-day-old neonate with renal failure. Longitudinal ultrasound images of the right and left kidney reveal bilateral renal enlargement with replacement of renal parenchyma by numerous, varying sized, noncommunicating cysts, findings suggesting bilateral MCDK.

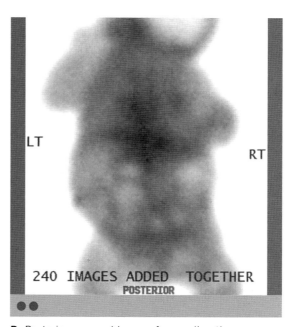

D. Posterior summed images from a diuretic renogram show an absence of renal uptake bilaterally, and large photopenic regions in the bilateral renal fossae corresponding to the enlarged, kidneys identified in image C, confirming a diagnosis of bilateral MCDK, a birth defect which is incompatible with life.

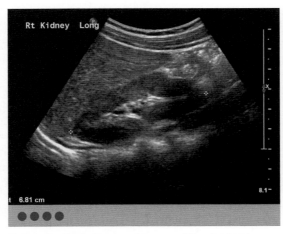

E. Longitudinal ultrasound image of the right kidney shows normal renal morphology.

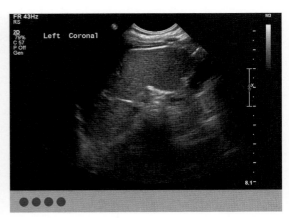

F. Longitudinal ultrasound image of the left renal fossa shows an absence of the left kidney.

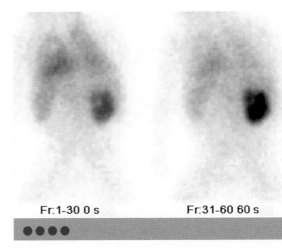

G. Radionuclide renogram to exclude renal ectopia shows absence of uptake within the left kidney and normal uptake within the right kidney, confirming left renal agenesis demonstrated on antecedent ultrasound (images E,F). Note the absence of mass effect and the presence of background activity, in comparison with images from MCDK (image B).

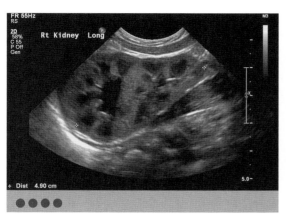

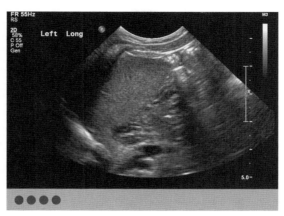

H. Longitudinal ultrasound image of the right renal fossa shows an abnormal morphology of the right kidney which, in conjunction with absence of a kidney in the left renal fossa (image I), either represents left renal agenesis with a duplex right renal collecting system or, more likely, crossed-fused renal ectopia. Diuretic renogram (image J) is obtained to evaluate renal function.

I. Longitudinal ultrasound image of the LUQ shows bowel filling the left renal fossa and absence of the left kidney.

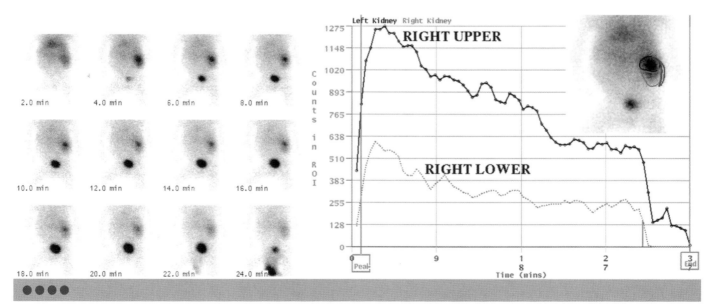

J. Posterior images from a radionuclide renogram with corresponding time-activity curve show an absence of uptake within the left renal fossa. Uptake pattern on the right may represent either a duplex right renal collecting system or cross-fused renal ectopia with hydronephrosis in the upper moiety/renal unit. VCUG (image K) establishes the diagnosis.

513

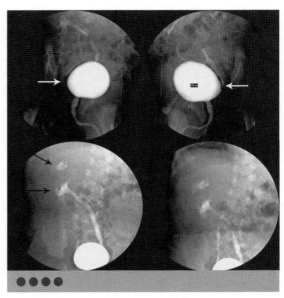

K. Fluoroscopic images from a VCUG on the same patient show reflux of contrast into normally located bilateral ureters (*white arrows, top row*) and contrast within the upper collecting system of both a cross-fused ectopic left kidney (*black arrows, lower left*) and a normally located right renal moiety.

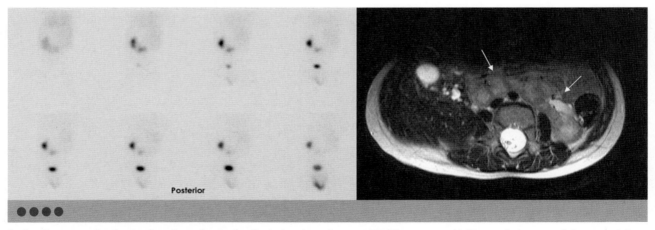

Posterior

L. Another example of cross-fused renal ectopia: Posterior views from an MAG3 renogram (*left*) reveal absence of tracer uptake in the right renal fossa. Uptake in the normal left kidney and in the cross-fused ectopically located right (inferior) kidney is a classic scintigraphic appearance of cross-fused renal ectopia which is confirmed on T2 MRI images (*arrows, right*).

Grace S. Phillips, MD and Marguerite T. Parisi, MD, MS Ed

PRESENTATION

An 11-month-old infant with hydronephrosis.

FINDINGS

Posterior images from MAG3 renogram (image A) demonstrate normal function of the lower pole and absence of uptake in the obstructed, dysplastic upper pole of the left kidney, consistent with a duplex collecting system. There is a rounded defect within the urinary bladder at the left ureterovesical junction. There is normal right renal function. Ultrasound images (image B) confirm a normal right kidney and a duplicated left renal collecting system. As seen on scintigraphy, there is a markedly dilated upper pole collecting system and a nonhydronephrotic lower pole moiety on the left. There is a dilated distal left ureter and a thin-walled cystic structure within the urinary bladder at the left ureterovesical junction, corresponding to an obstructive ureterocele of the left upper pole moiety.

DIFFERENTIAL DIAGNOSES

Differential diagnoses for scintigraphic findings of abnormal shape of renal uptake include:

- *Duplex collecting system*
- *Partial nephrectomy*
- *Renal scarring*
- *Renal mass*
- *Prominent column of Bertin: Typically seen on ultrasound*
- *Segmental MCDK*

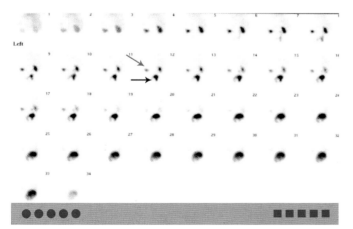

A. Posterior images from MAG3 renogram show normal function of the lower pole and absence of uptake in the obstructed, dysplastic upper pole of the left kidney (*red arrow*), consistent with a duplex collecting system. There is a rounded defect within the urinary bladder at the left ureterovesical junction (*black arrow*), consistent with a ureterocele. There is normal right renal function.

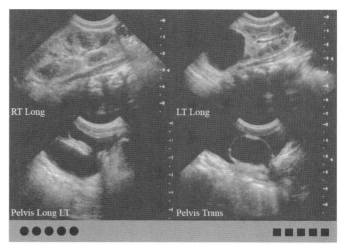

B. Ultrasound images confirm a normal right kidney and a duplicated left renal collecting system. As seen on scintigraphy, there is a markedly dilated upper pole collecting system and a nonhydronephrotic lower pole moiety. There is a dilated distal left ureter and a thin-walled cystic structure within the urinary bladder at the left ureterovesical junction, corresponding to an obstructive ureterocele of the left upper pole moiety.

COMMENTS

Duplex collecting system is the most common renal anomaly and occurs in approximately 1 in 160 people. A duplex collecting system results during embryology when two separate ureteric buds are present on the mesonephric duct. The orifice of the lower moiety ureter is typically more cephalad and lateral to the ureter draining the upper moiety. Reflux into the lower moiety is the most common abnormality in those with duplex system. However, reflux into the upper moiety and/or simultaneous reflux into both moieties may also occur. The upper moiety may be dysplastic or "obstructed," and associated with a

---

PEARLS

- The role of scintigraphy in those with a duplex collecting system is in assessing renal function, including evaluation for obstruction, VUR, and scarring of the upper and lower moieties, and in determining the need for heminephrectomy.

- As with other abnormalities on renal scintigraphy, ultrasound and/or VCUG may be helpful in better demonstrating anatomy.

- There is an increased incidence of VUR in patients with duplex renal collecting systems. The presence of VUR should in initially be assessed with fluoroscopic VCUG. In those with documented VUR, NM cystogram can then be used in follow-up as it is more sensitive yet imparts less patient radiation than the coventional, fluoroscopic VCUG.

ureterocele, as seen in images A and B. In some, the ureter associated with the upper moiety may insert distal to the bladder. In males, this ureter may insert into the posterior urethra proximal to the sphincter, or into the ejaculatory ducts or epididymis, which can cause epididymitis-orchitis. In females, the upper moiety ureter may insert into the bladder neck, uterus, or vagina (image E), resulting in enuresis.

The diagnosis of a duplex collecting system is typically initially made on ultrasound evaluation of the kidneys. VCUG has a role in evaluating for associated VUR. CT or MRU may be used to assess ectopic ureteral insertion. The role of renal scintigraphy and/or MRU is in assessing renal function and in determining the need for surgery.

ADDITIONAL IMAGES (C-E)

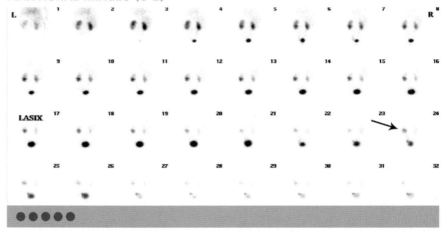

C. Posterior scintigraphic images from a patient with a known duplex left collecting system with normally functioning upper moiety and progressive accumulation of activity within a dilated left lower pole renal collecting system. VUR into the left lower moiety renal collecting system (*arrow*) is seen at 24 minutes.

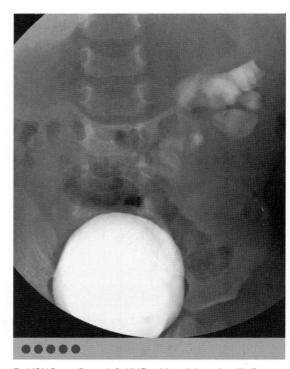

D. VCUG confirms left VUR with a "drooping lily" configuration, consistent with reflux into the lower pole moiety of a duplicated collecting system.

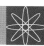

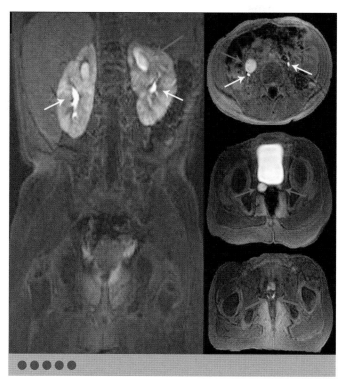

E. Magnetic resonance urogram in a 5-year-old with enuresis. There are bilaterally duplex renal collecting systems present with moderate dilatation of both upper (*red arrows*) and mild dilatation of both lower pole (*white arrows*) moiety collecting systems (coronal image, *left*). Axial images (*right*) demonstrate dilatation of dilated upper moiety ureters (*red arrows, top*) with ectopic insertion into the vagina (*bottom*). Lower moiety ureters (*white arrows*) are not dilated and insert in a more normal position (*not shown*).

Grace S. Phillips, MD and Marguerite T. Parisi, MD, MS Ed

PRESENTATION

A 10-year-old female child with spastic paraplegia and chronic emesis.

FINDINGS

Anterior views from a Tc-99m sulfur colloid gastric emptying study (image A) demonstrate radiotracer extending from the region of the stomach into the esophagus (*arrow*), consistent with gastroesophageal reflux (GER). Gastric emptying time was mildly delayed.

DIFFERENTIAL DIAGNOSES

- *Gastroesophageal reflux disease* (GERD)
- *Physiologic GER*
- *Achalasia*
- *Hiatal hernia*

COMMENTS

GER, or physiologic reflux, is a common phenomenon in the pediatric population and typically resolves by 12 months of age. GERD is differentiated from GER by the presence of a complication such as esophagitis. In infants, GERD may present with effortless emesis, increased irritability, failure to thrive, and/or reactive airways disease. In children, GERD may present with symptoms similar to the adult population, with poorly localized abdominal or chest pain, nonbilious emesis, reactive airways disease, or dysphagia. Other presenting symptoms include coughing, wheezing, and morning hoarseness. GERD may be associated with acute life-threatening events, repaired esophageal atresia, repaired duodenal atresia, mental retardation, cystic fibrosis, chronic lung disease of prematurity, asthma, and obesity. The etiology of GERD may be multifactorial and relate to an abnormal length or pressure or number of contractions of the lower esophageal sphincter; supradiaphragmatic location of the gastroesophageal junction; suboptimal relationship of the esophagus, stomach, and diaphragm; esophageal dysmotility; and delayed gastric emptying. GERD may also be seen in association with certain foods, medications, or hormones.

Intraesophageal pH study remains the gold standard for diagnosis of GERD. However, imaging evaluation of patients with suspected GERD is sometimes considered. An upper gastrointestinal (UGI) series may be performed to rule out structural abnormalities that may predispose patients to GERD, such as a hiatal hernia, disorders of esophageal peristalsis, swallowing dysfunction, and esophageal stricture or mucosal irregularity. However, UGI has relatively poor sensitivity

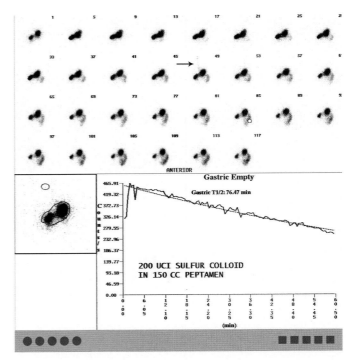

A. Anterior views from Tc-99m sulfur colloid gastric emptying study show radiotracer extending from the region of the stomach into the esophagus (*arrow*), consistent with GER. Gastric emptying time was mildly delayed.

and specificity for the diagnosis of GERD. Nuclear medicine gastroesophageal reflux (NM GER) study using Tc-99m sulfur colloid is more sensitive than UGI for detecting episodes of reflux, as images are acquired for 60 minutes or more after the initial ingestion of the radiotracer. NM GER is typically performed in conjunction with a gastric emptying examination; delayed gastric emptying may exacerbate GERD. Gastric emptying depends on a variety of factors. Most importantly,

PEARLS

- We consider the normal gastric emptying time in children to be 45% at 60 minutes and 60% at 90 minutes

- Atypical shape of the esophagus at scintigraphy may represent either achalasia, hiatal hernia, or colonic interposition graft.

- Evaluate for anatomical causes of emesis with UGI.

- Awareness of the normally expected radiotracer biodistribution may lead to identification of unanticipated but crucial findings that can alter patient management (images C, H, K).

- Consider non-GI causes of recurrent emesis.

gastric emptying of solids follows a linear function, whereas emptying of liquids follows an exponential course, which has a direct implication for how a nuclear medicine gastric emptying study is performed. Most institutions will evaluate gastric emptying of either solids or liquids, but not both, during a nuclear medicine gastric emptying study.

ADDITIONAL IMAGES (B-J)

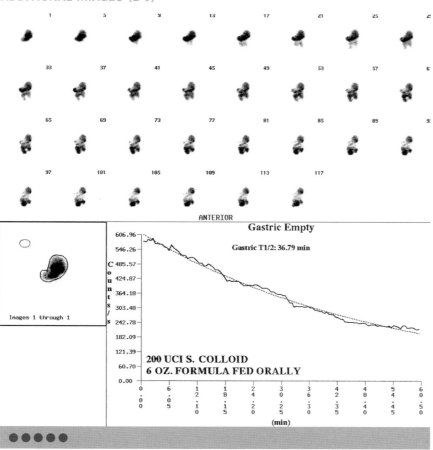

B. Normal Tc 99m sulfur colloid gastric emptying examination. No scintigraphic evidence of GER or delayed gastric emptying.

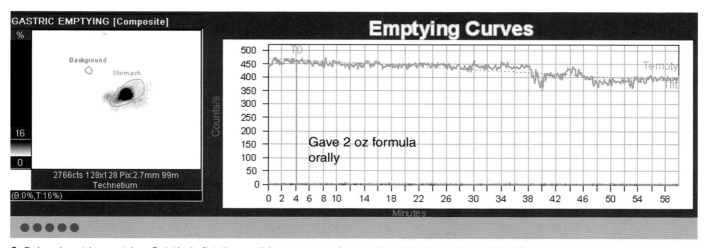

C. Delayed gastric emptying. Relatively flat time-activity curve, consistent with minimal gastric emptying from the stomach shown at 1 hour.

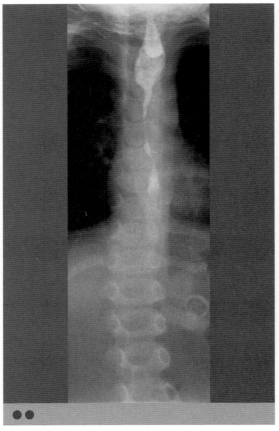

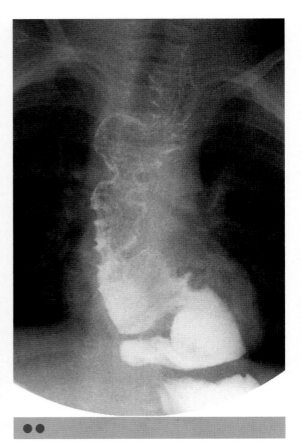

D. Esophageal stricture with an irregular, narrowed contour of the esophagus secondary to lye ingestion shown on UGI examination.

E. The patient underwent colonic interposition graft with poor motility and retention of contrast shown on follow-up UGI.

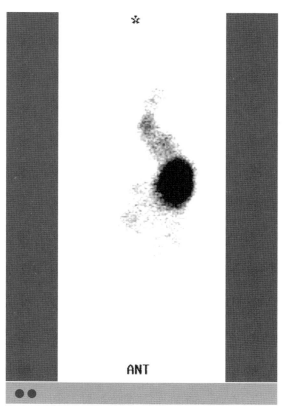

F. Irregular and wide column of activity seen in the expected region of the esophagus, consistent with GER after neoesophagus/interposed colon for lye ingestion.

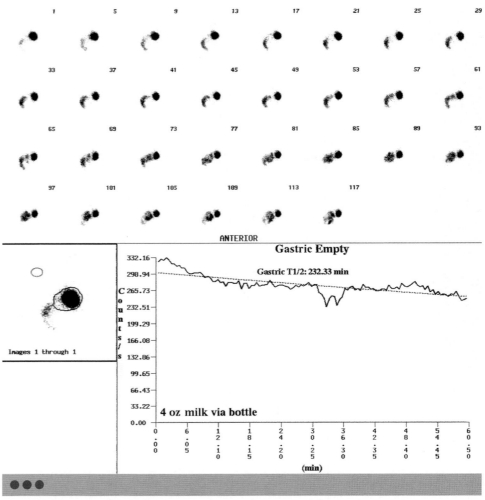

G. Significant delay in gastric emptying at 1 hour and no GER. Incidental note made of malposition of the ligament of Treitz and proximal small bowel loops located in the RUQ, consistent with malrotation.

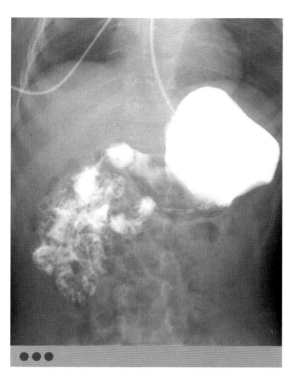

H. Correlative UGI image showing proximal bowel loops in the RUQ, consistent with malrotation.

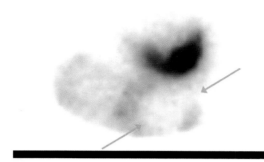

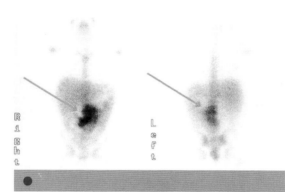

I. Top image from sulfur colloid gastric emptying study in a 14-year-old with AIDS shows paucity of activity centrally in the abdomen (*arrows*), suggestive of mass effect upon small bowel loops. Lower image shows corresponding increased activity on gallium scan within the mass (*arrows*), which was diagnosed as MAI by biopsy.

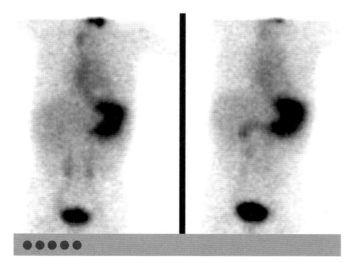

J. Intermittent radiotracer within the esophagus (*left*) incidentally identified during a Meckel scan, consistent with GER.

INDEX

Page numbers followed by *f* indicate figures.

The twentieth century has seen biology come of age as a conceptual and quantitative science. Biochemistry, cytology, and genetics have been unified into a common framework at the molecular level. However, cellular activity and development are regulated not by the interplay of molecules alone, but by interactions of molecules organized in complex arrays, subunits, and organelles. Emphasis on organization is, therefore, of increasing importance.

So it is too, at the other end of the scale. Organismic and population biology are developing new rigor in such established and emerging disciplines as ecology, evolution, and ethology, but again the accent is on interactions between individuals, populations, and societies. Advances in comparative biochemistry and physiology have given new impetus to studies of animal and plant diversity. Microbiology has matured, with the world of viruses and procaryotes assuming a major position. New connections are being forged with other disciplines outside biology — chemistry, physics, mathematics, geology, anthropology, and psychology provide us with new theories and experimental tools while at the same time are themselves being enriched by the biologists' new insights into the world of life. The need to preserve a habitable environment for future generations should encourage increasing collaboration between diverse disciplines.

The purpose of the Modern Biology Series is to introduce the college biology student — as well as the gifted secondary student and all interested readers — both to the concepts unifying the fields within biology and to the diversity that makes each field unique.

Since the series is open-ended, it will provide a greater number and variety of topics than can be accommodated in many introductory courses. It remains the responsibility of the instructor to make his selection, to arrange it in a logical order, and to develop a framework into which the individual units can best be fitted.

New titles will be added to the present list as new fields emerge, existing fields advance, and new authors of ability and talent appear. Only thus, we feel, can we keep pace with the explosion of knowledge in Modern Biology.

James D. Ebert
Ariel G. Loewy
Richard S. Miller
Howard A. Schneiderman

The Living Plant

second edition

Peter Martin Ray

Stanford University

Holt, Rinehart and Winston, Inc.
New York   Chicago   San Francisco
Atlanta   Dallas   Montreal
Toronto   London   Sydney

For Martin and Nigel

whose curiosity about nature
is yet to be satisfied

Text and cover design by Margaret O. Tsao

Preface

This book seeks to introduce you to what plants do and how they are equipped to do it. While almost everyone appreciates that plants are the ultimate suppliers of the food and much of the goods of mankind as well as of the animal kingdom as a whole, and thus constitute the foundation of the earth's ecosystems, plants go about their activities unobtrusively enough that even the most observant person is likely to be surprised at some of the things that take place inside a plant. Unlike much of the behavior of animals, few of the plant's major activities are directly evident to the senses. Consequently how plants make a living was grossly misunderstood both by learned men and by practical agriculturists from ancient times until the first half of the nineteenth century, when the results of experimental inquiry began to have their impact. How far we have come in understanding the functioning of plants is, indeed, a tribute to the principle of investigation by experiment and measurement.

Besides their economic and ecological importance to man, plants are also of great esthetic interest to human beings. Apropos of this subject most of us today have more or less frequent occasion to experiment, or to be experimented upon, and we are becoming more and more aware of how important trees and plants are to the difference between an agreeable or inspiring environment and an oppressive one. An appreciation of plant function and ecological adaptation, like a familiarity with plant classification and evolution, heightens our appreciation of and affection for the botanical component of the landscape and our awe of its more remarkable manifestations: the tall redwoods and giant sequoias, the diminutive arctic-alpine plants of the high mountains and the far north, the tough plants of the deserts and of the prairies, and the great broad-leaved forests of cold-temperate climates and of the tropics. It also gives a deeper feeling for a good field of corn or soy beans. As it is with music and art, understanding adds a great deal to our awareness and enjoyment of the botanical side of esthetic experience.

In the chapters that follow it is our goal to analyze the important principles known to be involved in the activities of plants and in the relation between these activities and the plant's environment. Attention is concentrated on the typical green land plant, let us say flowering plant; such plants are not only the most important in the everyday sense, they are also the most complex plants and offer the greatest diversity of problems. Studies of lower plants that have uncovered principles applicable to all green plants are, however, discussed extensively. For a comparative examination of the plant kingdom the reader is referred to Delevoryas, *Plant Diversification* in this Modern Biology series.

Familiarity with elementary chemistry and access to the biochemical material covered in Novikoff-Holtzman, *Cells and Organelles*, Modern Biology Series, are assumed.

Chapter 1 provides a general look at the functions and organs of a land plant, with some of the basic evidence for what different parts of the plant do. For those who have had previous contact with elementary biology much of this material should naturally constitute review. Chapter 2 considers the organization and function of plant cells, dealing only briefly, however, with matters of general cell physiology such as respiratory energy metabolism, which is covered more extensively in Novikoff-Holtzman, *Cells and Organelles*. In succeeding chapters each of the plant's specialized activities is explored more deeply, concluding with growth, development, and reproduction. Details of anatomical structure and the extensive terminology connected therewith are emphasized only insofar as they are important to an understanding of functional principles.

It is hoped that the reader will take away not only an appreciation of basic principles of function and ecological adaptation as they are presently understood, but also some notion of the important gaps that remain in our understanding of plant function and how current research is attacking them.

I wish to express my appreciation to the many individuals who have contributed data and illustrative materials, as cited with the individual figures, and to Olle Björkman, Winslow Briggs, David Fork, Harold Mooney, and Bruce Stowe for critical readings of the manuscript or parts thereof.

P.M.R.
Stanford, California
January 1972

Contents

ix

The
Living
Plant

chapter 1

The
Plant Way
of Life

The green plant is, first and foremost, a device for capturing the energy of sunlight and using it through the process of *photosynthesis*, to convert carbon dioxide into organic carbon compounds from which the substance of life can be manufactured. Much of the structure of plants can be understood as the equipment necessary to make photosynthesis successful in the environment in which the plant finds itself, and much of plants' behavior is directed toward ensuring that this equipment is at hand where and when it is needed.

Our understanding of how plants make a living had its beginnings in Joseph Priestley's discovery about 1770 that plants give off a gas (later to be called *oxygen*) that supports combustion and is fit for the respiration of animals. Priestley's results were rather erratic and aroused considerable controversy. The Flemish physician Jan Ingenhousz, a man unmistakably gifted in experimental insight, became interested in Priestley's findings and soon clarified them. In his classic *Experiments upon Vegetables*, published in 1779, Ingenhousz established that the gas discovered by Priestley is given off by plants only in the light and only by their green parts.

To Priestley and Ingenhousz the importance of this discovery seemed to be in revealing a beneficial role that plants play in "purifying" air that animal respiration has rendered unfit for breathing. They did not realize the role that carbon dioxide plays in the process nor its nourishing value for the plant. However, Ingenhousz noted that the release of bubbles of "pure air" by leaves in the light was most vigorous when the leaves were immersed in freshly pumped well water, and was poorest when they were immersed in recently boiled or distilled water. We can see in retrospect that this was because boiled or distilled water contains little carbon dioxide, whereas Ingenhousz's well water was enriched with bicarbonate, which served as a source of CO_2 for photosynthesis.

Lavoisier's discovery of chemical elements and the nature of combustion in 1785 showed that what Priestley and Ingenhousz had observed was a release of oxygen by plants in the light. Ingenhousz and others soon recognized that carbonic acid (CO_2) is taken up during this oxygen production and plants derive their substance from the carbon so absorbed. By 1804 Theodore de Saussure of Geneva had discovered by careful quantitative measurements that a plant in the light gains more weight than the difference between the weight of carbon dioxide it absorbs and the oxygen it releases, which he concluded must indicate that water is also used as a reactant in photosynthesis:

$$CO_2 + H_2O \xrightarrow{\text{Light}} \underset{\substack{\text{Organic} \\ \text{carbon}}}{(CH_2O)} + O_2 \qquad (1\text{-}1)$$

De Saussure also recognized that plants absorb from the soil, in addition to water, mineral elements (especially nitrogen) that are indispensable to their growth. He thus provided for the first time an accurate elementary picture of how plants obtain their nourishment. However, more than half a century elapsed before these simple facts became generally accepted.

The plant mode of nutrition, in which no organic carbon compounds need to be furnished by the environment, is called *autotrophic nutrition*. It contrasts with *heterotrophic* nutrition in which the organism must obtain at least some organic compounds (food) from its surroundings. The heterotrophic mode of life is followed not only by animals but by certain groups of plants, the most important being the *fungi*. These plants lack the green pigment *chlorophyll*, which is otherwise ubiquitous in the vegetable world and plays a central role in photosynthesis. In this book we shall not be concerned with the nongreen heterotrophic plants except as they affect the functioning of typical green plants. Information about fungi is presented in Delevoryas, *Plant Diversification* in the Modern Biology Series.[1]

Anyone who has not appreciated the vital importance of green plants and

---

[1]A complete listing of the Modern Biology Series appears in the front of this book.

of their remarkable process of photosynthesis should reflect a moment upon the fact that heterotrophic organisms, including man and animals quite generally, are eventually all dependent for their existence on the organic carbon compounds that autotrophic organisms synthesize, as well as on the oxygen that green plants return to the atmosphere as fast as it is used up by animals and by man's activities. Therefore man and animals owe not only the air they breathe, as Priestley and Ingenhousz conceived it, but also the substance of their bodies to green plants through their photosynthetic activity as summarized in Equation 1-1.

The simpler green plants, the *algae*, are found mainly in the oceans and in fresh water. Some of them consist of just a single chlorophyll-containing cell. Others are multicellular, and some kinds possess large and complex bodies (see Delevoryas, *Plant Diversification*). However, in their watery environment that furnishes at once the water, light, carbon dioxide, and minerals necessary for autotrophic life, few of the algae encounter such extreme problems in supply and demand of these essential commodities as do the plants that live on land.

In what follows we shall examine primarily how typical land plants solve these and other problems of autotrophic livelihood. We shall often consider comparable functions of algae, especially in the area of photosynthesis where experiments with algae have played a prominent role in developing modern understanding of the process. In this chapter we look briefly at the functions of the various parts of a land plant and how these functions are integrated to make a successful organism; in subsequent chapters we shall discuss in more detail the structural, physical, and chemical basis of each of the plant's important activities.

THE ORGANS OF A LAND PLANT

The body of a land plant is composed of two familiar and fundamental parts: the *root system*, which grows downward into the soil and serves to anchor the plant and hold it upright as well as to absorb water and mineral salts from the soil; and the *shoot system*, which grows upward into the air. The shoot (Figure 1-1) consists of green *leaves*, which are the structures adapted to carry on active photosynthesis, and are attached to the *stem* at points called *nodes* (the intervals between the leaves are *internodes*). The shoot system also produces specialized structures for reproduction (discussed in Chapter 10).

Growth in length of the shoot occurs at its tip and involves (1) production of new embryonic leaves, nodes, and internodes of microscopic size at the very tip or apex and (2) enlargement of the new leaves to full size, accompanied by elongation of the internodes to reach their mature length. The second process constitutes the visible growth of the shoot. It can readily be visualized by studying the stages of growth seen at successive nodes and internodes in the growing region as shown in the diagram in Figure 1-1.

The stem serves not only to support the leaves in the light but also to convey to them minerals and, in much larger amounts, water to replenish the water that is constantly evaporating from the leaves into the atmosphere. The invisible loss of water from plants into the air is called *transpiration*.

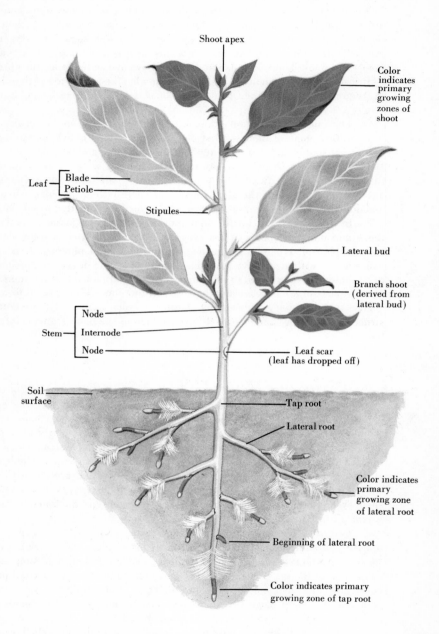

Shoot apex

Color indicates primary growing zones of shoot

Leaf — Blade
Petiole

Stipules

Lateral bud

Branch shoot (derived from lateral bud)

Stem — Node
Internode
Node

Leaf scar (leaf has dropped off)

Soil surface

Tap root

Lateral root

Color indicates primary growing zone of lateral root

Beginning of lateral root

Color indicates primary growing zone of tap root

Fig. 1-1 *Diagram illustrating typical external features and mode of growth of shoot and root systems. For simplicity the individual roots are represented as larger, in proportion to the shoot, and fewer in number than in an actual plant.*

In terms of quantity, transpiration is the most important exchange of materials between the plant and its surroundings, far exceeding the exchange of carbon dioxide and oxygen resulting from photosynthesis. The occurrence of transpiration was proved in 1727 (long before photosynthesis was known) by Stephen Hales, often regarded as the first person to make a substantial investigation of a plant function by means of experiment. For example, he enclosed a plant inside a glass vessel and found that liquid water, which must have come from the plant, condensed on the vessel walls. He measured the rate of transpiration in various ways, such as recording the continual loss in weight of an unwatered potted plant.

Leaves commonly lose into the air in a single day an amount of water exceeding their own weight. If the leaves are not to dry up, this loss must be made good by absorption of water by the roots and transport of this water to the leaves. The rapid loss of water by plant shoots seems to be a passive process, one that occurs simply because the leaves must be open to the atmosphere in order to absorb carbon dioxide from it efficiently enough to support photosynthesis.

Water absorption by the root is facilitated by the development of numerous *root hairs*, which are slender tubular extensions of the external cells of the root (Figures 1-1 and 5-8). They increase enormously the area of contact between root and soil and the volume of soil from which water can be drawn.

Growth in length of the root occurs in the zone between the root hairs and the tip of the root, a distance usually of a few millimeters or less. Longitudinal expansion or elongation of the cells in this zone actually drives the tip of the root forcibly through the soil. The very tip is provided with a protective structure called the *root cap* (Figure 1-1), which bears the brunt of the inevitable mechanical abrasion of the root tip; it is constantly regenerated from beneath. As the growing zone lengthens, the cells at its basal end, next to the nongrowing zone where root hairs are already found, become mature and cease to grow. Here new root hairs are formed and grow out into the soil.

Thus growth of the root continually adds to the root hair-bearing surface of the root and extends it through the soil. Individual root hairs have only a temporary existence. They finally die and are sloughed off along with other external tissues in the older part of the root which is beginning to grow in thickness.

The roots and most parts of the stem usually are not green; that is, they lack chlorophyll and they are incapable of photosynthesis. They have essentially heterotrophic nutrition and are "fed" by the leaves. Sugar, produced in the leaves by photosynthesis, is transported downward in the stem to the living cells within and to the tissues of the root. These cells require the sugar not only as a raw material for manufacturing and repairing their constituents but also as the substrate for respiration, the process by which the energy needed for such operations of manufacture and repair is made available to the cell. As an overall process respiration appears to be the reverse of photosynthesis; it involves the consumption of oxygen and the production of carbon dioxide and water from organic compounds such as sugar, which is the reverse of Equation 1-1. Thus roots and stems, like animals, require and consume oxygen from the air and give off carbon dioxide. Ingenhousz himself demonstrated that even green leaves consume oxygen when in darkness (as at night), showing that they too carry on respiration. In sunlight photosynthesis occurs much more rapidly than respiration; thus a net uptake of CO_2 and release of O_2 by plants is observed.

THE VASCULAR   The interdependent functioning of the leaves,
SYSTEM   stem, and roots, brought about through conduction of sugar downward and of water and min-
erals upward in the plant, is made possible by a specialized and microscopically
complex tissue system called the *vascular system*, which extends throughout the
root and shoot and is visible in the leaf as the familiar "veins."

The vascular system is composed of two distinct tissues that occur side by
side: the *xylem*, which conducts water, and the *phloem*, which conducts sugar.
The arrangement of these tissues in the two principal types of stems is dia-
gramed in Figure 1-2.

In the *herbaceous* type, such as in the soft stems of low-growing plants,
distinct *vascular bundles*, each composed of xylem and phloem, run through a
soft tissue (cortex and pith). The bundles occasionally branch, and some of the
branch bundles run out through the leaf petiole into the blade of the leaf and
become its system of veins. The bundles also extend downward into the roots
where they are found in a rather different arrangement (see Figure 5-8).

The *woody* stem is one that continues to grow in thickness; for example,
the trunk and branches of trees and shrubs. It actually begins life with a structure similar to the herbaceous stem, but gradually becomes transformed by
growth in thickness so that it possesses a solid central cylinder of xylem called
the *wood*, surrounded by an external layer of phloem. Outside the phloem a
tough protective tissue called the *cork* develops. The phloem and cork usually
can be stripped off together and comprise what we know as the "bark" of a tree.

If the bark is stripped off all the way around the trunk of a tree, the roots
become starved, quickly cease growing, and eventually die. This well-known

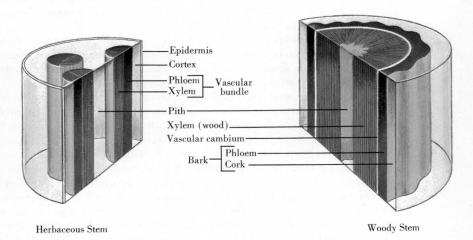

Epidermis
Cortex
Phloem } Vascular
Xylem } bundle
Pith
Xylem (wood)
Vascular cambium
Bark { Phloem
Bark { Cork

Herbaceous Stem   Woody Stem

Fig. 1-2   *Diagrams of structure of typical herbaceous and woody stems. Each is represented as a cylindrical segment that has been cut in half lengthwise. Vascular tissues are
shown in color, soft tissues (cortex and pith) and cork are represented as transparent. (Detailed cellular structure of herbaceous and woody stems is illustrated in Figures 8-8a and 8-
8d, respectively.)*

result indicates both the conducting function of tissues in the bark and the dependence of the roots on "food" coming down from the leaves. The leaves of a tree so treated continue, however, to be supplied with water for some time, indicating that water rises to them through the xylem. They wilt and die, however, as decline of the roots finally deprives them of the ability to absorb sufficient water.

The function of the vascular system of plants is in some ways analogous to the vascular or circulatory systems of animals in that it is the pathway of distribution of nutrients through the organism to sites of need. However, it is not a true circulatory system, despite the usually opposing traffic in xylem and phloem, because the two systems are not directly interconnected. Moreover most of the water that moves up in the xylem evaporates into the air rather than returning downward in the phloem. And nowhere in the system is there to be found any visible source of motive power for the propulsion of the fluids that move through the microscopic conducting channels of the xylem and phloem. There is nothing comparable with the various kinds of "heart" that activate the vascular systems of animals. The means by which substantial flows of liquid are brought about through the vascular system of plants are examined in Chapters 5 and 7.

Another difference between plant and typical animal vascular systems is that the plant system does not serve to bring oxygen from the air to the cells as it commonly does in animals. The oxygen supply mechanism in plants is discussed in Chapter 2.

In addition to serving as a vital avenue of conduction, the vascular system of plants also carries a major part of the burden of supporting the plant mechanically. Mechanical support is no mean problem in a large tree, not only because of its weight but also because of the great forces that wind can exert upon its large area of leaves and branches. A tree is basically held up by its wood. Actually, cells and tissues specialized for mechanical support are developed within both the xylem and phloem of most land plants. In some cases, mechanical tissues also arise outside the vascular system. On the other hand, the support of the soft parts of the plant body does not depend entirely on mechanical tissues, as will be discussed in Chapter 2.

Possession of a well-developed vascular system is one of the important features that distinguish the principal groups of land plants from algae and also from the most primitive land plants, the mosses and liverworts (see Delevoryas, *Plant Diversification*). It should be clear why the vascular system contributes so much to the success of plants on dry land and to their ability to attain large size. It is now becoming clear that at least some mosses and large algae have also developed cell systems that are specialized for long-distance transport of products of photosynthesis (Chapter 7).

SUGGESTED READING

Asimov, I. *Photosynthesis*. New York: Basic Books, 1968. Chapter 1.

Clark-Kennedy, A. E., *Stephen Hales*, D.D., F.R.S. Cambridge, England: Cambridge University Press, 1929. Chapter 4.

Hales, S. *Vegetable Staticks*. Reprint, with foreword by M. A. Hoskin. New York: American Elsevier, 1969. (Originally published 1727)

Kormondy, E. J., *General Biology, a Book of Readings*. Vol. 1. *Molecules and Cells*. Dubuque, Iowa: W. C. Brown, 1966. Chapters 26-27 (abridged original writings of de Saussure and Ingenhousz).

Nash, L. K., *Plants and the Atmosphere*. Cambridge, Mass.: Harvard University Press, 1952.

Reed, H. S., *Jan Ingenhousz, Plant Physiologist, with a History of the Discovery of Photosynthesis*. New York: Ronald Press, 1949.

Whittingham, C. P., *The Chemistry of Plant Processes*. New York: Philosophical Library, 1965. Chapter 1.

Plant Cells and Their Activities

All higher plants, like the higher animals, are built of units called cells. In a sense the cell constitutes the smallest truly living part of a plant because a cell (but no part thereof) can survive, grow, and reproduce itself indefinitely and in some cases can eventually give rise to a whole plant.

THE CELL WALL   The plant cell is almost always bounded by a visible jacket called the *cell wall*, which the cell deposits to the exterior of its external membrane. The cell wall of typical living cells (Figures 2-1, 2-3, and 2-4) is a thin, transparent, and seemingly delicate envelope, often less than 1 micron in thickness (1 micron = 0.001 mm). Animal cells do not possess a cell wall; it constitutes a structural characteristic of plant cells that is of great importance in their

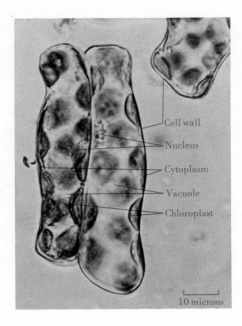

Cell wall

Nucleus

Cytoplasm

Vacuole

Chloroplast

10 microns

Fig. 2-1 *Living green plant cells, from leaf of privet (*Ligustrum*). Cells at left are palisade cells, cell at upper right is from spongy parenchyma (see Fig. 4-1). (Magnification 1000×. Photomicrograph by author.)*

function. The cell wall is composed primarily of polysaccharides — large molecules built up of sugar units joined together into long chains. The most characteristic polysaccharide of the cell wall in higher plants is *cellulose*, which is built from units of the sugar glucose ($C_6H_{12}O_6$). Cellulose is deposited in the cell wall as a meshwork of threadlike structures called *microfibrils*, generally 10 to 20 nm in diameter [1 nanometer (nm) $= 10^{-6}$ mm], that can be seen with the electron microscope (Figure 2-2). Each microfibril is a bundle of hundreds of cellulose strands, that is, individual chains of glucose units. This arrangement, which may be compared roughly with that of a cable, makes the microfibril surprisingly strong — about as strong as an equal amount of steel.

The cell walls of certain algae contain noncellulosic microfibrillar material, for example, mannan (a polysaccharide built up of the 6-carbon sugar *mannose*) and xylan (polysaccharide of the 5-carbon sugar *xylose*). The microfibrillar component of the cell walls of most fungi is *chitin* (a polysaccharide that is built of acetylglucosamine units; it is also the skeletal substance of arthropods).

Microfibrillar material makes up only a part of the dry matter of the cell wall. The remainder (the cell wall *matrix*) is material in which the microfibrils are embedded, rather like reinforcing rods in a matrix of concrete. The cell wall matrix consists of a complex of polysaccharides, called *hemicelluloses* and *pectic substances*, which are built up largely of sugars and sugar derivatives other than glucose. Cell walls also often contain an appreciable proportion of protein. This protein is found to be distinctively rich in the amino acids proline and hydroxyproline, as is the important connective tissue protein *collagen* of animal tissues. This resemblance has led to the suggestion that the hydroxyproline-rich protein of the plant cell walls is a structural protein. The cell wall matrix substances are highly hydrated, that is, physically combined with water.

The walls of adjacent cells are held together by a thin cementing layer called the *middle lamella* (Figure 2-3). The middle lamella is composed of non-cellulosic polysaccharides, especially pectin.

Traversing the cell wall and middle lamella and apparently connecting the protoplasm of adjacent cells are very fine strands of protoplasm called *plasmodesmata* (singular, plasmodesma), some of which show in Figure 2-3. Plasmodesmata are believed to transport materials from cell to cell, although there is as yet little direct evidence for their function. As we shall see later some important roles are assigned to this presumed transport function in plants.

Although synthesized by the cell, the polysaccharides and protein of the cell wall cannot as a rule be broken down into sugars and reused by the cell. Hence the cell wall is commonly regarded as an inert and nonliving structure. However, a number of cellular processes do appear to involve localized breakdown of the cell wall, or of its noncellulosic polysaccharides, by the cell (an example is noted in Figure 2-5).

Secondary Wall   The thin cell wall possessed by growing plant cells like that in Figure 2-3 and by unspecialized cells like those in Figures 2-1 and 2-4 is called a *primary* wall. In the differentiation of many specialized cells a thick additional wall called the *secondary* wall is deposited layer by layer by the cell upon its primary wall (Figure 2-5).

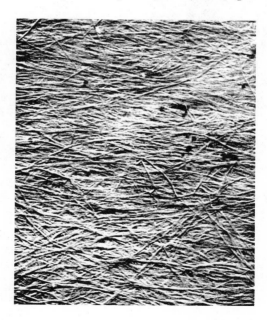

Fig. 2-2   *Electronmicrograph showing structure of the cell wall of a growing cell of the alga* Nitella axillaris *seen from the inner surface. The microfibrils of cellulose are 10 to 20 nm (1 nm = 10⁻⁹ meter) in diameter. Long axis of the cell corresponds with vertical direction in the illustration. (Magnification 24,000×. Courtesy of Dr. Paul B. Green.)*

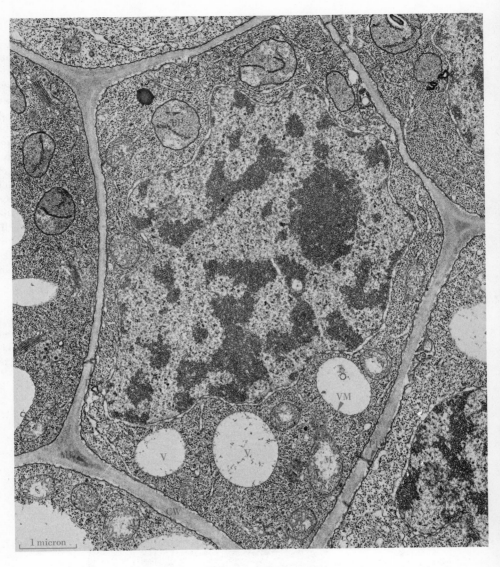

Fig. 2-3 *Cell from region of cell division in embryonic pea stem. (Magnification 14,500×.)*

CW   cell wall
D   dictyosome (Golgi body)
ER   endoplasmic reticulum
I   intercellular gas space
M   mitochondrion
ML   middle lamella
MT   microtubule
N   nucleus
NE   nuclear envelope
NL   nucleolus

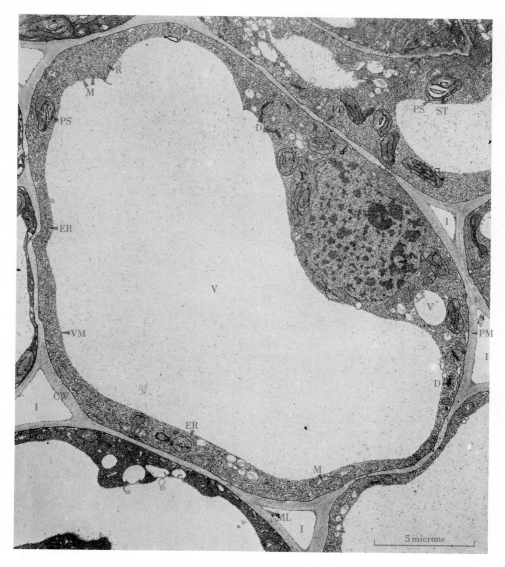

Fig. 2-4 *Vacuolate cell from a growing pea stem. (Magnification 5400×.)*

P   plastid
PD   plasmodesma
PM   plasma membrane
PP   proplastid
PS   amyloplast
R   ribosomes
SP   spherosome (lipid body)
ST   starch grain
V   vacuole
VM   vacuolar membrane

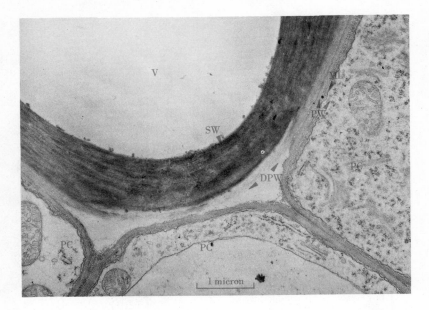

Fig. 2-5   *Secondary cell wall (SW) of a vessel cell (V) from an oat seedling. The primary walls (PW) of the vessel and of adjacent parenchyma cells (PC) are separated by the middle lamella (ML). Note the layered structure of the secondary wall due to its gradual deposition by this cell, and the region (DPW) in which the primary wall was largely broken down during differentiation of the vessel. (M) Mitochondrion. (Magnification 16,000×. Electron micrograph by the author.)*

The secondary wall typically has a quite different composition from the primary wall. It lacks pectic substances and contains considerably more cellulose, the microfibrils of which are usually deposited in a spectacularly regular orientation that confers great strength and rigidity. Secondary walls usually become impregnated also with a noncarbohydrate polymer called *lignin*, which is built up of benzene ring derivatives and adds further to the rigidity of the wall.

As it synthesizes the secondary wall, the cell refrains from depositing wall material upon certain areas of the primary wall where plasmodesmata occur. Thus there are left circular or otherwise shaped unthickened areas which from inside the cell look like depressions in the secondary wall; these depressions are called *pits* (an example is illustrated in Figure 2-6). Besides permitting the maintenance of protoplasmic connections between cells, pits serve other important functions to be explained in later chapters.

Plant cells cannot, as far as is known, break down their secondary walls. The rigidity of the secondary wall and the inability of the cell to attack it mean that the secondary wall cannot be expanded by growth as can the primary wall of a growing cell. This has been considered an important distinction between the secondary wall and certain thickened primary walls which can nevertheless extend during growth as, for example, the walls of sieve tube cells (Chapter 7), collenchyma cells (page 132), and epidermal cells (see below).

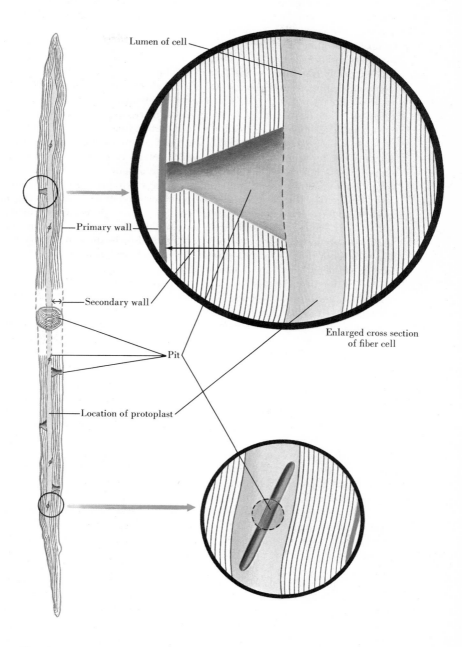

Lumen of cell

Primary wall

Secondary wall

Pit

Location of protoplast

Enlarged cross section
of fiber cell

Fig. 2-6   *A fiber cell in side view and (center) in cross section. Inserts show structure of wall layers and pits. Typical fibers are much more elongated than in the drawing, which omits the midpart of the cell in order to fit onto the page.*

The properties of the cell wall are crucial to many specialized functions in plants. For example, the strength and rigidity of the secondary wall are made use of in the cell called a *fiber* (Figure 2-6), a very elongated cell that may be found in the phloem or the xylem and that develops an extremely thick wall whose microfibrils are oriented nearly in the lengthwise direction, making the cell extremely resistant to extension. The fiber cell serves a specialized role of mechanical support analogous to the skeletal structures of animals. The rigidity of the secondary wall is also essential to the mechanism of water transport in the xylem to be discussed in Chapter 5; furthermore, its conducting cells bear a considerable fraction of the mechanical supporting function.

Another type of wall specialization that is of enormous importance to land plants is the deposition of wax layers which retard evaporative water loss. The *epidermis*, a single layer of cells at the surface of leaves and young stems, develops such a cell wall on its outer side, the waxy exterior layer being called the *cuticle* (page 52). During later growth in thickness of stems and roots the outermost tissue formed (see page 136) is called the *cork*; its cells lay down a secondary wall heavily impregnated with a waxy material called *suberin* that makes the walls not only waterproof but also very tough and resistant to mechanical abrasion. This cork tissue, which is many cells in thickness, constitutes the external surface of the bark of trunks and roots of trees.

The thin primary cell wall of unspecialized plant cells (called *parenchyma* cells) such as shown in Figure 2-4 is not in any sense rigid and will bend or crumple very readily. Yet it strongly resists stretching. By itself this primary wall offers little mechanical support for the cell or the plant. However, when the primary wall is stretched by the cell by turgor forces to be discussed subsequently, its mechanical role becomes very important.

PLANT CELL PROTOPLASM

Cells in the apical growing regions of a plant, as illustrated in Figure 2-3, are almost entirely filled with protoplasm. On the other hand, in a typical mature cell as shown in Figures 2-1 and 2-4 the protoplasm forms only a thin layer next to the cell wall, the entire central volume of the cell being occupied by a watery solution called the *vacuole* which may contain salts, sugars, organic acids, and/or amino acids.

The protoplasm is separated from the cell wall and from the vacuole by *membranes* of submicroscopic thickness called, respectively, the *plasma membrane* and the *vacuolar membrane* (see Figure 2-4). These membranes are highly permeable to water and small molecules such as oxygen, whereas they are virtually impermeable to larger molecules such as salts and sugars as well as to very large molecules like proteins. The plasma membrane permits the cell to maintain a composition different from that of its environment. Because of the vacuolar membrane, the chemical composition of the vacuole may be quite different from that of the protoplasm. Radioisotope tracer experiments show that vacuolated plant cells contain two distinct pools of many of the compounds such as sugars and organic acids that are vitally important in cell chemistry or *metabolism*. One pool is rapidly utilized by the cell in chemical reactions, whereas the second pool, although often much larger in quantity, is not directly accessible to the enzymes responsible for metabolic reactions and appears to represent substances that are held in reserve in the vacuole. This kind of internal separation of cell constituents into functionally separate pools is called *compartmentation.*

Rather commonly the protoplasm of plant cells engages in an easily visible movement or circulation within the cell, a behavior known as *streaming.* Streaming is dependent on normal functioning of the cell, and its occurrence is perhaps the best visible indication that the cell being observed is healthy. Neither the mechanism by which the protoplasm streams nor the functional importance of this activity is at all well understood (see page 22), but it is likely that streaming allows for better exchange of materials between the cell and its surroundings.

Several kinds of particulate structures or *organelles,* some of which are bounded by their own special membranes, are found within the protoplasm. Among these the *nucleus* (Figures 2-1, 2-3, and 2-4) is in a special category. Its DNA (deoxyribonucleic acid) specifies the synthesis of the cell's RNA (ribonucleic acid). By means of this activity the nucleus controls the synthesis of protein by the cell's *ribosomes,* RNA-rich particles that are found in the *cytoplasm,* which refers to the protoplasm outside the nucleus. Many of the cell's ribosomes are found attached to an internal membrane system within the cytoplasm, the *endoplasmic reticulum* (ER), which can be seen in Figures 2-3 and 2-4.

The processes of cellular RNA and protein synthesis are extensively discussed in Novikoff-Holtzman, *Cells and Organelles* and in Levine, *Genetics,* in the Modern Biology Series, and in Loewy-Siekevitz, *Cell Structure and Function* (Holt, 1969), and will therefore not be reviewed here.

ENERGY METABOLISM AND MITOCHONDRIA

A central process in cellular metabolism is *respiration,* the oxidation of sugar to CO_2 and water:

$$C_6H_{12}O_6 + 6O_2 \rightarrow 6CO_2 + 6H_2O + 686 \text{ kilocalories} \quad (2\text{-}1)$$

Glucose   Free energy

Respiration is the means by which cells obtain from sugar the useful chemical energy (adenosine triphosphate or ATP) needed for the maintenance of life and for growth. The ATP energy derived from respiration is used to drive energy-requiring processes within the cell, such as the synthesis of proteins or polysaccharides. In so doing the ATP is split into ADP (adenosine diphosphate) and phosphate, or into AMP (adenosine monophosphate) and two molecules of phosphate. Thus ATP acts as an *energy carrier* between respiratory reactions that release energy and other cellular processes that require energy.

As a result of much biochemical investigation we know that respiration in plant cells takes place in a manner essentially similar to respiration in the cells of animals and microorganisms. Two principal routes have been discovered by which cells can convert sugar into CO_2. These routes are summarized in simplified form in Figure 2-7. These processes are discussed in detail in Novikoff-Holtzman, *Cells and Organelles* and in Loewy-Siekevitz, *Cell Structure and Function;* we shall note here only some basic points that are necessary background for matters to be considered later.

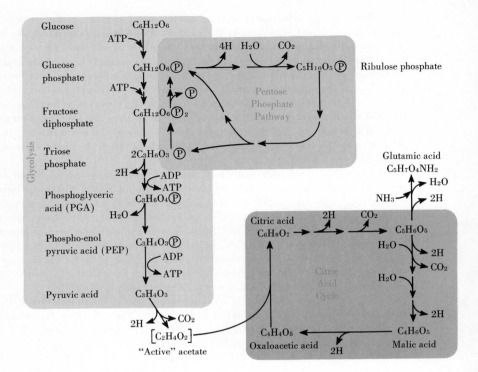

Fig. 2-7   *Carbon pathways of respiration summarized in simplified form with omission of many of the intermediate compounds.* $\textcircled{P}$ *represents phosphate group. Pairs of hydrogen atoms (2H) are transferred to a hydrogen acceptor (usually NAD or NADP) and are passed into the electron transfer chain (Equation 2-2).*

The enzymes responsible for the oxidation of pyruvic acid to CO_2 (the *citric acid cycle* or Krebs cycle pathway) are found to be attached to the membranes of the organelles called *mitochondria* (illustrated in Figures 2-3, 2-4, and 2-8). On the other hand, the enzymes required for the formation of pyruvic acid from glucose phosphate (the pathway called *glycolysis*) and those that are involved in the pentose phosphate or direct oxidation pathway are found free in the cytoplasm outside discrete organelles.

Oxidation of intermediates derived from glucose occurs, in both the direct oxidation pathway and in glycolysis and the citric acid cycle, by the removal of pairs of hydrogen atoms from particular intermediates by specific *dehydrogenase* enzymes. In most cases these enzymes transfer the hydrogen atoms to an essential hydrogen acceptor or "coenzyme" whose name is abbreviated NAD (nicotinamide adenine dinucleotide; some dehydrogenases utilize instead NADP, which is NAD phosphate). This hydrogen transfer *reduces* the coenzyme, producing $NADH_2$ (or $NADPH_2$). Carbon dioxide is formed at steps in which a carboxyl (—COOH) group of an organic acid that was produced by preceding dehydrogenase reactions becomes split off as CO_2.

By means of a separate enzyme system called the *electron transfer chain* or respiratory chain which is bound tightly to the membrane system within the mitochondria, the $NADH_2$ and $NADPH_2$ from dehydrogenase reactions are reoxidized to NAD and NADP by molecular oxygen. Electron transfer is the part of the respiratory process in which most of the chemical energy originally in glucose becomes released. The enzymes of the electron transfer chain in the mitochondria are able to trap a considerable fraction of this energy as ATP energy through the process known as *oxidative phosphorylation.* The overall reaction is

$$NADH_2 + \tfrac{1}{2}O_2 \xrightarrow{\text{Electron transfer chain}} NAD + H_2O$$

$$3ADP + 3H_3PO_4 \quad \overset{\text{Oxidative}}{\underset{\text{phosphorylation}}{\nearrow}} \quad \searrow \quad 3ATP + 3H_2O \qquad (2\text{-}2)$$

In the electron transfer chain hydrogen atoms (or electrons derived from them) from $NADH_2$ or $NADPH_2$ move successively from component to component along the chain and ultimately react with O_2 to form H_2O. The principal components of the electron transfer chain are *flavoprotein* enzymes (which accept hydrogen atoms directly from $NADH_2$); *cytochrome* enzymes including the final member of the chain (cytochrome a_3) which is the component that reacts directly with O_2; and quinones (*coenzyme* Q) which mediate electron transfer between flavoproteins and the cytochromes. Oxidative phosphorylation uses the release of energy in certain of these electron transfer steps to couple phosphate with ADP to make ATP which requires energy. The sequence of electron transfers in the respiratory chain is known (neglecting certain complications and questions) to be

$$NADH_2 \overset{*}{\rightarrow} \text{flavoprotein} \rightarrow \text{coenzyme Q} \rightarrow \text{cytochrome } b \overset{*}{\rightarrow} \text{cytochrome } c \overset{*}{\rightarrow}$$
$$\text{cytochrome } a \rightarrow O_2$$

in which the asterisks designate probable sites of ATP formation.

PLASTIDS   Much more conspicuous than the mitochondria are the *chloroplasts* (Figure 2-1) of a plant cell, which are the seat of photosynthesis. They are present only in the cells of the green parts of the plant; it should be noted that such cells, like the nongreen ones, contain mitochondria and carry on respiration. The structure of the chloroplast will be described in Chapter 3 in connection with the subject of photosynthesis.

Nongreen cells, like the one in Figure 2-4, frequently have colorless plastids (amyloplasts) that synthesize *starch* from sugar. Starch is a polysaccharide built up from glucose units joined together by a different form of linkage than occurs in cellulose. Unlike cellulose, starch is readily broken down to glucose by the cell; starch constitutes a reserve material that can be drawn on to supply glucose when needed for respiration or other processes. Like the synthesis of any polysaccharide, joining glucose molecules together to make starch requires energy which is furnished by ATP. In the mechanism of starch synthesis as

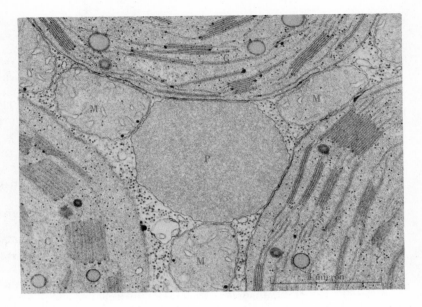

Fig. 2-8 *A microbody of the peroxisome type (P) in cell of a tobacco leaf. The peroxisome is surrounded by three mitochondria (M) and chloroplasts (C); note how the outer membrane of these organelles is double while the membrane of the peroxisome is single. This type of peroxisome is known to contain glycolate oxidase and catalase. (Magnification 29,000×. Courtesy of Dr. Eldon H. Newcomb; from Sue E. Frederick and E. H. Newcomb, Science, 163: 1353, March 21, 1969. Copyright 1969 by the American Association for the Advancement of Science.)*

presently understood, this energy input is effected by coupling ATP with glucose phosphate to produce the "sugar nucleotide" ADP-glucose (adenosine diphosphate glucose). This compound serves as a donor of glucose units for building up the polysaccharide chain. The enzyme (*starch synthetase*) that catalyzes chain synthesis is bound tightly to the starch grains or the surrounding plastid structure. The ADP that is left as a by-product of this reaction is reused by conversion to ATP in oxidative phosphorylation by the mitochondria.

Another class of plastids is *chromoplasts*, which synthesize and retain the brilliant orange, yellow, and red carotenoid pigments (see page 31) that are so characteristic of many flowers and fruits (and some other organs, for example, the carrot root for which the carotenoid class of pigments is named). Chromoplasts develop from previously existing green chloroplasts by a transformation in which the chlorophyll and the internal membrane structure typical of chloroplasts (page 33) disappear and masses of carotenoids accumulate.

In the last few years it has become clear that both chloroplasts and mitochondria contain their own DNA and ribosomes. There is evidence that RNA and protein are synthesized within the chloroplast and that at least some of this is coded for by chloroplast DNA. Interestingly enough the chloroplast ribosomes of higher plants resemble rather closely in size and biochemical properties the ribosomes of bacterial cells and differ distinctly from the somewhat larger ribosomes of the cytoplasm of plant or animal cells. This and other facts have led to the speculation that plastids originated from simple cells like those of blue-green algae to which plant cells became host.

OTHER PLANT CELL ORGANELLES

Microbodies (Glyoxysomes and Peroxisomes)

Microbodies are spherical organelles (Figure 2-8) about the same size as mitochondria but bounded externally by a single membrane (mitochondria have a double membrane); they contain a granular content (sometimes including a crystal or a local dense region) without any internal membranous structure comparable with that of mitochondria. The *peroxisome* contains oxidative enzymes that produce hydrogen peroxide, such as glycolic oxidase which oxidizes the 2-carbon organic acids, glycolic and glyoxylic acid. In addition, peroxisomes contain the enzyme *catalase* whose action decomposes the H_2O_2 produced by oxidases and prevents this toxic oxidant from being released into the cytoplasm. Peroxisomes appear to play a role in the glycolic acid metabolism that is associated with photosynthesis (page 45).

A special type of microbody called the *glyoxysome* contains the enzymes of the *glyoxylate cycle* by which fats are converted into carbohydrate during germination of many seeds (Chapter 10).

Dictyosomes or Golgi Structures

These distinctively shaped ("sheaf of wheat") organelles (Figure 2-3) seem to function in the packaging of cell products for secretion to the outside of the cell as the analogous structures do in animal cells. There is substantial indirect evidence that polysaccharides synthesized for export by many plant cells collect in the *vesicles* (membrane-bounded sacs shaped like minute bubbles) that are formed and pinched off at the margins of the dictyosomes, from which the vesicles migrate to and fuse with the plasma membrane, thereby discharging their contents to the cell exterior. The polysaccharide contents thus become part of the cell wall or of the extracellular mucilage that certain plant cells secrete. It has recently been found that enzymes responsible for synthesis of cell wall polysaccharides are carried by the Golgi membranes of plant cells.

Spherosomes

As their name implies, spherosomes are spherical organelles; they are about the same size as mitochondria (Figure 2-3), but are often more conspicuous than mitochondria under the light microscope because of refractile optical properties. Spherosomes are lipid bodies involved in the storage or transport of lipids in cells.

The term "spherosomes" is also sometimes applied to vesiclelike organelles that contain hydrolytic enzymes such as proteases, nucleases, and phosphatases that are capable of breaking down many cell constituents and structures. These organelles (which may merely be specialized small vacuoles or

Golgi vesicles) are thought to be equivalent to the *lysosomes* of animal cells (see Novikoff-Holtzman, *Cells and Organelles*). The existence and function of lysosomelike organelles in plant cells are suggested by various developmental phenomena of sudden autolysis (breakdown) of cell components. Examples are the breakdown of cell wall components and of the nucleus or entire protoplasm at the conclusion of differentiation of various specialized cells such as vessels and sieve tube cells (Chapters 5 and 7).

Microtubules   Microtubules are organelles that have the form of narrow, hollow, elongated tubes about 25 nm in diameter. They make up the spindle apparatus that functions during nuclear division (see Novikoff-Holtzman, *Cells and Organelles*).

Microtubules are often found in dramatic arrays in the cytoplasm of plant cells immediately next to the plasma membrane, running in a direction parallel to the principal direction of the microfibrils of the adjacent cell wall (Figure 2-9). This observation suggested that the microtubules play a role in the mechanism by which newly synthesized cellulose is oriented for deposition in a definite direction — an important feature of the developmental mechanics of plant cells (page 143).

The cytoplasm of plant cells also contains "microfilaments" which are thinner than microtubules and which may function as the propulsive organelles in protoplasmic streaming.

INTERCELLULAR   A conspicuous feature of most plant tissues is *GAS SYSTEM*   that any given cell is not in contact with neighboring cells at all points, but, particularly at its corners, adjoins seemingly empty *intercellular spaces* (see Figure 2-4). In intact tissue these spaces are typically filled with gas ("air") in contrast to the spaces between cells in animal tissues which are usually filled with liquid. Experiments show that the intercellular spaces of a plant tissue are not isolated gaps between cells but are connected together into an *intercellular gas space system* that penetrates throughout the tissue. The gas space system opens directly into the external air through special openings on the outside of the plant body (*stomates*, page 50, or *lenticels* which are porous regions in the otherwise impervious *cork* tissue comprising the outer bark described above).

The intercellular gas space system is the means by which oxygen for respiration is supplied to cells in the interior of a plant tissue. Diffusion of O_2 in water or in cell fluids is so slow that it would not be possible for cells deep within bulky tissues to obtain enough oxygen to support their respiration if oxygen had to reach them by diffusing through the cells from the outside of the tissue. With the rapidly respiring tissues of larger animals this is, of course, a critical problem that the circulatory system is designed to overcome. But it has been calculated that even in a potato, which is among the slowest respiring and hence least demanding of living tissues, the oxygen concentration would fall to zero

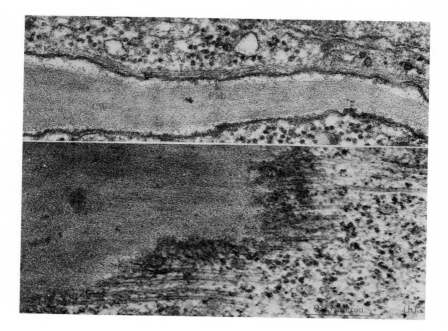

Fig. 2-9 *Cytoplasmic microtubules (M) in plant cells. (a) In growing cell from a pea stem microtubule is located in outer cytoplasm very close to plasma membrane (PM) and surface of cell wall (CW). (b) Microtubules are oriented parallel to the microfibillar material (cellulose) of the cell wall, as seen in a grazing section of a growing cell from root tip of timothy grass (Phleum). Plane of section in (b) is equivalent to a horizontal line cutting through cell wall and outermost cytoplasm in (a), thus microtubules appear to extend away from the cell wall although they are actually running closely parallel to its surface as in (a). Long axis of cell growth was perpendicular to the page in (a), vertical on the page in (b). (Magnification 75,000×. Micrograph (a) by the author; (b) courtesy of Dr. James R. Brennan.)*

scarcely 1 mm beneath the skin if diffusion through the cells from the outside had to supply oxygen to them. Cells deeper within the potato would have no oxygen and would be unable to respire at all.

Analyses show, however, that even in the center of a potato the oxygen concentration is never less than about half that at the very surface next to the outside air. This is because oxygen can diffuse about 300,000 times as fast through air as it can through tissue fluids. Because the intercellular gas space system provides an uninterrupted route for oxygen diffusion in a gas phase directly to the center of the tissue, cells in the center do receive adequate amounts of oxygen by diffusion. Experiments show that if the gas space system of a plant tissue is blocked, for example, by water, cells in the interior quickly become deficient in oxygen. This is why the roots of many trees die when they are flooded.

The gas space system is equally important in supplying CO_2 for photosynthesis. This will be considered in Chapter 4.

WATER BALANCE
OF PLANT CELLS

Whenever a membrane, such as a cell membrane, that is permeable to water but relatively impermeable to dissolved solutes separates two solutions of different solute concentration, there becomes apparent a physically inherent tendency for water to move through the membrane in the direction of the solution of higher solute concentration. This movement of water is called *osmosis*.

Osmosis is often assumed to be simply the diffusion of water molecules from the side of the membrane where their concentration is greater to the side where their concentration is less (that is, where the solute concentration is greater). Biophysical evidence indicates, however, that the mechanism of osmosis can be more complex, involving also *flow* of water through pores in the membrane if it possesses water-filled pores. In the case of one plant cell (the alga *Valonia*) it has been demonstrated that osmotic transport is entirely by diffusion and therefore that its cell membrane does not possess water-filled pores. Other plant cells are, however, much more permeable to water than is *Valonia*, and it seems probable that bulk flow contributes to osmotic transport through their membranes as it is known to do with certain animal cells and artificial osmotic membranes.

Osmosis poses general problems of water balance for cells. A cell in a medium more dilute than its own solute concentration tends to swell up through osmotic absorption of water, whereas in a medium more concentrated than itself the cell tends to shrink as a result of outward movement of water. In experimentation with animal cells a medium having the same solute concentration as the cells is always employed in order to avoid either swelling or shrinking and consequent physiological disruption. Problems of water balance in animals arise because the solute concentration in the external environment is frequently different from that of the animal. The animal must then possess special machinery either for getting rid of the excess water that enters or for counteracting water loss.

Plant cells handle the problem of water balance in a simpler way, which depends on the fact that they have inelastic cell walls. They are adapted to existence in a dilute environment from which they constantly tend to absorb water by osmosis. But they are restrained from swelling up by the cell wall. The result, as in pumping air into a tire, is that osmotic entry of water into the cell builds up hydrostatic *pressure* within the cell against its cell wall. The pressure within the cell is called *turgor pressure* and the cell possessing it is said to be *turgid* (Figure 2-10).

A basic principle of osmosis is that the movement of water through a membrane toward a more concentrated solution can be prevented by applying an appropriately great hydrostatic pressure to that solution. Pressure counteracts the tendency of solutes to cause osmotic entry of water into the solution, and the situation is then one of equilibrium so far as osmosis is concerned. When a plant cell is placed in a dilute medium, water simply continues to enter and stretch the cell until its turgor pressure has built up to the equilibrium value. At this point water uptake automatically ceases and the cell has come into water balance with the dilute environment without swelling appreciably and without itself doing any work.

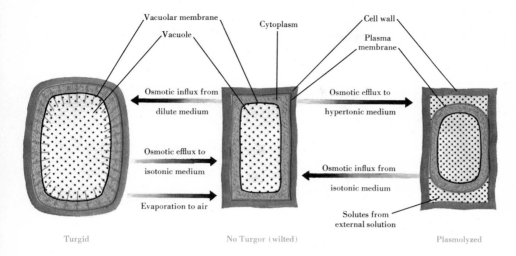

Fig. 2-10   *Osmotic states of a plant cell. Colored arrows denote internal pressure or turgor, dots represent dissolved solutes.*

Because the vacuole constitutes the bulk of the volume of most plant cells, the vacuole plays a dominant role in the cell's osmotic water balance. The solute concentration of the vacuolar solution determines how much turgor pressure will build up when equilibrium with a given dilute medium is reached. Calculation from thermodynamic principles and measurements made both with artificial instruments and with living plant cells show that the pressure in bars (1 bar $= 1$ kg/cm^2, or about equal to atmospheric pressure at sea level) that is required to bring about osmotic equilibrium between a solution and water across a semipermeable membrane is about 24 times the molar concentration of solute particles. Plant cell vacuoles are commonly 0.2 to 0.6 molar in solute concentration; hence they develop pressures up to 5 to 15 bars or about 75 to 220 lb/in.^{2} when in contact with water. That the cells do not burst under such pressures is because of the extraordinary strength of the cell wall (discussed in the first section of this chapter).

The distension of plant cells by turgor pressure is responsible for the crispness or rigidity of most soft tissues of plants, such as leaves and young stems, and is essential to their mechanical support. When turgor pressure is lost, these organs become limp and flabby and are said to *wilt*. The normal ability of the plant cells to maintain a turgor pressure through osmotic absorption of water eliminates the need for a rigid skeleton to support the soft parts of the plant.

Ordinarily, then, osmosis is not the cause of water-balance difficulties for plants. On the contrary, it is the means by which plant cells maintain their water content despite the loss of water to the air that is constantly occurring (Chapter 5).

The plant method of cellular water balance is not designed to cope with an external medium *more concentrated* than the cell itself. When placed into such a medium, the cell not only loses water until its turgor pressure drops to zero, but it then undergoes *plasmolysis* (illustrated in Figure 2-10). As the vacuole shrinks as the result of outward osmosis of water, the protoplasm and plasma membrane are pulled away from the cell wall, leaving part of the cell chamber to be filled with external solution. The fact that the protoplast and not the cell wall contracts shows that it is the cell membranes (plasma membrane, vacuolar membrane) and not the cell wall that are differentially permeable and involved in osmosis. The cell wall itself is rather permeable to solutes and hence does not act as an osmotic membrane.

Temporary plasmolysis is not destructive to the cell. The cell can be restored quickly to its normal turgid condition simply by returning it to a dilute medium or water. However, plasmolysis prevents normal water balance and other functions of the plant as a whole, and thus plants cannot tolerate prolonged exposure to a medium more concentrated than their own cells.

SUGGESTED READING

Beevers, H., *Respiratory Metabolism in Plants*. Evanston, Ill.: Row, Peterson, 1961.

Branton, D., and R. B. Park, *Papers on Biological Membrane Structure*. Boston: Little, Brown, 1968. pp. 1-44, 279-287.

Buvat, R., *Plant Cells. An Introduction to Plant Protoplasm*. New York: McGraw-Hill, 1969.

Esau, K., *Plant Anatomy*, 2d ed. New York: Wiley, 1965. Chapters 2 and 3.

Goldsby, R. A., *Cells and Energy*. New York: Macmillan, 1967. Chapter 4.

Jensen, W. A., *The Plant Cell*. Belmont, Cal.: Wadsworth, 1964.

Jensen, W. A., and R. B. Park, *Cell Ultrastructure*. Belmont, Cal.: Wadsworth, 1967.

O'Brien, T. P., and M. E. McCully, *Plant Structure and Development: A Pictorial and Physiological Approach*. New York: Macmillan, 1969. Chapter 1.

Whittingham, C. P., *The Chemistry of Plant Processes*. New York: Philosophical Library, 1965. Chapters 2-5.

chapter 3

Photosynthesis

Photosynthesis is the conversion of carbon dioxide to organic compounds in the presence of light. The immediate product of photosynthesis is usually sugar or starch and the process can most simply be written as the formation of glucose:

$$6CO_2 + 6H_2O \xrightarrow{\text{Light}} C_6H_{12}O_6 + 6O_2 \qquad (3\text{-}1)$$
$$\text{Glucose}$$

Both glucose and oxygen contain chemical energy in excess of what is contained in CO_2 and water. The most obvious demonstration of this fact is that glucose, like many carbon compounds, will burn in oxygen, giving heat energy in addition to CO_2 and H_2O. Respiration, as we noted in Chapter 2, is an oxidation of glucose to CO_2 and water in which this chemical energy becomes released partly in a form other than heat (ATP) that is useful to the plant or animal.

For the reverse process, the formation of glucose and O_2 *from* CO_2 and water, it is clearly necessary to *provide* energy. Not every source of energy will do; for example, heat itself. The secret of photosynthesis is that the plant cell has found a way to utilize *light* as the source of energy to make conversion of CO_2 to sugar possible.

Photosynthesis, therefore, can go on only in the light, and it has two basic aspects: (1) the conversion of light energy into chemical energy and (2) the conversion of CO_2 into organic compounds, which is called *fixation* of CO_2.

There are also two basic kinds of photosynthesis: (1) the oxygen-producing kind carried out by the chloroplasts of green plants as illustrated by Equation 3-1 and (2) the probably more primitive kind carried out by the photosynthetic bacteria in which no oxygen is produced, but instead some chemical available in the environment (such as H_2S) becomes oxidized as CO_2 becomes reduced to carbohydrate (see Sistrom, *Microbial Life*, Modern Biology Series, pages 61-67). In the 1930s, as a result of a comparative study of the photosynthetic metabolism of different kinds of photosynthetic bacteria, Cornelis Van Niel reasoned that the feature common to all kinds of photosynthesis must be the light-dependent production of some reducing agent or hydrogen donor, H_2X, which acts to reduce carbon dioxide to the carbohydrate level ("CH_2O"):

$$2H_2X + CO_2 \rightarrow (CH_2O) + H_2O + 2X \qquad (3\text{-}2)$$

In the case of green plant photosynthesis it seemed that the source of this hydrogen must be water and therefore that the oxygen produced during photosynthesis must be a by-product derived from water:

$$2H_2O + 2X \xrightarrow{\text{Light}} 2H_2X + O_2 \qquad (3\text{-}3)$$

If we sum this and Equation 3-2, labeling with (*) the oxygen atoms in Equation 3-3, we get

$$CO_2 + 2H_2O^* \rightarrow (CH_2O) + O_2^* + H_2O \qquad (3\text{-}4)$$

which differs from Equation 3-1 in indicating explicitly that the O_2 produced in photosynthesis is derived from water. This was virtually proved some years later by Ruben and Kamen by an experiment in which isotopically (^{18}O) labeled water or CO_2 was fed to photosynthesizing algal cells: $H_2{}^{18}O$ gave $^{18}O_2$, but $C^{18}O_2$ did not.

Hill Reaction   The first success in obtaining part of the photosynthetic machinery in functional form outside the living cell was achieved in England by Robert Hill about 1939. He isolated chloroplasts by centrifugation from ground-up leaves and found that they would produce O_2 in the light, *provided* they were supplied with a reducible substance (hydrogen or electron acceptor) such as ferric ions, ferricyanide, or quinone. This electron acceptor became reduced as oxygen was formed, the electron acceptor serving in fact as an X in Equation 3-3. We have here the part of the photosynthetic system that uses light to produce from water a reducing agent (electrons or hydrogen atoms) and O_2, but we have lost the CO_2-fixing part of it because nothing happens unless the artificial electron acceptor is added to dispose of the reducing agent.

This fragment of the photosynthetic mechanism is called the *Hill reaction* after its discoverer. It was found later that Hill-reaction chloroplast preparations can reduce NADP to NADPH$_2$:

$$2NADP + 2H_2O \xrightarrow[\text{Chloroplasts}]{\text{Light}} 2NADPH_2 + O_2 \quad (3\text{-}5)$$

This activity proved to require a special protein, *ferredoxin*, a nonheme iron protein (that is, protein with simple iron prosthetic group) whose reduced form is the most powerful biological reducing agent known (see page 104). Ferredoxin receives electrons generated by the photochemical process in the chloroplasts and hands these electrons on to NADP during the Hill reaction represented by Equation 3-5.

It turned out that NADPH$_2$ is the reducing agent utilized in photosynthetic CO_2 metabolism; that is, NADPH$_2$ serves as H_2X in Equation 3-2. Therefore NADP is the connecting link between the Hill-reaction part of photosynthesis (Equation 3-3) and the fixation of CO_2.

Photophosphorylation   The two molecules of NADPH$_2$ that are required by Equation 3-2 to reduce one molecule of CO_2 turn out to possess a little less than enough chemical potential energy to do the job. Ruben and Kamen suspected that ATP energy might also be needed, and this has proved to be the case.

Daniel Arnon and Albert Frenkel discovered that chloroplast preparations of the type that can carry out the Hill reaction, and comparable preparations from photosynthetic bacteria, have the ability to make ATP from ADP and phosphate in the light, provided certain electron carriers are added as cofactors. This process is called *photophosphorylation:*

$$ADP + H_3PO_4 \xrightarrow[\text{Cofactors}]{\substack{\text{Chloroplasts} \\ \text{light}}} ATP + H_2O \quad (3\text{-}6)$$

Under optimal conditions the Hill reaction and photophosphorylation proceed simultaneously and apparently coupled to one another:

$$NADP + ADP + H_3PO_4 \xrightarrow[\text{Light}]{\text{Chloroplasts}} NADPH_2 + ATP + \tfrac{1}{2}O_2 \quad (3\text{-}7)$$

One then has in the test tube the entire mechanism by which light energy is transformed into the forms of chemical energy that are needed to drive photosynthetic carbon metabolism.

PHOTOSYNTHETIC Because it was known (Chapter 1) that only the
PIGMENTS green parts of plants, particularly the leaves,
carry on photosynthesis, it has long been be-
lieved that their green pigment *chlorophyll* is involved in photosynthesis. The
kind of experiment by which we can demonstrate conclusively that chlorophyll
participates in photosynthesis is based on the fact that the chlorophyll molecule
absorbs red and blue light strongly while it absorbs green light only weakly. This
is expressed quantitatively as the *absorption spectrum* of chlorophyll, which can
be determined with an instrument called a spectrophotometer, and is plotted in
Figure 3-1.

We now determine the effectiveness of different wavelengths of light in
causing photosynthesis, for example, by shining equally intense beams of light

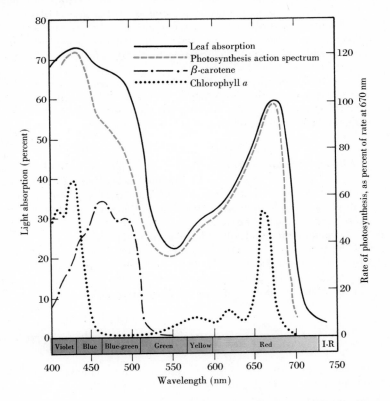

Fig. 3-1 *Comparison of action spectrum for photosynthesis by leaf of* Elodea densa *with
absorption spectrum of the same leaf and absorption spectra of typical chloroplast pigments. For the action spectrum a leaf was irradiated with equal quantum intensities of a
series of different wavelengths and the relative rates of photosynthesis were measured.
(Data courtesy of Dr. Max Hommersand, University of North Carolina.) Lower curves show
absorption spectra of chlorophyll* a *and of β-carotene (a typical carotenoid) obtained after
chemical extraction from the chloroplast. Note that the absorption spectrum of the leaf can
be largely accounted for as the sum of these two types of pigment absorption spectra.*

of a succession of different wavelengths upon a green plant and measuring the rate of photosynthesis at each wavelength. This type of experiment is called an *action spectrum*. The action spectrum for photosynthesis, illustrated by data plotted in Figure 3-1, proves to parallel closely the absorption spectrum of chlorophyll, reaching maximum values at the wavelengths where chlorophyll absorbs most strongly. We must conclude that it is *the light absorbed by chlorophyll* that activates photosynthesis. Chlorophyll serves therefore as the primary absorber of the light energy needed for photosynthesis.

The principal form of chlorophyll has the molecular structure pictured in Figure 3-2. This is called chlorophyll *a*. It occurs in all green plants but not in photosynthetic bacteria, whose photosynthetic pigments have a somewhat different structure and are called *bacteriochlorophylls*. The basis of chlorophyll's structure is the *porphyrin* ring system, composed of the four nitrogen-containing rings and their connecting carbon atoms. This means that chlorophyll is related to the cytochrome enzymes of the respiratory chain (page 19), and to hemoglobin, which are iron porphyrin (heme) proteins. Chlorophyll differs from heme in containing magnesium rather than iron, in the nature of the side groups, and in possessing the extra ring attached to its porphyrin nucleus.

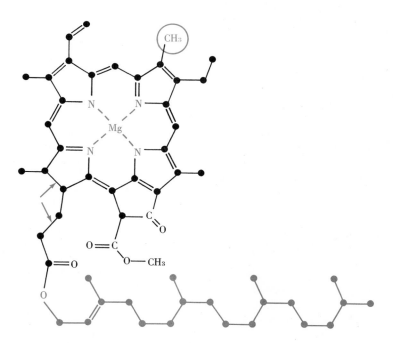

Fig. 3-2 *Structure of chlorophyll* a. *(Carbon atoms with only hydrogens attached are represented by black circles.) Absorption of light is due to the ring system of the molecule. The long* phytol *tail (color) makes the molecule insoluble in water and is important in binding the pigment in the membrane system of the chloroplast. Chlorophyll* b *differs in having an aldehyde group (-CHO) in place of the encircled methyl group (-CH₃). Chlorophyll* c *differs in possessing double bonds in positions indicated by arrows and in lacking the phytol side chain.*

Careful measurements of the absorption spectra of leaves and algal cells have revealed that chlorophyll *a* exists in the chloroplast in at least three principal forms which have absorption peaks at longer wavelengths (670 to 695 nm) than does extracted chlorophyll *a* (660 nm). These forms, which probably represent functional complexes of chlorophyll *a* molecules with one another or with proteins in the chloroplast, are named for their wavelengths of maximum absorption: chlorophyll *a* 673, *a* 683, and *a* 695 (chlorophylls *a* 673 and *a* 683 are usually the major components and occur in about equal amounts). This phenomenon explains why the absorption peak of the leaf in Figure 3-1 is at a somewhat longer wavelength than that illustrated for extracted chlorophyll *a*.

Chloroplasts contain in addition to chlorophyll *a* other pigments called *accessory pigments*. These are of three general types: (1) chemical variants of chlorophyll (chlorophylls *b*, c_1, c_2, *d*) whose presence is restricted to particular plant groups; (2) *carotenoids*, which are yellow pigments related to vitamin A and are found in all chloroplasts; and (3) *phycobilins*, which are red (phycoerythrin) or blue (phycocyanin) protein pigments that occur in the red and blue-green algae (see Delevoryas, *Plant Diversification*). The action spectra for photosynthesis by various algae prove that both carotenoids and phycobilins can act as absorbers of light for photosynthesis. Evidence indicates that the accessory pigments function by transferring the absorbed energy to forms of chlorophyll *a*.

STRUCTURE OF THE
CHLOROPLAST

What is there about chlorophyll in the chloroplast that enables it to convert light energy into chemical energy? When chemically extracted out of the chloroplast, chlorophyll loses all but the feeblest indications of its biological activity. The explanation is probably that the effectiveness of chlorophyll depends upon the way it is organized within the chloroplast.

Figure 3-3 shows a cross section of a chloroplast as seen with the electron microscope. Inside the chloroplast is an elaborate system of paired membranes, with the members of each pair connecting at their edges to form a flattened, disclike structure with a completely enclosed internal space. This structure is called a *thylakoid*. The thylakoid membranes prove to contain the chlorophyll and carotenoid pigments. In the chloroplasts of vascular plants (as in Figure 3-3) the thylakoids are stacked up to form aggregates somewhat like piles of coins; these stacks are called *grana* (sing., *granum*) and are often large enough to be visible with the light microscope, as in some of the chloroplasts in Figure 2-1. The grana are interconnected through the *stroma* region that separates them by less numerous lamellae that are extensions of some of the thylakoid membranes (see Figure 3-3). Chloroplasts of most algae do not exhibit the grana type of organization; their thylakoids run more or less from end to end. In the cells of blue-green algae, which do not possess distinct chloroplasts, comparable membrane structures bearing the photosynthetic pigments are simply found dispersed in the cytoplasm.

The dense aggregation of chlorophyll and accessory pigments within the thylakoid membranes appears to be important to the process of energy capture. It makes possible energy transfer between accessory pigments and chlorophyll *a*, a phenomenon noted previously. It also makes possible efficient transfer of energy between chlorophyll molecules themselves, which seems to be essential for efficient operation of photosynthesis as will be discussed subsequently (page 36). The enclosed nature of the thylakoid spaces is also believed to be important in the mechanism of photosynthesis, for example, by permitting a physical separation of the oxidizing intermediates of photosynthesis (that lead to O_2) from the reducing intermediates required for conversion of CO_2 to sugar (H_2X in Equation 3-2).

Face views of the thylakoid membranes (Figure 3-4) reveal the presence of a dense array of globular particles within each membrane. These particles are believed to be protein; they consist of two types, about 11 nm and 17.5 nm in diameter. It is thought that they may represent functional unit structures of photosynthesis (to be discussed later) and they have therefore been called "quantasomes."

The chloroplast is bounded on the outside by a *double* membrane somewhat comparable to that which delimits mitochondria. This external membrane shows osmotic properties and hence must be differentially permeable. The chloroplast membrane is delicate compared with the thylakoids and is easily disrupted. Such disruption allows essential enzymes and cofactors of photosynthesis to escape, particularly those concerned with the conversion of CO_2 into sugar. This explains why chloroplast preparations of the Hill-reaction type are unable to fix CO_2 (page 29). Photosynthetic CO_2 fixation appears therefore to occur in the stroma region outside the thylakoid spaces.

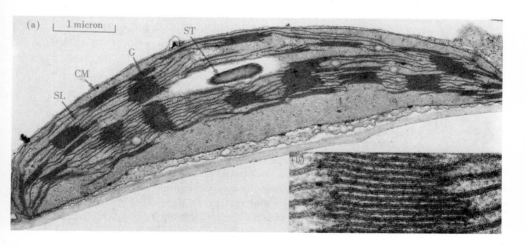

Fig. 3-3   *Electron micrographs of chloroplast of* Atriplex patula. *(a) Whole chloroplast showing grana stacks (G), stroma lamellae (SL), starch grain (ST), and chloroplast membrane (CM). (Magnification 16,700X.) (b) Single grana stack showing enclosed nature of the thylakoids and connections between thylakoid membranes and stroma lamellae. (Magnification 107,000×. Micrographs by author and Margery M. Ray.)*

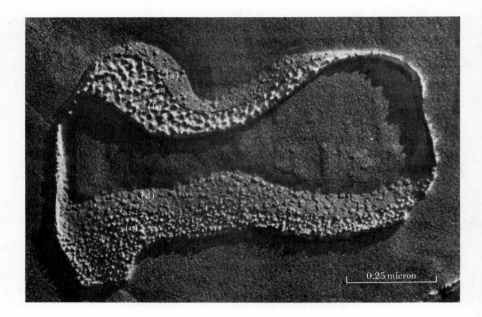

Fig. 3-4 *Particulate structure of thylakoid membranes of spinach chloroplast as revealed by the "freeze-fracture" method. The thylakoid suspension was quick frozen, the ice block was then split and a replica of the fractured surface was prepared and examined by electron microscopy. The illustration shows one complete thylakoid that passes obliquely through the ice surface and shows (a) outside surface; (b) 17.5 nm particles exposed by fracturing from outer surface; (c) 11 nm particles exposed by fracturing from the inner surface; (d) inner surface of thylakoid membrane (facing enclosed thylakoid space). (Magnification 100,000×. Courtesy of Dr. Roderic Park, University of California. See R. B. Park and A. O. Pfeifhofer,* Journal of Cell Science, **5:** *299, 1969).*

ENERGY CAPTURE AND CONVERSION Light energy is transmitted in units called *quanta*. Each quantum possesses a specific amount of energy determined by the wavelength of the light of which the quantum is a part. Absorption of light by a pigment such as chlorophyll amounts to the absorption by the pigment molecule of one quantum with its unit amount of energy.

Absorption of a quantum by a molecule raises the molecule (actually, one of its electrons) to an energetic "excited state" designated by an asterisk:

Absorption: chlorophyll + quantum → chlorophyll*

(3-8)

Decay: heat ←

The excited state is very short-lived (extremely small fraction of a second), and in the case of ordinary pigments it decays back to the normal state of the pigment molecule, releasing its energy as heat (or partly as light). The same thing happens with chlorophyll in solution. But somehow in the chloroplast the energy of the excited state is in part turned into chemical energy through some physical process and/or chemical reaction; this energy transformation is called the *primary process* of photosynthesis and is also referred to as the process of *quantum conversion*.

It is generally believed today that quantum conversion takes place by the reaction of an excited electron from chlorophyll with a specific enzyme or other electron acceptor located in or at the surface of the thylakoid membrane. This electron transfer *reduces* the electron acceptor and forms from the latter the *primary reducing agent*, whose formation represents conversion of physical into chemical energy. This can be written as

$$\underset{\substack{\text{Excited}\\ \text{state of}\\ \text{chlorophyll}}}{\text{Chl*}} \quad + \quad \underset{\substack{\text{Primary}\\ \text{electron}\\ \text{acceptor}}}{\text{X}} \quad \xrightarrow[\text{from Chl* to X}]{\text{Transfer of }(e^-)^*} \quad \underset{\substack{\text{Primary}\\ \text{reducing}\\ \text{agent}}}{\text{X}^-} \quad + \quad \underset{\substack{\text{Oxidized}\\ \text{chlorophyll}\\ (\text{"hole"})}}{\text{Chl}^+} \qquad (3\text{-}9)$$

This primary reducing agent is able, indirectly, to reduce NADP as will be explained below.

When the electron is captured by the primary electron acceptor, there is left behind a plus charge or "hole." This hole is equivalent to oxidizing power. At the surface of the thylakoid membrane the hole probably removes an electron from (oxidizes) a specific enzyme or substrate, producing from the latter the *primary oxidant*:

$$\underset{\text{"Hole"}}{\text{Chl}^+} \quad + \quad \underset{\substack{\text{Electron}\\ \text{donor}}}{\text{Y}} \quad \xrightarrow[\text{from Y to Chl}^+]{\text{Electron transfer}} \quad \underset{\substack{\text{Primary}\\ \text{oxidant}}}{\text{Y}^+} \quad + \quad \underset{\substack{\text{Normal}\\ \text{chlorophyll}}}{\text{Chl}} \qquad (3\text{-}10)$$

The primary oxidant removes electrons from water to form O_2 and is thereby disposed of:

$$Y^+ + \tfrac{1}{2}H_2O \rightarrow Y + \tfrac{1}{4}O_2 + H^+ \qquad (3\text{-}11)$$

The primary reducing agent must transfer its electron to some electron acceptor, such as any of the artificial electron acceptors that permit a Hill reaction to occur (page 28). The natural electron acceptor is apparently ferredoxin (Fd) from which electrons can be transferred to NADP, thus reducing it to $NADPH_2$:

$$2X^- \diagdown \quad \diagup 2Fd(Fe^{3+}) \diagdown \quad \diagup NADPH_2$$

$$\qquad (3\text{-}12)$$

$$2X \diagup \quad \diagdown 2Fd(Fe^{2+}) \diagup \quad \diagdown NADP + 2H^+$$

Each pair of coupled arrows in this equation represents a transfer of two electrons.

The sum of Equations 3-8 through 3-12 gives Equation 3-5, the Hill reaction using NADP as electron acceptor. This elementary explanation of the quantum conversion process is summarized by the diagram in Figure 3-5. According to this scheme one quantum gives rise to one hydrogen atom of reducing power for fixation of CO_2. Since as shown in Equation 3-2 four hydrogen atoms are required to reduce one molecule of CO_2 to the carbohydrate level, four quanta should be required to fix one molecule of CO_2. This is satisfactory from the energetic point of view, for 4 mole quanta of red light (40 kcal. per mole) are equivalent to $4 \times 40 = 160$ kcal of energy, whereas fixation of 1 mole of CO_2 requires 686/6 or only 114 kcal (see Equation 2-1). However, careful measurements that were made first by Robert Emerson in the 1930s and have been repeated and improved again and again over the years show that under the most efficient conditions that can be obtained with algal cells or leaves, one CO_2 is fixed for every eight to ten quanta that are absorbed. This suggests that two quanta may be required for each hydrogen atom of reducing power used in photosynthesis and therefore that two photochemical acts may be involved in the generation of each such hydrogen atom. Other evidence that this is the case is discussed below, but nevertheless each of the photo-acts can be described as a process similar to Equations 3-8 through 3-10 considered previously.

Photosynthetic   Robert Emerson and William Arnold discovered
Unit and   another unexpected feature of the photosynthetic
Reaction Center   machinery. They studied the utilization of light
energy by chloroplasts after exposure to brief flashes of intense light and determined that the maximum photosynthetic yield was equivalent to one quantum for about every 400 chlorophyll molecules. Because every chlorophyll molecule is equally capable of capturing a quantum and because during steady photosynthesis in low-intensity light quanta are utilized with an efficiency much greater than 1 in 400, Emerson and Arnold concluded that the system must consist of "photosynthetic units" each comprised of several hundred chlorophyll molecules from any of which the energy of an absorbed quantum can be funneled to one "reaction center" where the quantum conversion process takes place.

To make this argument fully persuasive would take us well beyond the scope of this discussion, but various independent lines of evidence have subsequently supported the concept of the photosynthetic unit as an aggregate of pigment molecules that are spread, as it were, as an antenna to provide the maximum probability of capture of a quantum for the reaction center that they collectively feed.

The reaction center itself has been detected in at least two ways. Measurements of changes in the absorption spectrum of chloroplasts or of green cells after brief flashes of light reveal a pigment, named P700 because its absorption peak is at or near 700 nm, which responds to illumination by becoming oxidized as required in Equation 3-9. P700 appears to be a long-wave absorbing form of chlorophyll *a* (similar to chlorophyll *a* 695 mentioned on page 32). It is found to occur in the ratio of 1 to about every 400 molecules of total chlorophyll, as expected if it is the reaction center of the photosynthetic unit.

A second method that reveals the quantum conversion process is electron spin resonance (ESR) measurement. This detects unpaired electrons such as occur when an organic molecule loses one electron as in Equation 3-9. Light is

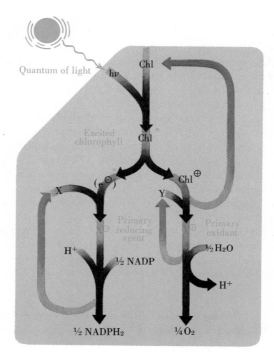

Fig. 3-5 *Elementary diagram of quantum conversion as an oxidation–reduction process involving loss of an electron from excited chlorophyll molecule. Note that by current thinking the formation of oxygen actually requires a second quantum conversion act (pages 37–41).*

found to induce in photosynthetic cells an ESR signal that corresponds to the oxidation of P700, again in the proportion of one oxidized pigment to about 400 chlorophylls.

TWO-PHOTOREACTION MECHANISM Much of the contemporary research activity in photosynthesis has grown out of an observation made by Robert Emerson about 1958. He had found earlier that when plants are illuminated only with light wavelengths on the upper side of the long-wave (red) absorption peak of chlorophyll (that is, with λ > 680 nm, see Figure 3-1) many more quanta had to be used to bring about fixation of a molecule of CO_2 than were required when using shorter wavelengths in the visible spectrum. His new finding was that if to a beam of such long-wave light he added a beam (of comparable intensity) of shorter-wave light (such as blue), then the quanta of long-wave red light became used as efficiently as if they themselves were of shorter wavelength. This phenomenon was called "enhancement" and became known as the Emerson effect. It sounds like an abstruse and academic observation, but Emerson and others realized that it might mean that photosynthesis requires two photoreactions only one of which can be sensitized by the long-wave forms of chlorophyll *a* (*a* 683 and/or *a* 695).

Emerson and others performed action spectrum experiments which indicated that the enhancement effect in the green alga *Chlorella* was due to chlorophyll *a* 670 and to chlorophyll *b*. In algae that do not possess chlorophyll *b* the enhancement effect was found to be attributable in each case to their principal accessory pigments, that is, phycocyanin and phycoerythrin in the case of blue-green and red algae, fucoxanthin (a carotenoid) and chlorophyll *c* in the case of brown algae, as well as to chlorophyll *a* 670. Examples of action spectrum data for enhancement in different algae are shown in Figure 3-6 and are compared with absorption data for the accessory pigments typical of these organisms.

These findings and other evidence led to the view that chlorophyll *a* 683 and *a* 695 are the principal light absorbers for one photoreaction (called System I) and that chlorophyll *a* 670 and accessory pigments (chlorophyll *b*, carotenoids, phycobilins) are the light absorbers for a second photoreaction (called System II, or the "short-wave" system since the absorption of its pigments does not extend to as long a wavelength as does that of System I, the "long-wave" system).

Photosynthetic Electron Transfer Chain

Hill (discoverer of the Hill reaction) and Bendall first proposed in 1960 the "series" explanation for the two photoreactions that is illustrated in Figure 3-7 and has since been adopted by most workers in the field. The diagram is plotted in relation to oxidation-reduction potential so as to show that System I is supposed to use quanta of light to generate a strong reductant (X^-) which can reduce ferredoxin (Fd) and thence reduce NADP to $NADPH_2$. This loss of an electron from System I leaves behind a weak oxidant that has been identified with the oxidized form ($P700^+$) of P700 mentioned above (page 36). P700 is apparently the reaction center for the photosynthetic units operative in System I. In this quantum conversion process P700 loses an electron to X exactly as explained in Equation 3-9. However, the resulting oxidized pigment $P700^+$ is much too weak an oxidizing agent to remove an electron from water to produce O_2.

The function of System II is to provide an electron to fill the "hole" in System I, in other words, to reduce $P700^+$. System II uses a quantum of light to generate a relatively weak reductant (Q^-) and a strong oxidant (Y^+) which is capable of oxidizing water to O_2 (Equations 3-10 and 3-11). Q^- is, however, a sufficiently strong reductant that it can donate an electron to $P700^+$ in System I. As of this writing the reaction center of System II has not been conclusively identified but is probably a relatively long-wave form of chlorophyll *a*. The metal manganese is specifically involved in oxygen production by System II. The participating manganese apparently serves to make the oxidized reaction center (Y^+ in Figure 3-7) a strong enough oxidant to remove electrons from H_2O.

Hill and Bendall placed Systems I and II relative to one another on the redox potential scale in Figure 3-7 primarily on the basis of their knowledge of the oxidation-reduction potentials of cytochromes *f* and b_6, which are characteristic components of chloroplasts in the discovery and characterization of which

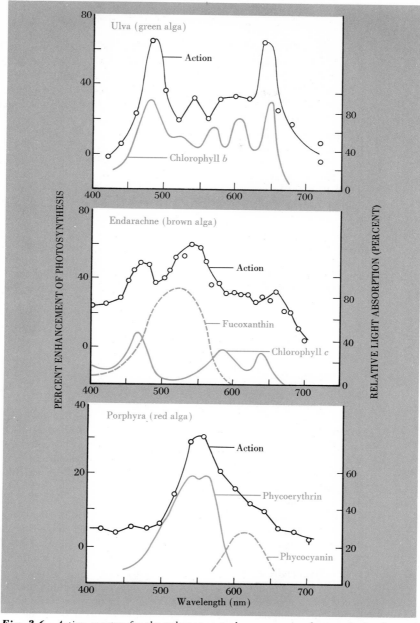

Fig. 3-6 *Action spectra for the enhancement phenomenon in photosynthesis of green, brown, and red algae, compared with absorption characteristics of their principal accessory pigments. Action spectra show the percent increase in photosynthetic action of light of a wavelength that is absorbed principally by chlorophyll a (680 nm in upper two curves, 436 nm in lower curve) which resulted from exposing the plants to different wavelengths of supplementary light. (Data of David C. Fork, from* Photosynthetic Mechanisms in Green Plants. *National Academy of Sciences, 1963, page 352). Absorption curves show fraction of absorbed light (of each wavelength) that is trapped by the given accessory pigment (this corrects the pigment's absorption spectrum for screening by chlorophyll a).*

Hill had played a major role. Hill and Bendall supposed that the cytochromes must be acting in electron transfer between System II and System I. According to the scheme electron transfer will be energetically "downhill," therefore spontaneous from Q^- via the cytochromes to $P700^+$. Subsequent investigation, which has mushroomed into literally hundreds of articles since the basic notions of Figure 3-7 were put forth, has substantiated these ideas and has provided evidence for the position of several other electron carriers in the Hill-reaction system as indicated in Figure 3-7. Despite the massive effort, however, opinion remains divided at the time of this writing regarding the exact role of a number of the chloroplast electron carriers, and even the identity of the two photosystems is disputed by some authors. Therefore the scheme given in Figure 3-7 should be regarded as an illustrative, tentative model rather than a conclusive description of the electron transfer mechanism in photosynthesis.

Techniques have been devised by which disrupted thylakoid membranes can be separated into two subfractions that contain principally System I and System II, respectively. From electron micrographic observations on these preparations it has been inferred that the 17.5 nm "quantasomes" (Figure 3-4) are characteristic of System I, and the 11 nm particles are a component of System II.

Photophosphorylation   The two-photoreaction scheme (Figure 3-7) offers an explanation for the energy source for photophosphorylation. The transfer of electrons through the electron transfer chain between Q^- and $P700^+$, which involves cytochromes, is sufficiently exergonic to generate ATP in the same way as the mitochondrial electron transfer chain does (page 19). It is evident from Figure 3-7 that if there is a phosphorylating (ATP generating) site between Q^- and $P700^+$, ATP will be formed as electrons flow from System II to System I during the reduction of NADP in the Hill reaction (Equation 3-7). ATP can also be formed *without* simultaneous reduction of NADP and evolution of oxygen (Equation 3-6). This is called "cyclic" photophosphorylation because it is due to a cyclical electron flow within the photosynthetic electron transfer chain. Cyclic photophosphorylation is induced by long-wave red light and is therefore due to operation of System I. As suggested in Figure 3-7, some of the electron transfer components of chloroplasts are thought to be involved specifically in this cyclic electron flow.

A lively argument has developed regarding the possibility that the formation of ATP by photophosphorylation occurs not during an electron transfer step (that is, a phosphorylating site as represented in Figure 3-7) but instead as a result of a hydrogen ion concentration difference between the interior of the thylakoids and the exterior. Light induces a demonstrable uptake of hydrogen ions by chloroplast preparations from the medium surrounding them; this uptake is due to operation of the chloroplast electron transfer chain. Several kinds of experiments suggest strongly that a hydrogen ion concentration difference between the chloroplast interior and its surroundings can cause phosphorylation by chloroplasts. However, both the "chemical" (phosphorylating site) and "chemios-

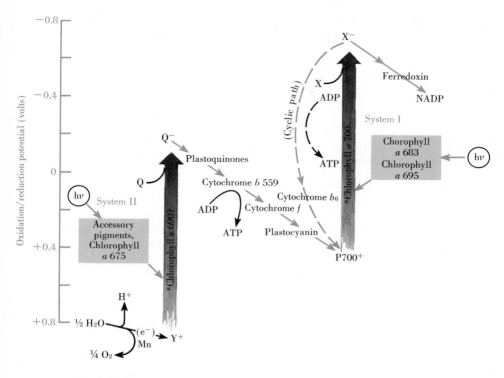

Fig. 3-7   *Energy and electron flow in photosynthesis as visualized in the two-photoreaction theory, showing positions of various electron carriers on the redox potential scale (more negative = more strongly reducing). Dashed arrow represents one possible route of electron flow in cyclic photophosphorylation. Opinions differ regarding the exact position of some of the electron carriers and sites of ATP formation.*

motic" (H^+ transport) theories of photophosphorylation have their adherents and supporting evidence, and it remains to be seen how this issue may be resolved.

PHOTOSYNTHETIC CARBON METABOLISM   Our knowledge about the means by which CO_2 is brought into organic combination in photosynthesis was gained largely through the use of radioactive tracers to follow the process within living plant cells. This approach was made necessary by the fact that photosynthetic carbon metabolism, unlike fermentation and respiration, until relatively recently resisted all attempts to isolate it in a functional condition outside living cells.

When $^{14}CO_2$ is supplied to green cells in the light, it becomes metabolized as does ordinary $^{12}CO_2$, and radioactivity appears in every compound into which CO_2 is being incorporated during photosynthesis. The problem of trying to identify what compounds become radioactive during photosynthesis in $^{14}CO_2$ was undertaken in the late 1940s by a group led by Melvin Calvin at the University of California. They used the unicellular algae *Chlorella* and *Scenedesmus* for most of their experiments and found that even within one minute radioactivity appears in a great variety of compounds inside the cells, including sugars and sugar phosphates, amino acids, and organic acids.

Primary CO₂ In order to determine what compounds are
Fixation Process formed directly from CO_2, Calvin and his collaborators had to devise methods of exposing photo-
synthesizing algae to $^{14}CO_2$ for only a few seconds. They then found that the first compound to become radioactive is *phosphoglyceric acid* (PGA), the 3-carbon acid that was already well known as an intermediate in glycolysis of sugar (Figure 2-7). It was further found that almost all the radioactivity in the PGA formed during a short period of exposure to $^{14}CO_2$ was located in the carboxyl (—COOH) group of PGA (see structural formulas at right side of Equation 3-13). Thus it appeared that this carboxyl group had been formed by adding CO_2 onto an "acceptor" molecule. Careful study of the other compounds that become radioactive during photosynthesis in $^{14}CO_2$ led to the conclusion that the CO_2 acceptor is a 5-carbon sugar phosphate, *ribulose diphosphate*. It takes on CO_2 and splits to give two molecules of PGA, and hence six organic carbon atoms where there were five before:

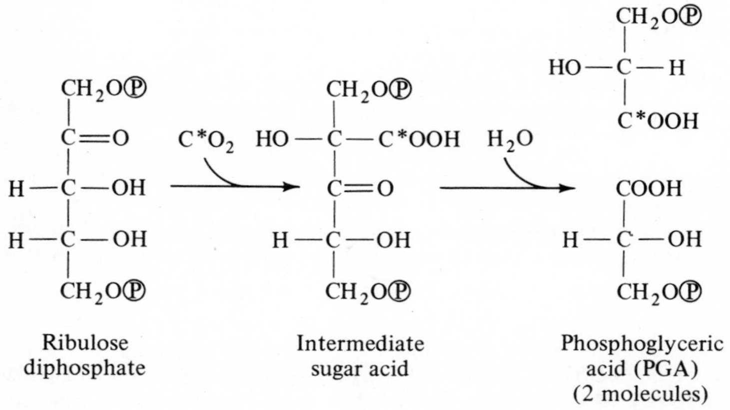

$$
\begin{array}{ccccccc}
& & & & & & CH_2O\textcircled{P} \\
& & & & & & | \\
& & & & & HO-C-H \\
CH_2O\textcircled{P} & & & CH_2O\textcircled{P} & & & | \\
| & & & | & & & C^*OOH \\
C=O & C^*O_2 & HO-C-C^*OOH & H_2O & & \\
| & \longrightarrow & | & \longrightarrow & & COOH \\
H-C-OH & & C=O & & & | \\
| & & | & & H-C-OH \\
H-C-OH & & H-C-OH & & & | \\
| & & | & & & CH_2O\textcircled{P} \\
CH_2O\textcircled{P} & & CH_2O\textcircled{P} & & &
\end{array}
\qquad (3\text{-}13)
$$

| Ribulose diphosphate | Intermediate sugar acid | Phosphoglyceric acid (PGA) (2 molecules) |

The asterisks show how the carboxyl group of one of the two molecules of PGA has been formed from CO_2. Reaction 3-13 is catalyzed by the enzyme *ribulose diphosphate carboxylase*. This reaction is notable in being rather exergonic, so it fixes CO_2 (goes from left to right) without need of an external energy input.

To complete the photosynthetic process, PGA must be converted into sugar. In addition the CO_2 acceptor, ribulose diphosphate, must be regenerated as fast as it is used up in the CO_2-fixing reaction shown above.

***Production
of Sugar
from PGA*** Formation of sugar was found to occur by a sequence of reactions that is practically the reverse of the early reactions of glycolysis (Figure 2-7), that is, the reverse of reactions by which sugar is converted into PGA during respiration. First PGA is reduced by hydrogen atoms from $NADPH_2$ to *triose phosphate* (3-carbon sugar phosphate) with the help of the enzyme *triose phosphate dehydrogenase*. To reduce PGA to triose phosphate, ATP energy (in addition to $NADPH_2$) must be added:

$$
\begin{array}{c}
\text{COOH} \\
| \\
\text{H}-\text{C}-\text{OH} \\
| \\
\text{CH}_2\text{O}\textcircled{P} \\
\text{Phosphoglyceric} \\
\text{acid (PGA)}
\end{array}
+ NADPH_2 + ATP \rightarrow
\begin{array}{c}
\text{CHO} \\
| \\
\text{H}-\text{C}-\text{OH} \\
| \\
\text{CH}_2\text{O}\textcircled{P} \\
\text{Triose} \\
\text{phosphate}
\end{array}
+ NADP + ADP + H_3PO_4 \quad (3\text{-}14)
$$

Calvin and his collaborators obtained evidence that conversion of PGA to triose phosphate is *driven by light*. This is explainable on the basis that the Hill reaction produces $NADPH_2$ and photophosphorylation produces ATP as discussed above, and these compounds drive Equation 3-14 from left to right. This is the point at which chemical energy and hydrogen derived from light are introduced into carbohydrates during photosynthesis.

The light-driven formation of triose phosphate from PGA (Equation 3-14) makes it possible for the early reactions of glycolysis to go in reverse, that is, upward in Figure 2-7, which leads to the production of 6-carbon sugars from triose phosphate.

***Formation of
CO₂ Acceptor*** Calvin and his co-workers deduced how the CO_2 acceptor (ribulose diphosphate) is formed by extensive study of how radioactivity goes into various sugar phosphates that become radioactive during photosynthesis in $^{14}CO_2$. It turned out that ribulose *mono*phosphate can be formed from triose and fructose phosphates by a rather complicated series of reactions that interconvert 3-, 4-, 5-, 6-, and 7-carbon sugar phosphates by transfer of 2-carbon units from one to another. Ribulose monophosphate is converted into the ribulose diphosphate needed as CO_2 acceptor by transfer of phosphate from ATP which is derived in turn from photophosphorylation. The net effect is a *cycle* in which ribulose diphosphate is used (in CO_2 capture) and regenerated (from other sugar phosphates) while as the cycle operates the excess of 6-carbon sugar phosphates that is produced gets siphoned off as the final products of photosynthesis such as sucrose or starch.

This photosynthetic carbon cycle has been named the *reductive pentose phosphate cycle*. It is depicted in much simplified form in Figure 3-8. This cycle is actually in large part a reversal of the pentose phosphate pathway of respiration (Figure 2-7). Most of the enzymes required for the photosynthetic cycle and the oxidative pentose phosphate pathway of respiration are the same but the carboxylation of ribulose diphosphate to PGA and its reduction to triose phos-

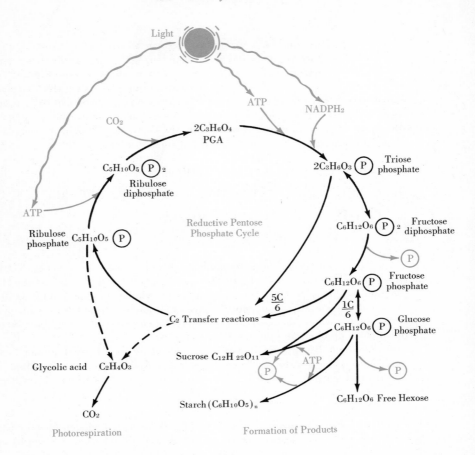

Fig. 3-8 *Simplified diagram of the carbon pathway of photosynthesis (reductive pentose phosphate cycle or C-3 pathway), omitting many intermediate compounds.* Ⓟ *denotes phosphate group. The fractions 5C/6 and 1C/6 indicate the proportion of carbon atoms that continue through the cycle and that are diverted to formation of ultimate photosynthetic products, respectively. Presumed origin of CO_2 in photorespiration (page 45) is also indicated.*

phate are different from the oxidative and decarboxylating processes of the respiratory pentose phosphate pathway.

The reductive pentose phosphate cycle as a whole is driven in the clockwise direction by (1) the input of ATP energy and reducing power at the step at which PGA is reduced to triose phosphate, (2) the utilization of ATP in the regeneration of ribulose diphosphate from its monophosphate, and (3) the splitting off (hydrolysis) of phosphate groups at certain steps. This hydrolysis is exergonic, and is indirectly at the expense of ATP energy because the phosphate groups being split off are ones that were previously introduced at step (2) just mentioned. In these ways the input of energy as $NADPH_2$ and ATP from the Hill reaction and photophosphorylation, respectively, drives the conversion of CO_2 into the carbohydrate products of photosynthesis.

Arnon's and Bassham's groups ultimately devised methods gentle enough to extract chloroplasts from leaves without breaking the chloroplast's outer membrane. Such chloroplasts (unlike the usual Hill-reaction chloroplast preparations) retain the capacity for photosynthetic CO_2 fixation, and $^{14}CO_2$ experiments show that they metabolize CO_2 by the same pathway as does the intact cell.

Photorespiration   The 2-carbon acid *glycolic acid* ($HOCH_2COOH$) rapidly becomes labeled when $^{14}CO_2$ is fed to photosynthesizing organisms. Most photosynthetic cells possess a glycolic oxidase enzyme system, which recent research shows is contained in a special organelle, the peroxisome (page 21), and can oxidize glycolic acid ultimately to CO_2. It appears that much of the glycolic acid that is formed during photosynthesis becomes rapidly reoxidized to CO_2 and this process contributes to a light-stimulated component of green cell respiration that is called "photorespiration." As much as 30 percent of the photosynthetically fixed carbon may thereby be "recycled" to CO_2 and the energy that was expended to fix it becomes in effect wasted.

The glycolic acid that is involved in photosynthesis probably arises by breakdown of ribulose diphosphate or of the 2-carbon intermediate in the reductive pentose phosphate cycle (page 43). The function of photorespiration may simply be to clean up and get rid of the carbon that becomes lost as glycolic acid from the photosynthetic cycle by this troublesome breakdown.

Certain plants, notably corn (maize) and sugar cane, various other tropical grasses, and members of a few other plant groups do not exhibit photorespiration. Consequently they waste none of their photosynthetically fixed CO_2 and as a consequence these plants are substantially more efficient in photosynthesis than normal plants are at high light intensities or low CO_2 concentrations. This helps make corn and sugar cane among the highest yielding of all crops relative to input of solar energy.

C-4 Photosynthesis   Radioisotope experiments with leaves of sugar cane, maize, and other plants that lack photorespiration indicate that their primary CO_2 fixation product is not PGA but the 4-carbon organic acid *oxaloacetic acid* which is familiar as an intermediate in the citric acid cycle (Figure 2-7). The CO_2 acceptor for this fixation process is the phosphate derivative of pyruvic acid, phosphoenol-pyruvate, abbreviated PEP (which is also an intermediate in glycolysis, see Figure 2-7):

$$
\begin{array}{c}
COOH \\
| \\
C\!-\!O \sim \textcircled{P} + C^*O_2 \xrightarrow[\;H_2O\;]{PEP\ carboxylase} \\
|| \\
CH_2
\end{array}
\qquad
\begin{array}{c}
COOH \\
| \\
C\!=\!O \quad + H_3PO_4 \\
| \\
CH_2 \\
| \\
^*COOH
\end{array}
\qquad (3\text{-}15)
$$

PEP   Oxaloacetic   Inorganic
                                          acid   phosphate

Because the high-energy phosphate group of PEP becomes split off, Reaction 3-15 is strongly exergonic and very effectively fixes CO_2.

During $^{14}CO_2$ feeding of corn or sugar cane leaves radioactive carbon appears rapidly in the C-4 acids malic (see Figure 2-7) and aspartic acid, which are formed directly from oxaloacetic by reduction, and addition of NH_3 in the case of aspartic which is an amino acid. Soon ^{14}C appears in PGA, apparently by transfer of carbon from one of these C-4 acids to a secondary acceptor which may be ribulose diphosphate, that is, a reaction like Equation 3-13 but with the added carbon atom coming from a C-4 acid. Isotope data indicate that conversion of PGA to sugar occurs by way of the same kind of reductive pentose phosphate cycle as is involved in normal photosynthesis.

This modified kind of photosynthesis in which 4-carbon acids formed via Reaction 3-15 are the primary CO_2 fixation products is called the "C-4 pathway" of photosynthesis, and plants possessing it are now commonly referred to as "C-4 plants," as against "C-3 plants" in which PGA (a 3-carbon acid) is the primary fixation product. The leaves of C-4 plants contain very high levels of PEP carboxylase (Equation 3-15) compared with C-3 plants. C-4 leaves also contain a special enzyme (pyruvate–phosphate dikinase) for ATP-dependent regeneration of the CO_2 acceptor PEP from the pyruvic acid that is released when carbon is transferred from C-4 acids to the reductive pentose phosphate cycle.

It is not clear from what has been said why C-4 plants lack photorespiration since as explained previously photorespiration seems to be a side result of operation of the reductive pentose phosphate cycle and this cycle is responsible

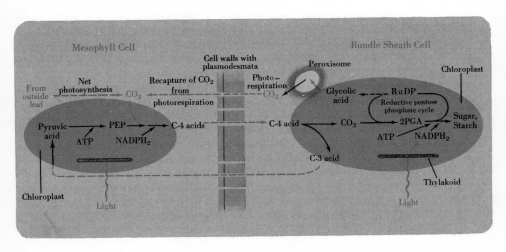

Fig. 3-9 *Diagram of C-4 pathway of photosynthesis, illustrating the concept that CO_2 is fixed into organic acids by mesophyll cell chloroplasts and reduced to carbohydrate by bundle sheath cell chloroplasts. Principal "C-4 acids" involved are malic or aspartic acids, in different plants. These acids are apparently transported from mesophyll to bundle sheath cells, and then probably decarboxylated yielding CO_2 which is refixed by ribulose diphosphate carboxylase and reduced to carbohydrate via the reductive pentose phosphate cycle (Fig. 3-8). The CO_2 that leaks outward from this process and the photorespiration associated with it can be recaptured by the mesophyll cells.*

for production of carbohydrate in C-4 plants. The key to this puzzle may lie in the observation that C-4 plants invariably possess an extremely distinctive type of leaf anatomy (Figure 4-10b) involving two types of photosynthetic cells (the "mesophyll" and "bundle sheath" cells) whose chloroplasts characteristically differ in size and/or structure. There are indications that CO_2 fixation into C-4 acids occurs primarily in the mesophyll cells, whereas the reductive pentose phosphate pathway operates primarily in the bundle sheath cells, producing carbohydrate from primary fixation products that have been imported, via plasmodesmata, from adjacent mesophyll cells. We visualize here a remarkable biochemical cycle, the two halves of which are carried out by separate cells as illustrated in Figure 3-9. Because the bundle sheath is entirely surrounded by mesophyll (Figure 4-10b), it is thought that the CO_2 released by photorespiratory side reactions of the pentose phosphate cycle in the bundle sheath can be completely recaptured by the CO_2 fixing mechanism (Equation 3-15) of the mesophyll cells. Apparently in this way the leaf as a whole gets around the problem of photorespiration.

The biological value of C-4 photosynthesis seems to be as an adaptation to conditions under which photorespiration is especially disadvantageous. This will be considered in Chapter 4 along with other ways in which plants have learned to modify their photosynthetic machinery adaptively in relation to environmental stresses.

SUGGESTED READING

Bassham, J. A., "The Path of Carbon in Photosynthesis," *Scientific American,* **206** (6):88–100, 1962.

Calvin, M., and J. A. Bassham, *The Photosynthesis of Carbon Compounds.* New York: Benjamin, 1962.

Clayton, R. K., *Molecular Physics in Photosynthesis.* New York: Blaisdell, 1965. Chapter 1.

French, C. S., "Photosynthesis," in *This Is Life,* W. H. Johnson and W. C. Steere (eds.). New York: Holt, Rinehart and Winston, 1962. pp. 3–33.

Fogg, G. E., *Photosynthesis.* London: English Univ. Press, 1968.

Hendricks, S. B., "How Light Interacts with Living Matter," *Scientific American,* **219** (3):174–186, 1968.

Hill, R., "The Biochemists' Green Mansions: the Photosynthetic Electron-Transport Chain in Plants," *Essays in Biochemistry,* **1**:121–151, 1965.

Kormondy, E. J., *General Biology, a Book of Readings.* Vol. 1, *Molecules and Cells.* Dubuque, Iowa: W. C. Brown, 1966. Chapters 29–34. (Abridged original papers of Van Niel, Hill, Ruben and Kamen, Calvin and Benson, Arnon, and Whittingham.)

Laetsch, W. M., "Relationship between Chloroplast Structure and Photosynthetic Carbon-fixation Pathways," *Science Progress (Oxford),* **57**:323–351, 1969.

Levine, R. P., "The Mechanism of Photosynthesis," *Scientific American,* **221** (6):58–70, 1969.

Rabinowitch, E. I., and Govindjee, "The Role of Chlorophyll in Photosynthesis," *Scientific American*, **213** (1):74–83, 1965.

Rabinowitch, E. I., and Govindjee, *Photosynthesis*. New York: Wiley, 1969.

Rosenberg, J. L., *Photosynthesis*. New York: Holt, Rinehart and Winston, 1965.

San Pietro, A., F. A. Greer, and T. S. Army (eds.), *Harvesting the Sun*. New York: Academic Press, 1967.

Walker, D. A., "Three Phases of Chloroplast Research," *Nature*, **226**:1204–1208, 1970.

Functioning of Leaves

In Chapter 3 we considered the phenomenon of photosynthesis at the cell and subcellular levels. This is most of the story in the case of unicellular algae which are exposed to light and can obtain the requisite CO_2 in quantity from the water that surrounds them simply by diffusion. Virtually the same can be said for multicellular algae — even massive ones like the kelps (see Delevoryas, *Plant Diversification*) because their pigmented, photosynthetic cells are located typically at the outside surface of the leafy organs (see Figure 7-6b) and thus are in almost direct contact with both light and the copious supply of CO_2 provided by sea water (which contains a high concentration of bicarbonate).

Logistical problems of a very different order confront the performance of photosynthesis by plants that live on land. Their source of

CO_2 is the atmosphere, which contains only about 0.03 percent CO_2 by volume. Because of this small concentration, the problem of ensuring an adequate supply to the cells for photosynthesis is severe; indeed, it is much more severe than the analogous problem of oxygen supply for respiration (page 22), since the atmosphere contains 21 percent oxygen, that is, almost 1000 times its concentration of CO_2. Leaves of land plants have therefore evolved features that tend to maximize the efficiency of gas exchange between them and the surrounding air. This has, however, brought on other severe problems, and it is the purpose of this chapter to study the gas and energy exchange problems of leaves and the mechanisms that plants have evolved for optimizing their photosynthetic performance in the face of what prove to be conflicting demands imposed by the terrestrial environment.

STRUCTURE The first principle of diffusional exchange is that
OF LEAVES for a given concentration difference the rate of
diffusion is inversely proportional to the length of
the diffusion path. Conforming with this, typical leaves are extremely thin (usually less than 1 mm thick), so that the path length for diffusion of CO_2 from the outside air to the cells is minimized. Second, by being furnished with an elaborately developed system of intercellular gas channels, leaves take maximum advantage of the fact (page 23) that diffusion of a gas such as CO_2 through gas (such as air) is much more rapid than diffusion over a comparable distance through liquid media such as cell contents.

The internal structure of a typical leaf of a moist-climate plant is illustrated in Figure 4-1. The bulk of the tissue consists of two layers: the *palisade layer* of elongated cells in the upper half of the leaf and the *spongy parenchyma* tissue of irregularly shaped cells in the lower half. The palisade cells are crowded with chloroplasts and appear to be specialized for efficiency in photosynthesis. Cells of the spongy layer usually possess fewer and smaller chloroplasts. Between the spongy parenchyma cells run large air spaces which actually extend up between every palisade cell and its neighbors. The elongated form of the palisade cells ensures that although almost every chloroplast is adjacent to an intercellular space for CO_2 absorption, there is at the same time a direct light path from the upper epidermis down through each photosynthesizing cell uninterrupted by air spaces that would scatter and diffuse the light.

The leaf is covered on both sides by a layer of cells called the *epidermis* whose cells fit tightly together without intercellular spaces. However, the epidermis is perforated by numerous small pores called *stomates* which are usually most abundant on the lower side of the leaf. Each stomatal pore is surrounded by two specialized epidermal cells called *guard cells*. The pore can be opened or closed by movements of the guard cells, as shown in Figure 4-2. When open, the pore affords a direct connection between the outside air and the air spaces of the internal tissue. There is, then, a direct route for diffusion of CO_2 *in air* from the outside, through the stomate, and via the air spaces of the spongy and then the palisade tissue to reach each palisade cell.

Despite their small size and separation from one another, the stomatal pores constitute a very efficient pathway for gas exchange — much more efficient

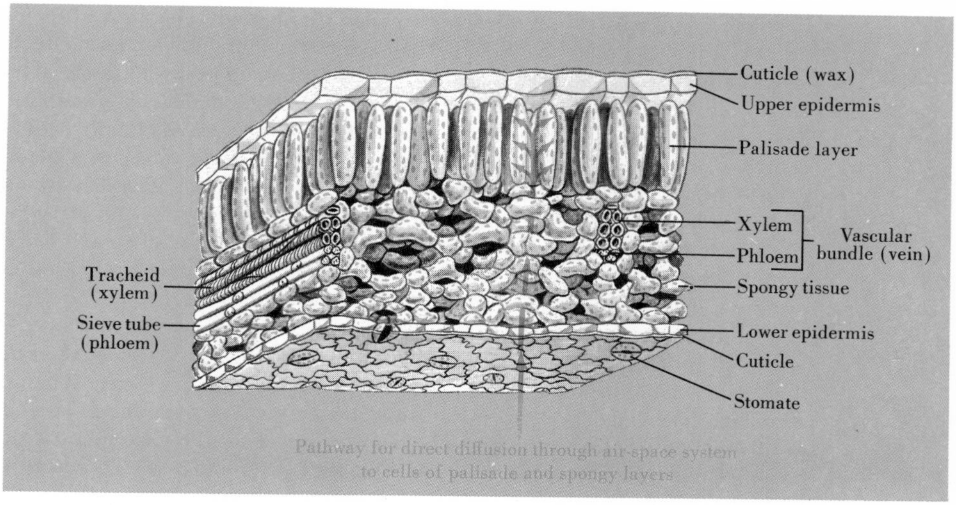

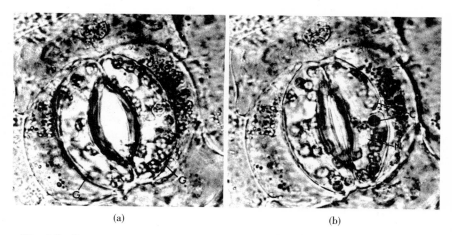

Fig. 4-1   *View of a small part of a leaf blade of the tobacco plant, seen from beneath, magnified about 200 times. Arrow in color shows pathway by which CO_2 diffuses through internal air-space system of leaf to reach individual palisade cells. Photomicrographs of palisade cells are shown in Figure 2-1.*

       (a)   (b)

Fig. 4-2   *Stomate in lower epidermis of leaf of* Rhoeo discolor. *(a) Living guard cells (G) and adjacent epidermal cells photographed after removing epidermis and mounting it in water so that stomate is open due to turgor pressure of guard cells. (b) Stomate has closed owing to loss of turgor of guard cells when epidermis was immersed in 0.4 M mannitol, which is almost equal to the solute concentration of the guard cells. N, nucleus; C, chloroplasts, many of which may be seen in guard cells but not in the other epidermal cells. (Magnification 700×. Photomicrographs by author.) Compare this with structure of stomate of a grass leaf illustrated in Figure 8-15f.*

than one might guess from the small fraction of the epidermal area (1 to 3 percent) that they occupy (Figure 4-1). The reason stomatal diffusion is so effective is basically that the stomatal channels are so short compared with the total path length for diffusion from the leaf tissue to the bulk air outside. This desirable efficiency of CO_2 absorption inevitably results, however, in an equally high efficiency of water loss, since it allows water vapor that evaporates from the leaf cells to diffuse rapidly into the drier air outside the leaf. This water loss is called *transpiration*.

Water loss requires replenishment, and for this purpose the leaf is heavily supplied with vascular bundles, the "veins," which branch and rebranch into ever finer divisions so that vascular tissue comes near to each leaf cell.

Furthermore, the epidermis is specialized to retard passage of water. The outer cell walls of all its cells develop an external layer of wax, called the *cuticle* (Fig. 4-1) which, like waxed paper, is relatively impervious to water. When the stomates close and cut off direct diffusion of water vapor from internal air space to the outside air, the cuticle greatly restricts water loss. Photosynthesis then becomes much reduced also, because the pathway for efficient CO_2 absorption has been closed off.

One must not get the idea that every leaf looks exactly like Figure 4-1. The kind of structure illustrated is representative for leaves of plants of relatively moist climates, but with considerable variations such as multiple palisade layers and specializations of structure in the vicinity of the vascular bundles. Stomates also vary considerably in structure among different plants, both in respect to the form of the guard cells and the presence, number, and nature of subsidiary cells (see, for example, stomatal apparatus of the grass leaf in Figure 8-15). More extreme specializations of leaf structure have evolved in the adaptation of vascular plants to arid climates, as discussed at the end of this chapter.

BEHAVIOR OF STOMATES Stomates exhibit two principal kinds of response: to light and to water stress. Stomates of typical moist-climate plants close in the dark and open upon illumination, and they close even in the light when the leaf suffers sufficiently great water shortage. These changes in stomatal opening may be observed directly under the microscope (as in Figure 4-2), but can more conveniently be measured indirectly either (1) in terms of the rate of transpiration (which is greatly reduced when the stomates close, as mentioned) or (2) by an instrument called a *porometer* that is attached to the leaf surface and is used to determine the rate of flow or diffusion of gas through the leaf under standard conditions. The time course of stomatal response to light and darkness measured in this way is shown in Figure 4-3a.

The opening of stomates is due to the development of a high turgor pressure within the guard cells. This is demonstrated by the fact that the stomate closes when the guard cells' turgor is reduced by treating them with an osmotic solution (as in Figure 4-2) or by puncturing them. As seen in Figure 4-2, stomatal opening occurs by a bending movement of the guard cells. Their cell walls are so shaped and thickened that distention of the cells by turgor results in their curving apart from one another. Stomates of the type developed by grass leaves

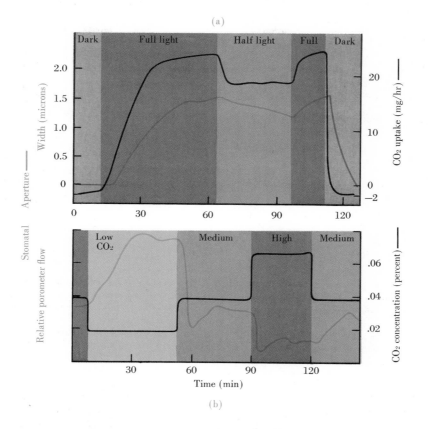

Fig. 4-3 *Timing of the responses to light and to CO_2 by stomates of a maize leaf. (a) Changes in photosynthetic rate of leaf (black line) and in width of stomatal openings (colored line) following changes in light intensity. Note initial lag in onset of measurable photosynthesis due to time required for stomatal opening to begin. (b) Changes in stomatal aperture (colored line) following step changes in CO_2 concentration of the air (black line). Note "overcompensation" by guard cells in course of adjustment to final stomatal width. Stomatal opening was measured with a porometer (in (a) the data were converted by calculation to corresponding values of stomatal pore width). (Data of Dr. Klaus Raschke, from Zeitschrift für Naturforschung, **20b**: 1261, 1965, and Planta, **68**: 115, 1966. Berlin-Heidelberg-New York: Springer 1966.)*

(Figure 8-15f) open by inflation, under turgor, of the thin-walled bulbous ends of the dumbbell-shaped guard cells. Expansion of these bulbs spreads the heavy-walled central part of the guard cells apart from one another, creating a slitlike opening.

The dependence of stomatal opening on turgor pressure makes the stomates responsive to water stress. Under a water deficit, turgor is reduced or lost (as in wilting) and the stomates automatically close. This is illustrated by data given in Figure 4-4, which shows how the degree of stomatal opening changed

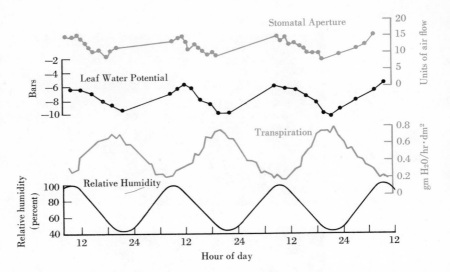

Fig. 4-4 *Variations in transpiration rate and stomatal opening in leaf of a castor bean plant when the relative humidity was varied cyclically over a three-day period with constant illumination, wind speed, and soil water. Water status of the leaf was measured in terms of its water potential (see Chapter 5), more negative values corresponding to increasing water deficits. Stomatal aperture was measured by porometer. Water potential of soil was low enough that higher transpiration rates induced partial stomatal closure, as can be seen in upper curve. (Data of R. Tinklin and P. E. Weatherley, from* New Phytologist, **67**: 605, 1968.)

when a water deficit was developed and relieved in a leaf by periodic changes in relative humidity and thus of transpiration rate. This stomatal behavior provides the leaves with powerful protection against desiccation by a purely passive mechanism, that is, requiring no expenditure of energy to be effective under the emergency conditions.

The opening response of stomates to light results from an increased solute concentration within the guard cells. This increase causes an osmotic uptake of water (page 24) which leads to an increase in the turgor pressure of the guard cells and thus to opening of the stomate. Stomatal opening has an action spectrum similar to photosynthesis (sensitive to both blue and red light). Guard cells always possess chloroplasts (in contrast with other epidermal cells — see Figure 4-2) and are capable of photosynthesis, but the rate at which their solute concentration increases upon illumination is much too rapid to be explained by photosynthetic production of sugar.

How an increase in solute concentration of the guard cells is induced by light is still a matter of dispute. The traditional view is that the change is caused by a conversion of starch to sugar. Some recent experiments support the idea that the increase results from active uptake of ions (especially K^+). There is also experimental evidence that guard cell behavior is hormonally conditioned: abscisic acid (page 167) causes stomatal closure and cytokinins (page 165) promote stomatal opening. These effects can modify the response of stomates to light and darkness, but how they are involved in normal stomatal behavior is still a matter for speculation.

The solute response of guard cells to light actually seems to be largely a result of sensitivity of the guard cells to CO_2. Treatment of a leaf with above-normal CO_2 concentrations causes stomatal closure and a dramatic reduction of transpiration, whereas stomatal opening may be induced in the dark by introducing CO_2-free air into the leaf. It is inferred that illumination causes stomatal opening as a result of the depletion of CO_2 within the leaf by photosynthesis (and especially CO_2 depletion within the guard cells by their own photosynthesis). This mechanism operates to adjust the gas exchange efficiency of the leaf in relation to the photosynthetic demand for CO_2 and can therefore be regarded as a feedback mechanism. This feedback serves to restrict gas exchange during periods of low demand for CO_2 (low light intensity) and prevents unnecessary transpiration, thus conserving the plant's supply of water.

Stomates commonly close also under high temperatures in the light, which causes a midday depression of photosynthesis and transpiration often found under summer conditions (as in Figure 4-7b). This may be explained by the sensitivity of stomates to CO_2 which tends to build up within the leaf at high temperatures as a result of the increase in respiration relative to photosynthesis. This phenomenon helps protect the plant against the excessively rapid water loss that tends otherwise to occur under midday summer conditions.

GAS EXCHANGE OF LEAVES

By consuming CO_2 in photosynthesis the palisade cells deplete the CO_2 concentration of the air around them *below* the CO_2 concentration of the air outside the leaf. As a result of this concentration difference, CO_2 diffuses from the external air to the palisade cells through the stomates and the intercellular gas channels as illustrated by the arrows in Figure 4-1.

As previously mentioned the external air contains at most about 0.03 percent CO_2. During photosynthesis most leaves can deplete their internal CO_2 concentration not more than to about 0.01 percent for reasons to be explained later. The maximum concentration difference that can drive diffusional CO_2 uptake by such a leaf is therefore about 0.02 percent.

The area of contact between leaf parenchyma cells and intercellar gas space is so great that evaporation of water from the cells normally keeps the internal gas space nearly saturated with water vapor. Therefore the water vapor concentration inside the leaf's gas space system equals the saturation vapor pressure of water at the temperature of the leaf,[1] equivalent to a water vapor concentration of 3 to 6 percent by volume over the temperature range of about 25 to 35°C that is most favorable for photosynthesis. On sunny days the air outside the leaf is usually far from being saturated with water vapor, the actual H_2O concentration often being of the order of 1 to 2 percent by volume. Thus a con-

---

[1]Saturation vapor pressure is the partial pressure of the vapor when in equilibrium with the liquid at a given temperature. For water, the saturation vapor pressure at 15°C is 12.8 mm of mercury or 1.7 percent of the volume of water-saturated air at sea level; at 25°C, 23.8 mm or 3.1 percent by volume; at 35°C, 42.2 mm or 5.5 percent by volume.

centration difference of as much as 2 to 4 percent commonly drives diffusion of water vapor *out of* the leaf into the external air. As fast as this vapor escapes, water evaporates from the cells inside the leaf, maintaining the state of virtual saturation of the intercellular gas spaces.

The rate of diffusion over a given path is proportional to the concentration difference between the ends of the path; for a unit concentration difference the rates of diffusion of CO_2 and water vapor are similar. Diffusion of both CO_2 and water vapor are occurring via the same path (stomatal pores), but from the previous estimates the concentration difference that is typically driving water vapor loss from the leaf is about 100 times greater than the maximum concentration difference that can be driving CO_2 uptake. Therefore, we predict that the rate of transpiration must be of the order of 100 times the rate of photosynthesis. This is confirmed by actual measurements, and indeed, except for very humid climates or certain special adaptations to be discussed later, the ratio of transpiration to photosynthesis is in practice typically even more unfavorable for reasons we shall consider shortly. The tremendous inequality between transpiration and photosynthesis means that water balance is one of the principal problems of a land plant.

DYNAMICS OF LEAF GAS EXCHANGE   To understand how stomatal behavior and the relevant environmental parameters control the rates of transpiration and photosynthesis and determine the transpiration–photosynthesis ratio, which is a measure of "water efficiency" of plant growth, it is helpful to represent each part of the gas exchange pathway in terms of a "diffusion resistance" analogous to an electrical resistance. The relationship between these resistances can then be written down as an electric circuit model that has conceptual and predictive value regarding the physiological performance of the entire system. The usefulness of such models results from the fact that for any circuit the resistances of successive components are additive and their sum, the total resistance of the circuit, is what determines the current or "flux" through the entire circuit for a given "driving force" across it. In Figure 4-5 circuits (a) and (b) represent the resistances involved in gas exchange by leaves and show the origin of the driving forces (concentration differences) that operate across them to cause fluxes of water vapor and CO_2, respectively, out of and into the leaf.

The boundary layer refers to that air adjacent to the leaf which is not mixed thoroughly with the bulk air beyond and through which molecules have to diffuse to exchange between the leaf and the bulk external air. The boundary layer is visible in Figure 4-6. The thickness of the boundary layer, and thus its resistance, is quite substantial in still air, but is reduced by air movement across the leaf and therefore decreases with wind velocity. For aerodynamic reasons, at equal wind velocities the boundary layer becomes thicker and its resistance greater the larger the leaf.

Diffusion through the epidermis is governed mainly by the resistance of the stomatal pores, which decreases as they open. In parallel with this is the resistance to diffusion directly through the cuticle which governs gas exchange

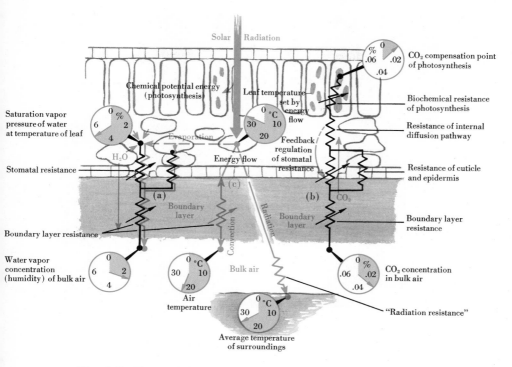

Fig. 4-5   *Circuit models and driving potentials for exchanges of gases (in black) and energy (in color) by a sunlit leaf. (a) Transpiration; (b) photosynthetic CO_2 uptake; (c) energy balance. Symbol $\sim\!\!\sim\!\!\sim$ represents a constant resistance (for a given leaf), $\sim\!\!\sim\!\!\!\nearrow\!\!\!\sim$ a variable resistance. The double-headed arrows for convection and radiation signify that the flux may go in either direction via these mechanisms depending upon whether the leaf is warmer or cooler than the air or than the surroundings.*

through the epidermis when the stomates are fully closed (their resistance then being infinite).

Transpiration   Because leaf cells immediately inward from the
Resistances   stomatal pores provide water vapor at saturation, the epidermal and boundary layer resistances essentially control water vapor exchange between leaf and bulk air as indicated in Figure 4-5a. The driving force for this exchange is, as previously mentioned, the difference between the saturation vapor pressure of water inside the leaf and the water vapor content of the outside air which is related to its relative humidity. Transpiration therefore decreases with increase in humidity of the ambient air and increases sharply with temperature since the saturation vapor pressure within the leaf increases rapidly with temperature.[2]

---

[2]See footnote 1.

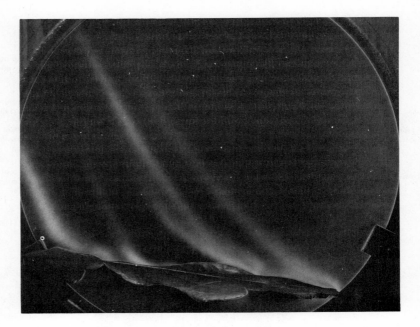

Fig. 4-6   *Photograph of a sunlit oak leaf taken with Schlieren optics to reveal the convective air stream flowing across and away from the leaf. Because of the sunlight it is absorbing, the leaf is warmer than the surrounding air and warms the air, which therefore becomes less dense and appears light in the photograph. The less dense air rises from the leaf surface in streams, carrying away heat (convective cooling of the leaf) and also water vapor released by transpiration (evaporative cooling of the leaf). The boundary layer of air moving across the leaf surface can be seen. (Courtesy of Dr. David M. Gates.)*

CO₂ Uptake Resistances   The path for photosynthetic uptake of CO_2 by the leaf (Figure 4-5b) involves resistances additional to those that govern diffusion of water vapor.

Carbon dioxide has to diffuse from the stomates through the internal gas space system of the leaf to the palisade cells and (through liquid) from the palisade cell surfaces to the chloroplasts. The latter resistance, which is potentially large because of the relative sluggishness of diffusion in liquid (page 23), is minimized, first, by keeping the liquid diffusion path length to a minimum by virtue of having each palisade cell face an air space on almost all sides. Second, leaf cells develop a high concentration of the enzyme *carbonic anhydrase*, which promotes uptake of CO_2 into aqueous solution and, indirectly, the equilibration of CO_2 and dissolved bicarbonate ion. This improves the efficiency of exchange between CO_2 in the leaf's gas spaces and at the chloroplasts, much as carbonic anhydrase is used by vertebrates to improve CO_2 exchange between the circulation on the one hand and the tissues or the lung air on the other.

$$CO_2 + H_2O \xrightleftharpoons{\text{Carbonic anhydrase}} \underset{\substack{\text{Carbonic} \\ \text{acid}}}{H_2CO_3} \rightleftharpoons H^+ + \underset{\text{Bicarbonate}}{HCO_3^-} \qquad (4\text{-}1)$$

The actual CO_2 concentration within the leaf at any instant depends upon the balance between the leaf's gas exchange resistance and the chloroplasts' capacity for photosynthesis under the conditions that prevail. In order to analyze CO_2 uptake explicitly it is helpful to represent the biochemistry of photosynthesis as a "biochemical resistance" (Figure 4-5b). To understand the meaning of this resistance and of the driving force shown for CO_2 uptake in Figure 4-5b we must consider what is meant by the CO_2 *compensation point.*

If we allow a fully illuminated leaf to deplete by its own photosynthesis the CO_2 content of a vessel of air in which the leaf is enclosed, we find that the leaf can reduce the CO_2 concentration only to a certain minimum, which we call the CO_2 compensation point. This is the concentration of CO_2 within the leaf at which the rate of photosynthesis equals the rate of respiration. For many plants the CO_2 compensation point ranges between 0.005 and 0.01 percent CO_2 at temperatures optimal for photosynthesis.

Net photosynthetic CO_2 uptake is possible only to the degree that the actual internal CO_2 concentration in the leaf exceeds its CO_2 compensation point. Thus with something of an abstraction we may regard the difference between actual internal CO_2 concentration and CO_2 compensation point as the driving force for a flux of CO_2 through the biochemical resistance of the photosynthetic mechanism. This resistance decreases with light intensity and temperature which promote the metabolic reactions of photosynthesis. The biochemical resistance is in series with the diffusion resistances. When it is introduced into the circuit model (Figure 4-5), the driving force for overall photosynthetic CO_2 uptake can be represented as the difference between bulk air CO_2 concentration and the leaf's CO_2 compensation point (see Figure 4-5b).

Consequences of Leaf Resistances

The current through a series of resistances is for practical purposes controlled by any one of the resistances that is large compared with the rest since the latter contribute relatively little to the total resistance. Thus much of the benefit for photosynthesis that can be obtained by opening the stomates will be achieved by opening them just enough that the total diffusion resistance for CO_2 is about the same as the biochemical resistance. With further reduction of stomatal resistance photosynthesis will increase more and more slowly because the biochemical and internal diffusion resistances will become largely controlling (assuming that boundary layer resistance is low). Transpiration, however, will continue to increase markedly with stomatal aperture because the internal resistances of the leaf are not involved (Figure 4-5a). Hence in this range of stomatal aperture further gains in photosynthesis become increasingly expensive to the plant in water loss. One might expect that the feedback response of guard cells to internal CO_2 discussed earlier would have evolved features that work to optimize this "cost effectiveness" of photosynthesis. In the case of maize leaves, for example, Klaus Raschke has found that the stomates behave as a control system that maintains a nearly constant internal CO_2 concentration of about 0.01 percent; this corresponds to an external diffusion resistance about twice the internal resistance of the leaf.

If the boundary layer resistance is high (still or slowly moving air), it may be possible to approach the desired internal CO_2 concentration only by opening the stomates fully so that their resistance is small compared with that of the boundary layer. In calm air, therefore, the rates of both transpiration and photosynthesis may be controlled by the large boundary layer resistance.

On the other hand, in wind, when boundary layer resistance becomes small, feedback regulation by the stomates according to the principle just explained will tend to lead to a stomatal resistance that is about the same as the internal resistance. Since internal resistance is not involved in transpiration, the resistance governing transpiration will then be about half that for photosynthesis; therefore the transpiration–photosynthesis ratio will be much higher than the value of about 100 that we calculated in the preceding section on the assumption of identical resistances for CO_2 and water vapor exchange. Under these conditions the stomatal resistance comprises a much larger fraction of the total transpiration resistance than of the total resistance governing photosynthesis; thus an increase in stomatal resistance will reduce transpiration more strongly than it reduces photosynthesis. Artificial reduction of stomatal opening by chemical agents or spray-on plastic films has therefore been advocated as a means of improving the efficiency with which agricultural water is utilized in arid regions. However, this benefit would have to be at the expense of a sacrifice in photosynthetic productivity. Only under severe stomatal curtailment of photosynthesis could the minimum value of transpiration–photosynthesis ratio (that for identical resistances for both processes) be attained — a minimum that is still a very large ratio as already emphasized.

To explain adequately how the rates of photosynthesis and transpiration are actually determined by environmental conditions and stomatal behavior, another important factor has to be considered: the temperature of the leaf, on which both photosynthesis and transpiration depend strongly. The temperature of a leaf is, in fact, seldom exactly the same as that of the air around it because of the role that leaves play in the interception and transformation of radiant energy from their environment.

ENERGY EXCHANGE OF LEAVES   Of the sunlight plus thermal (infrared) energy that is absorbed by a leaf, which we call its *radiation load*, only a small fraction (at most a few percent) is transformed by photosynthesis into chemical potential energy. The remainder accumulates as heat which tends to warm the leaf. Three principal mechanisms dissipate heat from the leaf: (1) emission of infrared radiation to the environment ("reradiation"), (2) convection to the surrounding air, and (3) transpiration. These mechanisms of energy dissipation are represented by a circuit model in Figure 4-5c. The rate of each increases in a characteristic way with leaf temperature; under a given radiation load the temperature of the leaf must rise or fall until the sum of the energy dissipation processes equals the radiation load. This is what determines the temperature of the leaf as compared with that of the air and the immediate surroundings of the leaf.

Infrared reradiation of heat from the leaf always accounts for a substantial fraction of the normal radiation load, roughly equal to the infrared radiation that the leaf is receiving from the surrounding environment other than from direct sunlight. The net exchange of infrared energy between the leaf and its surroundings is determined by the difference in temperature between the leaf and the average temperature of the surroundings. This temperature difference constitutes a driving force for a net flow of energy across what we may call the "radiation resistance" of the system (Figure 4-5c), which in effect expresses the capacity for absorption and emission of infrared radiation by the leaf and its surroundings. As can be seen in Figure 4-5c this net flow of infrared energy helps to dissipate heat derived from sunlight if the temperature of the sunlit leaf rises above the average temperature of its surroundings.

Convection is diffusion of heat through the boundary layer. Its rate is proportional to the temperature difference between leaf and air and inversely proportional to the thickness of the boundary layer. Its rate is therefore influenced by wind velocity and by leaf size in a manner closely comparable to the boundary layer effect on transpiration mentioned previously.

If the leaf is warmer than the air, as is normal for a sunlit leaf, diffusion of heat from the leaf warms the boundary layer which makes it less dense than the surrounding bulk air, as a result of which the boundary layer air rises. This creates a steady convective flow of air past the leaf which can be detected by special optics as illustrated in Figure 4-6. This flow is important because it determines the thickness of the boundary layer in still or slowly moving air and under these conditions sets the gas and heat exchange efficiency of the leaf. On the other hand, if any appreciable wind is blowing, its velocity determines boundary layer resistance to convection and gas diffusion.

For every gram of water that evaporates in transpiration, about 580 calories of heat disappear as latent heat of vaporization which cools the leaf. The contribution that transpirational cooling can make to the energy balance of a leaf at a given temperature is governed by the aforementioned parameters of transpiration rate, namely, exterior air humidity and both stomatal and boundary layer resistances (Figure 4-5a). The first two have, by contrast, no role in convective cooling. Favoring transpirational cooling are low stomatal resistance and low ambient humidity. High air temperature markedly favors transpirational cooling because the leaf's temperature will be warmer, thus increasing its internal water vapor concentration.

Consequences of Energy Balance for Leaf Function Because leaf temperature inevitably rises or falls until the leaf is in energy balance, that is, until the total fluxes of energy into and out of the leaf by the paths shown in Figure 4-5c have become equal, it is the energy budget of the leaf that determines, by its effect on leaf temperature, the rate of transpiration for given values of resistances and exterior humidity.

When transpirational cooling is restricted, much heat must be dissipated from a sunlit leaf by convection and consequently leaf temperature must rise well above air temperature. One beneficial result is that in cool air (transpiration modest) leaves tend to develop a temperature well above the air, which promotes their photosynthesis, whereas at high air temperatures transpirational cooling is strong and tends to hold leaf temperature from climbing when it is already above optimum for photosynthesis. In fact, leaves may actually be cooled by transpiration *below* air temperature in hot dry weather; under these circumstances convection is not helping at all and transpiration may come close to dissipating half the entire radiation load.

These benefits are available, however, only as long as the plant can obtain and transport to the leaves amounts of water equal to the evaporative demand that is operating with the stomates open. If it cannot, water stress develops in the leaf and its stomates begin to close, cutting down the proportion of the radiation load being borne by transpiration and forcing the leaf temperature to climb by as much as 5°C or more. This can be not only inhibitory to photosynthesis but injurious to the leaf if the air temperature is high. Under such circumstances factors that reduce the boundary layer resistance (small leaf size, wind) and thereby promote convective cooling are especially beneficial. Wilting of the leaf is also beneficial, because this reduces its angle of exposure to solar radiation and thus reduces its radiation load, thereby lowering its temperature.

The peculiar role of wind deserves attention. We think of wind as a drying influence, and indeed, when stomatal resistance is low, the effect of wind to decrease boundary layer resistance increases transpiration substantially. However, under water stress conditions when stomatal resistance is high, wind actually *decreases* transpiration. This is because, by reducing boundary layer resistance, wind increases the convective cooling of the leaf and reduces its temperature. This reduces the internal water vapor pressure of the leaf and therefore the driving force for transpiration without significantly reducing the transpiration resistance, since epidermal resistance is already large compared with that of the boundary layer.

When the radiation load is low, as in shade, transpirational cooling regularly reduces leaf temperature below air temperature. This cooling is significant enough (several degrees) to make it possible to distinguish real from plastic potted house plants by feeling their leaves. Under these circumstances leaves *gain* heat from the air by convection. At night the radiation of heat from leaves to the cold night sky adds to this cooling tendency. Under cool night air conditions, this cooling may be positively detrimental; for example, the nocturnal transport of photosynthetic products out of the leaf (Chapter 7) is a highly temperature-dependent process. The suppression of transpiration by stomatal closure during the night eliminates the evaporative component of cooling and may be among the reasons why closure of stomates at night is advantageous.

Performance under Actual Outdoor Conditions   Data in Figure 4-7 show examples of the dramatic daily changes in rate of photosynthesis and transpiration of plants outdoors under naturally varying environmental conditions. We can see from the foregoing analysis how such changes must be compounded out of the interactions between the biological (stomates) and the physical factors that determine driving forces for and resistances to exchange of CO_2 and water vapor. In Figure 4-7a, which shows data collected on a cool, relatively humid day, the stomates opened widely. Even then, however, the rate of photosynthesis was correlated strongly with stomatal aperture rather than sunlight through most of the day, suggesting that stomatal resistance was at least as great as the biochemical and internal diffusion resistances of photosynthesis. The divergence be-

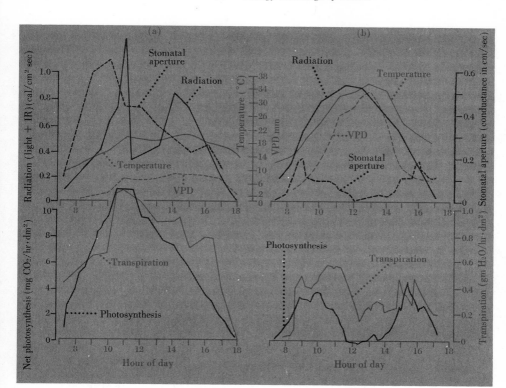

Fig. 4-7   *Daily cycle of photosynthesis and transpiration in the field by toyon, a California chaparral shrub* (Heteromeles arbutifolia), *in (a) cool weather with moist soil, and (b) hot dry weather under severe drought. Upper curves show changes in pertinent environmental variables (VPD = vapor pressure deficit, or difference in water vapor concentration between leaf and air expressed in millimeters of mercury), and in measured stomatal aperture. (The midday decrease of radiation in (a) was due to partly cloudy weather.) Note that the scales for plotting photosynthesis and transpiration differ by a factor of 100, so the data illustrate a transpiration-photosynthesis ratio of 100 or greater even under drought conditions. (Measurements by Dr. Harold A. Mooney, Stanford University.)*

tween the transpiration and photosynthesis curves in the latter half of the day shows the effect of the increasing water vapor concentration difference between leaf and air (VPD curve, showing the combined effects of changing temperature and humidity) that developed in the afternoon. In Figure 4-7b, which represents plants under severe water stress, the stomates at first opened only slightly, reflecting their response to water status of the plant. Under the hot daytime conditions midday closure of the stomates occurred and both photosynthesis and transpiration were restricted. The effect upon transpiration of the extremely desiccating midday conditions can be seen nevertheless in the divergence of the transpiration curve from those for stomatal aperture and photosynthesis in the late morning and midafternoon periods.

ADAPTATION OF LEAVES TO DIFFERENT ENVIRONMENTS   Because of the intimacy of their material exchanges and the intensity of their energy exchanges with the environment, leaves are the plant organs perhaps most involved in evolution of special adaptations to environmental variables such as light, water stress, and temperature.

Light Intensity   Even though we usually think of land plants as growing in sunlight, a variety of plants are adapted to growing in more or less shaded habitats including those where only skylight is received, or the even weaker light that has passed through other vegetation as on the floor of a dense forest. The leaves of these "shade plants" may be injured or killed if exposed to direct sunlight, whereas "sun plants" (adapted to growth in direct sunlight) grow very ineffectively or indeed may succumb under the low light intensities in which shade plants thrive.

Sun leaves are generally smaller and noticeably thicker than shade leaves, as illustrated by the diagrams in Figure 4-8. The most interesting difference between sun and shade leaves is in their photosynthetic characteristics, as shown in Figure 4-9. These curves illustrate the basic kinetic features of photosynthesis: (1) a light intensity called the *compensation point*[3] at which the rate of photosynthesis equals the rate of respiration, (2) a range of light intensities in which photosynthesis increases linearly with intensity and operates at maximum quantum efficiency, and (3) a "saturating" light intensity. Light saturation is the situation in which the rate of photosynthesis is limited by the rate of one or more of the enzymatic reactions that are driven indirectly by the quantum conversion process as explained in Chapter 3 or limited by the rate of diffusion of CO_2 to the chloroplasts by the mechanisms considered earlier in this chapter.

As illustrated in Figure 4-9, sun leaves exhibit a much higher saturating light intensity and a considerably higher light-saturating rate than shade leaves, which makes sense because shade leaves do not normally get access to these higher light intensities and thus can do without the means for utilizing them. Shade leaves, on the other hand, are just as efficient or more efficient at utilizing low light intensities, and because of lower respiration their compensation point is usually lower than that of sun leaves and thus they can keep in positive photosynthetic balance at lower light intensities than sun leaves can.

The leaves of certain plants are capable of "adapting" to high light intensity by modifying their structure and photosynthetic behavior; such an example is actually shown in Figures 4-8 and 4-9. During adaptation to high light the carboxylation enzyme, ribulose diphosphate carboxylase (page 42), increases several fold in parallel with the increase in light-saturation photosynthetic rate. Apparently the activity of the carboxylation enzyme limits the rate of photosynthesis under light saturation and must be increased to take advantage of higher light intensities.

---

[3]Not to be confused with the CO_2 compensation point explained on page 59.

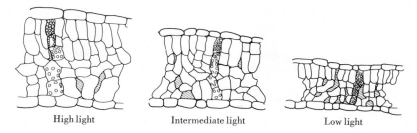

High light   Intermediate light   Low light

Fig. 4-8   *Diagrams of cross sections of leaves of scarlet monkey flower (Mimulus cardi-nalis) grown under three different light intensities. (Data of W. M. Hiesey, M. A. Nobs, and O. Björkman, Carnegie Institution of Washington Publication 628, 1971. Courtesy of Carnegie Institution.)*

Temperature   The light-saturated rate of photosynthesis increases strongly with temperature, but most plants cannot take maximum advantage of this in warm summer or tropical conditions because their net photosynthetic rate reaches a maximum ("optimum") at relatively low temperature (25 to 30°C), above which the rate declines sharply. This decline is connected with the CO_2 compensation point of photosynthesis,

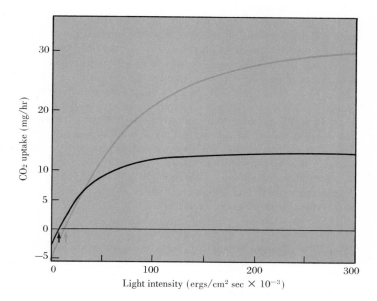

Fig. 4-9   *Photosynthetic rates of leaves of Mimulus cardinalis as a function of light intensity. One leaf (black line) was grown under low light intensity and the second leaf (color line) under high intensity as in Figure 4-8. (Data of W. M. Hiesey, O. Björkman, and M. A. Nobs, from Carnegie Institution Year Book 65, 1967. Courtesy of Carnegie Institution.)*

which as previously mentioned is relatively high (0.005 to 0.01 percent) even at the temperature optimum, and increases rapidly as temperature is raised above the optimum; it soon reaches 0.03 percent, at which point net photosynthesis in air has dropped to nil. The temperature dependence of the CO_2 compensation point appears to be due to the light-induced component of respiration referred to as "photorespiration" (page 45) which increases much faster with temperature than does photosynthesis and cuts into the latter severely at higher temperatures.

The rise in internal CO_2 concentration that inevitably results from a rise in CO_2 compensation point induces stomatal closure and is responsible for the midday closure previously noted that is seen under warm midday conditions as in Figure 4-7b. This has value in conserving water under conditions in which the cost of photosynthesis in terms of water loss would be greatest, but as already stated it prevents the plants in question from making full photosynthetic use of solar energy during warm weather.

Many grasses of tropical origin, such as sugar cane and maize and various other plants of hot climates, possess the C-4 pathway of photosynthesis and lack photorespiration as discussed in Chapter 3. Because of their lack of photorespiration, these C-4 plants show a negligibly low (less than 0.001 percent) CO_2 compensation point, which is in marked contrast to C-3 plants whose characteristics were under discussion in the previous paragraphs. They also show a peculiar type of leaf anatomy (Figure 4-10b) which, as explained in Chapter 3, we believe to be important in the ability of these plants to recover CO_2 lost in the photorespiratory side reaction of photosynthesis and in their capacity to remove, photosynthetically, virtually all the CO_2 from the internal gas space of the leaf. Because of their lack of overt photorespiration, these C-4 plants are not subject to the drastic rise in CO_2 compensation point with temperature that is observed in C-3 plants; thus their photosynthetic temperature optimum is raised well above 30°C. They can therefore use strong light at high temperatures at which typical C-3 plants are completely inactive photosynthetically.

In arctic and mountain habitats photosynthetic adaptation to low temperature is encountered. In general this involves an abnormally low temperature optimum for photosynthesis. Another adaptation commonly encountered in alpine plants is the development of copious hairs on the leaf surface, which increase boundary layer resistance. This reduces convection and causes in sunlight a considerable rise in leaf temperature above air temperature, to the advantage of photosynthesis at low air temperatures.

Water Stress   In many areas water stress is the most important factor affecting leaves and their ability to carry on photosynthesis and we see a variety of adaptations to cope with this. Some plants avoid the problem by simply shedding their leaves during the dry season, just as many cold-temperate trees and shrubs lose their leaves in adapting themselves to the winter (page 166).

However, many arid-climate plants keep their leaves through the dry season. Such leaves show an array of anatomical features seemingly designed to retard transpiration as much as possible: heavy layers of cuticular waxes; multiple-layered epidermis; stomates sunken beneath the surface of the leaf to in-

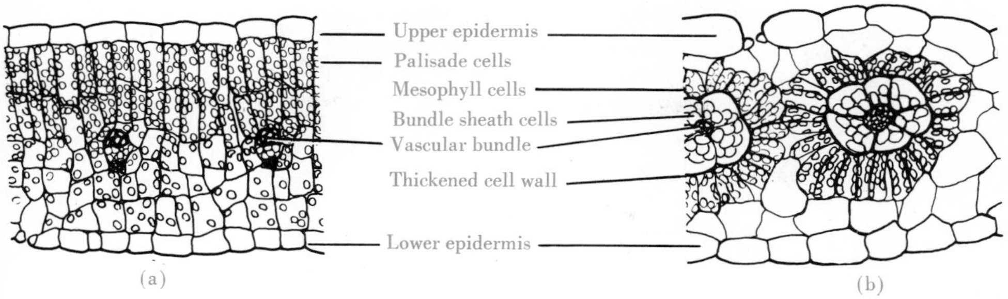

Upper epidermis
Palisade cells
Mesophyll cells
Bundle sheath cells
Vascular bundle
Thickened cell wall
Lower epidermis

(a)   (b)

Fig. 4-10   *Leaf structure of two species of saltbush* (Atriplex): *(a)* Atriplex patula, *which has C-3 photosynthesis; and (b)* Atriplex rosea, *which has C-4 photosynthesis and lacks photorespiration. Note the prominent bundle sheath cells with thickened cell walls and conspicuously larger chloroplasts. (Observations of O. Björkman, M. A. Nobs, and J. Boynton, from Carnegie Institution Year Book 69, 1971. Courtesy of Carnegie Institution.)*

crease the boundary layer diffusion distance without increasing the boundary layer thickness at the leaf surface which governs convective cooling; mechanisms of folding or rolling up under water stress so as to remove the stomate-bearing surface from contact with the air; small leaf size to minimize boundary layer resistance and thus maximize convective cooling when transpirational cooling is not available; and so forth. Figure 4-11 illustrates an example of leaf structure that shows several of these features.

Such leaves do transpire rather rapidly when the plant is supplied with water and the stomates are open; their specializations are effective mainly in minimizing water loss under water stress when the stomates are partially or completely closed. The leaves must be able to tolerate long-continued wilting conditions without damage; one feature that seems essential to this is the development of very heavy cell walls around many of the cells (Figure 4-11) so that the leaf is tough and leathery and does not, in fact, wilt visibly when its cells' turgor has been lost and its stomates have closed.

C-4 photosynthesis can serve to some extent as a metabolic adaptation to water stress. The very low CO_2 compensation point of C-4 plants means (by Figure 4-5) a larger driving force for CO_2 uptake relative to that for water loss than in a C-3 plant under the same conditions. Therefore under severe stomatal closure a C-4 plant uses water more efficiently relative to its photosynthesis than does a C-3 plant. This difference is augmented by the fact that under stomatal closure, leaf temperature will be maximal by the principles of energy exchange already discussed, so the CO_2 compensation point of a C-3 plant will tend to be exceptionally high and its driving force for CO_2 uptake especially weak.

A striking adaptation that leads to exceptionally efficient use of water is found in a variety of succulent plants such as cacti, *Agave*, and *Crassulaceae* (stonecrop, hen-and-chickens), many of which inhabit arid regions. They open their stomates at night, when conditions are least conducive to transpiration, and take in CO_2 from the air by converting it into the carboxyl groups of organic acids, especially malic and isocitric acid. During the day their stomates close, and behind this barrier the organic acids are split to release CO_2 which the cells

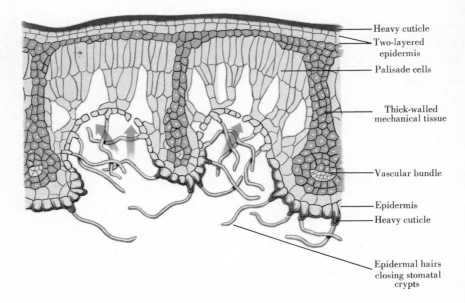

Heavy cuticle
Two-layered epidermis
Palisade cells

Thick-walled mechanical tissue

Vascular bundle

Epidermis
Heavy cuticle

Epidermal hairs closing stomatal crypts

Fig. 4-11   *Structure of leaf of* Banksia marginata, *an Australian arid-climate shrub. Arrows point to stomates, located exclusively in deep depressions infolded from the lower surface, the openings of which are occluded with numerous hairs that restrict air flow. Note the multiple upper epidermis with extremely thick cuticle and the ribs of heavy-walled cells which stiffen the leaf like I beams. (From diagram by M. A. Nobs, in Carnegie Institution of Washington Publication 623, 1963. Courtesy of Carnegie Institution.)*

immediately use for photosynthesis. As a result of this behavior the transpiration of these plants is actually greater at night than during the day (Figure 4-12), and in the aggregate is much less than that of ordinary plants; overall ratios of transpiration to photosynthesis as low as 30 have been measured. This permits these plants to continue photosynthesis and yet conserve over long periods the water that they store up in their fleshy leaves or stems when it is available.

Aquatic Habitats   The other extreme in leaf adaptation is that of vascular plants that have invaded the water. Here water conservation is, of course, no problem, but gas exchange to supply CO_2 still is. Two principal kinds of solutions to this problem are encountered. Submerged aquatic plants typically have extremely thin leaves, such as the leaf of *Elodea* (familiar from general biology laboratory observations) that is only two cells thick, or leaves that are very finely divided. These leaves make up for the low efficiency of CO_2 diffusion through liquid by having a short path length. On the other hand, aquatic plants whose leaves float on (for example, water lilies) or emerge from (for example, cattails, bullrushes) the water develop an elaborately organized and voluminous gas space system that serves to supply CO_2 to the photosynthetic parts and O_2 to the submerged organs by diffusion over long distances such as a meter or more.

Polluted Air   Because of the efficiency of their gas exchange arrangements, leaves are especially subject to the harmful effects of industrial pollutants such as sulfur dioxide and hydrogen fluoride, and of the peroxides and ozone that are generated photochemically from automobile exhaust in the formation of smog.

Sulfur dioxide is notoriously poisonous to plants for reasons that are still not well understood. In areas of high SO_2 emissions such as are produced by traditional methods of smelting metal ores, entire forests have been wiped out, and in many urban areas damage to plants from SO_2 derived from combustion of fuel oil and coal has become serious.

Smog oxidants attack the photosynthetic machinery of the chloroplasts and give rise to a toxicity that may kill most of the cells in the more effectively ventilated parts of the leaf, ultimately seriously weakening the entire plant. These effects have caused severe decline or complete abandonment of vegetable and orchard crops and extensive injury and death to trees in the native vegetation over vast areas in smog-afflicted districts such as the Los Angeles basin.

Different plant species, and even different strains of certain species, differ greatly in their sensitivity to air pollutants. Continuation or further increase of air pollution will inevitably impoverish seriously the vegetation of affected areas by eliminating the less pollution-resistant species, including many of the important trees which on account of their longevity are especially liable to the cumulative effects of airborne intoxicants.

Although the physiological basis for resistance to air pollutants is not yet understood, active programs for the breeding and dissemination of pollution-resistant strains of crop plants and species of street trees are underway. But whatever these efforts may do for agriculture or horticulture, they will hardly be able

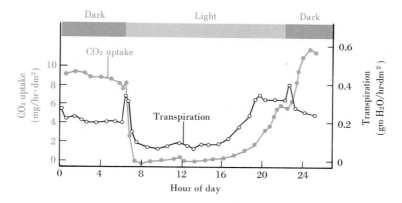

Fig. 4-12   *Daily cycle of CO_2 absorption and transpiration by a potted plant of* Agave americana *(century plant) under severe water stress. The transpiration curve reveals that the stomates closed soon after beginning of the light period and opened again in late afternoon, remaining open through the night. Note the accompanying nocturnal CO_2 uptake and lack of photosynthetic uptake of CO_2 during the day. (Data of T. F. Neales, A. A. Patterson, and V. J. Hartney, from* Nature, **219**: 470, 1968.)

to substitute for the ecological, economic, and recreational values of the countryside vegetation. Unless the breeding and propagation of smog-tolerant strains of *Homo sapiens* are also contemplated, one would think that the air pollution menace might best be combated at its source.

SUGGESTED READING

Esau, K., *Anatomy of Seed Plants*. New York: Wiley, 1960. Chapters 18 and 19.

Gates, D. M., "Heat Transfer in Plants," *Scientific American*, **213** (6): 76–84.

Gates, D. M., "Transpiration and Leaf Temperature," *Annual Review of Plant Physiology*, **19**:211–238, 1968.

Heath, O. V. S., *The Physiological Aspects of Photosynthesis*. Stanford, Cal.: Stanford University Press, 1969. Chapter 4.

Meidner, H., "Stomatal Control of Transpirational Water Loss," *Symposia of the Society for Experimental Biology*, **19**:185–203, 1965.

Meidner, H., and T. A. Mansfield, *Physiology of Stomata*. New York: McGraw-Hill, 1968.

Penman, H. L., and R. K. Schofield, "Some Physical Aspects of Assimilation and Transpiration," *Symposia of the Society for Experimental Biology*, **5**:115–129, 1951.

Salisbury, F., and C. Ross, *Plant Physiology*. Belmont, Cal.: Wadsworth, 1969. Chapter 6.

Slatyer, R. O., *Plant-Water Relationships*. New York: Academic Press, 1967. Chapter 8.

Sutcliffe, J., *Plants and Water*. New York: St. Martin's Press, 1968. Chapters 5 and 6.

Zelitch, I. (ed.), *Stomata and Water Relations in Plants*. New Haven, Conn.: Connecticut Agricultural Experiment Station, Bulletin 664, 1963.

chapter 5

Water Transport

Leaves inevitably transpire water vapor rapidly to the air when their stomates are open to allow efficient photosynthetic absorption of CO_2 (Chapter 4). Consequently, a most important function of the plant body is to keep the leaves supplied with water, that is, to maintain water balance in the leaves. As explained in Chapter 1 the principal parts of the plant body that serve this end are the xylem, the tissue through which water is transported through the plant body, and the root, which absorbs the required water from the soil.

It is possible to measure the rate of water absorption by the roots of a plant at the same time as the rate of water loss from its shoot is being measured. By this means it is found (Figure 5-1) that the increasing rate of transpiration that develops during the day is accompanied by a sim-

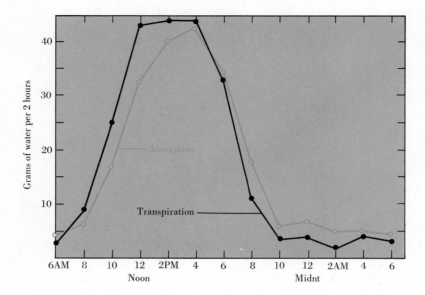

Fig. 5-1 *Transpiration and water absorption by a sunflower plant out of doors in the course of a summer day and the following night. (Data of P. J. Kramer, from* American Journal of Botany, **24:** *10, 1937.)*

ilar rise in water absorption. Actually, as may be seen in the Figure 5-1, changes in the rate of absorption typically lag somewhat behind changes in the rate of transpiration. It thus appears that water loss by the leaves sets in motion processes that result in water absorption by the roots. The lag between transpiration and absorption means that the water content of leaves falls during the morning and increases again in the evening.

WATER POTENTIAL In order to understand water transport it is extremely helpful to introduce the concept of *water potential*. Water potential is an expression of the energy status of water within cells or other parts of a transport system. Water will flow in the energetically downhill direction, that is, from where water potential is higher to where it is lower. Water potential differences constitute in effect the "driving forces" for water transport.

The concept of water potential is based upon the free energy of water, free energy being the thermodynamic parameter that determines the direction in which physical and chemical changes must occur and their ability to do work. Free energy is the sum of an energy and an entropy (randomness) component. For solutions, such as the contents of cells, water potential is determined primarily by two factors: (1) concentration of dissolved solutes, which by its effect on the entropy component reduces the water potential and (2) hydrostatic pressure, which by its effect on the energy component increases the water potential. Because of this, turgor pressure and concentration of cell solutes interact in determining the osmotic status of a cell, as explained on page 24.[1] In solid matrices such as cell walls or soils in which water is bound by hydrational forces, a hydrational or "matric" component also enters into the water potential.

The reference state or zero value for water potential is by convention taken to be pure water at atmospheric pressure. Relative to this reference state the water potential (ψ) of any part of the water transport system can be written as the sum of the solute concentration effect (s), turgor pressure (P), and matric effect (τ) in that part:

$$\psi = s + P + \tau \tag{5-1}$$

In this equation water potential is expressed in units of pressure, that is, force per unit area. The usual units are kilograms per square centimeter or *bars* (1 bar = 1 kg/cm^2). Turgor pressure (P) is an actual force exerted by cell contents upon each unit area of their walls (actually, turgor pressure is the amount by which pressure inside the cell *exceeds* the atmospheric pressure outside), whereas the solute (s) and matric (τ) components are thermodynamic effects on water potential that are *represented numerically* in pressure units. Expressed in bars the effect of solutes is (as stated somewhat differently on page 25) to reduce the water potential by approximately 24 times the total molar solute concentration (sum of all solutes present); being a lowering, s in Equation 5-1 is always a negative number (unless $s = 0$, the case where no solutes are present).[2]

Since water potential is the thermodynamically correct driving force for osmotic transport of water, we may now rephrase more accurately the explanation of plant cell water balance given on page 24. A cell will absorb water if and only if the water potential of its surroundings is higher than that of the cell. As a cell absorbs water its turgor pressure tends to rise, which raises its water potential. When the water potential of the cell has become equal to that of the external source of water, there will no longer be any driving force for water transport, that is, a state of osmotic equilibrium will be reached. In the case of a cell that is in contact with pure water at atmospheric pressure ($\psi = 0$), the water potential of the cell will become zero at equilibrium. Therefore by Equation 5-1 such a cell's turgor pressure must rise until it is equal and opposite to the (negative) solute effect of the cell's vacuolar solution (τ being negligible for typical cell sap) so that the sum of P and s is zero. Thus water potential considerations dictate the equilibrium turgor pressure of the cell.

At the earth's surface the water potential of pure water at atmospheric pressure is the *highest* water potential value that is encountered; solutes, matric effects, and evaporation into the air all tend to reduce the water potential and the pressure is, of course, atmospheric. Since land plants get their water more or

---

[1]It is advisable at this point to review the material on water balance of plant cells presented on pages 24–26 which is essential to a clear understanding of matters to be considered from this point onward.

[2]The solute concentration effect s used here is the negative of the traditionally employed "osmotic pressure" or "osmotic potential." Osmotic potential has the disadvantage that it must be *subtracted* from the other terms in defining ψ by an equation like 5-1, a subtraction that leads to much conceptual confusion.

less at the surface, and their water potential cannot be greater than that of their source of water, zero is the *maximum* value of water potential normally found in plants. When a plant is absorbing water from the environment, water potentials throughout the plant must be negative.[3] This situation may be vexing at first, but it should be understood and tolerated because pure water at atmospheric pressure is the only biologically convenient reference state for water potential values that can be chosen.

We are now in a position to analyze how water transport and absorption by plants are coupled to transpiration.

DYNAMICS OF WATER TRANSPORT

When transpiration is not occurring, the living cells in the leaf inevitably come into equilibrium with the practically pure water that is contained in the nearby xylem of the leaf veins, hence by the principles just considered the leaf cells will have a relatively high water potential and high turgor pressure. When the leaf begins to transpire, water evaporates from its cells. As their volume falls their turgor pressure drops rapidly, and therefore by Equation 5-1 their water potential falls. A water potential difference thereby develops between the leaf cells and the xylem. This water potential difference causes water transport from the xylem into the leaf cells.

Leaving aside for the moment the specific mechanisms by which water is transported through the vascular system, root, and soil, we may recognize that each of these components presents an inherent frictional resistance to water transport. These resistances are in series, as depicted in Figure 5-2, and we may regard water transport as a problem of current flow or flux through a system of resistances in the same way that the problem of leaf gas exchange was analyzed in Chapter 4.

The flux of water through the transport system will be determined by the driving force that is acting across the sum of the resistances of the successive parts of the system; this driving force is the difference in water potential between the leaves and the soil. Accordingly the fall in water potential of the leaf cells during transpiration sets up a driving force that causes water transport through the plant and absorption from the soil.

When transpiration begins (or increases), the leaf's water content and water potential must fall until the water potential difference becomes large enough (relative to the sum of resistances of the transport pathway) to cause a flux equal to the existing rate of transpiration. Once the required potential difference has developed, the leaf will be receiving water at the same rate that it is losing water to the air, so its water content and water potential will thereafter remain constant as long as transpiration does not change. This is called a *steady state* of transport. If the transpiration rate is reduced, the leaf cells will at that moment be absorbing water at the previously existing rate, that is, faster than they are now losing it. Consequently, their volume will increase, and hence their

---

[3]An exception to this statement can occur when it is raining, water at zero potential then falling on and being absorbed by the top of a tree: water potential can then become positive below the top of the tree for reasons that may be apparent from the subsequent discussion.

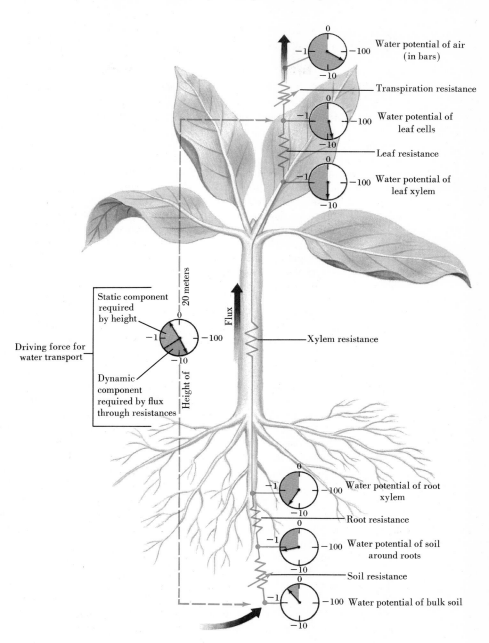

Fig. 5-2 *Diagram of components of plant water transport system represented as the analog of an electric circuit. The imaginary gauges illustrate an example of how the water potential varies through the transport pathway. Note that gauges are marked out in a scale that is logarithmic (except near 0) so as to be able to show the wide range of water potential values over the entire soil-plant-air system. The leaf and root resistances represent the aggregate values for all the leaves and for the entire root system, respectively.*

turgor pressure and water potential will rise until a new steady state of transport is attained. Examples of the timing of such adjustments are shown in Figure 5-3.

A vivid demonstration of the role that turgor and water potential play in maintaining water balance of the leaf is the phenomenon called "temporary wilting" which often occurs on warm bright days. The rate of transpiration may become so great that for the leaf cells to obtain water at an equal rate, their turgor pressure would have to fall to zero. As this happens the leaves droop and wilt. When conditions are changed so that transpiration is reduced, the leaves begin to regain turgor and rise, for there is actually a large driving force for water transport at this low leaf water potential. Temporary wilting is most commonly seen when the water potential of the soil is somewhat depressed (soil fairly dry) but it can be noticed in some plants even when the soil is saturated.

The actual site of evaporation within the leaf is, of course, the surface of the cell walls of internal parenchyma cells; at this site water potential is actually determined mainly by a matric effect on water potential (τ in Equation 5-1), which becomes increasingly negative as the cell wall material becomes dehydrated. Some investigators think that much of the water flux passes from the xylem to the evaporation sites via cell walls rather than through the parenchyma cells themselves. If this view is correct, the leaf transport resistance shown in Figure 5-2 would be due mainly to resistance to water flow in cell walls rather than through cell membranes. The overall dynamics of transport should be the same in either case because the water potential of the leaf parenchyma cells cannot help but become virtually the same as that of their cell walls.

Static Component of the Transport Problem   In performing water transport, work must be done not only against frictional resistance to water flow through the transport system but also against the force of gravity as water is raised above the ground. Raising of water therefore adds to the water potential difference that is required between the leaves and the roots. The work required for raising water is determined strictly by the height to which water has to be raised, no matter how slowly or rapidly it is being moved, and thus we can refer to this component of the required driving force as the "static component." The static component is dictated by the specific gravity of water and amounts to 1 bar of water potential difference for each 10 meters (33 ft) of height. For example, the water potential at the top of a tree 30 meters tall must be 3 bars lower than in its roots even when transpiration is almost completely shut down.

In contrast, the dynamic or frictional aspect of water transport requires a driving force proportional to the flux that is to be achieved. The static and dynamic components *add* to one another in determining the water potential that must be reached by the leaves for them to achieve water balance (a steady state of transport) under given conditions of transpiration and soil water potential.[4]

Measurements performed on various trees show that the dynamic and

[4]Transport equations can be made more general by defining water potential with inclusion of a gravitational potential term in Equation 5-1. Even though this is prevalent practice and is mathematically advantageous, the convention is initially confusing for many students and as the mathematical advantages are of no benefit at the present level of treatment, we eschew the convention here.

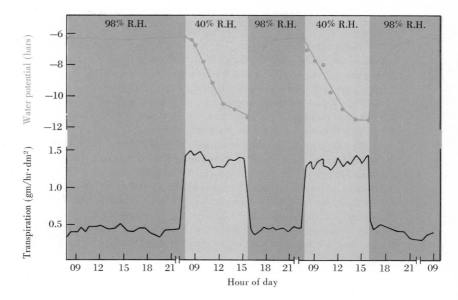

Fig. 5-3   *Changes in transpiration rate and leaf water potential of a castor bean plant under constant light, wind velocity, temperature, and soil water potential, when relative humidity of the air was changed suddenly from 98 to 40 percent and* vice versa. *The results show the time required for adjustment of leaf water potential to a new steady level following changes in transpiration rate, and thus indicate the time required for water transport in the plant to become equal to the new transpiration rate. (Data of R. Tinklin and P. E. Weatherley, from* New Phytologist, **67**: 605, 1968.)

static components of the required water potential driving force are approximately equal at maximum rates of transpiration. In other words, in the example of a tree 30 meters tall mentioned previously it might be found that the water potential of the leaves falls by 3 (static component) + 3 (dynamic component) = 6 bars below that of the soil during steady rapid transpiration under midday conditions.

Transport resistance might be expected to be greater in herbaceous plants since their stems contain relatively little vascular tissue (Figure 1-2, a compared with b). Indeed from a careful analysis of transport resistance in the xylem of the tomato plant it appears that at a moderate rate of transpiration the dynamic component of the water potential gradient in the stem must be about three times the static component. The resistance of the transport system would be enormously greater were it not for the specialized structure of the xylem to be examined in the next section.

THE XYLEM   The pathway by which water is transported to the leaves while they are transpiring may be detected by cutting off a shoot and immersing its cut base in a dilute solution of a dye. The dye rises rapidly in the xylem of the stem and soon travels out into the veins of the leaves. It moves in two types of water-transporting cells: *tracheids* and *vessel elements.*

The tracheid (T in Figure 5-4) is a long narrow cell extending in the direction of water movement. The functional tracheid is dead and has no protoplast or membranes; it is strengthened by a fairly thick secondary wall that was laid down by the cell's protoplast before it died. The wall possesses thin areas, either pits (BP in Figure 5-4b) or larger areas of primary wall upon which a secondary wall was not deposited; through these areas water can pass from one tracheid to the next, where the ends of two tracheids overlap.

The thin pit membrane (primary cell wall) offers much less resistance to water flow than do cellular osmotic membranes (plasma and vacuolar membranes). Moreover the elongated form of tracheids minimizes the number of pit barriers to be traversed as water moves through the xylem and, as can be seen in Figure 5-4b, maximizes the number of pit channels through which water can flow from each tracheid into the one above it. These features plus the lack of cytoplasmic contents to impede water flow through the cell interior give a system of tracheids much less resistance to water transport than a comparably sized piece of living tissue possesses.

In the xylem of more primitive vascular plants such as ferns and conifers the tracheid is the only type of water-conducting cell. The wood of fir (shown in Figure 5-4a and b) is an example of this type of xylem.

The xylem of flowering plants possesses not only tracheids but also multicellular water-conducting structures called *vessels* (V in Figure 5-4), made up of individual cells termed "vessel elements" (VE in Figure 5-4d). Like tracheids vessel elements are dead cells with a secondary wall, but unlike tracheids the vessel element has one or more open holes at each end, called "perforations," by which it connects with adjacent vessel elements. The result is a multicellular tube, the vessel.

Vessel elements develop as separate cells. A secondary wall is not deposited on the end wall areas that are to become perforations. As the vessel cells mature the cytoplasm, nucleus, and cellular membranes suddenly break down (autolysis) and the primary walls in the unthickened end wall areas disappear, thus creating open holes. These holes eliminate all resistance to water flow between the successive cells that make up the vessel, and a vessel is therefore an even more efficient water-transporting device than a series of tracheids. A vessel still offers some frictional resistance to water flow, governed like flow through any pipe, by its diameter and by the viscosity of water. Resistance decreases sharply with diameter, and consequently the more advanced flowering plants have evolved extremely wide vessels (for example, the upper ones in Figure 5-4c) which absolutely minimize the transport resistance of the xylem.

Individual vessels extend for a limited distance—from a few centimeters to more than a meter in some cases — and finally end in a blind cell from which water must pass into adjacent vessels through pits in the walls in the same manner as water is transferred from one tracheid to another.

The xylem also contains various types of living cells. Experiments performed well before the turn of the century established, however, that movement of water in the xylem is not caused by activities of the living cells that it contains, for these may be killed without stopping water transport. It appears instead that removal of water from the xylem by the leaves causes water transport in the xylem.

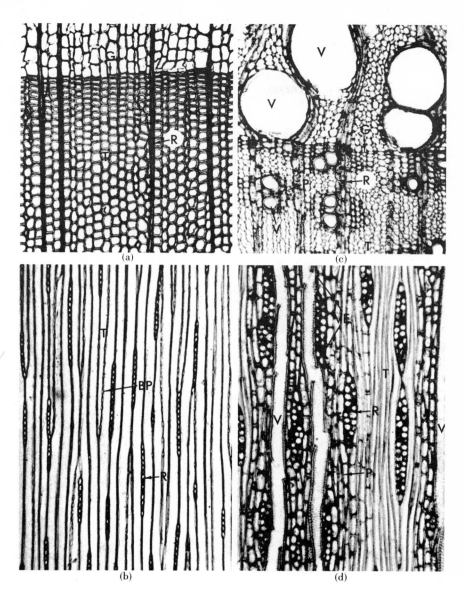

Fig. 5-4. *Photomicrographs of cross sections (above) and longitudinal sections (below) of wood of balsam fir,* Abies balsamea, *(a) and (b); and sassafras,* Sassafras albidum, *(c) and (d). G, growth ring (end of season's growth; wood above (G) was formed at beginning of new growing season, see page 137). R, ray (rows of living cells running from center of tree toward outside); P, wood parenchyma (other living cells in wood); T, tracheids; V, vessel. In (b), BP indicates wall at tip of tracheid where many bordered pits occur; note that individual tracheids are longer than the segment of wood illustrated. In (d), VE indicates length of a single vessel element, the perforations by which it connects with adjacent elements being visible at the ends of this and other vessel elements in the section; note pits in side walls. Longitudinal sections were cut in the plane formed by the bottom of (a) and (c), thus the rays are seen in end view, and relatively narrow vessels of the "late wood" appear in (d). Note how much wider are the vessels formed early in the growing season, (top of (c). (All magnifications 85×.)*

MECHANISM
OF WATER TRANSPORT
IN XYLEM

As explained previously leaf cells develop a capacity to remove water from the xylem when they are losing water by evaporation. Withdrawal of water from a vessel or tracheid tends to collapse the xylem cell, but this is opposed by the nearly rigid secondary thickenings of its cell wall with the result that what we may call for the moment a "suction" is set up inside the xylem cell. By "suction" we mean a pressure below the atmospheric pressure of about 1 bar that the cell's contents are under in the undisturbed state.

The situation that develops within the xylem when cells of the leaf remove water from it is somewhat analogous to that within a drinking straw when you apply suction by mouth to one end: by reducing the pressure at the leaf end of the xylem a pressure gradient is set up within the system. Because of this pressure gradient, water tends to flow hydraulically through the vessel and tracheid channels from the roots (where pressure is highest, that is, nearest to atmospheric pressure) toward the leaves (where pressure is lowest). The gradient of pressure within the xylem is equivalent by Equation 5-1 to a gradient of water potential. [Xylem sap is normally very dilute, so s (and also τ) are negligible.] A flow of water along the xylem can occur to whatever extent the actual gradient of pressure exceeds the statically required water potential gradient of 1 bar per meter of height (page 76).

Tension-Cohesion
Mechanism

There is an important difference between the reduced pressure at the leaf end of the xylem system and the suction that you impose by mouth on the end of a straw by reducing the air pressure in your mouth. By pumping air out of a system the pressure can be reduced *at most* by 1 bar; this would be when all of the air was pumped out leaving a vacuum that exerts no force on the walls. Therefore if plants really transported water by applying suction to the xylem, they could raise water a *maximum* of 10 meters or 33 ft because a water potential drop of 1 bar below that at ground level is inescapably required at this height for the static gravitational reasons already explained. The fact that trees reach and transport large amounts of water to heights much greater than 10 meters, indeed to more than ten times this height in the case of some California Redwoods and Australian Eucalyptus trees, shows that simple suction cannot account for the water transport phenomenon. This can engender the dismaying feeling that such a rise of sap in tall trees is impossible.

The solution to this classic biological enigma is the tension-cohesion principle of xylem water transport, which depends upon the fact that functional tracheids and vessels are entirely filled with water. Water molecules attract one another strongly by forces such as hydrogen bonds that are responsible for water being a liquid, and for similar reasons water also interacts strongly with the polysaccharide materials of the cell wall. The resulting behavior is called *cohesion*, which means that the water molecules within a water-filled xylem cell cannot readily be pulled away from the wall or apart from one another to create a space inside the cell. Consequently, if some water is drawn out of a xylem cell through its wall, the remaining water becomes in effect "stretched," generating a pulling force among the water molecules and between them and the walls. Such a force field is the opposite of an ordinary pressure; it is a pulling force per unit area of the walls rather than a push on them. This state of *negative* pressure is called a *tension* because it is analogous to the tensional force in a wire or rope when you pull on it. However, under tension in a liquid the pulling force is transmitted in all directions just as the pushing force of a positive pressure is exerted in all directions.

The capacity for development of tension in the xylem depends upon the following features in addition to cohesion: (1) Rigidity of the secondary wall thickenings prevents the pulling force of tension from collapsing the xylem cells. (2) Because of the narrowness of the pores by which water passes through xylem cell walls (pores in pit membranes or other unthickened wall areas), bubbles of air cannot be sucked into the cell from outside under normally prevailing tensions: to push gas through these narrow pores would require the action of enormous forces against the surface tension forces of water. Exclusion of air from the xylem cells is important because a gas always exerts *positive* pressure, which prevents a state of tension from existing.

The possibility of developing negative pressure or tension in the xylem greatly extends the range of water potential differences that may be generated for water transport as compared with the difference of only 1 bar that can be created by suction. Existence of tension in the xylem appears to be indispensable for water transport to the tops of tall trees.[5] The way in which this state of tension is presumed to arise according to the explanation just given is illustrated diagrammatically in Figure 5-5.

Measurement of Tension and Flow in Xylem   Although there has long been indirect evidence that tension develops in the xylem during rapid transpiration (for example the observation that tree trunks shrink in diameter during the day and expand at night), only recently has a method been invented by which tensions in the xylem sap can actually be measured. P. F. Scholander and his collaborators introduced a pressure chamber method that is illustrated and explained in Figure 5-6. By this method they found tensions that increased with height in the theoretically expected manner in the xylem of tall redwood and Douglas fir trees in coastal California. They also confirmed the tension-cohesion theory in certain other situations in which the tension was predictable in theory.

Unfortunately the pressure chamber method is destructive; that is, the plant part has to be cut off to obtain the measurement and since only one measurement can be obtained from a single shoot, changes with time can only be fol-

---

[5]Pressure P in Equation 5-1 for water potential is defined as the difference between actual pressure and external atmospheric pressure (this definition is required by choice of the reference or zero state of water potential as that of pure water at atmospheric pressure). Therefore subatmospheric positive pressures (ordinary suction) correspond to values of P between 0 and about −1 bar; the exact numerical value of P that corresponds to *zero* force on the walls of the container or the null point of absolute pressure depends, of course, on the actual prevailing atmospheric pressure (less at altitudes above sea level or during low pressure weather cycles). True negative pressures or tensions, that is, a pulling force on the walls, correspond to P values *more negative* than this null point of about −1 bar.

lowed by the crude method of "sampling" different shoots from a large shrub or tree.

The pressure chamber method is also a method for determining the water potential of a leaf or shoot, since for reasons mentioned above the pressure in the xylem equals its water potential. Different, nondestructive methods exist for

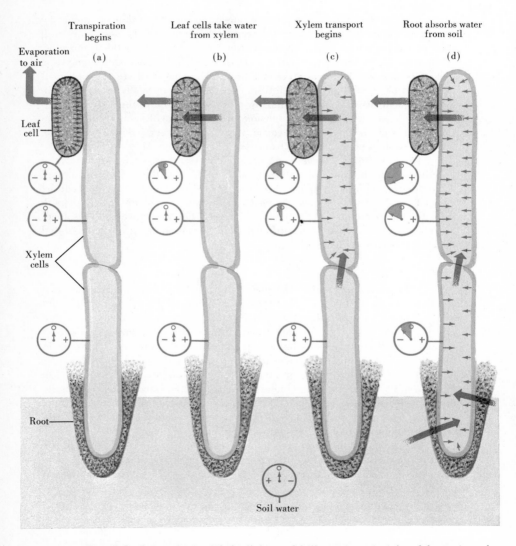

Fig. 5-5 *Extremely simplified cellular model illustrating principles of the tension-cohesion mechanism of water transport. The gauges represent imaginary sensors of water potential. Dots indicate solute concentration and small colored arrows represent turgor pressure (directed outward) or tension (directed inward). Large block arrows show water flow. Successive stages following the onset of evaporative water loss from the initially fully turgid leaf cell (diagram a) are represented.*

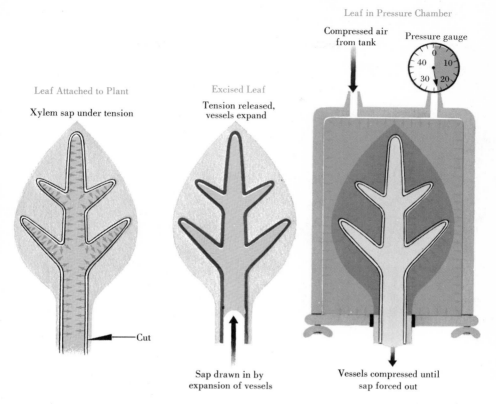

Leaf in Pressure Chamber

Compressed air
from tank

Pressure gauge

Leaf Attached to Plant

Xylem sap under tension

Excised Leaf

Tension released,
vessels expand

Cut

Sap drawn in by
expansion of vessels

Vessels compressed until
sap forced out

Fig. 5-6   *Diagram explaining Scholander's pressure chamber method of measuring tension in the xylem. Leaf is cut off plant, immediately placed into chamber, and pressure is increased until sap begins to emerge from cut ends of vessels, which are now being compressed from the outside to the same extent that they were previously being contracted by pull from within. The procedure is normally carried out with a small branch rather than a single leaf, which is illustrated (with grossly exaggerated vascular elements) for simplicity of representation. A feature not shown in the diagram is that when tension is released by excision, xylem sap is absorbed by leaf cells and this is returned to the xylem when the cells are compressed by the imposed pressure. (See P. F. Scholander et al., Science, **148:** 339, 1965.)*

determination and monitoring of leaf water potential as used to obtain the water potential data shown in Figures 4-4 and 5-3. These methods actually measure the saturation vapor pressure of water in the leaf, which is related to the leaf's water potential as will be explained later in the chapter.

The *velocity* of xylem sap flow can be measured in an intact plant by the "heat pulse" method illustrated and explained in Figure 5-7. Such measurements show a dramatic variation of sap flow rate in trees with time of day, conforming in general with the transpiration curve as exemplified in Figure 5-1. The heat pulse method reveals also that in some broadleaved trees the velocity of sap flow is very large compared with what one would predict from the transpiration rate and the cross-sectional area of the xylem. It seems that in these trees xylem

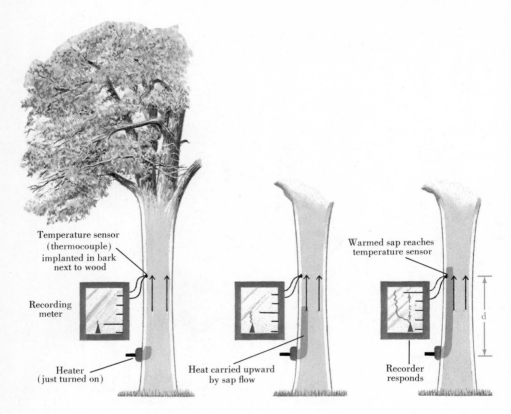

Fig. 5-7   *Heat pulse method for measuring the flow rate of sap in the xylem of an intact plant. From the chart produced by the recording thermometer we read off the time required for the warmed sap to travel the distance* d *between the heater and the temperature sensor located above it. (In actual use the sensor is placed much closer to the heater than implied in the diagram.)*

sap flow is largely confined to a narrow zone of wood just under the bark in which because of its small cross-sectional area a much larger flow velocity is needed to supply the volume demands of transpiration than would be required if the entire cross section of the wood were functional for water transport.

Problems with the Cohesion-Tension Mechanism

Existence of tension in a conducting element depends as previously stated upon its being completely filled with liquid water; if it contains any gas at all, its contents cannot be under tension because a gas always exerts positive pressure. Tension is therefore an unstable state, for both warming of xylem sap and freezing of it tend to cause dissolved air to come out of solution, and various agencies such as mechanical disturbance and ionizing radiation tend to cause formation of gas bubbles. Any conducting element in which a gas bubble forms is thrown completely out of action as far as the tension-cohesion mechanism is concerned. Experiments indeed show that when air is introduced artificially into the xylem, the resistance to flow increases enormously. Microscopic observations indicate that some of the xylem elements in an intact plant contain air bubbles and that the proportion of such blocked elements increases under water stress.

That vascular plants are able to get by despite the seeming precariousness of the tension-cohesion mechanism can be attributed first of all to the huge redundancy ordinarily built into their transport systems by the enormous number of individual cells that are involved (see, for example, Figure 5-4) and to the fact that the cell walls that separate the conducting elements from one another do not allow gas bubbles to pass through, as mentioned above, even though they let liquid water flow rather freely. This compartmentation prevents a gas bubble that forms in one place from spreading through the whole transport system and inactivating it.

Plants that have vessels almost invariably possess tracheid pathways in parallel with the vessels as illustrated in Figure 5-4d. At the cost of higher resistance these tracheids can take over the burden of water transport through any parts of the vascular system in which the vessels become accidentally blocked by "gas embolisms."

Finally, many plants continuously generate new, water-filled xylem elements in their stems and roots by the process of secondary growth (to be discussed in Chapter 8) and thus are able to replace vascular elements that have been knocked out of action by gas embolisms. This may explain the high sap flow rates observed in the outer and most recently formed part of the wood in some trees.

An interesting problem is presented, however, by palm trees, which during their long life span do not add any new vascular elements whatever to the stem except at the top where the tree is growing in height. Palm trees often greatly exceed 33 ft in height and must therefore sustain continuous tensions in their xylem, so it is hard to see how they could avoid succumbing to air embolisms unless they possessed some kind of active mechanism for removing air bubbles from the xylem sap. No such mechanism is known, however.

THE ROOT   Water transport through the xylem to the leaves is accompanied by absorption of water from the soil by the roots. Although the xylem is continuous between the stem and the roots and it extends down to near the tip of each root, it does not open directly into the soil. It is, instead, surrounded on all sides by living tissues of the outer part of the root as illustrated in Figures 5-8 and 6-3a. The absorption of water from the soil and its transfer into the xylem occur in these living tissues.

Water absorption by the root is tied to water transport in the xylem. This may be explained by noting that transport of water through the xylem toward the leaves draws water from the xylem cells in the root, which reduces, as explained previously, the pressure of water in these cells and therefore their water potentials. The resulting water potential difference between soil and root xylem causes a transport of water from the soil across the intervening tissues in which a water potential gradient becomes set up somewhat as the water potential gradient is established in the xylem. As illustrated in Figure 5-8 this transport apparently is a combination of osmotic flow through the membranes of living cells and hydraulic flow in the cell wall space between the cells except at the level of the *endodermis* where the cell wall pathway is blocked by a waxy impregnation called the "Casparian strip" whose function will be considered in Chapter 6.

The vascular tissues of the root are so arranged that in cross section we can see several "arms" of xylem extending outward from the center with strands of phloem located between them; at the ends of the xylem arms no phloem lies exterior to the xylem as it always does in the stem (see Figure 1-2). This arrangement makes it possible for water moving inward from the epidermis to enter the xylem directly without having to cross the phloem in which a separate conduction phenomenon in a different direction is occurring (Chapter 7).

Solute-Induced Water Transport and Root Pressure

The roots of many plants have the ability by themselves to absorb water from the soil and transport it into the xylem. In detached roots this transport can build up a striking positive pressure in the xylem called "root pressure." When the rate of transpiration of an intact plant is very low, as at night under high humidity, enough pressure can develop inside the xylem because of transport by the roots to force liquid water out of the leaves, usually through special pores at the edges of the leaf. This process, called *guttation*, produces part of the "dew" that appears on grass during the night.

Water uptake by detached roots results from transport of mineral ions from the soil into the xylem by the living cells of the root (Chapter 6). When water flow due to transpiration is not occurring, these ions can accumulate in the xylem, building up its solute concentration. This reduces the water potential in the xylem and causes water transport into the xylem by osmosis across the living cells.

The amount of water moved into roots by solute-generated transport is much less than the amounts typically lost by transpiration, so this transport contributes very little to the supply of water to the leaves when they are transpiring rapidly. Under these conditions no positive pressure can build up in the root, so root pressure does not assist in raising water to the tops of trees during normal transpiration. And the roots of some trees, notably conifers, exhibit no solute-generated water transport or root pressure whatever. Therefore the cohesion-tension mechanism is believed to dominate the dynamics of water transport; the significance of solute-induced transport by roots may be as a mechanism for moving needed mineral ions from roots to shoots during periods of low transpiration.

Transport Resistance of Root

A considerable part of the total resistance to water transport through the plant appears to be caused by the living cells of the root because of the high resistance of osmotically effective cellular membranes (compared with resistance to hydraulic flow in dead xylem cells) that was noted previously. Plants compensate to some extent for the high transport resistance of cellular

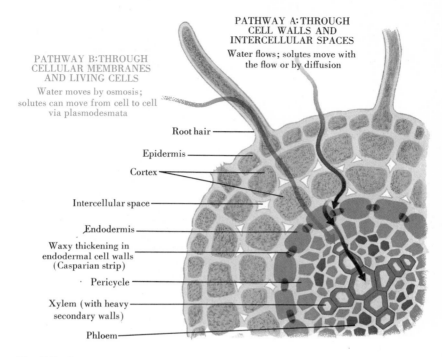

PATHWAY A:THROUGH
CELL WALLS AND
INTERCELLULAR SPACES
Water flows; solutes move with
the flow or by diffusion

PATHWAY B:THROUGH
CELLULAR MEMBRANES
AND LIVING CELLS
Water moves by osmosis;
solutes can move from cell to cell
via plasmodesmata

Root hair

Epidermis

Cortex

Intercellular space

Endodermis

Waxy thickening in
endodermal cell walls
(Casparian strip)

Pericycle

Xylem (with heavy
secondary walls)

Phloem

Fig. 5-8 *Diagrammatic cross section of a root, showing pathways of uptake of water and
nutrients. Living cells, enclosed by differentially permeable cell membranes, are shown stippled. Note how waxy thickenings in cell walls of endodermis block off pathway A all the
way around the vascular core of the root. For simplicity the cortex is shown as being only
two cells thick, although in typical roots it is much thicker. Thickness of cell walls of living
cells is exaggerated in the diagram. (See Figure 8-4 for cross sections of an actual root,
showing typical proportions of and relations between tissues.)*

membranes by proliferating enormously the extent of root surface in contact
with soil. The root system typically branches and rebranches much more extensively than the shoot, and even a small plant such as wheat develops miles of
total root length. Second, the root epidermis (which does *not*, like the epidermis
of the shoot, produce a waxy cuticle) develops elongated tubular extensions, root
hairs, from many of its cells that greatly increase the surface area.

Although dead roots, in which the osmotic membranes of the cells have
been destroyed, offer much less resistance to water movement than do living
ones, it is not possible for the plant to eliminate these living tissues in the interest of increased efficiency of absorption. For one thing the myriad of root
hairs makes it possible for the roots to tap a sufficiently large volume of soil to
supply the plant with the water it needs, and the functioning of the root hairs
depends upon the fact that they have differentially permeable cellular membranes and can absorb water by osmosis. Moreover, growth of the root as a
whole often seems to be essential to adequate water absorption. This is because
of water transport properties of the soil which will be discussed in the next section.

WATER TRANSPORT The water potential of soil is related to the soil's
IN THE water content and in normal soils is determined
SOIL mainly by the matric effect on water potential
(page 73).

As water is taken up from the soil by the roots and root hairs, the soil's
water potential at the root surface is reduced and water tends to flow toward the
surface from the bulk soil under this water potential difference. In wet soils this
works well to supply the roots with a water volume that meets their demands.

As the soil dries out, either from evaporation or from moisture depletion
by plant roots, its water potential decreases due to the fact that the remaining
water is more and more tightly bound to the soil particles. Since the plant cannot
obtain water unless its water potential is less than that of the soil, the plant's
water potential must decrease correspondingly.

An adverse complication arises from the fact that the resistance of a soil
to water flow *increases* as soil water potential falls. This means that as a soil
dries out, water movement through it becomes very slow; as the root-hair zone
exhausts the water available in its vicinity, little moves in from adjacent soil
even though it contains water. In order to get adequate water the root may have
to grow continually into new soil and form new root hairs.

As plants deplete the soil of water and reduce its water potential, a point is
eventually reached at which the plant cannot absorb water except when the
turgor pressure of the leaf cells has fallen to zero and the leaves have wilted. At
this point the water potential of the soil has become equal to the osmotic effect
of the leaf cells' solutes (*s* in Equation 5-1); the turgor pressure (*P*) of the leaves
cannot rise above zero in these circumstances because the water potential of the
leaves cannot become greater than that of the soil from which they get their
water. The leaves therefore *stay* wilted, even when transpiration is not occurring. This "permanent wilting point" represents essentially the limit of soil dry-
ness and water potential beyond which the plant's method of maintaining water
balance ceases to be effective.

Soils differ greatly in the amenities of water supply that they can furnish
plants; these differences are principally a function of soil texture.

Course-textured sandy or gravelly soils can hold relatively little water
when saturated, so that after a rain the water disappears rapidly from the root
zone by percolation downward, evaporation, and plant water uptake. Therefore
except in very rainy climates these soils often reach the permanent wilting point
and the kind of vegetation that inhabits them must be able to tolerate this; for
example, often found are pines, oaks, and other plants with tough reinforced
leaves as described on page 67.

Clay soils consist of much finer particles (page 107) and can hold considerably more water. As a clay soil dries out, however, it tends to become tough and
difficult for roots to penetrate and it also develops a large resistance to water
transport. Indeed the dense texture of clay soils impedes water permeation even
when the soil is wet, so that much of the precipitation that could be used for
plant needs may be lost as runoff. Therefore clay soils tend to be disadvantageous for plant growth in arid or semiarid climates, although they are satisfactory in the humid climates that exist in many tropical regions.

Loam soils are those that consist of sand and/or clay plus a substantial proportion of organic matter that arises in a manner to be discussed in Chapter 6. This organic matter confers a light, spongy texture that favors water and root penetration and permits retention of substantial amounts of water above the wilting point. Loams are therefore generally the most favorable soils for plant growth.

A *saline* (salty) condition develops in soils in regions of low precipitation, such as in the southwest United States, in places where a large inflow of ground water, for example, by irrigation, disappears largely by evaporation rather than percolation or runoff. The salts contained in the ground water accumulate to high concentrations in the surface layers of the soil. This results in a substantial osmotic effect of solutes (s, Equation 5-1), so the soil's water potential is very negative even when waterlogged. Ordinary crop plants may find themselves very near the permanent wilting point in such a soil. Because partial or complete stomatal closure is inevitable for much or all of the time, photosynthesis, growth, and crop yield are severely reduced, and plants can suffer desiccation injury or death.

Similar conditions occur naturally in coastal salt marshes and in extreme form around the "dry lakes" or basins in which surface water evaporates in desert areas. Here we find native plants that are able to grow in saline soils because they possess the ability to accumulate abnormally high salt concentrations in their cells, reaching solute effects of as much as −100 bars in some instances. These plants thereby develop a water potential lower than that of the saline environment and can remove water from it while maintaining an appreciable turgor pressure in their cells.

REGULATION OF WATER TRANSPORT

In this discussion we have regarded transpiration as a process whose rate is fixed by environmental conditions and have attempted to explain how water loss from the leaves creates water potential forces that generate a compensating flux through the transport system. In other words, water transport is regulated by transpiration. That this expectation is correct in principle can be seen by the following considerations.

The water potential of water vapor in air is related to its water vapor concentration. The lowest water potentials reached by most functioning plants, for example, at the permanent wilting point, still correspond to water vapor concentrations within a few percent of saturation. The water vapor concentration in the outside air, on the other hand, is typically far below saturation as discussed in Chapter 4. Therefore the water potential difference that exists across the leaf-air boundary is typically much greater than the entire water potential difference within the plant. In a steady state of transport the flux through these two resistances (transpiration and plant) must be the same; because the potential drop across the former is much greater than across the latter, it follows that when expressed in comparable terms the transpiration resistance must be much greater than the sum of all transport resistances within the plant (see Figure 5-2). This situation is evidently necessary in order for the leaves to be maintained in the air at a high enough water potential and water content for them to function effectively in photosynthesis, and this maintenance is in turn made possible by the evolution of the efficient low-resistance water transport machinery that we have discussed above.

By the principles considered in Chapter 4, however, the flux through any series circuit is essentially governed by whichever resistance is large compared with the rest. Therefore transpiration resistance inevitably controls water transport within the plant and transpiration rate is independent of internal water flow or water potential, except as these factors can influence the transpiration resistance or other physical parameters of transpiration.

But for one regulatory capability plants would, in consequence of the foregoing, be totally at the mercy of environmental conditions in regard to their water balance and survival. Their mechanisms for maintaining water balance would indeed collapse completely at the wilting point, beyond which rapid changes of water potential due to turgor pressure changes are no longer possible. The saving feature in this precarious state of affairs is, of course, the stomatal mechanism, which (as discussed earlier) responds to wilting conditions, either temporary or permanent wilting, by closure, causing an enormous increase in transpiration resistance and thereby reducing the transpiration rate dramatically. Stomates thus afford a means by which the capacity of the plant for water transport and absorption can and does powerfully regulate the rate of transpiration, at least under water stress conditions.

Even wilted plants, however, lose some water by evaporation through the cuticle, and many plants from moist climates soon become injured or killed at the permanent wilting point. Desert plants, however, are able to tolerate months or even years at the permanent wilting point in a soil from which water can hardly be extracted and in an environment that is maximally conductive to water loss. Many of them apparently succeed in this situation by means of leaf adaptations (discussed in Chapter 4) that minimize transpiration when the stomates are closed. It has even been suggested that some such plants may maintain water balance by taking up water vapor from the air at night by virtue of the extremely low water potential that their leaves develop.

Succulent plants, cacti, *Agave*, and some others store up large amounts of water, when obtainable from the soil, in special water storage tissue in their leaves or stems. They conserve this water over long periods of drought while still engaging in gas exchange to support photosynthesis, by making use of biochemical and stomatal adaptations (discussed on page 67). Such plants are therefore rarely in a state of water balance called for by a flow circuit like that shown in Figure 5-2.

Even in relatively moist environments many primitive plants such as mosses, lichens, and ferns succeed in habitats that seasonally become much too dry for their poorly developed powers of water absorption, transport, and retention. Instead of trying to maintain water balance, they simply shrivel and dry up, coming to look almost as dead as a piece of paper. But their cells are not dead, and when moisture returns they swell up and return, sometimes within minutes, to a functional state. To survive adverse conditions simply by being tough enough to tolerate them is in a way less effective than to have equipment and behavior for circumventing the conditions, as many vascular plants do; the latter can get ahead during periods when the less well equipped are "out of business." However, just as with human problems, there is something to be said for both methods of dealing with adversity.

SUGGESTED READING

Fogg, G. E. (ed.), "The State and Movement of Water in Living Organisms," *Symposia of the Society for Experimental Biology*, **19,** 1965.

Knight, R. O., *The Plant in Relation to Water*. New York: Dover Publications, 1965. Chapters 4, 6, and 7.

Kramer, P. J., *Plant and Soil Water Relationships: A Modern Synthesis*. New York: McGraw-Hill, 1969.

Nobel, P. S., *Plant Cell Physiology*. San Francisco: Freeman, 1970. Chapter 2.

Rose, C. W., *Agricultural Physics*. New York: Pergamon Press, 1966. Chapter 8.

Scholander, P. F., H. T. Hammel, D. Bradstreet, and E. A. Hemmingsen, "Sap Pressure in Vascular Plants," *Science*, **148:** 339–346, 1965.

Slatyer, R. O., *Plant-Water Relationships*. New York: Academic Press, 1967. Chapter 7.

Sutcliffe, J., *Plants and Water*. New York: St. Martin's Press, 1968. Chapters 3, 4, and 7.

Zimmerman, M. H., "How Sap Moves in Trees," *Scientific American*, **208** (3): 132–142, 1963.

Zimmerman, M. H., "Sap Movements in Trees," *Biorheology*, **2:** 15–27, 1964.

chapter 6

Mineral Economy

Apart from their requirements for light and water, the most conspicuous demand plants make upon their environment is for the various chemical elements other than carbon, hydrogen, and oxygen that are indispensable to their life. These "mineral elements" are normally absorbed by the roots from the soil.

Many of the commonly occurring mineral elements, and a considerable list of not-so-common ones, are needed by both animals and plants. The functions that these elements perform are to a considerable extent similar in both types of organism. The requirements of plants for minerals appear somewhat more conspicuous than those of animals, because animals eat organic food and this food usually contains the necessary elements (calcium in milk, iron in meat, and so on). The need for organic food dominates the dietary habits of animals, whereas with plants, which have no such need, the requirement for inorganic minerals is paramount. Traced back through the food chain, much of the dietary mineral element intake of land animals is derived ultimately from mineral salts that were absorbed from the soil by plants.

Curiously enough certain of the most abundant elements, notably sodium and chlorine which are required (as Na^+ and Cl^-) in large amounts for the well-being of higher animals, are needed in trace amounts, at most, by plants. On the other hand at least one element, boron, that serves no known function in the animal body is absolutely essential to plants.

The most widely employed method of establishing what elements a plant requires is to grow it in water culture, in which its roots, instead of growing in soil, are suspended in a vessel of distilled water to which has been added appropriate inorganic salts containing a variety of elements. If the omission of a particular element from the salts used results in poor growth and in symptoms of disease, the element in question can be considered essential.

THE ESSENTIAL By the water culture method it was established
MINERAL ELEMENTS before the end of the last century that plants require the elements nitrogen, phosphorus, potassium, calcium, magnesium, sulfur, and iron. Nitrogen, the mineral element they require in largest amounts, is obtained from the soil as nitrate (NO_3^-) or as ammonium (NH_4^+) ions. Plants obtain sulfur as sulfate (SO_4^{2-}) and phosphorus as phosphate (PO_4^{3-}); the remaining elements mentioned are absorbed as their simple ions (K^+, Ca^{2+}, Mg^{2+}, Fe^{2+}, or Fe^{3+}). The amounts of these elements that are required by growing plants are large enough for ill effects usually to appear within a few days after a plant is deprived of one of them, and the necessity for them can be detected by very simple technique.

During the present century it has been found that plants suffer or even die if deprived of any of several elements that are much less abundant in nature than those mentioned above, and that are required in such small amounts that mere contaminating traces are often sufficient to supply the needs of plants when ordinary chemicals are used to make up culture solutions. Thus these requirements escaped the notice of earlier investigators. These elements include boron, manganese, zinc, copper, and molybdenum. They are called *trace elements* or *micronutrient elements* to distinguish them from the *macronutrient elements*, those previously mentioned elements that are required in large amounts and for which the requirement is easily detected.

The amounts of the various elements typically required for good growth of plants in water culture solutions are shown in Table 6-1. The amount of iron required is not much greater than of some of the trace elements; hence iron is now generally listed as one of the micronutrient elements even though the requirement for it is easy to detect.

At the end of Table 6-1 are listed three common elements, chlorine (Cl), sodium (Na), and silicon (Si). In soil-grown plants these elements occur in amounts comparable to the macronutrient elements. Unlike the case with macronutrients, however, it is possible, by using water-culture solutions to which Na, Si, and Cl are not added, to obtain plants in which the amounts of these elements have been vastly reduced without any apparent ill effects.

Table 6-1   Mineral Elements Required by Green Plants

Element	Approx. Level Needed[a]	Role in Plant Function
		MACRONUTRIENTS
Nitrogen (N)	15	In proteins, coenzymes, nucleic acids, etc.
Potassium (K)	5	Activates certain enzymes in glycolysis; important in cell membrane potentials
Calcium (Ca)	3	Structure and permeability properties of membranes; structure of middle lamella
Phosphorus (P)	2	In nucleic acids, coenzymes, ATP, metabolic substrates
Sulfur (S)	1	In proteins; in coenzymes for carbohydrate and lipid metabolism
Magnesium (Mg)	1	In chlorophyll; Mg^{2+} a required cofactor for many enzymes
		MICRONUTRIENTS
Iron (Fe)	0.1	In enzymes of electron transfer chain (cytochromes, ferredoxin), nitrogenase, etc.; essential for chlorophyll synthesis
Boron (B)	0.05	Unknown (possibly in cell wall formation in meristems and/or in sugar translocation)
Manganese (Mn)	0.01	Formation of O_2 in photosynthesis; cofactor for various enzymes
Zinc (Zn)	0.001	In several dehydrogenases of respiration and nitrogen metabolism; in carbonic anhydrase
Copper (Cu)	0.0003	In respiration (cytochrome oxidase) and photosynthesis (plastocyanin; ribulose diphosphate carboxylase)
Molybdenum (Mo)	0.0001	In nitrate reductase; in nitrogenase (N_2 fixation)
Cobalt[b] (Co)	<0.00001	For symbiotic N_2 fixation; for blue-green algae and (as part of vitamin B_{12}) for various other algae
Chlorine (Cl)	0.05	Cl^- activates O_2-producing system of photosynthesis
Sodium[b] (Na)	0.05	Required by *Atriplex* (saltbush) and probably by other saline-habitat plants, sugar beet, and blue-green algae; role unknown
Silicon[b] (Si)	0.1	Essential for *Equisetum* (horsetail) and probably for rice and some other grasses and sedges; required by diatoms for cell wall formation
Iodine[b] (I)	0.001	Required by certain brown and red algae; role unknown

[a] Milligram atoms (millimoles of a salt containing the element) per liter of nutrient solution. These figures are extremely approximate and vary considerably with the species.

[b] These elements are not as yet known to be required *generally* by plants, as are the other elements listed in the table.

With a number of plant species, however, it has been proved that chloride ion (Cl⁻) is required in small but definite amounts for healthy growth. The Cl⁻ requirement is difficult to detect because it is harder to reduce contamination by Cl⁻ to low enough levels than it is, for example, to get rid of contamination by the trace metals. The amount of Cl⁻ found to be required is actually considerably larger than the requirements for some of the trace metals (see Table 6-1).

Beneficial effects of sodium on higher plant growth have been obtained mainly in plants with a reduced supply of potassium, in which sodium is thought to make the limited amount of potassium "go farther" in the plant. A specific and vital requirement for small amounts of sodium has been demonstrated, however, for the "saltbush," *Atriplex*, a shrub that in nature grows in salty soils and accumulates very large quantities of NaCl (see page 105). There are indications that other plants adapted to salty habitats require sodium. Careful experiments with sugar beet also indicate that sodium is probably required by this species. It seems likely that sodium is more generally required by plants but in such trace amounts that it has not yet been possible to reduce contamination enough to produce disease symptoms and hence to detect the requirement.

Both sodium and chlorine are needed by certain algae, and silicon is required absolutely for growth of the unicellular algae called *diatoms*, whose cell walls are built of silica (SiO₂). Certain vascular plants, notably the horsetail (*Equisetum*) and many grasses (for example, rice) and sedges, take up particularly large amounts of silica and deposit it in cell walls and special siliceous structures. A number of workers have found that depriving these plants of silicon leads to poor growth and symptoms of disease, so that silicon may be considered an essential element for them.

Several marine algae have been reported to require iodine (I), an element that is accumulated in large amounts by certain species. Another curiosity of algal nutrition is the requirement of a variety of unicellular algae for cobalt (Co) as a constituent of vitamin B₁₂. Animals require cobalt for the same function, but it has not been possible so far to detect any requirement for cobalt by higher plants, with the interesting exception of symbiotic nitrogen fixation which will be discussed later.

IMPORTANCE OF MINERAL ELEMENTS IN FUNCTION   Biochemical studies of cell metabolism have shown that most of the required mineral elements are needed as parts of, or for the activity of, particular enzymes in important metabolic processes. Table 6-1 lists some of the important roles that mineral elements are known to serve in plants. The roles of nitrogen and phosphorus in metabolism are of course so numerous that a detailed listing would be impractical.

The external symptoms of mineral element deficiency are often quite distinctive for different elements and reflect to some extent both the functions that they serve and the ability of the plant to translocate and reutilize them (discussed in Chapter 7). For example, nitrogen is required for chlorophyll synthesis and a nitrogen deficiency invariably shows as a strong yellowing or *chlorosis*, which occurs in the older leaves since nitrogen is moved from older to growing parts under shortage conditions. This is also true of magnesium deficiency because magnesium is required for chlorophyll formation, but the chlorosis is usually less marked and the affected leaves show other disease features. On the other hand, deficiency of iron causes strong chlorosis because iron is required in reactions by which chlorophyll is synthesized, but in this case (a common ailment of house plants) chlorosis is most pronounced in the young leaves because iron is not moved from mature leaves to growing points.

Other deficiencies that affect the growing points most strongly are those of Ca^{2+}, which is apparently required for normal cell wall formation and growth in meristems, and of boron, which deficiency leads to abnormal growth and finally death of the shoot tips. This has been ascribed variously to involvement in cell wall formation and in translocation of sugar to the growing region, but the exact manner in which boron functions in plants is still unknown.

Deficiency of phosphorus does not destroy the growing regions (since phosphorus is mobile) nor does it cause chlorosis but results in generally stunted growth often accompanied by a conspicuous red or purple pigmentation of the leaves due to anthocyanin pigments which contain sugars. This symptom may be due to an inhibited ability of the plant to utilize its sugar by the central metabolic processes that require conversion of sugar into phosphate derivatives (Figure 2-7).

ABSORPTION OF MINERAL IONS   It is natural to suppose that since minerals occur in the soil and the plant's roots are located in the soil, the required minerals simply diffuse into the roots or flow along with the water that the roots absorb from the soil. Study of ion uptake by living plant tissues and by isolated roots has shown, however, that they take up ions vigorously when no absorption of water is occurring, and that they can absorb an ion even when the concentration and electrochemical potential[1] of this ion inside the tissue is greater than in the external medium. This would be impossible by diffusion, which always goes in the direction of decreasing electrochemical potential. Movement of ions *against* electrochemical gradients requires energy and takes place by a mechanism called *active transport*.

There is extensive evidence that the energy required for active transport comes from respiration; for example, poisoning the respiration or depriving the tissue of oxygen greatly reduces or stops active transport. With various algal cells and aquatic higher plants a light-stimulated component of ion uptake, dependent upon energy coming directly from photosynthetic reactions, is also detected.

Active transport is believed to be brought about by enzymelike entities called *carriers* which are located in or on the membranes. A carrier can combine with an ion on one side of the membrane and transport the ion to and release it on the other side. One striking indication that specific carriers are involved in

---

[1]Electrochemical potential is a measure of the energy status of an ion (analogous to water potential for water discussed in Chapter 5) which takes into account the effects of both concentration and electrical forces on passive diffusion of the ion.

active transport is the competing effect of chemically similar elements. Elements in the same group of the periodic table, for example K^+ and Rb^+, or Ca^{2+} and Sr^{2+}, often inhibit each other's uptake. Apparently the carrier for one of these ions acts for the other one also, not being able to "tell the difference," but does not act on the chemically dissimilar ions of elements from different groups of the periodic table. Carriers may, however, distinguish between some elements in the same periodic group, for example, between Ca^{2+} and Mg^{2+} or between Na^+ and K^+.

In a plant cell carriers may be located either at the plasma membrane, or at the vacuolar membrane, or at both. To distinguish experimentally the transport of ions through the plasma membrane from that through the vacuolar membrane is difficult. The clearest information has been obtained using certain "giant" algal cells that are millimeters in length or diameter, from which one can directly obtain samples of cytoplasm and vacuolar contents for chemical and isotopic tracer analysis and can insert microelectrodes separately into the cytoplasm and vacuole to measure electrical potential differences. Results indicate the existence of active transport mechanisms at both plasma and vacuolar membranes, at least in respect to the three major ions K^+, Na^+, and Cl^- (Figure 6-1).

Higher plant cells give evidence for the existence of two carrier mechanisms for uptake of certain ions such as K^+, one a "high-affinity" mechanism that absorbs ions vigorously even at low external concentrations and is highly specific for K^+, the other a relatively unspecific "low-affinity" mechanism that operates to a significant extent only at a much higher concentration of ions and transports either Na^+ or K^+. It is believed by some workers that the high-affinity mechanism is located at the plasma membrane, whereas the low-affinity mechanism is located at the vacuolar membrane and serves to transport ions from cytoplasm to vacuole. Others, however, consider both mechanisms to be located in the plasma membrane.

Also somewhat unsettled is the nature of the energy coupling between respiration or photosynthesis and the ion transport machinery. Its energy requirement could, of course, be met by ATP from respiration or from photophosphorylation. There is especially good evidence that light-stimulated K^+ uptake by giant algal cells depends upon photophosphorylation, because K^+ uptake is prevented by inhibitors of photophosphorylation.

On the other hand, some investigators think that ion uptake by plant cells is driven not by ATP but by the flow of electrons across mitochondrial or chloroplast membranes during operation of the electron transfer chains of respiration or photosynthesis. Light-stimulated Cl^- uptake by giant algal cells is blocked by agents that prevent photosynthetic electron flow but is not prevented by inhibitors of photophosphorylation, which conforms with the hypothesis just mentioned. It is not clear, however, how electron flow in chloroplasts or mitochondria can cause ion transport through the plasma or vacuolar membranes.

A major goal in the investigation of active transport is to isolate carriers and determine their mode of action. This goal seems within reach in the case of certain bacterial transport systems and of the ATP-splitting enzyme (ATPase) that may be involved in coupled Na^+-K^+ transport through animal cell membranes. Whether ion carriers of plant cells are similar to these systems is yet to be learned.

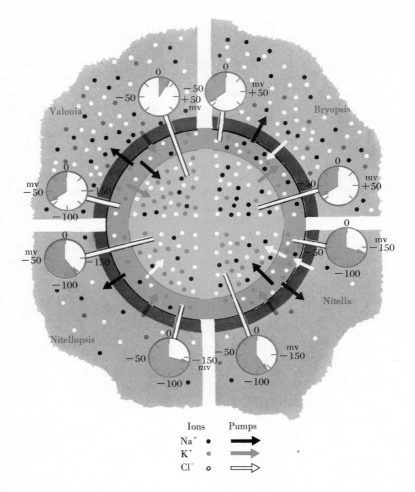

Fig. 6-1   *Ionic relations of giant algal cells. Each quadrant represents a different cell, including two marine algae (above), a brackish-water alga (lower left), and a fresh-water alga (lower right). Gauges indicate electrical potential (in millivolts) of cytoplasm and of vacuole, relative to external medium. Relative concentrations of Na⁺ (black circles), K⁺ (colored circles), and Cl⁻ (open circles) are shown for vacuole and cytoplasm as well as external solution. Arrows of corresponding colors show the active transport pumps for different ions that must be operating across plasma and vacuolar membranes to maintain the observed concentration ratios. (Data from J. Gutknecht and J. Dainty, Oceanography and Marine Biology Annual Review, **6**: 163, 1968.)*

MINERAL ION   TRANSPORT   BY ROOTS   In order for minerals to reach the shoot, ions absorbed by the root from the soil must enter the xylem. It appears that the root moves ions into the xylem by the same type of active transport mechanism as is used by an individual cell to accumulate ions from its surroundings. Under some circumstances the concentration of ions within the xylem of the root may become many times the concentration in the external medium. Absorption of ions into the xylem can be greatly reduced by poisoning the respiration or depriving the roots of oxygen.

The conducting cells of the xylem (tracheids and vessel elements) are dead cells with no metabolism and no membranes and hence by themselves are not capable of actively transporting ions or of retaining concentrations greater than those of the surrounding medium. The vascular cylinder of the root is, however, enclosed by a special layer of cells called the *endodermis* (see Figure 5-8). The cell wall between each endodermal cell and the next develops a conspicuous waxy thickening, the Casparian strip, which appears to block the passage of solutes from one side of the endodermis to the other via this cell wall route. Therefore ions can leave the vascular cylinder only by passing through the *protoplast* of an endodermal cell, whose differentially permeable plasma membrane greatly retards diffusion of ions. Rapid loss of ions from the xylem is thereby prevented.

By what means are ions actively transported by the root from the soil into the dead xylem cells? Most students of this problem favor the idea that the ions that are transported into the vascular system are in fact absorbed actively through the plasma membrane of cells of the outer part of the root (epidermis and cortex), then transported inward from cell to cell through cortex and endodermis via plasmodesmata (protoplasmic connections between cells, see page 11), and finally released into the xylem from cells located inward from the endodermis. This is called the *symplast theory* of ion uptake. The term "symplast" refers to a system of cells whose protoplasts are interconnected as shown in Figure 6-2.

SPECIAL ADAPTATIONS FOR MINERAL UPTAKE

A peculiar feature of the roots of many plants — good examples being many of the principal forest trees such as pines, oaks, and beeches — is the

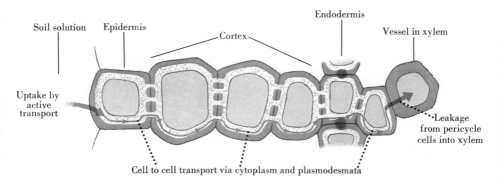

Fig. 6-2   *Diagram illustrating the symplasmic transport concept of ion uptake into xylem of a root. Note how the symplasmic pathway by-passes both cell vacuoles and cell walls. Plasmodesmata are represented much larger, relative to cell size, and fewer in number, than in actuality; their detailed structure is not shown. Diagram of entire root cross section, for comparison, is shown in Figure 5-8.*

association of many of their root tips with fungi which grow upon the root surface and penetrate to varying degrees into the interior. Such roots are called
mycorrhizas. Figure 6-3 shows the structure of a mycorrhiza as compared with
an uninfected root. Many of the mushrooms commonly found on forest floors are
involved in mycorrhizas. The fungus obtains organic nutrients from the host
plant; there is evidence that the host plant also benefits, so the mycorrhizal association can be regarded as an example of the kind of symbiosis called "mutualism," that is, beneficial for both partners.

In soils poor in mineral nutrients it is observed that pine trees grow much
better when fungi that form mycorrhizas are present. Apparently the fungus
absorbs mineral ions more efficiently than do the tree's own roots, and the
fungus thus aids the tree in the competition for scarce minerals. Radioisotope
experiments show that minerals such as phosphorus that have been absorbed by
the fungus are indeed transferred from fungus to the host plant.

Another nutritional relationship that has intrigued people for centuries is
presented by the insect-catching plants such as pitcher plants, sundew, and
Venus' flytrap (Figure 6-4). The insects that these plants capture by means of
their specialized leaf structures become attacked by digestive enzymes released
by the plant and the digestion products are ultimately absorbed by the plant.
Insectivorous plants are green and photosynthetic, and it is found that they grow
perfectly well without any insect meals so long as they are supplied with adequate amounts of the required mineral elements. However, their native habitats

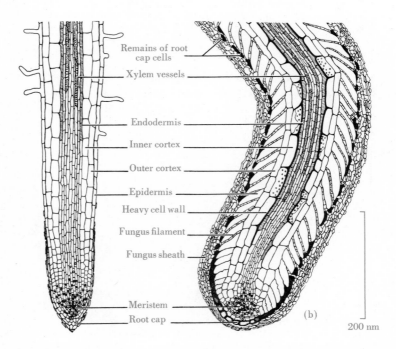

Remains of root
cap cells

Xylem vessels

Endodermis

Inner cortex

Outer cortex

Epidermis

Heavy cell wall

Fungus filament

Fungus sheath

Meristem

Root cap

(b)

200 nm

Fig. 6-3   *Uninfected (a) and mycorrhizal (b) root tips of* Eucalyptus. *(Diagrams by G. A.
Chilvers and L. D. Pryor, from* Australian Journal of Botany, **13**: 245, 1965.)

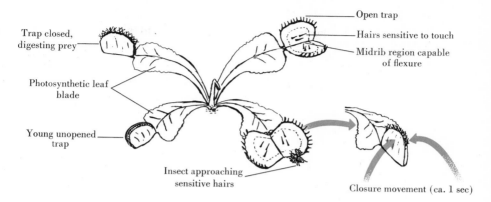

Trap closed, digesting prey

Photosynthetic leaf blade

Young unopened trap

Open trap

Hairs sensitive to touch

Midrib region capable of flexure

Insect approaching sensitive hairs

Closure movement (ca. 1 sec)

Fig. 6-4   *Capture of insect by a young plant of Venus' flytrap* (Dionaea muscipula). *(Approximately natural size. Drawing by Martin F. Ray.)*

are very depleted in minerals and under these conditions their growth is benefited greatly by availability of insects. It seems clear that the insectivorous habit is to be regarded as a specialized way of obtaining essential mineral nutrients.

UTILIZATION OF NITROGEN BY PLANTS   Like all organisms, plants need a wide variety of organic nitrogen compounds for their metabolism and growth: amino acids, purine and pyrimidine bases, B vitamins, porphyrins such as chlorophyll and the heme group of cytochromes. Plants make these from inorganic nitrogen and the carbohydrate that is produced in photosynthesis. Ammonium (NH_4^+) is the form of inorganic nitrogen that can be combined directly with carbon compounds such as a number of the intermediates in respiration (Figure 2-7) to yield certain amino acids and other organic nitrogen compounds.

Under field conditions the principal nitrogen source available to plants is nitrate (NO_3^-), to which the nitrifying bacteria of the soil rapidly convert any ammonium or urea nitrogen that enters the soil from decay and excretion or that is added as fertilizer. Plants can utilize nitrate because they possess a special enzyme system (not found generally among animals) for reduction of nitrate to ammonium:

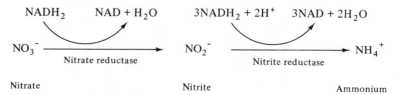

$$NADH_2 \quad NAD + H_2O \qquad 3NADH_2 + 2H^+ \quad 3NAD + 2H_2O$$

$$NO_3^- \xrightarrow[\text{Nitrate reductase}]{} NO_2^- \xrightarrow[\text{Nitrite reductase}]{} NH_4^+$$

Nitrate   Nitrite   Ammonium

Nitrate reductase contains molybdenum as a component essential to its catalytic activity. This appears to be why Mo is required by plants; in molybdenum-deficient plants nitrate cannot be reduced and a nitrogen shortage results.

Ammonium is utilized directly to form only a few organic nitrogen compounds, the principal of these (in terms of quantity) being the amino acid *glutamic acid* which is formed by adding ammonia to one of the organic acid intermediates of the citric acid cycle of respiration (Figure 2-7). The enzyme that catalyzes this reaction, glutamic dehydrogenase, requires zinc for its activity; this is one of the reasons why Zn is an essential element for plants. Nitrogen can readily be transferred from glutamic acid to various other carbon skeletons by a type of enzymatic reaction called *transamination*, and in this way amino acids such as alanine, aspartic acid, glycine, and serine are formed from intermediates in respiration and closely related processes.

Other amino acids are made from these fundamental ones by special biosynthetic pathways. Here we encounter another important difference in nitrogen metabolism between plants and typical animals. Plants can make all of the 20 amino acids that are required for protein synthesis, as of course they must since they have no source for these compounds other than biosynthesis. Animals on the other hand typically lack the enzymes for some of the special pathways for amino acid biosynthesis, so that even though they can make simple amino acids such as glutamic acid or alanine from carbohydrate and ammonium, they must obtain several of the derivative amino acids in their diet or they are unable to synthesize protein.

A similar difference between plants and animals is seen in the case of the B vitamins, which are nitrogen-containing components of various coenzymes such as NAD that are essential to enzyme action and metabolism. Even though plants are self-sufficient for vitamins (and are, of course, the source of vitamins for animals), one finds that when the roots from a plant are removed and an attempt is made to grow them separately in a sterile culture medium, it is necessary to supply not only sugar and the usual required mineral salts but also certain of the B vitamins such as thiamine and nicotinic acid in order to keep the roots growing. Thus it appears that roots lack biosynthetic ability for these vitamins but are normally supplied them by the shoot.

So far as is known the mechanism of protein synthesis by the cytoplasmic and chloroplast ribosomes of plant cells is basically similar to that worked out for animal and bacterial cells, respectively (see Novikoff-Holtzman, *Cells and Organelles* or Loewy-Siekevitz, *Cell Structure and Function*). Certain special features of protein synthesis during plant growth will be discussed in Chapter 8.

NITROGEN FIXATION   One important respect in which the synthetic powers of plants are inadequate is that plants are generally unable to make use of the great store of nitrogen, N_2 gas, in the air. A number of lower plants, chiefly certain bacteria and blue-green algae, do have the ability to convert N_2 gas into combined forms of nitrogen useful to themselves and to other plants. This process is called *nitrogen fixation*.

From the practical point of view the most important nitrogen fixers are special soil bacteria, called *Rhizobium*, which inhabit structures called "nodules" on the roots of plants of the legume family, including many important crop plants such as peas, beans, clover, alfalfa, and peanuts. A variety of other plants, for example, the widespread alder tree and shrubs of the genus *Ceano-*

thus, bear root nodules containing other nitrogen-fixing microorganisms (not *Rhizobium*).

The relationship between root-nodule organisms and the host plant is another example of mutualism: the host plant supplies the nodule microorganisms with organic carbon (sugar) while the microorganisms supply the host plant with usable nitrogen, probably amino acids. As a result the host plant can flourish in soils that are completely lacking in any combined nitrogen (nitrate or ammonium) in which ordinary plants could not grow.

Root-nodule organisms occur in the soil and they infect the roots of a host plant when it grows in the soil. The infection stimulates the development of a nodule which otherwise does not form. Curiously neither the host plant *nor* the microorganism by itself can fix nitrogen; this ability arises only when the two are associated. However, there are a number of heterotrophic soil bacteria that fix nitrogen while living independently (*Azotobacter*, *Clostridium*, and so on), and some photosynthetic bacteria are also known to fix nitrogen.

Probably the most important of the free-living nitrogen-fixing organisms are blue-green algae. Only certain species of blue-green algae have the capacity to fix nitrogen, and all of these species possess occasional distinctively different cells called *heterocysts* (Figure 6-5). It is suspected that the heterocysts are cells that are specialized for N_2 fixation. This segregation of function may be necessary because N_2 fixation is typically inhibited by O_2 and therefore seems incompatible with normal green plant photosynthesis.

Nitrogen fixation by blue-green algae is important in aquatic habitats and in flooded land. It is believed, for example, that blue-green algae are largely responsible for providing the nitrogen needs of rice (a crop that is grown on flooded land) throughout large areas of southern Asia where adequate fertilization is not practiced. Curiously a few vascular plants have evolved specialized chambers in

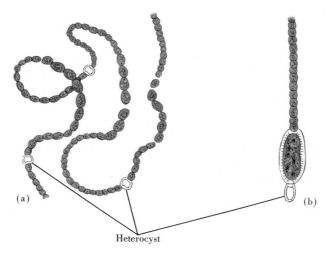

(a)   (b)

Heterocyst

Fig. 6-5   *Nitrogen-fixing blue-green algae, showing unpigmented* heterocyst *cells that may be the sites of nitrogenase action. (a)* Nostoc; *(b)* Cylindrospermum. *Large subterminal cell in (b) is a reproductive spore.*

their leaves that house N_2-fixing blue-green algae, which presumably provide combined nitrogen for the host plant.

Biological fixation of nitrogen is a remarkable process because N_2 is, chemically, among the most inert substances in nature. Only by employing very high temperatures and pressures can the chemist get N_2 to react with anything. Nitrogen-fixing organisms possess a special enzyme system, *nitrogenase*, that is capable of reducing N_2 to NH_4^+ by using a hydrogen donor such as pyruvic acid and ATP as an energy source. The electrons needed for the reduction are transferred to nitrogenase by the iron-protein *ferredoxin* (see page 29) which was originally discovered as a component of the nitrogenase system.

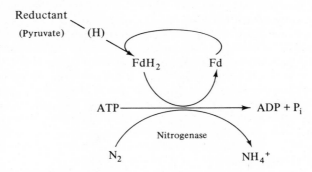

Nitrogenase itself has proved to consist of two distinct proteins, one containing iron only and the other containing both iron and molybdenum. Both of these metals are essential to nitrogen fixation.

Cobalt is also required in very small amounts for effective nitrogen fixation by root nodules, even though the host plant (legume, alder, and so on) grows well without Co when combined nitrogen is available. The Co requirement seems to be for growth of the symbiotic microorganism; free-living nitrogen-fixing bacteria and blue-green algae also require cobalt.

REGULATION OF MINERAL NUTRIENT ECONOMY The inability to make all of its nitrogen compounds from ammonia or amino nitrogen means that an animal always has some form of nitrogen left over, in excess of its capacity to reuse it, from the constantly occurring biochemical breakdown (turnover) of its cellular proteins and other nitrogenous constituents as well as from surplus nitrogen compounds that have been ingested. Disposal of this waste nitrogen is one of the principal aspects of excretion by animals (see Griffin-Novick, *Animal Structure and Function* in the Modern Biology Series).

Plants, which can make use of ammonium for synthesis of all their nitrogen compounds, normally reuse all the nitrogen from their turnover processes. Plants therefore do not need to excrete nitrogen, and they have no excretory machinery comparable with the elaborate mechanisms that have evolved in the animal kingdom.

Almost the only circumstance in which waste ammonium tends to accumulate in a plant is when it grows for so long in the dark that it exhausts its supply of carbohydrates and is forced to utilize its protein in respiration, for example, a seed germinating in darkness. The left-over ammonium is then trapped by combining it with glutamic or aspartic acids to form the amides *glutamine* or *asparagine*. This nitrogen can be reutilized later when light becomes available and photosynthesis begins to produce sugar.

Plants exhibit notable regulatory behavior in the utilization of nitrate nitrogen. The nitrate reductase system proves to be substrate inducible. When a plant is grown on ammonium as nitrogen source, nitrate and nitrite reductases are not made, but if the plant is transferred to a nitrate medium, these enzymes are rapidly formed. Substrate induction serves to adjust the level of the nitrate reductase system so that it can handle whatever nitrate is available from the environment.

The second important function that excretion serves in animals is to regulate the ionic composition of body fluids by eliminating amounts and kinds of mineral ions that have been absorbed in excess. Although plants lack a specialized excretory system, they nevertheless have certain means for regulating their ion balance. As illustrated in Figure 6-1 aquatic algae possess a sodium pump, rather comparable to that of animal cells, which expels Na^+ through the plasma membrane to the exterior and in certain cases also from the cytoplasm into the vacuole, thus maintaining the concentration of Na^+ in the cytoplasm at a relatively low level. Higher plants on the other hand tend to accumulate Na^+, although because of carrier characteristics mentioned above, K^+ is taken up preferentially over Na^+ when the outside concentration of these ions is low.

Regulation of the ion content of land plant tissues must be effected at the level of uptake by the roots. Roots show regulatory ion transport behavior tied to their salt status. When grown in media of low ion concentration, they avidly absorb all the nutritionally important ions using carriers of high affinity. If such roots are provided with luxury levels of mineral nutrients, however, they absorb ions rapidly at first, but gradually shut down their ion transport pumps to a level of activity that maintains the ionic concentrations within the plant at moderate (in some cases rather closely regulated) values as the plant grows. The mechanism of this kind of regulation is not at all well understood.

Among plants that have specialized for inhabiting saline (salty) habitats such as coastal salt marshes or desert salt flats and dry lakes we find many, such as *Atriplex* mentioned previously, that carry out an extraordinary accumulation of NaCl in their cells, to concentrations in some cases in excess of $2 M$ (12 percent). This permits them to obtain water from their high-salt environment (page 89). Moreover some plants that grow in saline habitats, such as the tamarisk tree (*Tamarix*) that is widely planted in desert areas, have evolved salt-excreting glands on their leaves which expel excess NaCl that has been absorbed by the roots and transported upward in the xylem, much as marine birds dispose of excess NaCl via salt-secreting glands (see Griffin-Novick, *Animal Structure and Function*).

The carriers for nitrate uptake show in some instances a substrate inducibility similar to that which controls the level of nitrate reductase. Under natural or primitive agricultural conditions luxury levels of nitrate are rarely if ever available to plants, which therefore had in the past no need to develop mechanisms to prevent excess nitrate uptake. In modern competitive agriculture, however, it has become widespread practice to attempt to maximize crop yields by literally force feeding with excessive nitrogen fertilization. Under these conditions more nitrate is sometimes absorbed than can be reduced by the nitrate reductase system at maximal levels of induction, and nitrate then accumulates in the tops of the plants and can actually be passed on in the produce to consumers in toxic quantities. Much of the nitrogen that is supplied at this level cannot be absorbed or utilized by the crop and becomes a serious cause of water pollution.

MINERAL NUTRIENTS IN THE SOIL

Mineral nutrition of plants is one of the principal determinants of natural productivity both on land and in aquatic habitats. As implied previously nitrogen is the element that is most often limiting to plant growth in natural or primitive agricultural ecosystems. This is not only because nitrogen is the element required in largest amount, but also because nitrogen is the one element that is not obtainable in quantity from the breakdown (weathering) of parent rocks from which soils and the mineral nutrients of natural waters are ultimately derived. The "nitrogen capital" of a natural ecosystem is therefore largely a biological product, accumulated as a result of the past nitrogen fixation that the ecosystem has supported (or that some other system has, in case of an aquatic ecosystem whose minerals are washed in from elsewhere). Hence we have the importance of nitrogen fertilization in efforts to raise productivity artificially as commented upon above.

The availability of required elements other than nitrogen is conditional in the first instance upon the chemical composition of the local parent rocks, or of rocks some distance away in the case of alluvial soils, and of the minerals of natural waters. Not astonishingly there are regions whose soils are deficient individually for any one to, in some cases, several of the macroelements. Most often encountered are deficiencies of potassium, and/or phosphorus; these elements are therefore included with nitrogen in the usual "NPK" general fertilizers. Severe deficiencies of calcium with excess of magnesium occur in regions of "ultrabasic" ("serpentine") parent rocks, and in many such areas one can observe a highly distinctive "serpentine flora" of species that have evolved the ability to obtain calcium from soils that are completely sterile for ordinary plants.

Considering the minute amounts of micronutrient elements that plant growth requires it is surprising to learn that stubborn agricultural problems in various places have proved to be due to deficiencies of boron, manganese, zinc, copper, or molybdenum. In one area of California, for example, sickly growth of fruit trees is due to zinc deficiency and can be cured by the simple expedient of driving a galvanized (zinc plated) nail into each tree trunk. Because of the importance of molybdenum in N_2 fixation and NO_3^- reduction (pages 101, 104), serious shortage of nitrogen is encountered in certain Australian soils that are deficient in molybdenum. This problem can be ameliorated by applying as little as an ounce of molybdenum per acre.

Soil Development and Function

The nutrient status of terrestrial ecosystems depends profoundly upon what goes into the development and exploitation of the local soil; the prevalent mineral deficiencies of ecological and agricultural significance are actually due more often to soil conditions than to defects in composition of the parent rocks. Soil development and maintenance involve a complex combination of physical, chemical, and biological processes.

Weathering of rock minerals yields soluble mineral nutrient ions and also minute aluminum silicate fragments (clay particles) that have the capacity to bind cations (positive ions) such as Na^+, K^+, Mg^{2+}, and Ca^{2+}. These ions thus can be retained in substantial amounts in soil in a manner that prevents them from being readily washed away by rain water, but the nutrient ions are available to plants because the binding is reversible. The production of plant debris resulting from growth of vegetation and attendant N_2 fixation feeds a wide variety of decomposer microorganisms whose activities both release previously utilized minerals in available form and generate a residue of relatively stable organic matter called "humus" which retains important elements such as nitrogen and phosphorus in insoluble, slowly available form. This organic matter provides additional binding sites for retention of mineral nutrient ions and also improves the texture and water-retention properties of the soil (page 89).

Through these processes a local ecosystem generates a "capital" of all the mineral nutrients, which is continually reutilized or "cycled" over a time scale of years, and at any one time greatly exceeds what would be available by immediate weathering of parent rock minerals or (in the case of nitrogen) the immediately occurring nitrogen fixation. Physical factors that affect the relevant biological and chemical processes strongly influence the extent of development of the nutrient capital. For example, arid or arctic conditions that inhibit growth of vegetation and accompanying accumulation of organic matter and nitrogen fixation result in soils poor in all the mineral nutrients, and the same tends to be true if any one of the major nutrients is in serious deficiency in the parent rock.

Another factor that strongly conditions the nutrient status of the soil is acidity or alkalinity. Alkaline soils often develop from calcareous (limestone) rocks; under alkaline conditions iron and phosphorus form very insoluble salts and consequently become unavailable to ordinary plants even when substantial amounts are present. Various wild plant species have evolved the ability to obtain adequate amounts of nutrients from calcareous soils and may be recognized as making up the distinctive vegetation of limestone regions.

Alkaline conditions typically exist also in the saline soils that can develop in arid regions (page 89); here the problem for crop plants is aggravated by the high concentration of Na^+ which displaces nutritionally important cations such as K^+ and Ca^{2+} from soil binding sites and permits them to be washed away. Boron accumulates in some alkaline soils and proves to be severely toxic to plants at levels above those needed for nutritional purposes (Table 6-1). These problems of arid-climate agriculture are very difficult to overcome.

Acidity tends to develop, on the other hand, in soils of regions of high precipitation or of standing water such as bogs and swamps. Under these conditions most of the cations become leached away as fast as they are released by weathering, their places on the clay and humic acid ion-binding sites being taken by H^+ ions, thus making the soil acidic. Acidification is also encouraged by the accumulation of certain kinds of plant debris, such as the leaf detritus from coniferous forests, microbial decomposition of which produces more humic acids than can be neutralized by the cations that the material contains. Acidity tends in turn to prevent binding and retention of nutrient ions, and acidic conditions also inhibit nitrogen fixation and microbial release of nutrients from debris. Thus acidic soils have a generally poor nutrient status. In addition, acidic conditions make certain of the nutrient elements abnormally available, especially iron and manganese, and have the same effect for aluminum which is not a required element but can become toxic to plants when available in excess, as can manganese. For these and other reasons acidic soils are unfavorable for the great majority of plant species. Certain plants, notably many members of the heather family (Ericaceae) including rhododendrons and azaleas, are specifically adapted to growth in highly acid soils and tolerate their low nutrient levels and toxic influences. However, they are accustomed to what are in effect luxury conditions for iron and when grown in neutral garden soils often need application of iron-rich fertilizers in order to thrive.

Because the mineral nutrient capital of an ecosystem is in a dynamic state, it is readily depreciated by any agencies or practices that break the nutrient cycle, such as erosion, failure to return organic matter to the soil, overcropping, destruction of vegetation, and so on. The consequences are a drastic decrease in productivity; because of the slow and interdependent nature of the processes that contribute to building the nutrient capital, degradation of the nutrient status of a soil cannot be easily or quickly reversed. On the other hand, sound management can do a great deal to conserve favorable soil conditions, and some such practices, like manuring to return nitrogen and organic matter and liming to counteract the tendency to acidification, have been known for a long time. Today we understand to considerable depth the principles involved in maintaining favorable soil conditions, but because of economic pressures for maximum immediate productivity for immediate profit, we witness the pursuit of practices such as excessive ammonia fertilization, mentioned previously, that actually conflict with long-term conservation of soil physical characteristics and nutrient status and also injure other aspects of the ecosystem.

These matters comprise an important part of the plant physiological foundations of agriculture and of ecosystem function, which is considered in depth in Odum, *Ecology*, in the Modern Biology Series.

SUGGESTED READING

Anderson, A. J., and E. J. Underwood, "Trace Element Deserts," *Scientific American*, **200** (1):97-106, 1959.

Gilbert, F. A., *Mineral Nutrition of Plants and Animals*. Norman, Okla.: University of Oklahoma Press, 1949.

Harley, J. L., *The Biology of Mycorrhiza*, 2d ed. London: Leonard Hill, 1969.

Hewitt, E. J., and C. V. Cutting (eds.), *Recent Aspects of Nitrogen Metabolism in Plants*. New York: Academic Press, 1969.

Lloyd, F. E., *The Carnivorous Plants*. Waltham, Mass.: Chronica Botanica, 1942.

Russell, E. W., *Soil Conditions and Plant Growth*, 9th ed. New York: Wiley, 1961.

Scott, G. D., *Plant Symbiosis*. New York: St. Martin's Press, 1969.

Stewart, W. D. P., *Nitrogen Fixation in Plants*. London: Athlone Press, 1966.

Stewart, W. D. P., "Nitrogen-fixing Plants," *Science*, **158**:1426–1432, 1967.

Stiles, W., *Trace Elements in Plants*, 3d ed. Cambridge, England: Cambridge University Press, 1961.

Sutcliffe, J. F., *Mineral Salts Absorption in Plants*. New York: Pergamon Press, 1962. Chapters 1 and 3.

Treshow, M., *Environment and Plant Response*. New York: McGraw-Hill, 1970. Chapter 13.

chapter **7**

Long-Distance Transport of Nutrients

Critical to the functioning of the plant as a whole is the transport, not only of water, but (1) of mineral elements from the roots, where they are absorbed, to the shoot, where they are needed in metabolic processes and (2) of organic carbon from the leaves, where it is produced by photosynthesis, to the nongreen parts, where it is needed for respiration and biosynthesis. In this chapter we consider how the plant body accomplishes these kinds of transport, which are often referred to as *translocation*.

TRANSPORT OF MINERALS By applying to the roots radioactive isotopes of mineral elements such as radioactive potassium or radioactive phosphorus, it has been shown that the mineral ions absorbed by the roots move upward to the aerial parts of the plant via the xylem, this being the pathway followed by the radioactivity. The means by which mineral ions are actively transported by the root into its xylem were considered in Chapter 6. In the xylem the mineral ions appear to be carried along passively by the flow of water, and as the ions arrive in the top of the plant they are absorbed by the living cells. The rate of water flow in the xylem is usually rapid enough (several centimeters per minute) for radioactive minerals to reach the top of a small plant in a matter of minutes after they are applied to the roots. Movement all the way to the top of a tree takes, of course, considerably longer.

Under ecologically natural nitrogen-limiting conditions it appears that much or all of the nitrate that is absorbed by plants becomes reduced to ammonia and converted into organic nitrogen compounds (page 101) within the roots. Organic nitrogen compounds are therefore translocated through the xylem to the shoot. If we collect and evaporate a sample of xylem sap, we can detect the presence of some of the common amino acids such as alanine, leucine, glutamic and aspartic acids, and the related amides (glutamine and asparagine, page 105). Certain plants have developed specialized nitrogen transport compounds, notably the *ureides* or urea derivatives, which are found in xylem sap. Under moderate nitrogen fertilization nitrate uptake begins to exceed reduction by the roots; nitrate is then translocated in the xylem sap and is reduced by the inducible nitrate reductase system of the leaves (page 105). Under heavy fertilization the capacity of the latter system can be exceeded and nitrate accumulates in the leaves (as discussed in Chapter 6).

What happens to the minerals after they have reached the top depends upon the particular element. For example, phosphorus and sulfur will move out of the leaves by which they were first absorbed and go into other parts of the plant, particularly the growing parts. This process has been elegantly demonstrated by use of radioactive isotopes. Nitrogen, potassium, and magnesium are likewise very mobile elements within the plant. This mobility permits plants to withdraw their private mineral capital from old parts such as leaves prior to shedding; the yellowing of leaves before they fall reflects breakdown of chlorophyll and is accompanied by almost total breakdown of their protein, with return of this nitrogen to the shoot. The mobile minerals thus can be largely reused or recycled internally over many years without having to be entirely recycled through the ecosystem for each step of growth. As noted in Chapter 6, however, certain elements, especially calcium and iron, seem to move out of leaves only to a minor extent. The needs of growing tissues for calcium and iron must be largely supplied by concurrent uptake and translocation from the roots, and considerable recycling of these elements via the ecosystem presumably occurs during plant growth.

Transport of mobile elements such as phosphorus from leaves to other parts of the plant may readily be detected by applying radioactive phosphate to the surface of a leaf. In experiments of this type it is found that radioactivity travels in the *phloem* rather than the xylem. Export of minerals from leaves shares many features with transport of organic substances produced by photosynthesis, which also travel via the phloem.

THE PHLOEM Phloem (pronounced "flow-em") almost always accompanies xylem tissue, running parallel with the xylem strand (see Figures 1-2, 5-8). Phloem is characterized by the presence of elongated cells with porous sievelike areas in their cell walls, particularly at their ends. In flowering plants these cells are called *sieve-tube elements* and their end walls are *sieve plates* (Figure 7-1a). Sieve-tube elements occur end to end along a phloem strand, the sieve plates of adjacent elements connecting them together into a *sieve tube* in a manner analogous to the joining of vessel elements to form a vessel in the xylem. This structural feature long ago suggested that the sieve-tube elements might be the actual conducting cells of the phloem. Lower vascular plants such as conifers and ferns do not possess identifiable sieve tubes, but their phloem contains *sieve cells* that apparently perform the same transport function, much as tracheids serve in the xylem of these plants the same role that vessels do in flowering plants.

Despite the analogy between tracheids or vessels on the one hand and sieve cells or sieve tubes on the other, the conducting cells of the xylem and phloem contrast profoundly in almost every possible way. Sieve cells and sieve-tube elements do not possess a heavy, lignified secondary wall like that of xylem elements, but on their walls, especially in the sieve areas, there is deposited a distinctive glucose polymer called *callose* that is chemically distinct from both cellulose and starch. And unlike the conduits of the xylem, sieve cells and sieve-tube elements are living cells with an intact, osmotically effective plasma membrane. The transport function of these cells depends upon their vitality, for phloem transport does not occur through a section of stem that has been killed, for example, by scalding it with steam, whereas water transport through the xylem is not prevented.

Remarkably, the living sieve-tube element lacks a nucleus; during the development of a sieve-tube element, the nucleus that was originally present in the cell breaks down and disappears at the time the element matures. Each sieve-tube element is accompanied by one or more closely associated cells with prominent nuclei called *companion cells* (Figure 7-1).

Electron microscope investigation has indicated that the sieve-tube element is also remarkable in possessing very few mitochondria and almost no other cytoplasmic organelles except plastids. Furthermore, as illustrated in Figure 7-1b, the originally present vacuolar membrane and normal distinction between vacuole and cytoplasm disappears. The main volume of the sieve tube is occupied by an aqueous solution, often containing a more or less fibrous proteinaceous material called "slime." The few mitochondria and other organelles that are present are associated with the external plasma membrane. In contrast the companion cells are packed with mitochondria, plastids, dictyosomes, endoplasmic reticulum, and ribosomes. It thus appears that the sieve-tube elements may depend upon the companion cells for general metabolic activities as well as for nuclear functions.

Electron micrographs show, as illustrated in Figure 7-1b, that the plasma membranes of adjacent sieve-tube elements are connected through the sieve-plate pores and therefore impose no osmotic barrier to transport of solutes from cell to cell.

That the sieve-tube elements do indeed function in transport of organic substances from leaves has been proved by the use of radioactive tracers. If a leaf is enclosed in an illuminated chamber while still attached to the stem of the

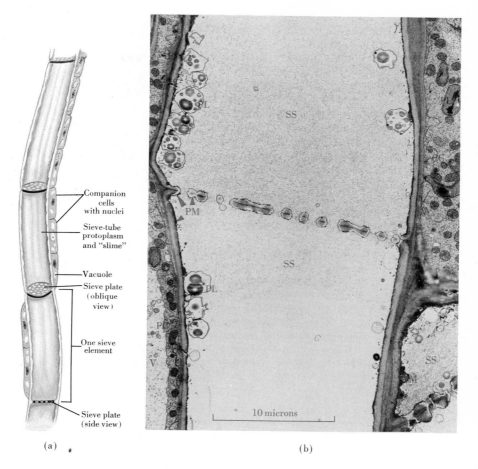

(a)

(b)

Fig. 7-1 *Sieve-tube elements and associated cells in phloem. (a) Sieve tube and com-*
*panion cells of squash (*Cucurbita pepo*). (b) Electron micrograph of adjoining ends of two*
sieve-tube elements of the tobacco plant, showing the large pores that connect the adjacent
cells. CC, companion cell; PC, phloem parenchyma cell; M, mitochondrion; N, nucleus;
PM, plasma membrane; PL, plastid; SS, sieve-tube sap, containing slime protein which
shows as a fibrous material; V, vacuole. Note absence of separate cytoplasm and vacuole
in the sieve-tube cells. (Magnification 3300×. Electron micrograph by R. Anderson and
J. Cronshaw, from Planta, **91:** *173, 1970. Berlin-Heidelberg-New York: Springer 1970.)*

plant and radioactive $^{14}CO_2$ or ^3H_2O is introduced into the chamber, the leaf
forms radioactive products of photosynthesis, and these become transported out
of the leaf and down through the stem (Figure 7-2). Radioactivity is found to be
localized in the phloem of the stem, and in some cases has been seen by autoradiography to occur specifically in the sieve-tube elements rather than in the
other types of cells that are found in the phloem (Figure 7-3).

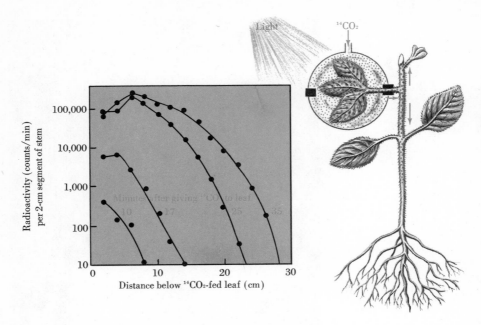

Fig. 7-2 *Method for measuring translocation of radioactive products of photosynthesis (color dots) from a single leaf that is fed radioactive CO_2 (or radioactive H_2O). The movement of radioactivity down the stem can be seen from the radioactivity profiles plotted at different times after supplying $^{14}CO_2$ to the leaf. The apparent velocity of translocation in this soybean plant was about 48 cm per hour. (Data of Donald B. Fisher, from* Plant Physiology, **45:** 107, 1970.)

In order to determine what substances are being transported, we must find out what is in the sieve tubes. If we cut into the actively conducting part of the phloem with a knife, sap exudes which is being forced out of the cut sieve tubes. Another, more ingenious method of obtaining sieve-tube sap takes advantage of the fact that the insects called *aphids* feed on the phloem. From the outside of the stem the aphid inserts a slender feeding tube (the aphid's mouth parts) directly into a single sieve-tube element, thus obtaining for itself a steady supply of what the leaves are exporting via the phloem. By a delicate operation we can cut off the body of a feeding aphid while leaving its mouth parts in position. Pure unaltered sieve-tube sap then exudes from the cut end of the mouth parts, evidently being forced out from within the sieve tube under pressure (see Figure 7-4).

Sieve-tube sap, obtained by either method, proves to be a sweet, concentrated solution of sugar, usually between 10 and 25 percent sugar. In the majority of plants that have been examined the principal sugar in the sieve-tube sap is *sucrose* (cane sugar), formed of one molecule of glucose joined to one of fructose. Simple sugars such as glucose and fructose are not present except in traces. Sucrose therefore appears to be the principal material that is transported. This conclusion is supported by experiments of the type described previously in which radioactive CO_2 or H_2O is fed to a photosynthesizing leaf attached to the plant: the radioactivity appears to travel down the stem as sucrose, although it is rapidly converted into other compounds after it leaves the sieve tubes and enters other living cells of the stem.

In some plants, such as ash and elm trees, compound sugars built of three or four simple sugar units are transported in the sieve tubes. Certain plants also translocate sugar alcohols (mannitol or sorbitol) in their phloem. By the aphid feeding technique it has been proved that relatively small amounts of amino acids and mineral ions also are found in sieve-tube sap and are presumably being transported. In view of the dependence of root growth upon vitamins supplied by the shoot (page 102) it must also be presumed that vitamins are translocated in the phloem, although possibly in such trace amounts as not to be readily detectable.

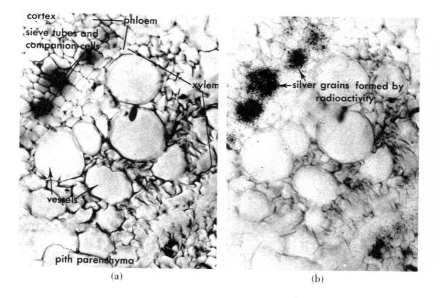

(a)   (b)

Fig. 7-3   *Cross section of vascular bundle of a cucumber leaf petiole, demonstrating transport by the phloem of radioactive products of photosynthesis. The leaf was fed tritium-labeled water, H^3HO. After photosynthesis for 30 min the petiole, through which products were being transported, was frozen, dried, and sectioned transversely, and the sections mounted in contact with a photographic emulsion. Radioactivity in the tissue, from organic compounds containing tritium, caused formation of silver grains in emulsion, making a "radioautograph." In (a) the microscope is focused on the tissue section so the cells can be seen clearly. In (b) the microscope is focused on the emulsion covering the section so the silver grains indicating the presence of radioactivity can be seen while the cells are out of focus. Notice that the radioactivity is concentrated in a few sieve tubes and companion cells of the phloem, and is not present in the xylem. (Magnification 320×. Data of R. S. Gage and S. Aronoff, from* Plant Physiology, **35:** 65, 1960.)

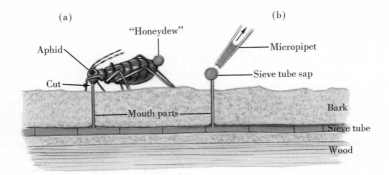

Fig. 7-4 *Aphid mouth-part method of obtaining sieve-tube sap. At (a), aphid has inserted mouth parts into sieve tube and is obtaining sap which emerges in chemically altered form as "honeydew" after passing through its gut. When the feeding tube is cut at arrow, pure sieve-tube sap exudes (b), and can be collected by a micropipet. (See T. E. Mittler,* Journal of Experimental Biology, **35:** 74, 1958; *M. H. Zimmermann,* Science, **133:** 73, 1961.)

MECHANISM OF PHLOEM TRANSPORT Two principal methods have been employed to measure the rate of phloem translocation. The classical method is to measure the growth of a root, fruit, or tuber, whose increase in dry weight is due mainly to organic compounds imported via the phloem. From the rate of increase in dry weight per day we can calculate, using measured values for the total cross section of sieve tubes in the supplying stem and the concentration of sugar in sieve-tube sap, that translocation of sugar in the sieve tubes must occur at velocities of 50 to 200 cm per hour. Measurement of the transport of labeled products of photosynthesis from leaves in the type of experiment shown in Figure 7-2 gives similar velocities, although the results are fraught with more complications of interpretation. Martin Zimmermann at the Harvard Forest has also measured the velocity of phloem translocation in ash trees by following the movement, down the trunk, of daily fluctuations in composition of sieve-tube sap (ratio of sucrose to other sugars which as mentioned above are translocated by ash trees) and obtained rates of 30 to 70 cm per hr.

The measured velocities are enormously greater than could occur by diffusion, so it is evident that simple diffusion of sugar through the sieve tubes is not the mechanism of translocation. Beyond this negative conclusion, however, there is no general agreement about the mechanism by which phloem translocation takes place. This is remarkable when we consider that the phenomenon has been known and studied since the latter part of the last century and is of central importance in plant function. The reasons the problem remains unsolved can be appreciated if we examine some of the currently competing explanations of phloem transport.

All the proposed mechanisms fall into two categories, namely, those that envision a mass transport (bulk flow) of the sieve-tube sap and those that envision a transport of sugar and other solute molecules without a bulk flow of the sap, for example, by an active transport carrier mechanism. It will be obvious that if solutes are moved by sap flow, then any different solutes that are present should be carried along at the same rate, and water should also move at the same rate. Experiments using radioactive ^3H_2O show that it is indeed translocated from leaves via the phloem, but multiple-label experiments using ^3H_2O, ^{14}C-sugar, and $^{32}PO_4^{-3}$ have given different velocities of transport for these substances. However, this kind of experiment is inconclusive because the different substances exchange at different rates between the sieve tubes and tissues adjacent to them, thus making determination of transport velocity inaccurate.

Under a mass flow all substances must move in the same direction, and mass flow mechanisms would therefore be disproved if it could be demonstrated that materials moved in opposite directions through a single sieve tube. This result has indeed been claimed in experiments in which different tracers were fed to two leaves and both tracers were then detected in single sieve tubes in the region of stem between the two treated leaves by autoradiography and by the aphid feeding technique. However, these experiments are inconclusive because the second tracer found in the sieve tube could have gotten there by moving up in a different sieve tube, then exchanging laterally into and moving back down in the given sieve tube.

It appears that any materials that enter the sieve tubes are translocated by them regardless of utility to the plant, for example, foreign substances such as dyes, and even virus particles, for which specific transport mechanisms seem most unlikely. This is easily understandable, however, on the basis of a mass flow mechanism; they just get carried along in the stream.

The most widely favored hypothesis as to what would cause a mass flow is that it is due to an osmotically generated gradient of turgor pressure along the length of the sieve tube. At the supply end, the leaf (where sugar is produced), sugar must be transported *into* the sieve tube, which will tend to raise the concentration and thus the osmotic solute action of the sieve-tube sap, leading to water absorption and a high turgor pressure by the principles considered in Chapter 5. Sugar must on the other hand be released from the sieve tube at the delivery end such as in the root or a fruit, which will tend to lower the solute concentration in the sieve tube and lead to osmotic loss of water and a lower turgor pressure. Because of the resulting pressure difference between the supply and delivery ends of the sieve tube, the sugar solution will simply flow hydraulically from element to element through the sieve-plate pores.

This *pressure flow hypothesis* is shown diagrammatically in Figure 7-5. It attractively explains why phloem translocation always goes from regions of supply ("sources") to regions of demand ("sinks") for sugar without the need for any special mechanism to determine direction; for example, sugar is translocated downward to the roots but also upward from leaves to fruits and to the growing regions of the shoot, which are nutritionally dependent upon the mature leaves and thus constitute sinks.

That turgor pressure exists in sieve tubes and that sap can flow through them is proved by the experiments with aphid mouth parts already described. The expected gradient in sugar concentration through the sieve tubes has been demonstrated by sampling the sieve-tube sap along the length of the trunks of trees.

According to the pressure flow hypothesis the long-distance translocation

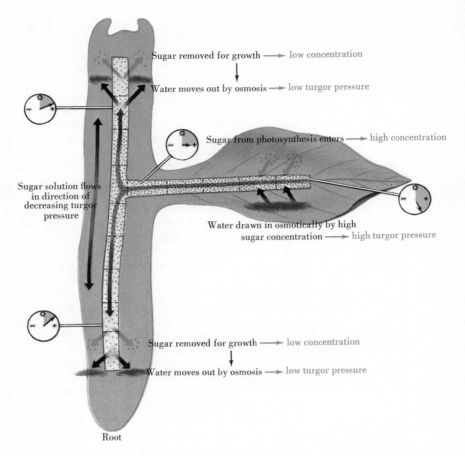

Sugar removed for growth ⟶ low concentration

Water moves out by osmosis ⟶ low turgor pressure

Sugar from photosynthesis enters ⟶ high concentration

Sugar solution flows in direction of decreasing turgor pressure

Water drawn in osmotically by high sugar concentration ⟶ high turgor pressure

Sugar removed for growth ⟶ low concentration

Water moves out by osmosis ⟶ low turgor pressure

Root

Fig. 7-5 *Schematic diagram explaining the pressure flow theory of translocation in sieve tubes. Dots represent sugar concentration; imaginary gauges measure the level of turgor pressure.*

of sugar in the phloem is a passive physical process. Living cells are required, however, because the development and retention of the turgor pressure that drives the process are completely dependent upon the sieve tube being sur-rounded by an osmotically effective plasma membrane. Furthermore in view of the high concentration of sugar that exists in the sieve tubes by comparison with that in the leaf cells that supply this sugar it is necessary to conclude that sugar is actively transported into the sieve tubes by an energy-driven carrier mecha-nism.

Despite the simplicity and completeness of the pressure flow hypothesis as an explanation of phloem translocation, reasons are continually being ad-vanced why it cannot be correct. Some of the tracer evidence against mass flow was mentioned above. Other investigators feel that the pressure forces are too small or the resistances of the sieve-plate pores too large for translocation to occur at the measured rates. Electrically driven sap flow (electro-osmosis), dependent upon active transport of ions, has been invoked as an alternative mechanism. Some interpret electron micrographs of sieve tubes as showing that the sieve-plate pores are completely blocked with plugs of proteinaceous material (slime), precluding any mass flow at all. However, sieve tubes are remarkably responsive to injury and the function of slime may be to plug up the sieve plates and prevent loss of sugar when a localized injury occurs, which seems to be exactly what happens when we try to fix a specimen of phloem for electron microscopy.

Another school of workers contends that protoplasmic strands extend from end to end through each sieve-tube element and connect through the sieve-plate pores with similar strands in adjacent sieve-tube elements. They believe that a streaming or peristalsis carries material from cell to cell along these strands. Electron micrographs indicate to others, however, that these strands are composed merely of slime protein rather than of cytoplasm, and none but the most ardent advocates of the theory has been able to observe any streaming in sieve tubes.

We may see in this sketch of the continuing controversy over the mechanism of phloem transport some likeness to the political arena with its never-ending conflict of claims and advocacy. The reasons for dispute are at least in part similar, namely, that the available evidence does not admit of unequivocal interpretation and it is difficult to experiment upon the subject unambiguously. In the case of phloem this is because of the reactiveness of sieve tubes toward injury and their embedded location always surrounded by other cells and tissues, which has so far made it impossible to study the translocation phenomenon in isolation.

TRANSLOCATION IN NONVASCULAR PLANTS

Many of the kelps or brown algae (see Delevoryas, *Plant Diversification*) that inhabit coastal waters attain a size comparable to that of land plants and support attachment organs at the ocean bottom far removed from the floating leaflike organs that are specialized for photosynthesis, in some cases by distances as great as 100 meters. The stems of these plants are found to contain chains of cells that resemble to a remarkable degree the sieve tubes of vascular plants (Figure 7-6). Radioisotope evidence, although still meager, supports the idea that these cells function to transport products of photosynthesis to the deeply submerged organs. Isotope evidence for translocation of organic material has also been obtained in the case of certain red algae.

Rather convincing radioisotope evidence has been published that long-distance translocation of photosynthetic products takes place in the stem of the large moss *Polytrichum* via specialized cells that are interconnected by numerous plasmodesmata. The stem also possesses a distinct tissue of living cells that have long been regarded as possibly adapted for water transport, which seems necessary since these plants grow into the air for distances of several to many centimeters.

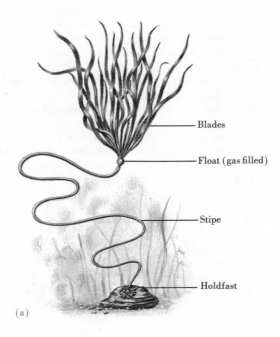

Blades

Float (gas filled)

Stipe

Holdfast

(a)

Cortex   Medulla   Trumpet filament   Epidermis

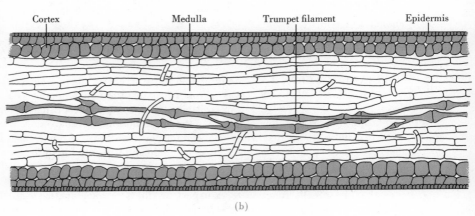

(b)

Fig. 7-6 Nereocystis, *a kelp (large marine brown alga) that possesses "sieve filaments" for translocation of photosynthetic products from the "blades" (leaf-like photosynthetic organs) through the "stipe" to the "holdfast" that attaches the plant to the ocean bottom. The stipe can grow to as much as 40 meters in length, and the blades themselves attain a length of more than 3 meters, as shown in (a). (b) Longitudinal section of a blade, showing photosynthetic cell layers (epidermis and cortex) and sieve filaments (trumpet filament). (Courtesy of Dr. Nancy L. Nicholson.)*

These observations suggest that the customary distinction between vascular and nonvascular plants in regard to translocation functions may be unnecessarily sharp. At the same time they call further attention to the functional significance of translocation mechanisms for any large organism and thus emphasize the importance of the elaborate translocation tissues that have been evolved by the vascular plants.

SUGGESTED READING

Biddulph, S., and O. Biddulph, "The Circulatory System of Plants," *Scientific American*, **200** (2):44-49, 1959.

Crafts, A. S., *Translocation in Plants*. New York: Holt, Rinehart and Winston, 1961. Chapter 6.

Esau, K., *Plants, Viruses and Insects*. Cambridge, Mass.: Harvard University Press, 1961.

Esau, K., "Explorations of the Food Conducting System in Plants," *American Scientist*, **54**:141-157, 1966.

O'Brien, T. P., and M. E. McCully, *Plant Structure and Development*. New York: Macmillan, 1969. pp. 80-86.

Richardson, M., *Translocation in Plants*. New York: St. Martin's Press, 1968. Chapters 4 and 5.

Zimmermann, M. H. "How Sap Moves in Trees," *Scientific American*, **208** (3):132-142, 1963.

Zimmermann, M. H., "Translocation of Nutrients," in *Physiology of Plant Growth and Development*, M. B. Wilkins (ed.). New York: McGraw-Hill, 1969. Chapter 11.

Plant
Growth
and
Development

Unlike many animals, plants typically continue to grow throughout their lives and either encounter no apparent limit in size or, if they remain of restricted size, do so because they continually discard old parts as they replace them with new ones through new growth.

The two principal aspects of plant growth are *primary* growth, the growth in length of shoots and roots, and *secondary* growth, the subsequent growth in thickness of stem and root.

The general plan by which each of these kinds of growth is accomplished is that new cells are continually produced by cell division in a special tissue called a *meristem;* on the periphery of the meristem, cells derived from it enlarge, often to many times their original size, and bring about visible increase in size of the plant. As these cells reach full size they cease to grow, and become part of the mature, nongrowing tissues of the plant. Plant growth thus depends on localized zones of cell division and cell enlargement, in contrast with the plan of growth of most animals in which the body increases in size and number of cells throughout. Only in the very earliest stages in the life of a plant does it grow in the latter fashion.

Cell growth, or *irreversible increase in size*, occurs in both the zones of cell division and of cell enlargement. Cell division is an additional process that *accompanies* growth in the former but not the latter zone. The difference between growth with and without cell division is illustrated in Figure 8-1. Normally, in the meristem after a cell has grown to about double its original size, cell division occurs. Although cell division merely partitions the cell and does not result in any actual growth, the occurrence of cell division and of the synthetic processes associated with it doubtless prepares the daughter cells for further growth. Furthermore cell division provides for the possibility of unlimited growth of the plant by continually multiplying the number of cells.

Cell division occurs in two steps: *mitosis*, the division of the nucleus into two nuclei, which is considered in Novikoff-Holtzman, *Cells and Organelles* in this series so will not be described here; and *cytokinesis*, the division of the resulting binucleate cell into two uninucleate cells. In plants cytokinesis occurs by formation of the *cell plate*, a thin membrane-bounded layer of polysaccharide material that forms by fusion of vesicles from the Golgi and/or endoplasmic reticulum across the spindle between the daughter nuclei toward the end of mitosis (Figure 8-1a). The cell plate quickly grows outward until it reaches the cell wall. The daughter cells deposit new primary cell wall material on each face of the cell plate, and thus each daughter cell soon possesses its own complete cell wall. The cell plate becomes the middle lamella separating the two cells.

Two very important developmental processes, *morphogenesis* and *differentiation*, normally accompany growth. Morphogenesis is development of the shape of cells and organs. Differentiation is the gradual acquisition of different

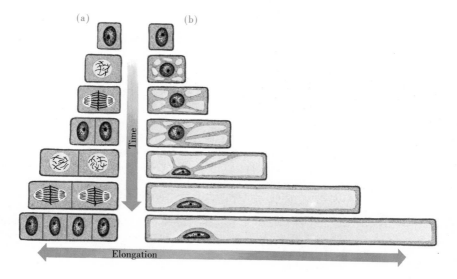

Fig. 8-1 *Diagram illustrating growth of plant cell with (a) and without (b) cell division. Lightly stippled material is cytoplasm; clear areas are vacuoles.*

structural features and different functions by the cells that originally were all part of the relatively uniform and unspecialized cell population of the meristem.

We shall examine first how growth, cell division, morphogenesis, and differentiation take place during plant development and will then consider the mechanisms of these phenomena.

PRIMARY GROWTH OF THE ROOT A diagram of the young part of a typical root, seen in longitudinal section, is shown in Figure 8-2. Just beneath its tip, under the protective root cap, is its meristem. Rows of cells are seen leading back from the meristem toward the older part of the root. These rows have been produced by continued growth and repeated division, in the lengthwise direction, of the cells in the meristem in the manner illustrated in Figure 8-1a. Cell divisions in the meristem add new cells both to the body of the root and to the root cap (to make up for the wearing away of the root cap as the root grows through the soil).

If we follow back any one of the rows of cells beginning at the tip of the meristem (Figure 8-2) we come to a point beyond which the cells become noticeably and progressively larger. This region is called the *elongation zone* of the root and its significance may be appreciated by studying the diagrams of actual growth and division of cells in a root given in Figure 8-3. These data show that cell division takes place throughout the apical region of the root in which the cells are of relatively uniform size, but not in the elongation zone which therefore differs from the meristem by the absence of cell division. The tissue within the meristem elongated a total of about 50 percent during the 6-hr period of the record in Figure 8-3. On the other hand the uppermost of the cells initially mapped (numbers 26 to 38), which lay within the elongation zone, elongated to almost ten times their initial size during the same period. Therefore growth in size is much more rapid during the cell enlargement phase (elongation zone) than in the meristem where growth is accompanied by cell division. Some cells, such as numbers 23, 24, and 25, passed from the meristem to the elongation zone during the 6-hr period recorded in Figure 8-3, while the cells numbered 26 to 38 actually reached mature size, leaving the elongation zone and becoming part of the nongrowing part of the root where root hairs are initiated (root-hair zone).

Another important fact that may be deduced by examining Figure 8-3 is that *none* of the cells that were mapped within the meristem will remain indefinitely as part of the meristem. Every cell shown is separated from the tip of the meristem (the curved line at the bottom of each diagram) by several cells, like those at the tip of the meristem in Figure 8-2; these are not shown in Figure 8-3 because they could not be recorded accurately by the method used to obtain the diagrams. These tipmost cells, like the cells mapped, are growing and dividing, causing the cells behind them (those that appear in Figure 8-3) gradually to become separated farther and farther from the tip of the meristem. Therefore every meristem cell shown in Figure 8-3 will eventually find itself in the position of cells 23, 24, and 25; or, more exactly, the progeny of every meristem cell will, because each meristem cell will itself have grown and divided into many cells before that time arrives, especially if it is a cell now located near the tip of the meristem.

Returning to Figure 8-2 we see that the only cells that will remain *indefinitely* part of the meristem are those cells located at the *very tip* of the meristem where the files of meristem cells appear to converge. When one of these tipmost cells divides, one of the daughter cells may remain permanently a part of the meristem while the other daughter cell begins the slow but sure progression through the meristem and eventually, after having divided into many cells, ends up as part of the mature tissues of the root.

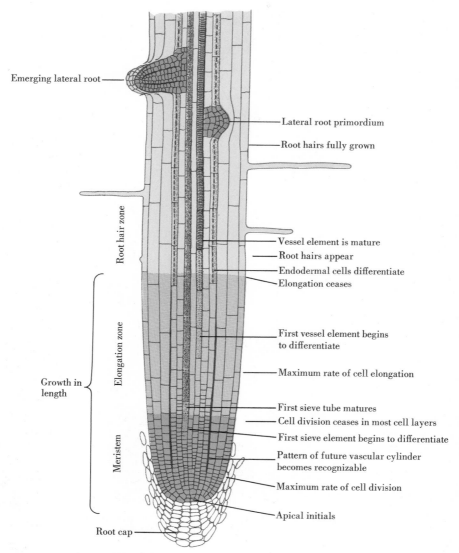

Emerging lateral root

Lateral root primordium

Root hairs fully grown

Root hair zone

Vessel element is mature
Root hairs appear
Endodermal cells differentiate
Elongation ceases

Elongation zone

First vessel element begins
to differentiate

Maximum rate of cell elongation

Growth in
length

First sieve tube matures
Cell division ceases in most cell layers
First sieve element begins to differentiate
Pattern of future vascular cylinder
becomes recognizable

Meristem

Maximum rate of cell division

Apical initials

Root cap

Fig. 8-2   *Diagram of zone of primary growth of a root as seen in longitudinal section. The number of cells is much greater in typical roots than in this diagram, which has been made as simple as possible. Differentiation only of the first-formed sieve tube and vessel is shown.*

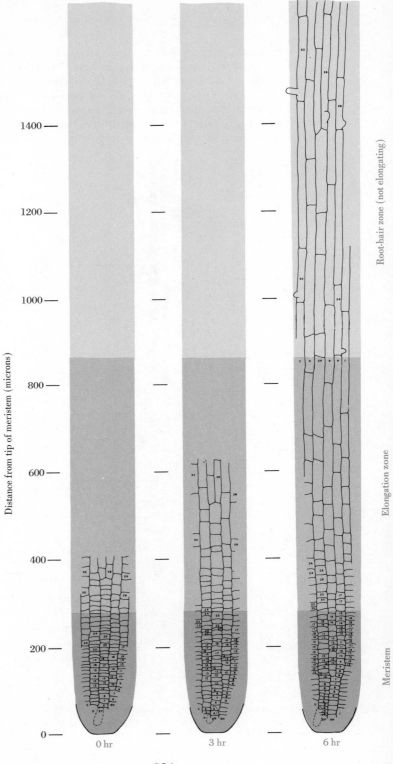

Over a period of time all the meristem cells and hence all the cells of the root can in this way be traced back to the tipmost cells of the meristem, which are called the *apical initials*. The part of the meristem in which they are located is called the *apical meristem*.

Although the apical initials are indirectly the source of all the cells of the root, it should be emphasized that the apical initials are *not* the principal site of cell multiplication. This takes place throughout the meristem, as is evident in Figure 8-3, and in fact it has been demonstrated that the frequency of cell division in the middle part of the meristem is considerably greater than in the vicinity of the apical initials. This apical region of relative inactivity in DNA replication and mitosis has been called the "quiescent center" of the apical meristem.

The cells of the root cap arise by division of initials that may be the same as those of the root meristem or may be located just ahead of the latter toward the root cap, depending upon the details of organization in the apical meristem region.

CELL DEVELOPMENT AND DIFFERENTIATION The growth of a cell in the elongation zone involves not only enlargement of the cell to mature size but also development of its protoplast from the type that occurs in the meristem to the type that is characteristic of mature cells. Cells in the meristem are filled with protoplasm, and the nucleus occupies a considerable proportion of the cell's volume (see Figure 2-3). Vacuoles are small and may not be visible. As the cell enters the elongation phase (Figure 8-1b) these vacuoles enlarge by uptake of water and become conspicuous. With further growth they fuse, leaving the nucleus suspended in the center of the cell by cytoplasmic strands. The nucleus finally moves to a peripheral position, commonly leaving an uninterrupted central vacuole by the time growth has ended. This kind of organization, as explained in Chapter 2, is typical of most mature plant cells (Figure 2-4).

Accompanying this protoplasmic development structural *differentiation* of cells for specialized functions occurs. Cellular differentiation actually begins within the meristem. Very near the tip of the meristem some differences in size and shape of cells become apparent (Figure 8-2), as do differences in protoplasmic density, size of nucleus and vacuoles, and so on. These differences tend to become more and more pronounced as growth of the cells continues, and therefore become increasingly evident farther back from the tip of the root where the cells have passed further through the developmental process.

Fig. 8-3 *Cellular behavior during growth of the root of timothy grass (*Phleum pratense*). Diagram at left shows the cells on the external surface of the tip portion of this root as they appeared at a certain time. Middle and right-hand diagrams show these same cells 3 and 6 hr later. Any cell that either divided or formed a root hair during the 6-hr period is marked with a number. The two daughter cells of a cell that divided are both marked with the same number. The line at the bottom shows the tip of the meristem where cells were not in focus. During the 6-hr period the root rotated so that cell row C largely disappeared from view, while row I came into view. (From R. H. Goodwin and C. J. Avers,* American Journal of Botany, **43:** *479, 1956.)*

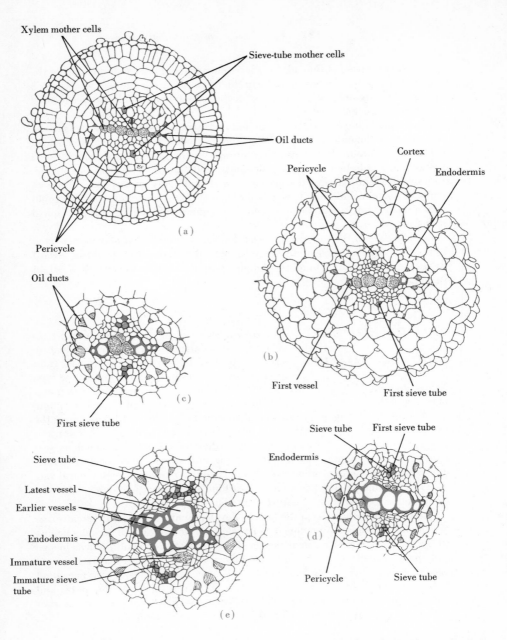

Xylem mother cells

Sieve-tube mother cells

Oil ducts

Pericycle

(a)

Cortex

Pericycle

Endodermis

Oil ducts

(c)

First sieve tube

(b)

First vessel

First sieve tube

Sieve tube

First sieve tube

Endodermis

Sieve tube

Latest vessel

Earlier vessels

Endodermis

Immature vessel

Immature sieve
tube

(d)

Pericycle

Sieve tube

(e)

Fig. 8-4 *Tissue differentiation as seen in transverse sections of the young root of the carrot plant. Sections a-e were cut successively farther back from the tip of the root and hence represent successively later stages of differentiation. The cortex and epidermis, although present, are not shown in diagrams (c) to (e). Mature xylem and phloem cells are indicated with heavy walls. Oil ducts are specialized structures formed in tissues of carrot and certain other plants. (a) Within meristem, 0.2 mm from tip of root; (b) in elongation zone, about 1.5 mm from tip of root; (c–e) successively farther back into root hair zone. In (e) primary differentiation is complete and secondary growth (which gives rise to the "carrot") is about to begin. (Magnification 280×. From K. Esau, Hilgardia, **13**: 175, 1940.)*

The first specialized cells to develop mature structure are sieve-tube elements. The first sieve-tube elements differentiate at a level at which cells in other tissues of the growing root are still actively dividing, that is, within the meristem (Figure 8-2). The new sieve-tube elements add onto existing sieve tubes leading forward from the older part of the root, and so serve to bring early into the developing tissues food-conducting channels to supply their needs. These first sieve-tube elements continue to elongate as the tissues surrounding them grow in length.

Considerably farther back, usually within the zone of elongation, the first tracheids or vessel elements of the xylem begin to develop mature structure; they too add onto the existing strands in the older part of the root. Cells of other specialized tissues, for example, the endodermis as shown in Figure 8-2, commonly begin to differentiate in the zone of elongation. However, differentiation of tissues does not become completed until after elongation has ceased.

The course of cellular differentiation can be appreciated better in transverse sections, as illustrated with the young carrot root in Figure 8-4. Differentiation of vascular tissue is *progressive*. Rather than occurring in all cells more or less at the same time, it begins with the maturation of particular phloem and xylem cells and proceeds by gradual maturation of more and more specialized cells in each tissue. In the root the first phloem and xylem cells always differentiate at the *outer* edge of the groups of cells destined to become phloem or xylem, respectively (Figure 8-4b). Further differentiation occurs progressively inward toward the center. The completion of differentiation (parts (d) and (e) of Figure 8-4) occurs in the root-hair zone, that is, after elongation has ended.

The earliest-formed xylem cells show interesting structural features that permit these conducting cells to differentiate within elongating tissue despite the fact that the secondary wall is rigid and inextensible. These cells develop localized secondary wall thickenings of ringlike or of helical form, as illustrated in Figure 8-5. From the thin primary wall between these thickenings the wall

First formed vessels   Primary walls   Secondary thickenings   Pit   Most recent vessel

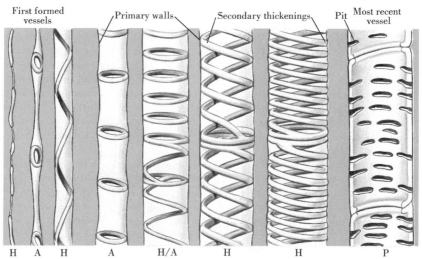

H   A   H   A   H/A   H   H   P

Fig. 8-5 *Types of vessel elements in the primary xylem: A, annular; H, helical; H/A, transitional between annular and helical; P, pitted. The sequence from center to left illustrates the effect of continued elongation on earlier formed vessels and tracheids.*

matrix material actually becomes removed at completion of differentiation when the cytoplasm is undergoing autolytic breakdown, leaving a loose microfibrillar residue. The result is a tube that is reinforced by the ringlike or helical thickenings but can readily be stretched as the tissue elongates. As growth continues the ringlike thickenings become separated farther and farther from one another, and the helical thickenings become pulled out into steeper and steeper helices. In the stem where maturation of xylem begins very early in the elongation zone, the first-formed xylem cells are often stretched so much by subsequent elongation that the cells collapse and helical thickenings are torn apart (as shown at the left in Figure 8-5). The earliest-formed sieve-tube elements, although capable of continued growth as mentioned above, also normally become stretched to the point of collapse by subsequent elongation and their function is taken over by the sieve tubes that differentiate later.

Xylem elements that mature after elongation has ceased, on the other hand, usually develop a continuous, pitted secondary wall (at right in Figure 8-5), which is stronger than a ring- or helically thickened wall but would prevent the tissue in which it is embedded from elongating.

It is important to notice that tissue differentiation entails not only functional and structural modification of cells but formation of an anatomical pattern. Formation of the pattern is actually a very early event in the course of differentiation, as illustrated by Figure 8-4a. This section was taken within the meristem beyond the point at which any vascular element had matured. Yet from their size and appearance the cells that will become the principal xylem elements can already be recognized, even though most of them will not develop mature structure until after this segment of the root has passed through the elongation phase and has ceased to elongate. It is tempting to think that these cells become committed or *determined* at this early stage to differentiate later into vessels or tracheids, by analogy with determination phenomena that control the fates of cells during animal development. But this may not be entirely warranted.

PRIMARY GROWTH OF THE SHOOT

The developmental plan just examined with regard to the root also applies, in general terms, to the shoot. The growing region of the shoot is at its tip and consists of an apical zone of cell division behind which lies the zone of cell enlargement in which the embryonic leaves and stem internodes produced at the apex grow to mature size. Owing to the intermittent formation of leaves and other appendages and the consequent modification of the stem into nodes and internodes, the development of the shoot is considerably more complex than that of the root.

The zone of cell division at the apex of a shoot (within its "terminal bud") is illustrated in Figure 8-6. The central mound or cone of meristematic tissue at the very tip of the stem is called its *apical meristem*. However, the developing stem below and the young leaves to either side are also regions of active cell division, that is, meristematic. Notice that the apical meristem of the shoot is not covered by any cap analogous to the root cap; but it is protected by the overarching young leaves and often by bud scales outside of these.

The apical meristem gives rise on its flanks to new embryonic leaves, called *leaf primordia*. Two leaf primordia just emerging from the apical meristem show as bumps on either side of the meristematic dome in Figure 8-6.

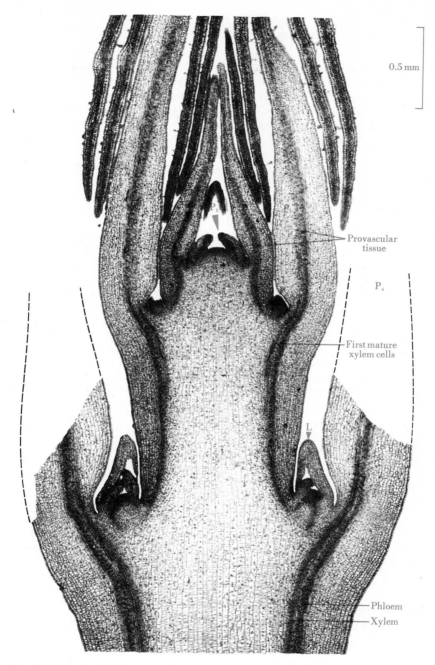

Labels on figure:
- Provascular tissue
- P_4
- First mature xylem cells
- L
- Phloem
- Xylem
- 0.5 mm

Fig. 8-6 *Longitudinal section of shoot tip of lilac (*Syringa vulgaris*), showing apical meristem (A) and successively older leaf primordia P_1, P_2, P_3, and P_4. L, lateral or axillary bud primordium. Provascular tissue denotes strands of elongated cells that will subsequently complete their differentiation into mature xylem and phloem, forming vascular bundles. Dark structures at top between P_1, P_2, and P_3 are sections of the blades of leaf primordia that are folded in the bud in such a way as to cut across the plane of section. (Magnification 43×.)*

Formation of leaf primordia occurs at regular intervals and in a regular pattern around the apical meristem. Cell division in the apical meristem also continually adds cells to the stem beneath it. The way in which new leaf primordia and stem arise from the apical meristem is illustrated in Figure 8-7. The leaf primordia and the young stem undergo a characteristic development involving growth and extensive cell division. The leaf primordia elongate markedly so that they soon tower above the apical meristem, and they later extend sidewise to form the leaf blade. The stem thickens and slowly lengthens. Progressive stages can be seen by examining the successive leaf primordia out from the apical meristem in Figure 8-6 and the successively lower (older) portions of the stem associated with each leaf primordium.

Accompanying the growth of leaf primordia and stem, differentiation of the vascular tissues occurs. This process begins with the early appearance of elongated cells in strands (Figure 8-6), which lay out the pattern of bundles that the vascular system will follow. From these elongated cells sieve-tube elements differentiate, beginning on the side of each strand nearest the outside of the stem; and later vessel elements and/or tracheids differentiate, beginning on the side of each strand nearest the inside of the stem.

As the young leaf and young stem internode enlarge, cell division gradually ceases and these organs enter a phase of cell enlargement. Internodes elongate throughout their length, and leaves expand throughout their area (with some exceptions to be noted later). The distinction between meristematic and cell enlargement phases of growth tends to be less sharp in leaves and internodes than was illustrated for the root. Cell division continues in some leaves until they have reached half their final mature size; but by this time cell division is lagging far behind the rate of growth, so the average size of the cells is increasing steadily even though some are still occasionally dividing. During this phase of growth chloroplasts grow and develop photosynthetic capability, and differentiation of vascular tissue, epidermis, stomates, and so on progresses. But as in the root such differentiation processes usually attain completion only after mature cell size has been reached and growth in size of the leaf or internode has ceased.

At this time in the stem *fibers* (page 16) differentiate conspicuously in the phloem and sometimes elsewhere, strengthening the shoot mechanically (Figure 8-8a). Because of their heavy secondary walls, fibers cannot be formed earlier since they would prevent elongation, like vessels or tracheids with continuous secondary walls. However, a distinct kind of mechanical tissue, called *collenchyma*, differentiates earlier to serve the needs of growing shoots. It consists of bundles of living cells, located usually in the cortex (Figure 8-8a), which develop extremely thick *primary* walls that afford mechanical support for the organ but can nevertheless be extended by the collenchyma cells during growth.

Intercalary Growth   Certain plants, notably the grasses, possess *intercalary* shoot meristems that allow growth in length to occur in regions other than the tip of the shoot. For example, there is an intercalary meristem at the base of each grass leaf which continually adds new cells to the leaf and allows it to elongate (see Figure 10-5). Thus after a lawn is mowed its regrowth is not mainly by formation

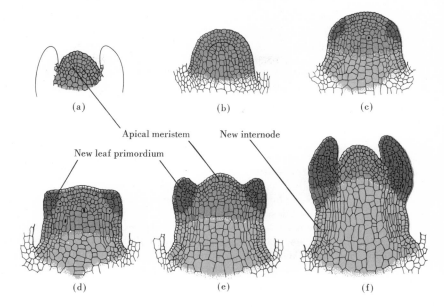

(a)   (b)   (c)

Apical meristem   New internode

New leaf primordium

(d)   (e)   (f)

Fig. 8-7   *Sequence of diagrams showing development of leaf primordia and internode from the apical meristem of St.-John's-wort* (Hypericum) *seen in longitudinal sections. In the first diagram only, adjacent already-formed leaf primordia are shown in outline. (Magnification 150×.) All tissue derived from the apical meristem during this cycle of growth is indicated in color. (After W. Zimmerman,* Jahrbücher für wissenschaftliche Botanik, *68: 289, 1928.)*

of new leaves but by the lengthening of the old leaves that have been cut off short. Since the intercalary meristem of each leaf is basal, it does not get cut off. This growth pattern permits grasses to tolerate grazing by herbivorous animals and was presumably evolved as an adaptation to the activities of such animals. Intercalary growth also occurs in many of the large marine brown algae or kelps, for example, *Nereocystis* (shown in Figure 7-6a) which elongates in the upper part of its stipe and at the base of each blade. The intercalary mode of growth enables these plants to replace continuously their photosynthetic tissue as the latter gets eroded at the tip by wave action.

BRANCHING   Along with the formation of leaf primordia and stem internodes at the shoot tip as illustrated in Figure 8-6, small apical meristems appear in the angles between leaf primordia and stem. These develop into *axillary buds* which normally remain dormant until well after growth of the adjacent leaf and internode has been completed. These buds can later grow out to produce lateral branches of the shoot. Alternatively they may develop into specialized shoots such as rhizomes or tubers (underground shoots) or flowers.

The root system normally branches even more extensively than the shoot does, but its branches originate in a fundamentally different way. No lateral root primordia analogous to axillary buds are formed at the root apex. Instead, back of the elongation zone cell division resumes in local spots in the cell layer (called the *pericycle*) just inward from the endodermis as illustrated in Figure 8-2. The resulting nest of dividing cells gradually becomes organized into a root apical meristem and the root so generated literally bores its way out through the endodermis, cortex, and epidermis.

Regeneration of   Many plants are able to supplement the mecha-
Meristems   nisms of branching, just mentioned, by forming
"adventitious" buds or roots, which means buds or roots that arise in locations and in fashions other than the normal subapical modes of branching described above.

Adventitious roots can be formed on a piece of stem that has been detached from the plant, as in the propagation of plants by cuttings. Adventitious roots arise on the shoot during normal growth of some plants, for example, the "prop roots" of maize and of various tropical trees; these serve to strengthen the supporting and absorptive functions of the root system. The initiation of an adventitious root is by local inception of cell division followed by development of the nest of dividing cells into a root apical meristem in a manner somewhat comparable to that involved in normal branch root formation (Figure 8-2), except that this initiation can take place in a variety of tissue locations.

Adventitious buds may form on roots as a means of vegetative propagation, or of regeneration if the shoot has been removed, for example, the familiar regeneration of a dandelion if its top is cut or pulled off. Many trees form adventitious buds in the bark of their trunks as a means of shoot regeneration if the crown has been damaged or destroyed, or as a supplemental mode of shoot formation during normal growth. Adventitious buds are initiated, somewhat like adventitious roots, by inception of cell division in tissues that may be mature and have long since ceased cell division, as contrasted with axillary meristems which are formed as derivatives of the shoot apical meristem as explained above.

The leaves of some plants can form adventitious roots and buds; this is indeed the usual means by which African violets (*Saintpaulia*) are propagated horticulturally.

SECONDARY   In the majority of vascular plants development of
GROWTH   the *primary tissues* of the stem and root is followed by the formation of additional *secondary tissues*, which increase the thickness of the axis. Secondary growth is brought about by the development of two distinct layers of meristematic tissue within the stem or root, the *vascular cambium* and the *cork cambium*. Their activity not only increases the thickness of the axis but profoundly modifies its structure. We shall consider first how these meristems arise and function in the stem.

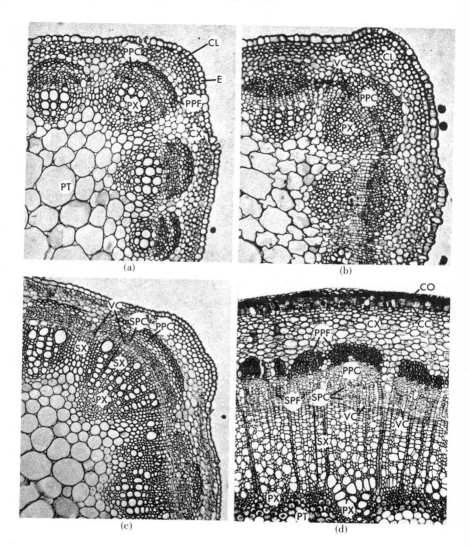

Fig. 8-8 *Photomicrographs of cross sections of stems, showing how secondary growth occurs. (a–c) Stem of alfalfa* (Medicago), *showing (a) primary structure; (b) formation of vascular cambium within and between vascular bundles; (c) formation of secondary xylem and phloem by cambium. (Magnification 100×.) (d) One-year-old stem of tulip tree* (Liriodendron) *illustrating more advanced stage of secondary growth, in which cork cambium has begun to produce cork, and extensive layers of secondary xylem and phloem have been formed. (Magnification 65×.) CC, cork cambium; CL, collenchyma in cortex; CO, cork; CX, cortex; E, epidermis; PPC, primary phloem conducting tissue; PPF, primary phloem fibers; PT, pith; PX, primary xylem; SPC, secondary phloem conducting tissue; SPF, secondary phloem fibers; SX, secondary xylem; VC, vascular cambium.*

The vascular cambium is the meristem that adds to the vascular tissue. It forms initially between the primary xylem and primary phloem of each vascular bundle of the stem, usually not long after elongation of that portion of the stem has ceased. Its presence first becomes evident by the occurrence of cell divisions in the radial (inward to outward) direction which multiply the number of cells separating the already-formed primary xylem and phloem from one another (Figure 8-8). It then becomes apparent that the innermost of these new cells are enlarging and differentiating into vessels, tracheids, and other cells of the *secondary xylem*, while the outermost of the new cells are differentiating into sieve-tube elements, companion cells, and other cells of the *secondary phloem*. The secondary xylem and phloem tissues are thus formed in contact with the primary xylem and phloem, respectively.

The zone of dividing cells also spreads into the parenchyma tissue that separates the vascular bundles from one another (Figure 8-8), and there the vascular cambium also begins to form secondary xylem to the inside and secondary phloem to the outside. Once this is taking place all the way around the stem, a continuous cylinder of vascular tissues replaces the formerly more or less separate vascular bundles. The positions previously occupied by vascular bundles can be identified, however, by the strands of primary xylem and phloem lying at the internal and external edges, respectively, of the cylinder of secondary vascular tissue.

While these changes are occurring in the vascular tissue, a somewhat similar meristematic activity begins in one of the cell layers near the outside of the stem, usually in one of the outer cell layers of the cortex. This meristem is called the *cork cambium* because it gives rise to cork cells. Differentiation of cork cells, which occurs to the outside of the actively dividing layer, involves the formation of a secondary wall containing impervious layers of waxes of a chemically resistant nature, called *suberin*. Cork tissue is very compact, without intercellular spaces. It not only retards water loss from the stem, taking over this function from the epidermis which soon peels off, but also, because of its toughness and resilience, provides effective and important protection against mechanical damage for the underlying delicate conducting and meristematic tissues.

The cork cambium also sometimes adds cells toward the inside, as does the vascular cambium, but the tissue produced is of a parenchymalike nature and is not especially important.

Secondary growth occurs in the roots of most of the plants that exhibit secondary growth of the stem; and in the case of plants having storage roots (carrot, turnip, and others) it is more conspicuous there than in the stem. Secondary growth in the root begins somewhat differently in that the vascular cambium initially follows a sinuous course corresponding with the outer edge of the primary xylem (see Figure 8-4). By more rapid addition of secondary xylem in the "bays" between the xylem arms the xylem is soon brought into the form of a cylinder, after which further secondary growth is practically the same as in the stem.

Figure 8-9 illustrates the way in which cell division in the vascular cambium, followed by transverse enlargement and differentiation of the cells derived by cell division in the cambium, adds new cells to the secondary xylem and phloem. Those cells within the vascular cambium that remain permanently a part of the meristematic zone are called the cambial *initials*. On either side of

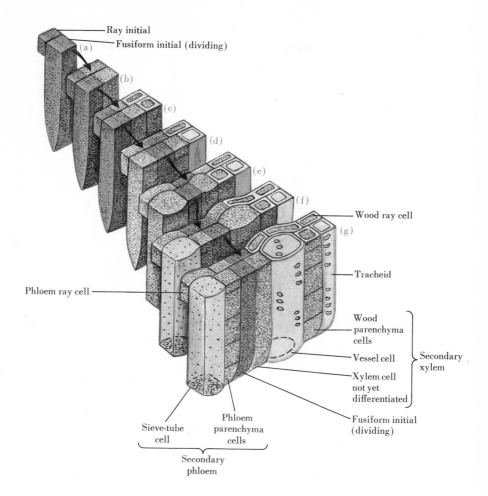

Ray initial

Fusiform initial (dividing)

(a)

(b)

(c)

(d)

(e)

(f)

Wood ray cell

(g)

Tracheid

Phloem ray cell

Wood
parenchyma
cells

Vessel cell

Secondary
xylem

Xylem cell
not yet
differentiated

Fusiform initial
(dividing)

Sieve-tube
cell

Phloem
parenchyma
cells

Secondary
phloem

Fig. 8-9 *Diagram illustrating how cambial initials give rise to cells of secondary xylem and phloem. Upper surface of segments of the diagram shows cells cut in transverse section. Outside of tree is toward lower left; inside is toward upper right. Beginning at upper left each segment of the diagram shows what happens between successive divisions of a fusiform initial. The newly forming cell wall during each division is shown with a dotted line. Arrows and solid color lines show where each such wall is to be found after the next division has occurred. The concomitant formation of a ray from a ray initial is also shown. Shapes of cells are stylized in this diagram. For simplicity not more than one un-differentiated cell is shown to either side of the initial, whereas in an active cambial zone there will be several undifferentiated derivatives on either side of the initials and cell divisions may be occurring in some of these derivatives as well as in the cambial initials themselves.*

the zone of initials plus immediate derivatives is a narrow zone of cell enlargement in which the derivative cells are growing, in the transverse direction, to their mature widths. Then follows a zone of differentiation, in which secondary walls or other structural features of mature cells are formed, and the protoplasts disappear from those types of cells that die at maturity. These developmental stages resemble those involved in primary growth but, as can be seen in Figures 8-8 and 8-9, they occur over a very short distance and involve only a few cells at a time.

The secondary phloem and xylem are not only composed of entirely different types of cells, but within each of these tissues there is (especially in flowering plants) a markedly heterogeneous cell population (for example, Figure 5-4). Moreover this heterogeneity develops in a pattern that is distinctive for different plant groups and species and evidently is controlled genetically. To explain how these many types of cell development are induced and regulated at such close quarters offers an intriguing problem.

In one respect very marked differentiation is apparent within the vascular cambium itself. The cambial initials are of two types: (1) *fusiform* initials, of very elongated shape similar to the elongated conducting cells and fibers to which they give rise (Figure 8-9) and (2) *ray* initials, which are short and block-shaped (Figure 8-9) and give rise to *ray cells*, which become elongated in the radial rather than the longitudinal direction. These radial rows of cells, called *rays*, remain alive and apparently function in transport of food materials inward from the phloem to living cells in the xylem and pith. The ray cells also commonly store up as starch large amounts of surplus photosynthetic products for breakdown and use in the spring flush of bud and cambial growth.

The types of cells formed by the cambial initials vary to a considerable extent with the seasons. The xylem cells formed during the spring, when cambial activity is most intense, are generally larger and thinner-walled than those formed in the summer. When the cambium begins activity the following spring, the new large thin-walled xylem cells contrast sharply with the dense wood of the previous summer. This conspicuous boundary between one season's growth and the next is called a "growth ring" or "annual ring" (see Figure 5-4).

As secondary growth continues year by year in a tree trunk or root a time is reached at which the living ray and parenchyma cells within the primary xylem and the older layers of secondary xylem undergo rather sudden degenerative changes. The cells produce dark-colored tannic products, and often grow into and block any vessels that are present; finally all the living cells in the area die. This creates the dark "heartwood" portion of a tree trunk which is readily distinguishable from the lighter-colored "sapwood" in which living cells are still present. As the tree grows the heartwood zone spreads out from the center, taking over successive annual rings and leaving a relatively thin layer of sapwood inward from the vascular cambium. The heartwood represents xylem that has become superfluous for transport and reserve storage functions and from which the nitrogen and other nutrients tied up in the living cells may profitably be withdrawn for reutilization elsewhere. The heartwood may, however, still be important for the mechanical support of the tree, and the chemical changes that occur during the sapwood to heartwood transition may serve to generate products that discourage invasion of this dead tissue by wood-rotting microorganisms.

***Circumferential
Growth of the
Bark***
The increase in diameter of the cylinder of wood by secondary growth of a trunk or root continually stretches in the circumferential direction all tissues outside the vascular cambium. We can see the consequences of this in the development of the furrows and ridges in the bark of older trees and in the annual rupturing and peeling of the outer layer of bark from certain trees such as birch and Eucalyptus. Were it not for mechanisms of adjustment to this stretching, the bark would crack all the way in to the phloem which would damage these delicate conducting tissues and expose them and the vascular cambium to desiccation and entry of disease organisms.

Within the secondary phloem, parenchyma cells (often ray cells) elongate and divide in the circumferential direction, expanding the phloem to keep pace with the increase in circumference of the tree. Thus growth and cell division are not confined to the vascular and cork cambium regions during secondary growth.

The external cork tissue is made up, as explained previously, of dead cells and cannot itself grow to accommodate increase in circumference. However, the notable elastic properties of cork cell walls, properties that are made use of in man's employment of cork as a commercial and industrial material,[1] permit the cork to stretch elastically to a considerable extent before it cracks to produce furrows or peels off as mentioned above. Meanwhile, inward from the existing layer of cork a new cork cambium becomes initiated within the secondary phloem and gives rise to a new continuous layer of cork underlying the external corky layer that is being stretched and cracked. Therefore the cork cambium is not, like the vascular cambium, a permanent meristem but one that is replaced periodically by regeneration from cells of the older secondary phloem, somewhat as adventitious buds and roots may be initiated in mature tissue. This behavior causes the formation of discrete layers of corky bark in trees like birch and Eucalyptus and accounts for the characteristic scaly nature of the bark of many other trees, each "scale" being the cork that was produced by the activity of one cork cambial zone.

***Secondary
Growth in
Monocotyledons***
The preceding account describes in general how secondary growth occurs in nonflowering vascular plants and flowering plants, with the exception of the great group of Monocotyledons, which includes the grasses, orchids, palms, and bulb-forming plants such as tulips, daffodils, lilies, and onions. Most monocots engage in no secondary growth whatever, as we can readily verify by inspecting a stalk of corn or the trunk of a palm tree. Therefore, as noted in Chapter 5, the primary (apically produced) vascular system of a monocot has to remain functional for the entire life of the plant, whereas the primary vascular system of other plants is commonly completely superseded by the secondary vascular tissues during subsequent growth.

---

[1]Cork of commerce is the outer bark of the cork oak, *Quercus suber*, native to the Mediterranean region.

A very few monocots have, however, evolved a mechanism for secondary growth. Such plants include the picturesque Joshua tree (*Yucca brevifolia*) of the southwest deserts and the "dragon tree", *Dracena*, that is often planted as an ornamental in subtropical and mediterranean climates. These trees develop a cambiumlike meristematic cell layer within the trunk, which produces corky bark to the outside and to the inside produces *both* xylem and phloem, in a succession of vascular bundlelike arrangements similar to that found in a herbaceous plant (that is, rather like the vascular bundles in Figure 8-8a). This cambium therefore functions morphogenetically in a manner fundamentally different from the cambia of ferns, conifers, and broad-leaved trees.

MOLECULAR AND CELLULAR ASPECTS OF GROWTH

Let us now inquire into the mechanisms that underlie the kinds of developmental phenomena described above.

Growth of whole plants is, of course, tied to photosynthesis, and from the point of view of agricultural or ecological productivity plant growth is often equated with net photosynthesis. Although this is true in an overall sense, it is easy to find situations in which a great deal of growth occurs without any or without an equivalent amount of photosynthesis, for example, the germination of a seed in darkness or the spring flush of growth of a deciduous tree. These kinds of growth are, of course, achieved at the expense of the reserve photosynthetic products previously stored by the plant. The overall coupling between growth and photosynthesis is imposed by the dependence of biosynthetic processes in the meristems and zones of cell enlargement upon organic substrate (sugar) imported from the leaves via the mechanisms of translocation discussed in Chapter 7.

From the point of view of molecular biology, growth is the operation of the pathways of intracellular transfer of genetic information, summarized in Figure 8-10, upon which all biosynthesis of cell constituents and structures is founded. The processes of information transfer are thoroughly discussed in Novikoff-Holtzman, *Cells and Organelles*, Levine, *Genetics*, and Ebert-Sussex, *Interacting Systems in Development* in this series, and need not be reviewed in detail here.

Prior to each mitosis meristematic growth requires a round of replication of the mother cell's DNA, which duplicates all the genetic information that the cell possesses, so that a copy of this information can be passed via the chromosomes (and cell organelles to the extent that they contain their own DNA) to each daughter cell. On the other hand growth during the cell enlargement phase does not require nuclear DNA replication. However, in some tissues of a good many plants DNA replication does continue, *without mitosis*, during the cell enlargement phase of growth, resulting in polyploid cells, that is, cells possessing some multiple of the basic diploid chromosome number. This striking phenomenon may help the occurrence of differentiation processes by multiplying the number of genes available for transcription in each cell, but it does not seem to be generally essential to development in plants because the cells of many tissues complete growth and differentiation without becoming polyploid.

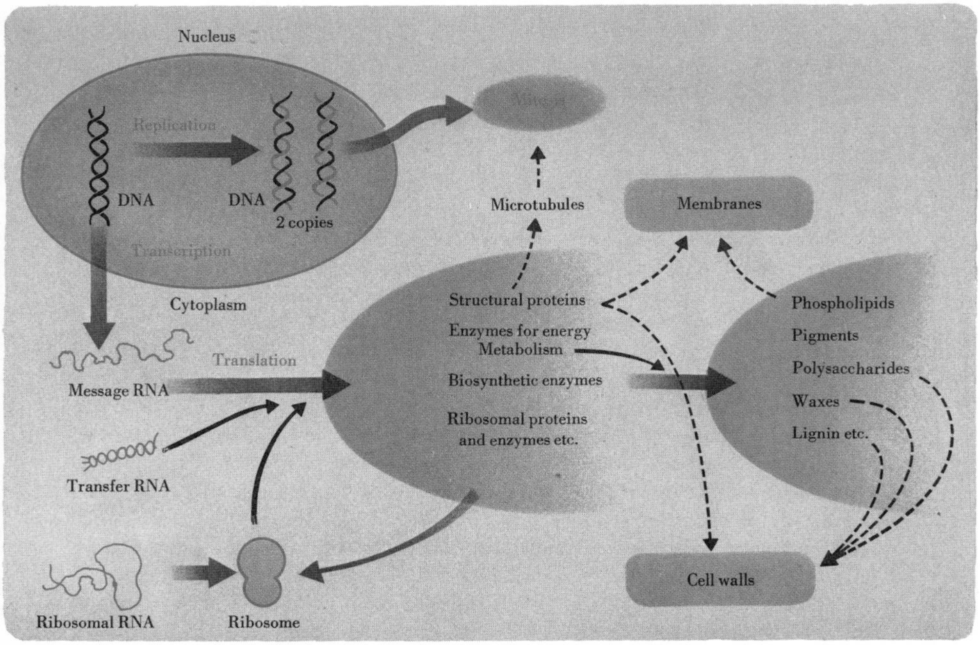

Fig. 8-10   *Diagram of intracellular pathways of genetic information transfer involved in growth and differentiation. The lists of classes of cell proteins and nonprotein constituents are, of course, not complete and are meant just to call attention to some of the major components that contribute to plant cell development. Analogous information transfer occurs to some extent in chloroplasts and mitochondria but is not represented in the diagram.*

During typical meristematic growth each daughter cell acquires, after the completion of each cycle of cell growth and division, a biochemical composition and complement of cell organelles equivalent to that possessed by the mother cell from which it arose. Therefore a complete reduplication of all cell components must be achieved by biosynthesis in the course of each division cycle. This involves first of all the production of a unit-cell equivalent (1) of soluble, ribosomal, and messenger RNA by transcription (by RNA polymerase) of DNA and (2) of all cell enzymes and structural proteins by translation (by the cell's ribosomes) of messenger RNAs. In addition, there must occur biosynthesis of a complete cell complement of membrane phospholipids, cell wall polysaccharides, and other secondary cell constituents that are derived by the action of biosynthetic enzymes. Regulatory mechanisms evidently exist in meristems to balance all of these syntheses relative to one another and in relation to the import of primary substrate (sugar and mineral nutrients) from outside the meristem. The nature of this control is not yet known, but it doubtless involves a regulation of transcription since this is the primary control point for all biosynthetic pathways. There is indeed evidence that inception of bud growth during sprouting of potatoes involves a dramatic increase in the capacity of the cells' DNA to support transcription, which probably reflects the activation or "derepression" of many genes.

In the cell enlargement phase of growth synthesis of protein and RNA normally continues but lags far behind the volume increase of the cell, which is due (as explained on page 127) mainly to increase in volume of the vacuole rather than of cytoplasm. Indeed in some instances, such as the growth of flower petals, the amounts of RNA and protein per cell actually fall during the cell enlargement phase of growth. This relative uncoupling of volume increase from biosynthesis may be why growth in size can proceed so much more rapidly in the cell enlargement phase than in meristems (noted on page 124). However, cell growth in the cell enlargement phase does apparently require the synthesis of some RNA and protein species, because this growth can be blocked by antibiotics that inhibit transcription or translation. Growth is also very sensitive to inhibitors and uncouplers of respiratory energy metabolism, as would be expected if growth depends upon biosynthesis.

The one kind of biosynthesis that almost invariably goes hand in hand with increase in cell size in the cell enlargement phase of growth is synthesis of primary cell wall material. This is necessary in order to maintain, as the cell expands, a cell wall thick enough to withstand without rupture the turgor forces operating from within the cell and between cells in a tissue. Cells that cannot continue to synthesize a cell wall, such as sieve-tube elements, become stretched during further growth to the point of collapse as mentioned earlier.

Cell Wall In order for any growth in size to occur in either a
Expansion meristem or a cell enlargement zone, it is essential that the cell wall, despite its ability to restrain turgor forces, undergo an extension or expansion in surface area. Ability to undergo surface expansion is a characteristic of the primary cell wall as contrasted with the secondary wall (page 14). The wall expansion that is required for growth in size depends upon turgor pressure, therefore growth can be prevented by conditions that cause a reduction in turgor, for example, by a medium that has a solute concentration close to that of the cell. Wall expansion during growth can thus be considered a physical stretching of the cell wall under the forces exerted by turgor pressure. This stretching in turn reduces the cell's turgor pressure and (by Equation 5-1) its water potential, generating a driving force for osmotic uptake of water into the cell, which increases its volume. To maintain a turgor pressure sufficient to extend the cell wall and thus bring about continued growth in volume, it is essential that the cell's solute concentration be maintained, against the dilution caused by water uptake during growth, by absorption of solutes by the growing cell or by solute production in photosynthesis.

Despite its biophysical character, extension of the primary wall during growth is under tight metabolic control of the cell, for wall expansion and growth in size stop in a matter of minutes if respiratory energy metabolism is interfered with. The capacity of the primary wall to expand in growth is evidently due to some kind of energy-dependent biochemical input from the cytoplasm. Two principal hypotheses exist as to how the growing cell acts on its cell wall to cause it to become extensible. One is that extension is due to degradation of wall polymers (polysaccharides, protein) by hydrolytic enzymes released into the wall by the cytoplasm, whereas the other considers that introduction of newly synthesized wall polymers into the wall structure permits it to expand. These hypotheses are not mutually exclusive, and either of them can afford an explanation, by Figure 8-10, of why cell enlargement depends upon RNA and protein synthesis. However, the actual biochemistry by which growing plant cells permit their cell walls to expand is still unsettled.

CELL   The shape of a plant cell is determined by the
MORPHOGENESIS   shape of its cell wall enclosure, and the mechanisms of cell wall growth just considered are
therefore basic to morphogenesis in plants. Plant cells utilize two methods of achieving specific morphogenesis during their growth, *anisotropic* wall expansion and *localized* wall expansion.

The principal strengthening elements of the cell wall are the cellulose *microfibrils* (page 10 and Figure 2-2). When the microfibrils are laid down in random orientation within the wall, the cell tends to grow equally in all directions and hence approximately as a sphere (Figure 8-11a). When, however, the microfibrils are deposited with a preferred orientation in one direction, as in Figure 8-11b, they strengthen the cell wall preferentially in that direction, and thus the growing wall expands primarily at right angles to the principal direction of the microfibrils. The result is that the cell *elongates* into the form of a cylinder. Elongation is, of course, the typical form of cell enlargement in roots and stems as well as parts of other organs. We may say that cell elongation results from *anisotropic* mechanical structure, that is, varying with direction, which causes anisotropic expansion of the wall to occur under the turgor forces that stretch it during a growth.

The following evidence suggests that cytoplasmic *microtubules* (page 22) determine the orientation in which cellulose microfibrils are deposited during cell wall synthesis. (1) When oriented deposition of cellulose is occurring, as in

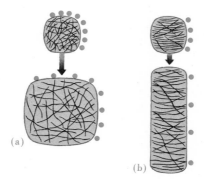

(a)

(b)

Fig. 8-11   *How orientation of cellulose microfibrils in the cell wall determines morphogenesis. Microfibrils are represented by lines. They are shown as more widely spaced after the cells have grown (lower cells in diagram), to indicate that the entire wall has expanded, as shown by displacement of markers (colored dots) placed on cell surface during growth. (The preferentially transverse orientation indicated for the cells in (b) is illustrated by the electronmicrograph in Figure 2-2.)*

elongating cells or in the deposition of the highly ordered cellulose of the secondary wall (page 14), arrays of microtubules are found in the adjacent cytoplasm, running in the same direction as the microfibrils that are being deposited (Figure 2-9). (2) When microtubules are disrupted by the drug *colchicine*, which interacts specifically with the subunit protein (tubulin) of the microtubules, cellulose deposition is not prevented but its orientation is disrupted and becomes random. Control of the anisotropic aspect of plant cell morphogenesis thus apparently is based on the ability of the cell to control the orientation of cytoplasmic microtubules. The mechanism by which microtubules may determine the orientation in which microfibrillar material is deposited is not yet understood.

The second aspect of plant cell morphogenesis is seen in the development of cells such as root hairs, which acquire their distinctive shape through the occurrence of extremely localized cell wall expansion restricted just to the hemispherical tip of the cell (Figure 8-12). In this kind of morphogenesis the expansion of the cell wall may be simply isotropic (not directional) in the tip region where expansion is occurring, but by precisely restricting the region that is permitted to expand a very elongated cell results. This kind of cell elongation is referred to as "tip growth" and it is simply an extreme case of the principle that morphogenesis may be accomplished by *variation in the rate of growth with position* in the cell. This focuses attention upon the fact that it is not only the directionality but also the *rate* of the process of cell wall expansion that is under extremely local, specific control of the cell.

These geometrical aspects of plant cell development are intriguing because it is not at all obvious from the known pathways of information transfer (Figure 8-10) how local and directional processes of the kind just explained could be specified within the cell.

The classical object for investigating genetic control of these processes is

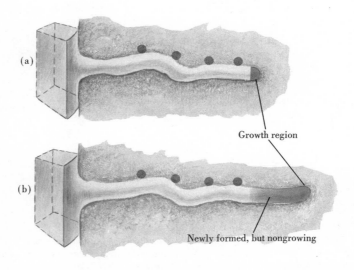

(a)

Growth region

(b)

Newly formed, but nongrowing

Fig. 8-12 *Diagram of tip growth as seen in a root hair. Note that in contrast to Figure 8-11, markers applied along the length of this cell do not separate during its elongation.*

the alga *Acetabularia*, a uninucleate giant cell that grows as illustrated in Figure 8-13. The "stalk" elongates by localized tip growth. By means of a precise pattern of outgrowths that emerge around the tip of the stalk the "hairs" and "cap," which consist of radial arrays of cell projections, develop. The fine details of this development are under nuclear control, as shown by the fact that if the cell's nucleus (which is located in one of the rhizoids) is replaced by the nucleus of a different species of *Acetabularia*, the cap that forms will be characteristic of the species from which the nucleus was derived, as is discussed further in Ebert-Sussex, *Interacting Systems in Development* in this series.

By means of excision (surgical removal) experiments with *Acetabularia* it has been established that the capacity for cap morphogenesis is due to a "morphogenetic substance," now considered to be messenger RNA, that is released by the nucleus and is transported specifically to the tip of the stalk where it accumulates. This reveals an inherent *polarity* within the cell that is as essential to the occurrence of normal morphogenesis as is the morphogenetic "message" itself. The message might specify enzymes for building up the cell wall at the tip in some particular way. There is indeed evidence that the cell walls of the cap contain much larger amounts of glucose and galactose polysaccharides than the stalk and that enzymes for the production of these polymers increase at the time of cap formation. However, in order for synthesis of wall constitutents to expand the cell wall in a precise, species-specific pattern, phenomena of orientation and localized deposition have again to be invoked.

In a variety of tip-growing cells such as root hairs, pollen tubes, and fungus filaments, we can observe with the electron microscope a conspicuous accumulation, in the hemispherical tip region, of vesicles derived from the Golgi

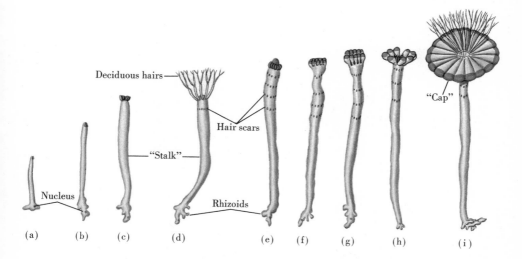

Fig. 8-13 *Development of the giant uninucleate cell of the green alga* Acetabularia. *Germling (a) has arisen from a fertilized egg. Elongating regions of the "shoot" are shown with color. Note lateral expansion of older part of stalk that accompanies elongation. (After drawings by Lois Eubank Egerod, in* University of California Publications in Botany, **25**, *1952. Originally published by the University of California Press; reprinted by permission of The Regents of the University of California.)*

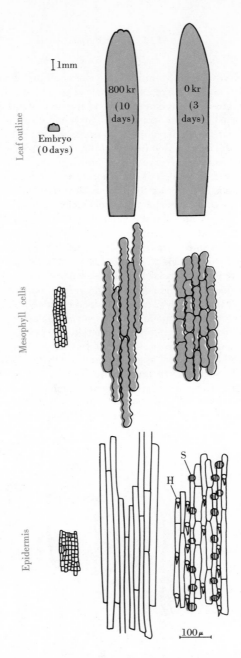

Fig. 8-14 *Cell growth and morphogenesis in the first foliage leaf during germination of normal wheat seeds and of seeds that were given a dose of gamma radiation sufficient to prevent cell division. Left-hand column shows the outline of the embryonic leaf and the size and shape of its mesophyll cells (internal tissue of leaf) and epidermal cells as they appear in the seed. Center and right-hand columns show leaf outline and cell sizes and shapes after the leaf had grown to a length of 17 mm, which required 3 days in the germination of normal seeds ("0 kr," right-hand column) and 10 days in the germination of seeds that had received 800 kilorads of gamma radiation (center column). Because of the*

146

dictyosomes and/or the endoplasmic reticulum. These vesicles contain carbohydrate similar to that which is being added to the growing cell wall, and the apparent fusion of such vesicles with the wall has been seen in many instances. The localized growth of the tip may therefore be due simply to a directional transport of these vesicles toward the tip from their sites of production within the cell, which leads to a locally intense action on the cell wall specifically in the tip region. The nature and control of this transport mechanism, like that involved in morphogenetic polarity in *Acetabularia*, remain to be discovered.

Tissue and Organ Morphogenesis We might think that the local rate and direction of growth in meristems, upon which morphogenetic phenomena such as emergence and elongation of leaf primordia depend, would be dictated by the frequency and direction of cell division. The experiment illustrated in Figure 8-14 indicates, to the contrary, that the directionality of growth is built into the cells (that is, determined by their wall structure as explained above) and persists even when cell division is completely blocked.

Cell division in meristems is usually symmetrical and follows along with the principal direction of growth, as shown in Figures 8-1a and 8-14. But in some important morphogenetic processes, such as the formation of the stomatal cell complex in the leaf epidermis illustrated in Figure 8-15, cells divide very asymmetrically, and/or in a direction different from the major axis of growth. It has been found that prior to these asymmetric mitoses a band of microtubules forms in the peripheral cytoplasm approximately in the location of the future cell plate. These microtubules may function to position the mitotic spindle and thereby to determine where the cell plate will be formed.

The genetic specification of morphogenesis in meristems presents questions even more challenging than those raised by the geometrical aspects of single-cell development, for we witness in the kinds of phenomena just discussed a coordinated and specifically patterned modulation of growth and division among numerous cells in a population. These cells are all derived ultimately from the same group of apical initials and evidently all possess the same genetic information. One indication that they do is the fact that adventitious bud and root apical meristems can arise from the mature derivative tissues (discussed on page 134). Moreover, since adventitious buds can arise from root tissues and vice versa, there can be no difference between the genetic information possessed by the cells of shoot and root apical meristems.

That single vegetative plant cells from different organs carry the totality of genetic information of the species has been shown dramatically with the carrot

---

absence of cell division, the increase in cell length between left and center columns reflects the approximately 25-fold elongation that occurred during growth. Cells in right-hand column are shorter, even though the same amount of elongation occurred, owing to the cell division that accompanied normal growth. Note the failure of stomatal complexes S and hair cells H to differentiate in epidermis of irradiated leaf, since this morphogenesis requires cell division. Observe, nevertheless, the normal morphogenesis of the irradiated leaf as a whole and even of the sinuous outline of its mesophyll cells. (Data of Alan H. Haber, from American Journal of Botany, **49:** *583, 1962.)*

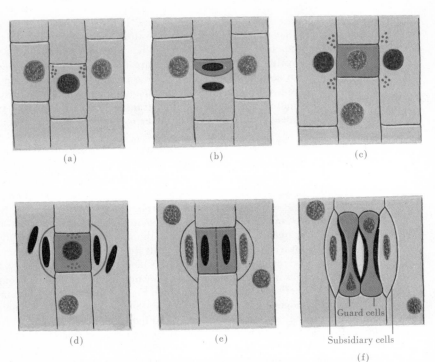

Fig. 8-15   *Development of the stomatal complex in epidermis of leaf of wheat, illustrating the role of preprophase bands of microtubules (colored dots) in determining the positions of mitosis and cell plate formation that bring about the specific morphogenesis. Note that between each successive cell division all cells get longer because of elongation growth. (See J. D. Pickett-Heaps and D. H. Northcote,* Journal of Cell Science, **1:** 121, 1966.)*

plant. When tissues from the leaf, stem, and root are grown in liquid culture in certain growth media, it is observed that individual cells in large numbers develop into embryolike plantlets in a manner very similar to the development of a normal plant embryo from a fertilized egg (Figure 10-1). These vegetative embryos will grow into mature plants that complete the life cycle by producing flowers and seed, and therefore express all the plant's genetic potentialities.

The profound differences in morphogenetic function of shoot and root apical meristems must therefore be ascribed to regulatory forces operating within each type of meristem to control which aspects of the genetic instructions are expressed in its development. An indication of such forces is seen in surgical experiments on shoot apical meristems which indicate that already-formed leaf primordia tend to inhibit the initiation of a leaf primordium nearby. This effect apparently determines the regular, species-specific pattern in which leaf primordia become initiated on the flanks of the apical meristem. From experience with hormone effects to be discussed in Chapter 9 we infer that these morphogenetic forces are probably of a hormonal nature. For example, the type of hormone called *auxin* can induce vascular differentiation and is produced by buds; in situations such as grafting and adventitious bud formation buds induce differentiation of vascular elements in adjoining nonvascular tissue. Thus it seems that auxin production by the shoot tip and leaf primordia could contribute to establishing the anatomical pattern that is formed during normal growth.

The actual details of the control systems that operate within meristems to bring about normal morphogenesis are not yet understood. These control forces must be rather strong and self-perpetuating, because a shoot apical meristem never transforms itself into a root apical meristem or vice versa, even though tissues derived from each of these meristems are capable of giving rise to the other as discussed previously.

There must be some level of genetic information that specifies root development as against vegetative shoot, leaf, flower, or secondary growth, and so forth. At present we have no evidence of how "organ-specific" genes might cause specific morphogenesis, but it seems possible that they act as regulators of genes that are involved with production of growth-regulatory substances and with the biochemical and biophysical mechanisms of cellular growth and morphogenesis outlined above.

DIFFERENTIATION   It should be clear from this discussion that differentiation of the specialized mature tissues of plants does not in general depend upon any kind of irreversible commitment ("determination") or permanent loss of developmental potentiality of the cells involved, except insofar as the overt structural specialization itself involves irreversible changes such as secondary wall deposition or loss of nucleus or cytoplasm. Plant cell differentiation differs rather fundamentally in this respect from differentiation in animal systems, in which the commitment to a given kind of differentiation, once made, is usually virtually irreversible (see Ebert-Sussex, *Interacting Systems in Development*).

Differentiation of animal cells generally requires induction of synthesis of *tissue-specific proteins* that are responsible for specialized functional capabilities, for example, hemoglobin in red blood cells and actin and myosin in muscle. This induction depends upon an activation of the transcription of genes that code for the tissue-specific proteins in question, genes that are evidently inactive in embryonic cells as well as in other types of differentiated tissue in which different tissue-specific proteins are being produced. Tissue-specific gene transcription is therefore regarded as a key to cellular differentiation.

It has been found in certain instances that the complement of protein species differs between different plant organs such as roots, leaves, and flowers, but the functional meaning of these differences is not known. Perhaps the clearest example in plants of induction of synthesis of proteins that are specific to a particular specialized function is encountered in the differentiation of chloroplasts. This subject is of interest and importance from several points of view and merits special attention.

Chloroplast   Growing algal cells typically contain fully differ-
Differentiation   entiated chloroplasts which grow and divide
along with their host cell while performing the
process of photosynthesis. The cells of vascular plant meristems on the other hand normally lack visible chloroplasts and photosynthetic capability but con-

tain precursor organelles called *proplastids* that are rather similar to mitochondria in size and appearance and evidently grow and divide as the meristematic cells divide (see Figure 2-3).

During cell enlargement and differentiation of leaves, proplastids grow enormously and differentiate into photosynthetically competent chloroplasts with formation of the pigments and elaborate thylakoid membrane system discussed in Chapter 3. This differentiation is accompanied by a massive synthesis of the enzymes of photosynthetic carbon metabolism such as ribulose diphosphate carboxylase and NADP-linked triose phosphate dehydrogenase (page 42), which are virtually absent from nongreen meristematic cells. Initiation of synthesis of chloroplast-specific proteins during differentiation can be prevented by inhibitors of transcription and therefore presumably depends upon an activation of transcription of chloroplast-specific genes.

Chloroplast development is under both internal and environmental control. Existence of internal controls is shown by the lack of chloroplast differentiation in meristems, in tissues of most roots, and in the epidermis of the shoot (except for stomatal guard cells, where chloroplasts do differentiate). Environmental control is exerted by light. In the dark, proplastids in young leaf cells grow not into chloroplasts but into nongreen plastids called *etioplasts* (Figure 8-16a), which usually develop a curious internal tubular membrane structure called the "prolamellar body" and which lack almost entirely the photosynthetic enzymes mentioned above. Illumination induces the synthesis of photosynthetic enzymes and pigments as well as transformation of the prolamellar body into the thylakoid membrane system (Figure 8-16b and c). The nature of the photoregulatory system that controls chloroplast-specific gene activity and biosynthesis will be discussed in Chapter 9.

Chloroplasts contain (page 20) both DNA and their own ribosomes, which are smaller than cytoplasmic ribosomes and biochemically more like bacterial ribosomes. It appears that at least some of the chloroplast-specific proteins are coded for by chloroplast DNA and synthesized by chloroplast ribosomes via a pathway of information transfer *within the plastid* like that represented for nuclear DNA and cytoplasmic ribosomes in Figure 8-10. This situation is termed *genetic autonomy* of chloroplasts. The controls of chloroplast development mentioned above may be exerted partly at the level of plastid (or proplastid) gene transcription. Nuclear functions are also involved, however, in chloroplast development because synthesis of plastid pigments depends upon enzymes that are coded for by nuclear genes. Differentiation of a chloroplast from a proplastid or an etioplast is blocked in nuclear mutants that are defective for pigment synthesis.

Tissue Differentiation Processes The proteins that are involved in photosynthetic functions are actually organelle-specific rather than tissue-specific. And except for them, it is difficult to point to particular proteins that are truly specific to the specialized functions of the major types of differentiated plant cells that have been discussed previously in the way that hemoglobin and actomyosin are, say, to red cells and muscle cells, respectively. The "slime" proteins of sieve-tube elements may be an example. But the functions of the

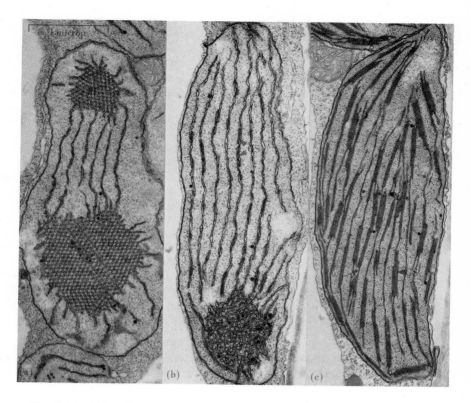

Fig. 8-16   *Light-induced development of the chloroplast in leaf of oat seedling. (a) Etioplast as found in dark-grown leaf; PL, prolamellar body. (b) After 2 hr exposure of leaf to light; note disorganization of prolamellar body from which is proliferating the lamellar membrane system with beginning of formation of grana stacks (GS). (c) Differentiated plastid after 24 hr exposure to light. (Magnification 21,000×. Electron micrographs by the author and Dr. Margery M. Ray.)*

major specialized plant tissues, such as xylem, phloem, epidermis, endodermis, collenchyma, and so forth, seem to be due more to the specialized *structure* of their cells which involves principally cell wall components (polysaccharides, lignin, waxes) than to functionally unique proteins. The primary role of genetic information in differentiation of these structural specializations presumably is, as indicated in Figure 8-10, to specify enzymes for biosynthesis of the appropriate structural components. These components may be tissue-specific, at least in some cases such as the epidermal cuticular waxes or the suberin of cork cell walls, and accordingly the required biosynthetic enzymes may be tissue-specific proteins, the activation of genes coding for which becomes central to the occurrence of the differentiation process.

An example of these principles may be seen in the case of lignin formation in differentiating secondary cell walls, which is due to oxidative action of the enzyme *peroxidase* upon phenolic (benzene ring with —OH attached) compounds. Peroxidase activity is found to rise to a high level in cells that are about to differentiate into vascular cells with secondary walls, such as the cells in the central part of the young carrot root in Figure 8-4a. Indeed the tissue-specific localization of peroxidase is one of the longest-known biological examples of enzyme localization; it can be demonstrated spectacularly with simple staining procedures.

The deposition of cell products such as waxes or wall polymers in cell-specific *locations* and *orientations* is, however, just as important to useful cell differentiation as is the synthesis itself. The fact that the patterns of deposition of one and the same wall component, such as the secondary cell wall constituents, can vary so dramatically and importantly among different cell types shows, moreover, that the pattern of deposition is not due to the nature of the product but is under developmental control of the cell. Thus differentiation involves a geometrical aspect closely analogous to the control of growth and morphogenesis discussed above. For example, bands of microtubules collect in the positions in which bands of secondary wall polymers are to be deposited in the differentiation of locally thickened vessels like those to the left in Figure 8-5. And then localized breakdown of the wall occurs which removes not only the end walls but, as mentioned on page 129, much of the material between the localized thickenings of the side walls. To explain how these subtle, but vital, localized and patterned actions of enzymes and organelles within cells can be specified genetically by the known routes of information transfer (Figure 8-10) provides an exciting challenge for developmental biology.

SUGGESTED READING

Cutter, E. G., *Plant Anatomy: Experiment and Interpretation.* Reading, Mass.: Addison-Wesley, 1969. Chapters 7, 8, 9, and 11.

Esau, K., *Anatomy of Seed Plants.* New York: Wiley, 1960. pp. 114-121, 180-187, 217-256.

Gemmell, A. R., *Developmental Plant Anatomy.* New York: St. Martin's Press, 1969.

Gibor, A., "Acetabularia: A Useful Giant Cell," *Scientific American,* **215** (5):118-124, 1966.

Goodenough, U. W., and R. P. Levine, "The Genetic Activity of Mitochondria and Chloroplasts," *Scientific American,* **223** (5):22-29, 1970.

Green, P. B., "Cell Walls and the Geometry of Plant Growth," *Brookhaven Symposia in Biology,* **16:**203-215, 1963.

O'Brien, T. P., and M. McCully, *Plant Structure and Development: A Pictorial and Physiological Approach.* New York: Macmillan, 1969. Chapters 3-7.

Steward, F. C., *Growth and Differentiation in Plants.* Reading, Mass.: Addison-Wesley, 1968. Chapter 1.

Sussex, I. M., "Plant Morphogenesis," in *This Is Life,* W. H. Johnson and W. C. Steere (eds.). New York: Holt, Rinehart and Winston, 1962.

Torrey, J. G., *Development in Flowering Plants.* New York: Macmillan, 1967. Chapters 5-8.

Wareing, P. F., and I. D. J. Phillips, *The Control of Growth and Differentiation in Plants.* New York: Pergamon, 1970. Chapters 1-3.

chapter **9**

Regulation
of Growth
and
Development

Growth in plants serves more than just to increase stature and amount of functional equipment. It allows the plant to orient itself as favorably as it can with respect to its environment, even though it lacks any proper organs for locomotion. The two best-known orientation responses are *geotropism*, the response to gravity, and *phototropism*, the response to direction of illumination. Study of these responses led to the knowledge that plant growth is influenced by hormones, a concept that has gone far toward explaining how plants regulate and control their development.

AUXIN AND If a growing plant
TROPIC RESPONSES is placed horizontally, we may observe within a few hours that the growing zone of the root bends until the root tip

154

becomes directed again vertically downward and the growing zone of the stem bends vertically upward (Figure 9-1). Roots are said to show *positive* geotropism, bending toward gravity, and shoots have *negative* geotropism. The tropic curvatures are brought about by *unequal growth* on the two sides of the axis; for example, in a horizontally placed stem the lower side of the zone of elongation grows more than the upper side and so causes an upward curvature of the growing zone.

When a shoot is illuminated from one side, the growing zone of the stem bends toward the direction of illumination. This response is positive phototropism. Leaves also commonly orient with respect to light, usually turning until their surfaces are nearly at right angles to the direction of illumination. Leaves of many arid-climate plants on the other hand orient edgewise to the sun, which minimizes their radiation load advantageously in these circumstances (see page 62).

Another less well-known orientation response is the growth curvature of stems and/or tendrils of climbing plants in response to contact.

Of the various growth curvatures or tropisms phototropism has been the most intensively studied. Long ago Charles Darwin, founder of the theory of organic evolution, and his son Francis discovered that the seedlings of grasses could be prevented from bending to light if the very tip of the young shoot (tip of the coleoptile, see Figure 9-2a) were covered with an opaque cap, even though the growing zone and normal region of phototropic curvature lay largely below the tip. They concluded that only the tip could perceive light, and that upon illumination a stimulus formed in the tip is transmitted down into the growing zone where it causes curvature. Much later it was found that some substance

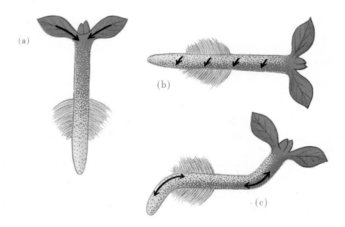

Fig. 9-1 *Geotropism in a seedling, illustrating the hormonal explanation. Auxin-producing region is shown in color and the distribution of auxin in shoot and root is shown by color dots. When the seedling is turned horizontally (b), auxin is transported to the lower side. As shown by arrows in (c) auxin promotes elongation of cells in the shoot so that the lower side grows more rapidly and causes upward curvature; and it inhibits elongation of cells in the root so that the upper side grows more and causes downward curvature.*

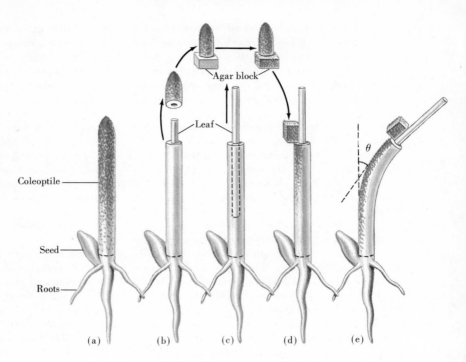

Fig. 9-2 *Went's curvature bioassay for auxin. A 3-day-old oat seedling (a) is decapitated (b), and the leaf inside is pulled up (c). An agar block containing auxin (here
illustrated as obtained by placing the coleoptile tip in contact with the block for about an
hour) is applied to one side of the leaf so that it contacts the cut surface of the coleoptile
(d). Auxin from the block becomes transported down the coleoptile and causes that side to
grow faster than the opposite side, resulting in curvature (e). The angle of curvature, θ,
can be used to determine the amount of auxin in the agar block. The actual procedure is
slightly more complicated than pictured here.*

coming out of the tip would, if applied to one side of a grass seedling from which
the tip had been cut off, cause greater elongation in the tissues below on that
side and hence a curvature.

Figure 9-2 illustrates the method that Frits Went developed about 1927 to
detect and measure this substance by the amount of curvature it produced when
applied to one side of a decapitated oat seedling. By this method of *bioassay* it
could be shown that sidewise illumination of the tip causes more of the "growth
substance" to be emitted from the dark side than from the light side, thus
causing greater growth on the dark side than on the light side and hence a
bending toward the light (Figure 9-3). Similarly, lateral exposure to gravity was
found to result in an accumulation of growth substance on the lower side of the
stem, which accelerates growth on that side thus causing the stem to bend upward (Figure 9-1). The "growth substance" was later named *auxin*.

Went's method of assay made it possible to purify and isolate auxin and
thus to identify the material chemically as *indoleacetic acid* (IAA).

$$\text{CH}_2\text{--COOH}$$

Indoleacetic acid (IAA)

Indoleacetic acid in very minute amounts promotes growth; one millionth of a milligram is sufficient to produce a conspicuous curvature if applied to one side of a decapitated oat seedling. Since auxin is produced in the tip, travels down into the zone of elongation, and there brings forth a response (growth), it is regarded as a chemical messenger or *hormone*.

Auxin is probably produced by and promotes growth in the shoots of all higher plants. Production of auxin is usually centered in the shoot tip and particularly the young leaves. The hormone is transported down the shoot by a special transport mechanism that is called the *polar transport system* because it moves auxin through tissue strictly in the basal direction regardless of the tissue's orientation relative to external influences such as light or gravity. Polar transport takes place through the general parenchyma tissue of young organs such as coleoptiles, but there is also evidence that transport of auxin through the vascular system occurs in some cases. The mechanism of polar transport is not at all well understood as yet, but the process may be cited as another manifestation of fundamental developmental polarity of the kind discussed in Chapter 8 (page 145).

Mechanism of   It has proved very difficult to establish just how
Tropic Responses   lateral light or gravity causes a lateral inequality

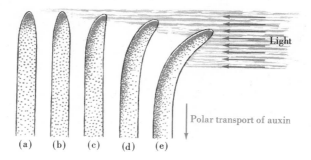

Fig. 9-3 *Phototropism in coleoptile of a grass seedling, illustrating the hormonal explanation. Auxin-producing region is shown by color, while distribution of auxin within coleoptile is indicated by color dots. Note that the difference in auxin concentration on the two sides arises at the tip, which is the light-sensitive site, and moves down the coleoptile because auxin is transported toward the base. As a result curvature begins just below the tip and progresses toward the base of the coleoptile. The events illustrated would occur in about 2 hr in a coleoptile 2 cm high. The difference between auxin concentrations on the two sides in response to light is exaggerated in the diagram.*

of auxin concentration to appear in the plant. Apparently this inequality results from a lateral transport of auxin that is induced by the physical stimulus
and may be in fact a sidewise deflection of the polar transport of auxin just
discussed. (We should beware of the common misconception that auxin molecules simply fall to the lower side of the stem under gravitational force; the
force is in fact much too small for any such effect.) But how light or gravity
causes lateral transport still eludes us almost completely.

In the case of phototropism it is not even proved what pigment is responsible for perception of light, although it definitely is not chlorophyll; phototropism occurs only in response to wavelengths in the blue, violet, and ultraviolet part of the spectrum and is totally insensitive to red light which
chlorophyll absorbs strongly (Chapter 3). The action spectrum for phototropism
(Figure 9-4) resembles the absorption spectrum of carotenoids such as β-caro-
tene (see Figure 3-1); it has in addition a peak in the near ultraviolet at 360 nm
which resembles the absorption spectrum of flavin pigments (for example, the
vitamin riboflavin). It seems possible that both types of pigments are involved,
but the nature of the photoact remains unknown. The photoreceptor pigment
most likely does not act directly on auxin; the photoreceptor for phototropism by
the fungus *Phycomyces* appears to be the same as in higher plants, but auxin is
not involved in the growth response of the fungus. This and other evidence indicate that phototropism is not due to inactivation of auxin by light, although such
a mechanism is still frequently presented by textbook writers.

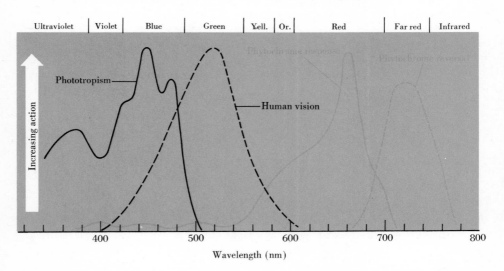

Fig. 9-4   *Action spectra for phototropism in oat seedlings, for phytochrome-induced
hypocotyl hook opening in bean seedlings, and for its reversal, compared with the spectral
sensitivity of human (rod cell) vision. Note that plants are phototropically sensitive to
ultraviolet light that the human eye cannot see, and that phytochrome response peaks in
the red region, to which human sensitivity is poor. Observe the resemblance between the
action spectrum for phototropism and the absorption spectrum for β-carotene shown in
Figure 3-1. (From data of K. V. Thimann and G. M. Curry,* Comparative Biochemistry, **1**:
243, 1960 *and R. B. Withrow, W. H. Klein, and V. Elstad,* Plant Physiology, **32**: 453,
1957.)*

Equally intriguing is the question of how gravity is sensed in the geotropic response. The classical theory is that large amyloplasts (plastids containing starch grains, page 19, which can be observed to fall to the lower side of the cells possessing them, are the gravity-sensing organelles ("statoliths"). For example, in roots large amyloplasts are usually found in the cells of the root cap but not in the meristem or elongation zone, and if the root cap is cut off, geotropism does not occur even though the root keeps on growing. Although the "statolith" theory of geoperception has been denied on several grounds, no realistic alternative has been proposed and the classical theory survives. How lateral displacement of amyloplasts may cause lateral transport of auxin is, however, still understood little better than at the level of speculation.

As illustrated in Figure 9-1 the geotropic response of roots is opposite to that of shoots. The explanation for this brings up an unexpected feature of auxin action: it turns out that auxin powerfully *inhibits* growth of root cells; indeed, inhibition of root growth occurs at auxin concentrations even lower than those that promote growth in stems. Therefore transport of auxin to the lower side of a horizontally placed root *reduces* the growth rate on the lower side and causes the growing zone to bend downward (Figure 9-1) so that root growth is directed toward gravity, a response of obvious functional value.

GROWTH-CORRELATION MECHANISMS INVOLVING AUXIN

Synthesis of auxin by and polar transport from young leaves at the shoot tip provides a means by which elongation of the internodes, which is dependent on auxin, can be regulated in proper relation to expansion of the leaves and development of new leaf primordia and internodes at the apical meristem. This is an example of a *growth-correlation* mechanism, a kind of developmental regulation that is vital to any organism that possesses diverse organs and growing zones.

Several other growth-correlation mechanisms in plants are known or suspected to involve auxin. One is the growth of fruits in relation to growth of seeds (to be discussed in Chapter 10). Another is growth activity in the vascular cambium. This is stimulated by auxin, an effect that involves promotion of cell division rather than simply of cell enlargement as in the previously considered auxin effects. The stimulation permits secondary growth of the stem to be coupled to the auxin-producing primary growth of the shoot tips, as is developmentally desirable. Other hormones (cytokinins, gibberellins) may also be involved in normal cambium function as we shall see later.

An important effect of auxin that also involves cell division is to provoke the initiation of branch roots and of adventitious roots from the root and the shoot (page 134). This effect tends to correlate the degree of branching of the root system with the extent of bud development in the shoot. Moreover, because of downward polar transport, auxin tends to accumulate just above any site of damage in the stem or root system; this accumulation promotes initiation of adventitious roots at the site of damage, thus promoting regeneration of lost roots and increasing the chances of survival of the aerial parts of a plant after an injury below or at ground level.

The root initiation effect of auxin has proved to be of great horticultural usefulness in the propagation of plants by cuttings. Treatment of cuttings at the time of preparation with auxins related to IAA is now quite general practice. It can greatly increase both the total number of roots formed and the percent of cuttings that root, increasing both the vigor and the total yield of vegetatively propagated progeny.

The important role of auxin in cell division is shown most impressively with tissue cultures. If we remove from a stem or other organ a piece of living tissue and place it upon a sterile nutrient medium (usually solidified by adding agar), the cells may begin to grow and divide vigorously, provided the medium contains the necessary constituents (sugar, minerals, and sometimes vitamins and other growth factors). Such growth usually produces a rather disorganized, haphazard mass of cells called a *callus* (Figure 9-5). Auxin is generally required in order for this kind of cell multiplication to occur rapidly, as can be seen from the results illustrated in Figure 9-5.

In addition to its growth and morphogenetic (root initiation) effects, auxin also exerts influences on differentiation. For example, it promotes differentiation of xylem and phloem tissue in stems and roots. This may serve to correlate vascular differentiation with growth and morphogenesis at the apical meristem as suggested on page 148.

Apical Dominance

Although axillary buds are initiated in the apical meristematic zone (page 133), they typically remain inactive for a prolonged period while the main shoot continues to grow. But if the main shoot tip is cut off, lateral buds immediately begin to grow out to form branch shoots, thus making up for the

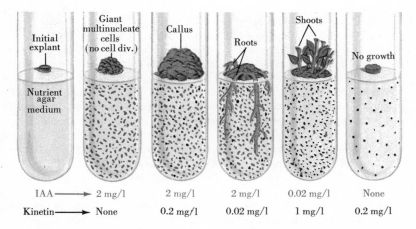

IAA	2 mg/l	2 mg/l	2 mg/l	0.02 mg/l	None
Kinetin	None	0.2 mg/l	0.02 mg/l	1 mg/l	0.2 mg/l

Fig. 9-5 *Growth responses of a plant tissue culture to auxin and kinetin. The initial explant is a small piece of sterile tissue derived from the pith of tobacco stem and placed on a nutrient agar medium, as shown at left. After several weeks the kinds of growth illustrated occur on media supplemented with the indicated levels of growth factors. (See F. Skoog and C. O. Miller, Symposia of the Society for Experimental Biology,* **11:** *118, 1957.)*

loss of the shoot's growth zone (Figure 9-6). This inhibition of axillary bud growth by the main shoot tip is called *apical dominance*. It provides for rapid initiation of lateral bud growth when the shoot tip is damaged or removed by some accident.

If auxin is applied to the cut end of a shoot from which the growing tip was removed, it can substitute for the inhibitory effect of the tip and prevent the lateral buds from growing (Figure 9-6c). This suggests that auxin coming down from the normal growing shoot tip inhibits the growth of lateral buds.

Various experiments indicate that the role of auxin in apical dominance is probably not as a direct inhibitor of lateral buds and that other growth factors are involved (pages 165 and 169). The exact mechanism of the apical dominance phenomenon is not, in fact, yet understood, and a good deal of evidence suggests that competition between buds for nutrients translocated from the leaves and roots may be important in apical dominance.

Synthetic Auxins and Herbicidal Action Various synthetic chemicals with structures resembling IAA to the extent of having a ring system containing double bonds and a side chain bearing an acid group, exert auxin activity on plants. It is thought that cells sensitive to auxin must have a more or less specific "receptor" site that combines with molecules of this general structure, inducing the physiological response.

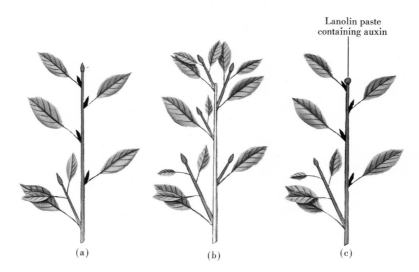

Lanolin paste
containing auxin

(a)   (b)   (c)

Fig. 9-6 *Apical dominance and the effect of auxin. Growing, auxin-producing buds are shown in color, auxin being transported down the stem is indicated in lighter color and nongrowing lateral buds are shown in black. In (a) all lateral buds except the lowest are inhibited by the shoot tip, since when the tip is removed in (b) the lateral buds begin to grow. The lowest lateral bud in (a) has previously escaped from inhibition because it is so far removed from the tip. If the shoot tip is removed but immediately replaced by auxin in (c), lateral bud growth is prevented as if the tip were still present. Note that this auxin does not inhibit the lateral branch that was already growing.*

As we have seen auxin is involved in so many subtle regulatory phenomena in plant development that it is perhaps not surprising that when auxins are applied to plants in high concentrations, they may disrupt normal growth and morphogenesis leading to physiological breakdown and finally death. Plants possess inactivation mechanisms that prevent IAA, their native hormone, from accumulating to excessive levels within the tissues, but these mechanisms do not work on many of the foreign, synthetic compounds that mimic the action of IAA. Therefore some of these compounds have come into widespread use in agriculture and horticulture as weed killers (herbicides), especially "2,4-D" (2,4-dichlorophenoxyacetic acid) and the closely related trichloro compound "2,4,5-T." These herbicides are exceptionally useful because, for reasons still not well understood, they are of only limited toxicity to plants of the grass family but extremely effective against most broad-leaved plants. Therefore they are used to kill broad-leaved weeds in cereal grain crops and in lawns, virtually eliminating the necessity of weeding.

GIBBERELLINS   Gibberellins are compounds that in minute quantities accelerate shoot growth; they were first discovered as products of the fungus *Gibberella*, after which they are named. Several gibberellins have been isolated from higher plant tissues and are certainly plant products. They comprise a family of over 30 substances with closely related chemical structures somewhat distantly resembling the steroid structure of several animal hormones.

Gibberellin A₃ (GA)

A striking effect of gibberellins is seen with single-gene "dwarf" mutant strains whose growth is greatly stunted by comparison with normal (nondwarf) plants of the same species. Many dwarf mutants are extremely sensitive to gibberellin and can be made to grow essentially like normal plants by applying it (Figure 9-7), whereas treatment of this kind of dwarf with auxin gives no comparable effect. Dwarf corn seedlings consequently can be used in a specific bioassay for gibberellins.

The existence of gibberellin-sensitive dwarf mutants strongly implicates

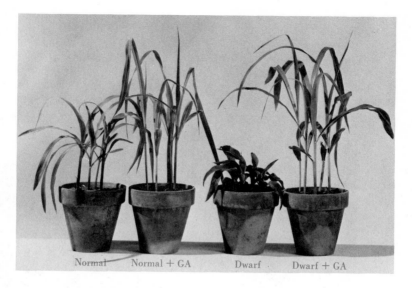

Fig. 9-7 *Effect of gibberellin (GA) on normal and dwarf corn plants. The plants were 3 weeks old when photographed; treated plants had been given 10 μg of gibberellin A_3 every other day beginning on the seventh day. Note that the dwarfs responded much more markedly to gibberellin than did the normals, and that gibberellin caused the dwarfs to grow just as rapidly as the treated normal plants. (Dwarf plants were genetically similar to normals except in being homozygous for the recessive gene* dwarf-1.)

involvement of gibberellins in the regulation of shoot growth in normal nondwarf plants. It was at first thought that dwarf mutants were defective for synthesis of gibberellins. However, dwarf peas synthesize the gibberellins normally found in peas but are unresponsive to these even though they respond strongly to most other gibberellins; so the genetic defect that is involved seems to be a rather subtle one.

An important role of gibberellin within the normal plant seems to be to alter the balance between internode growth and leaf development so as to bring on different forms of growth to suit the requirements of the plant at different seasons or for different purposes. For example, many plants go through a stage of development in which several to many leaves are produced with little if any elongation of the stem; this form of growth (Figure 9-8a) is called a "rosette." Then, often before the onset of reproduction, the stem begins to elongate so that the leaves that mature thereafter become separated by typical elongated internodes (Figure 9-8c). By applying gibberellin we can induce the rosette form of growth to change into the elongated form (Figure 9-8b). The requirement of gibberellin for the elongation of internodes enables the plant to regulate its own growth form by altering its production of gibberellin, a decrease leading to the rosette form and an increase leading to the elongated form.

Gibberellin promotes shoot growth mainly by accelerating the rates of cell elongation and cell division in the subapical meristem region where young internodes are developing (page 130). Certain kinds of experiments indicate that the effects of auxin and gibberellin are complementary, the full stimulation of elongation by either of these hormones requiring the presence of adequate amounts of the other.

Another dramatic effect of gibberellins is to induce synthesis of hydrolytic enzymes such as amylase (hydrolyzes starch) and protease (hydrolyzes protein) during germination of cereal seeds such as barley and wheat. This effect has

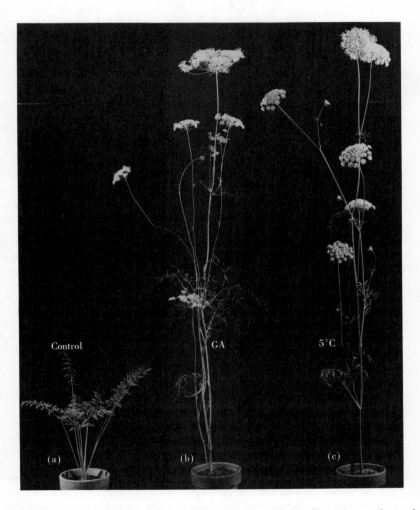

Fig. 9-8   *Rosette form of growth (a) and its transition ("bolting") to elongated growth (b and c) in flowering of the carrot plant. Plant (a) was kept at greenhouse temperature under long days (19 hr light per day); plant (b) was kept under the same conditions but was treated with 10 μg of gibberellin A₃ per day for 9 weeks; plant (c) had been kept at 5°C for 8 weeks and was then allowed to grow in the greenhouse along with (a) and (b). Induction of flowering by cold temperature is called* vernalization *(see page 193). (Photograph courtesy of Dr. Anton Lang; see* Proceedings of the National Academy of Sciences, **43:** 709, 1957.)*

been studied extensively because of the interest in hormonal control of enzyme synthesis as a molecular explanation of the mechanism of action of hormones (to be discussed at the end of this chapter). This gibberellin effect is exerted on specific cells within the cereal seed called *aleurone cells* (Figure 10-3); its physiological importance in seed germination will be considered in Chapter 10.

CYTOKININS Cytokinins were discovered as factors, additional to auxin, necessary in minute amounts for cell division in certain types of plant tissue cultures (Figure 9-5). The best characterized natural cytokinin is *zeatin*, a derivative of the purine base adenine of DNA and RNA. Various other artificially produced adenine derivatives such as *kinetin* are highly active and are often used in experiments with cytokinins. Because of their extremely potent activity as cell division stimulants in tissue culture test systems, it is inferred that cytokinins participate in the regulation of cell division in normal growth. For example, cytokinins in conjunction with auxin greatly promote cambial cell division activity in certain organs such as pea stems and radish roots (as is involved in formation of the edible radish).

$$HN-CH_2-CH=\overset{\underset{\displaystyle |}{CH_3}}{C}-CH_2OH$$

Zeatin

$$HN-CH_2-\text{(furan ring with O)}$$

Kinetin

Cytokinins have proved to exhibit a variety of actions not obviously related to their originally visualized role as cell division factors. For example, cytokinins promote leaf expansion, in which auxin and gibberellin are usually not effective. Perhaps the most curious effect of cytokinins is to oppose aging of leaves, preventing the breakdown of protein and chlorophyll that normally occurs as a leaf gets old or when it is detached from the plant. Cytokinins can thus control *senescence* (the complex of aging processes that ultimately lead to death) and may serve as a "juvenile hormone" of plants. In a number of plants the same kind of effect is exerted instead by gibberellins. This kind of overlap is sometimes encountered between effects of chemically quite different growth regulators.

Cytokinins exert some effects opposite to those of auxin. Cytokinins counteract the inhibition of lateral bud growth by auxin; that is, they promote bud outgrowth. Cytokinins tend to induce tissue cultures and isolated plant parts to form adventitious buds, whereas auxin tends to induce initiation of roots (Figure 9-5). How these "morphogenetic" effects of cytokinin and auxin actually operate is unknown, but they are of great interest because of the leads they may provide toward understanding the control of complex morphogenesis in chemical terms.

Cytokinins are found in xylem sap and are apparently being translocated from the root to the shoot. This provides a means of correlating the growth and longevity of buds and leaves with the development and vigor of the root system. It also provides a possible mechanism for initiation of adventitious buds when the shoot is broken off, as happens, for example, at the upper end of a dandelion root after its top is pulled off.

The complementary effects of auxin and cytokinin allow us to visualize how interaction between different hormones may regulate developmental processes in subtler and more complex ways than could be achieved with a single regulating hormone.

DORMANCY, ABSCISSION, AND ABSCISIC ACID   Normally the development of a plant is geared to the seasons in a way that permits the plant to survive periods of unfavorable environmental conditions such as frost or drought. This adaptation almost always involves temporary cessation of growth and suppression of metabolism, bringing the plant into a state known as *dormancy*. Dormancy is usually accompanied or followed by the senescence and shedding of parts that would be intolerant of or detrimental under unfavorable conditions. For example, the leaves of deciduous trees fall, as a result of the process of *leaf abscission*, and the entire above-ground shoot dies down in the case of herbaceous perennials. Moreover onset of dormancy commonly involves development of specialized resistant structures that protect the dormant growing points, for example, the scale-covered winter buds of trees (Figure 9-9) and the various underground survival organs of perennial herbaceous plants, including scale-enclosed buds, bulbs, and tubers.

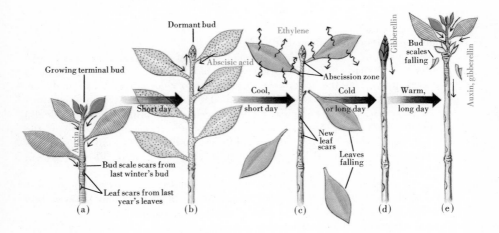

Fig. 9-9   *Typical seasonal cycle of growth and dormancy of a woody shoot in cold-temperate climate, illustrating current interpretation of its hormonal control. Note that exposure to a period of cold weather (in d) is shown as causing both disappearance of abscisic acid and induction of gibberellin production.*

Drought dormancy, for example in drought-tolerant perennial grasses which make up the grassland vegetation that inhabits many seasonally arid areas, seems to be induced directly by a state of water shortage and is terminated by the occurrence of sufficient rainfall. On the other hand, the winter dormancy and leaf abscission of cold-temperate vegetation typically develop in autumn well before onset of the winter temperature conditions that this dormancy permits the plants to tolerate. Therefore such winter dormancy is not a *consequence* of cold weather conditions but a state that anticipates and prepares plants against these conditions. It is known that dormancy and leaf fall in many cold-temperate plants are induced by the short days of autumn, which provide a reliable advance warning of the coming winter. This kind of response to the length of the day, called *photoperiodism*, is also of basic importance in reproduction and will be examined in Chapter 10.

Once it is induced, winter dormancy of cold-temperate plants persists until it is terminated by an appropriate environmental signal. Frequently the signal that is effective is cold temperature itself. Depending upon the species, from a few weeks to several months at temperatures near freezing may be required to break bud dormancy. With other plants, for example, the European beech tree, long days (as occur in spring) are effective in breaking dormancy. By such responses, attuned suitably to the local climatic cycle, the plant can "know" that winter has passed and will begin to grow again at a time when favorable temperatures have returned for the duration of the growing season.

Role of Hormones in Dormancy   Plants contain chemical *growth inhibitors* that act in a manner opposite to that of the promotive hormones discussed previously. There is evidence that inhibitors accumulate during induction of dormancy in various cold-temperate climate plants and decline under conditions that break dormancy, suggesting that a growth inhibitor is responsible for the induced state of dormancy. This inhibitor appears to be made in the leaves when they are exposed to short days and is translocated thence to the buds where it prevents growth. In the case of dormancy in the European field maple this inhibitor was identified as the compound *abscisic acid*.

Abscisic acid

Abscisic acid has been demonstrated to occur in a wide variety of plants, and it must be regarded as a natural hormone that has a negative effect on growth. Application of small amounts of abscisic acid to buds induces dormancy under conditions in which the buds would otherwise keep growing. Despite being inhibitory to growth, abscisic acid is not toxic and its effects are reversible even after lengthy exposures to the hormone, unlike the effects of overdoses of auxin or of treatment with many other chemicals that inhibit growth.

Inhibition of bud growth by abscisic acid can be prevented by simultaneous treatment with gibberellic acid, and gibberellic acid treatment can also break natural bud dormancy in some cases. Therefore natural bud dormancy may be regulated by a hormonal balance between gibberellins and abscisic acid. This interpretation of the dormancy cycle is illustrated in Figure 9-9.

Abscisic acid suppresses the previously discussed induction by gibberellin of amylase synthesis in barley seeds, further indicating an antagonistic action of the two hormones. However, some abscisic acid effects involve an interaction with auxin or cytokinins. For example, cytokinins are known to promote stomatal opening, whereas abscisic acid promotes stomatal closure and in effect antagonizes the effect of cytokinins (page 54). There are evidently multiple possibilities for regulatory interaction between abscisic acid and other plant hormones.

Control of Leaf Abscission   Abscisic acid promotes leaf abscission in certain test systems, and it was actually with the aid of such a test that the compound was first isolated and named.

Leaf abscission occurs by formation of a localized zone of cell wall breakdown, involving the action of cellulases, at the base of the leaf petiole. Leaf abscission is another feature of plant development that is under multiple growth-regulator control. Auxin coming from the leaf blade normally *inhibits* development of the abscission zone, for if the blade is cut off, the petiole will abscise within a day or two, but this may be prevented by applying auxin. Auxin similarly inhibits development of abscission zones in fruit stalks, and commercially important reductions in the loss of fruit by premature abscission are achieved by spraying fruit trees with auxin. On the other hand, various substances other than abscisic acid accelerate abscission, notably the gas ethylene to be discussed in the next section, and even auxins promote abscission under some circumstances. As in the case of apical dominance it has proved difficult to unravel these complexities and achieve an unequivocal description of how natural leaf abscission is regulated.

ETHYLENE   Long ago it was noted that exposure of plants to low concentrations of domestic illuminating gas produced stunting, lateral swelling of the stem, loss of normal geotropic behavior, leaf abscission, and other symptoms. This was traced to *ethylene* ($CH_2{=}CH_2$) which is present in illuminating gas. Considering the abnormal character of most of these effects it is surprising indeed to learn that plants themselves *produce* ethylene in minute but measurable quantities. Because ethylene is active at extremely low concentrations (well below 1 part in 10 million of air), the small ethylene production by plants is nevertheless sufficient to provoke physiological responses.

Ethylene's effects on development are mostly inhibitory, for example, inhibition of auxin transport (thus loss of geotropic response) and inhibition of cell elongation accompanied by sidewise expansion of the cells, which is indicative of interference with the mechanisms that are involved in the anisotropic aspect of morphogenesis discussed on page 143.

Treatment with auxin *stimulates* the production of ethylene by plant tissues. Thus it is suspected that a number of the effects of auxin are actually due to ethylene. For example, overdoses of auxin cause inhibition of stem elongation accompanied by lateral swelling of the cells; this effect has been proved to result from auxin-induced ethylene formation. Stimulated ethylene production is probably responsible for cases of promotion of leaf abscission by auxin. There is evidence that the inhibition of growth of roots and of axillary buds by auxin is actually due to auxin-induced ethylene production, and further that this is the basis for the difference between the geotropic response of roots and of shoots, whose elongation is less sensitive to inhibition by ethylene.

Ethylene is involved importantly as a growth regulator in fruit ripening (Chapter 10).

PHOTOMORPHOGENESIS AND PHYTOCHROME

Plant development can be profoundly modified by light, quite apart from the previously described bending toward lateral illumination (phototropism). In the dark chlorophyll does not form, chloroplasts do not develop, and leaves do not expand but remain small and rudimentary; and the internodes elongate many times more than normal, so that the plant soon becomes very tall and spindly (Figure 9-10). This complex of symptoms is called *etiolation*. It is a response of great value to the plant, for it causes a buried or heavily shaded shoot to elongate rapidly, unencumbered with bulky and in the circumstances useless leaves, until it emerges and reaches light, which restores the normal pattern of development.

The effect of light in reversing etiolation involves two kinds of action. At the biochemical level light is required for the last step in chlorophyll synthesis, the conversion of yellowish "protochlorophyll" to green chlorophyll. In the dark protochlorophyll accumulates; exposure to light causes rapid conversion to chlorophyll. At the level of morphogenesis light acts to *promote* expansion of the leaves and to *inhibit* elongation of the internodes. This phenomenon is called *photomorphogenesis* and is independent of the direction of illumination.

The action spectrum of photomorphogenesis reveals that plants are *most* sensitive to *red* light, which, as we saw earlier (page 158), is quite without effect in phototropism. Hence plants perceive light by different pigments in these two types of responses. Furthermore, the receptor pigment is neither chlorophyll nor protochlorophyll, because although red light (wavelength about 660 nm) is highly active, blue light (which chlorophyll and protochlorophyll also absorb) is rather ineffective.

Red/Far-Red Interaction

The photomorphogenic response shows an extremely peculiar feature: the effect of red light (or of white light, which gives the same effect) is completely prevented if far-red light (wavelength about 730 nm, barely visible to

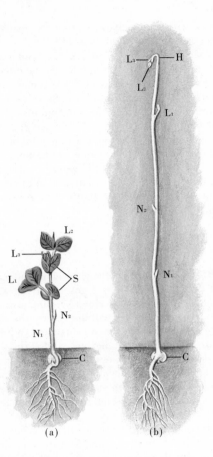

Fig. 9-10 *Pea seedlings grown for 9 days at 25°C (a) in light and (b) in darkness (etio-lated). Notice extreme differences in leaf expansion and in stem elongation as seen in positions of successive leaves L₁, L₂, L₃, and of nodes N₁ and N₂ at which only scale leaves are formed. C, cotyledons; S, stipules; H, hook-shaped part of growing region of stem in (b); note absence of hook in (a) (see page 185). (Half natural size.)*

the human eye) is given soon after the exposure to red (or white) light. Suppose, for example, that a dose of red light, which will promote leaf expansion strongly, is given. If this is followed immediately by a dose of far-red light, the response to the preceding dose of red light is prevented and the leaves do not expand. Processes that red light inhibits, such as stem elongation, are stimulated by far-red: the effect of far-red always being antagonistic to that of red.

Figure 9-11 illustrates the photomorphogenic response in dark-grown bean seedlings. The experiments were set up by placing the group of plants briefly in a continuous spectrum extending from red at the left to infrared at the right. Figure 9-11a shows the effect on plants not previously exposed to light: red light of wavelengths less than 700 nm induced leaf expansion whereas wavelengths greater than 700 nm did not. In Figure 9-11b all the plants were first exposed to red light, so that without further treatment their leaves would have expanded like those on the left in Figure 9-11a. But after the exposure to red light, the plants were placed in the spectrum for a short time. We can see that far-red light of wavelengths around 730 nm specifically inhibit leaf expansion, preventing the response to the previous dose of red light.

The action of red versus far-red light seems to be completely reversible, for if red light is given again after exposure to far-red, the red light effect (promotion of leaf expansion) is obtained. In fact, the plant can be stimulated repeatedly by alternating doses of red and far-red, and the subsequent response is always to the last kind of light given.

S. B. Hendricks and H. A. Borthwick of the U. S. Department of Agriculture, who have investigated these light effects extensively, proposed the following explanation for the remarkable antagonistic action of red and far-red light. The receptor pigment involved in developmental responses, which they

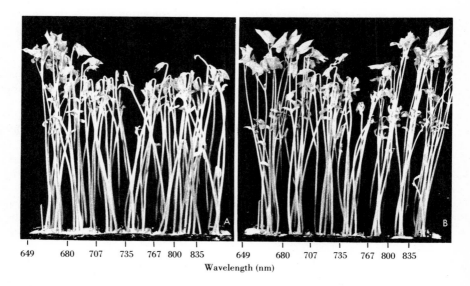

649   680   707   735   767 800 835   649   680   707   735   767 800 835
                                    Wavelength (nm)

Fig. 9-11   *Developmental effects of red and far-red light on bean seedlings. In (a) the seedlings were grown in the dark and then placed in a continuous spectrum extending from red at left to infrared at right with particular wavelengths falling where indicated. Red light (wavelengths below 700 nm) caused leaf expansion and unhooking of the shoot tip, while in light of wavelengths above 700 nm the seedlings look as if they had remained in the dark. In (b) all the seedlings were first given a dose of red light and immediately afterward were placed in the spectrum. In the far-red wavelength region (700 to 750 nm) the effect of the red-light treatment was reversed and the leaves did not expand, whereas longer wavelengths (infrared) had no reversing action and the leaves expanded owing to the preceding red treatment; in the red part of the spectrum the leaves, of course, expanded also. (From H. A. Borthwick and S. B. Hendricks, Science, 132: 1223, 1960. Copyright 1960 by the American Association for the Advancement of Science. Courtesy of Sterling Hendricks, United States Department of Agriculture.)*

subsequently called *phytochrome*, exists in two forms, one of which absorbs strongly in the red region of the spectrum (at wavelengths around 660 nm) and was called P_R; P_R is the form that accumulates in the plant in darkness. As a result of absorbing light P_R becomes converted into a distinct form, P_{FR}, whose absorption spectrum differs in that it absorbs strongly in the far-red region of the spectrum at wavelengths around 730 nm. P_{FR} has some kind of biological activity that promotes leaf expansion and inhibits stem elongation; hence red light by converting P_R to P_{FR} causes the photomorphogenic response,

$$P_R \underset{\substack{\text{Far-red light} \\ \text{(for darkness)}}}{\overset{\text{Red light}}{\rightleftarrows}} P_{FR} \longrightarrow \text{Developmental responses}$$

But absorption of light by P_{FR} converts it back to P_R. Hence far-red light which P_{FR} absorbs strongly will undo the action of red light. However, because the process is reversible a further treatment with red light will again make possible the developmental response.

The relative sensitivities of P_R and P_{FR} to light are such that in white light or sunlight the majority of the P_R becomes converted into P_{FR}; hence the red-sensitive response is the normal response to daylight.

Isolation and Identification of Phytochrome The action spectra for a phytochrome response and its reversal (Figure 9-4) show the absorption characteristics of P_R and P_{FR}. By delicate spectrophotometric methods it has been possible to detect phytochrome within plant tissue as a pigment that undergoes the expected reversible shift between maximum absorbancy at 660 and 730 nm when irradiated with red and far-red light. With the help of this assay the pigment has been extracted and purified and proves to be a blue *protein* closely related to the biliprotein pigment phycocyanin of the blue-green and red algae (page 38). The light-absorbing portion of the phytochrome molecule apparently undergoes a reversible change in structure upon illumination, somewhat analogous to the changes that light causes in rhodopsin and other visual pigments of animals.

The Diversity of Phytochrome Responses A wide variety of developmental phenomena other than leaf expansion and stem elongation are known to be regulated by phytochrome, as evidenced by opposing responses to red and far-red light, a feature which is diagnostic for the involvement of phytochrome as explained previously.

Germination of many seeds, straightening of the hook-shaped shoot of many seedlings (as can be seen in Figure 9-11), and photoperiodism are phytochrome-mediated developmental responses to light which will be discussed in Chapter 10. Phytochrome also influences phototropism and geotropism by affecting their sensitivity to blue light and to gravity, respectively, and phytochrome can influence the day–night movements of leaves known as "nyctinasty" (Chapter 10). In certain algae phytochrome acts as photoreceptor pigment for an orientation response of chloroplasts in which the (flat) chloroplast faces the light at low light intensities but at higher intensities the chloroplast rotates within the cell until it is edge-on to the light.

Various biochemical phenomena are also regulated by phytochrome, for example, formation of protochlorophyll and of carotenoids in leaves; of anthocyanin and flavonoid pigments in flowers, stems, and in the ripening coloration of the tomato fruit; synthesis of ascorbic acid in mustard seedlings; and of various phenolic compounds in a variety of seedlings.

The growth and differentiation of chloroplasts (page 150) is an important biochemical and morphogenetic phenomenon that is under phytochrome control. Stimulation of protochlorophyll and carotenoid formation is involved, these components participating in the light-induced formation of normal thylakoid structure. P_{FR} also induces synthesis of a wide variety of chloroplast enzymes and a marked increase in total chloroplast protein. These changes accompany phytochrome-induced leaf expansion but they are separate phenomena since leaf expansion occurs in mutants whose chloroplast development is blocked.

Photoconversion of P_R to P_{FR} is extremely sensitive to light, almost down to the level of moonlight, but in a number of the responses mentioned there is evidence for the participation of a "high-energy reaction" requiring much higher light intensities. This feature has been thought to indicate existence of a photomorphogenic pigment other than phytochrome, but it may be that high-energy responses are due actually to P_{FR} serving as a photoreceptor for photochemical reactions.

The diversity of phytochrome responses suggests that this pigment system can be evolutionarily coupled to almost any morphogenetic or biochemical facet of development if adaptively useful behavior is created thereby.

Some of this coupling is achieved by making use of the growth hormones previously discussed. For example, the effect of long days (perceived by phytochrome, see Chapter 10) to induce stem elongation of rosette plants comes about by increased production of gibberellins by the plant, and there is evidence that the influence of P_{FR} on stem elongation in the etiolation response involves a change in sensitivity to the plant's own gibberellins. Likewise the induction of dormancy by short days (probably a phytochrome response) may be brought about by production of abscisic acid as discussed above. Effects of P_{FR} on both auxin and ethylene production have been found in certain plants, and there are reasons to think that the shoot hook-openings (page 185) and leaf expansion responses to P_{FR} involve ethylene. The expansion of leaf tissue can be stimulated by cytokinins, as mentioned previously, but it seems unclear whether cytokinins are involved in phytochrome-induced leaf expansion.

Phytochrome action itself seems to be localized at the site of irradiation; in the case of the chloroplast rotation in algae mentioned above response can be observed in a small part of one cell when such a part is irradiated. In instances in which a photomorphogenic effect due to phytochrome is transmitted from one plant organ to another, as in cases discussed above or in the flowering response to be considered in Chapter 10, it is clear that the transmission is brought about by a growth regulator other than phytochrome. Therefore even though phytochrome is one of the major growth regulators of plants, it cannot be regarded as a hormone because this term refers to a regulatory agent that is at least potentially transmissible.

MODE OF ACTION
OF GROWTH REGULATORS

The various kinds of growth hormones and regulators discussed serve to modulate and control the expression of genetic information upon which development ultimately rests. This is particularly obvious in qualitative "morphogenetic" effects such as those of cytokinins on bud initiation, auxins on root initiation, and phytochrome on leaf and chloroplast development.

Much interest centers around the idea that growth regulators cause their effects by activating specific gene function, that is, by inducing transcription of particular genes that code for proteins specially involved in one or another particular aspect of development. In many plant test systems it has been found that promotive growth regulators stimulate the synthesis of RNA and protein, as assayed by incorporation of radioactivity when the tissue is fed isotopically labeled nitrogen bases or amino acids, respectively.

The best-studied case of specific enzyme induction by a plant growth regulator involves the aleurone cell layer of cereal seeds (mentioned on page 164) in which gibberellins dramatically induce the production and secretion of amylase as well as of a variety of other hydrolytic enzymes. This induction requires synthesis of RNA, presumably message RNA coding for the enzymes in question. Phytochrome (P_{FR}) causes in a variety of plants a comparably striking induction of phenylalanine ammonia-lyase, the key enzyme for entry of carbon into the "phenolic system" of pathways. This enzyme induction effect appears to be how phytochrome stimulates, as noted above, the synthesis of various phenolic compounds and of anthocyanins (which are derived from phenolic compounds). From indirect evidence the induction of phenylalanine ammonia-lyase by phytochrome is interpreted as an activation of specific gene transcription. This interpretation is not proven for either the gibberellin–amylase or the phytochrome–phenylalanine ammonia-lyase systems and in fact some of the evidence suggests that the growth regulators may in fact be acting in these systems to promote translation, the second major site of potential hormonal control over expression of genetic information (Figure 8-10).

One potential method of selecting what message RNAs may be translated is by means of the transfer RNAs that are required by the ribosomes in order to "uncode" the message (see Figure 8-10 and Levine, *Genetics*). If a given transfer RNA were missing, none of the messages that require this particular transfer RNA for their translation could be translated, that is, the corresponding proteins could not be made. A striking discovery is that the natural cytokinins, zeatin and several closely related adenine derivatives, occur as constituents of specific transfer RNAs. This suggested the possibility that the cytokinin hormones act on development by permitting these specific transfer RNAs to be synthesized, thus allowing expression of the message RNAs that require these particular transfer RNAs for translation. This possibility is in controversy because, among other things, the cytokinin constituents of transfer RNAs are apparently not formed by the incorporation of free cytokinin molecules like zeatin. Even so it seems likely that cytokinins play some role in regulation of transfer RNAs and thus of specific gene translation.

It is as yet difficult to point to very many protein synthesis and enzyme induction effects that convincingly account for important physiological actions of plant growth regulators. This may be viewed both as an indication of enormous opportunity for future research and also perhaps as a hint that other possible modes of action of growth regulators deserve exploration.

The most rapid growth regulator responses, such as the elongation rate response to auxin and certain of the responses to phytochrome, occur in a matter of minutes, whereas growth regulator-induced enzyme increases generally occur on a time scale of hours. Therefore the view is growing that at least in some responses the immediate action of growth regulators is not necessarily at the level of gene function or even of translation, but may occur at membranes and influence critical transport processes. Such effects may lead to activation or repression of genes in the longer time scale of development and thereby work indirectly an influence on the total expression of genetic information.

In the case of simple promotion of cell growth rate, as in the classical effects of auxin and gibberellin, the conclusion is unavoidable, as explained on page 142, that the developmentally critical target of hormone action is the cell wall, which must be made more extensible either by increased synthesis or by degradation of pre-existing structural material. Unfortunately although inductive effects of auxin on both synthetic and degradative enzymes for wall polymers are known, neither effect apparently occurs quickly enough to account for the auxin effect on cell enlargement. This tends to suggest that the immediate action of auxin may actually be on transport of such enzymes or their products into the cell wall.

CONCLUSION It is now clear that plants produce a powerful array of specific growth-regulating factors — auxin, gibberellin, cytokinin, abscisic acid, ethylene, phytochrome, and others less well established and not discussed here — which have multiple effects on a variety of target tissues and interact with one another both cooperatively (auxin and gibberellin in stem elongation, auxin and cytokinin in cell division) and antagonistically (auxin versus cytokinin in bud growth and bud induction; abscisic acid versus gibberellin in bud dormancy). The production and action of these growth regulators are often influenced by environmental factors such as light and temperature. By this means development can be controlled and modified adaptively in relation to environmental stresses, hazards, and cues; in effect different aspects of the genetic capabilities of the organism can thus be called into action at an advantageous time and place. We shall see further illustration of this principle in the next chapter which considers the regulation of reproductive activity of plants.

It is inferred that interplay between growth regulators is involved in control of the subtle aspects of morphogenesis and differentiation during development of tissues and organs from the meristems that give rise to them (Chapter 8). This role of hormones is suggested by effects such as those of auxin on vascular cell differentiation, of auxin and cytokinin on activity of the vascular cambium, and of ethylene on geometry of cell enlargement. A detailed causal explanation for the determination of form and structure during plant growth cannot, however, yet be given and is one of the major challenges to further research.

SUGGESTED READING

Butler, W. L., and R. J. Downs, "Light and Plant Development," *Scientific American*, **203** (6):55-63, 1960.

Chouard, P., et al., *The World of Plants. Encyclopedia of the Life Sciences*, Vol. 3. Garden City, New York: Doubleday, 1965. pp. 36-44, 74-94.

Darwin, C., and F. Darwin, *The Power of Movement in Plants*. New York: Da Capo Press (Reprint), 1966. (Originally published 1881.) Chapters 8-11.

Fogg, G. E., *The Growth of Plants*. Baltimore: Penguin Books, 1963. Chapters 6 and 9.

Fox, J. E. (ed.), *Molecular Control of Plant Growth*. Belmont, Cal.: Dickinson, 1968.

Galston, A. W., and P. J. Davies, *Control Mechanisms in Plant Development*. Englewood Cliffs, N.J.: Prentice-Hall, 1970.

Hendricks, S. B., "How Light Interacts with Living Matter," *Scientific American*, **219** (3):174-186, 1968.

Laetsch, W. M., and R. E. Cleland, *Papers on Plant Growth and Development*. Boston: Little, Brown, 1967.

Leopold, A. C., *Plant Growth and Development*. New York: McGraw-Hill, 1964.

Van Overbeek, J., "The Control of Plant Growth," *Scientific American*, **219** (1):75-81, 1968.

Wareing, P. F., and I. D. J. Phillips, *The Control of Growth and Differentiation in Plants*. New York: Pergamon, 1970. Chapters 4-8, 11-13.

Went, F. W., "Plant Growth and Plant Hormones," in *This Is Life*. W. H. Johnson and W. C. Steere (eds.). New York: Holt, Rinehart and Winston, 1962. pp. 213-253.

Wilkins, M. B. (ed.), *The Physiology of Plant Growth and Development*. New York: McGraw-Hill, 1969. Chapters 1-7, 14-15.

Flowering Plant Reproduction

Land plants reproduce both *asexually* and *sexually*. Asexual reproduction, which produces offspring genetically identical with the parent, is generally accomplished by shoots specialized for this function, for example, rhizomes (underground stems), tubers, and bulbs, organs that are also employed for survival through unfavorable seasons as discussed in connection with dormancy on page 166).

Most land plants reproduce sexually by means of *flowers*, which are highly modified shoots. The new plant arises as a result of fertilization of an egg cell in the flower by a sperm that is brought via pollen usually from a different plant.

DEVELOPMENT OF SEED In the flower ***AND FRUIT*** the egg cell is produced inside a saclike structure called the *embryo sac.* This contains a number of haploid cells that are derived, as illustrated by diagrams a and b and 1 to 4 in Figure 10-1, from a meiotic (reduction) division of one of the diploid cells within a microscopic organ called an *ovule* which is to become a seed and is contained within the externally visible "ovary" of the flower (see Figure 10-2). Meanwhile pollen grains, each of which contains two haploid sperm nuclei, are formed in the stamens of the flower. Upon opening of the flower, wind, insects, or other animals transfer pollen to the stigma; here each pollen grain germinates, sending forth a *pollen tube* which grows down through the style to meet one of the ovules and there discharges its sperm nuclei into the embryo sac. There ensues a remarkable phenomenon called *double fertilization* in which one sperm fuses with the egg to form the diploid *zygote* while the second sperm nucleus fuses with two other (haploid) "polar nuclei" of the embryo sac to form the *primary endosperm nucleus,* which is therefore triploid (three sets of chromosomes).

The zygote develops into an embryo plant through a specific embryological sequence, as illustrated by diagrams 5 to 13 in Figure 10-1. Concomitantly the primary endosperm nucleus multiples extensively within the embryo sac by mitosis, giving rise to triploid *endosperm* tissue surrounding the growing embryo (Figure 10-1d). The ovule itself is meanwhile growing and its outer folds of tissue are differentiating into the protective *seed coats* as illustrated in diagrams c, d, and e. And while all this is taking place, the surrounding ovary is developing into a *fruit* (Figure 10-2).

The growing endosperm is a locus of intense biosynthetic activity for nutrients such as amino acids and vitamins, and growth factors such as cytokinins and gibberellins which presumably benefit the developing embryo. Young liquid endosperm such as coconut milk or the endosperm of corn grains in the "milk" stage provides a rich source of cytokinin-type growth factors that can be used to stimulate growth of plant tissue cultures (page 165) and to encourage development of "embryos" from vegetative plant cells in culture (page 147). Later the maturing endosperm tissue may accumulate large amounts of carbohydrate, protein, and/or lipid reserves to be used subsequently for growth of the embryo during seed germination. In the development of many seeds, however, the growing embryo ultimately digests away the surrounding endosperm largely or completely and stores its food reserves in its first leaves (cotyledons) (Figure 10-1e).

A hormonal mechanism operates to correlate development of the seed with growth of the fruit. The primary stimulus for fruit growth seems to be auxin coming (1) from the pollen and (2) from the developing embryo or endosperm. Many flowers can be induced to develop without fertilization into (seedless) fruits by applying auxin to them. In other cases gibberellin will induce development of fruits without fertilization, and since endosperm tissue is, as mentioned above, a source of gibberellins this type of hormone may also be involved in regulation of normal fruit growth.

FRUIT RIPENING With completion of the development of the seeds the fruit *ripens,* which usually involves changes that in one way or another promote dispersal of the seeds from the parent plant; for example, in the case of edible fruits the ripening process makes the fruit at-

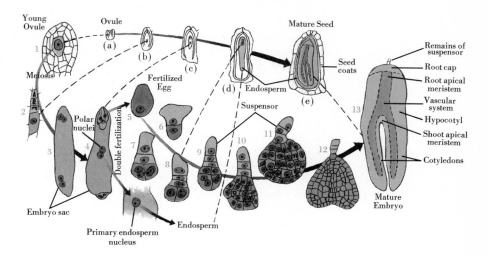

Fig. 10-1 *Development of embryo and seed of a flowering plant, as recorded for* Kunzea capitata, *an Australian shrub. Sketches (a) to (e) show development of seed from ovule at a magnification of about 50-fold (ovules are contained within ovary of flower, as in Figure 10-2 except that in this species there are several ovules within the ovary). Diagrams 1 to 4 show origin of embryo sac from one of four haploid cells (diagram 2) produced by meiosis of a diploid cell in center of ovule (diagram 1). Diagrams 5 to 13 show development of fertilized egg (within embryo sac) into mature embryo of seed. Magnification is about 500× in diagrams 1 and 5 and decreases through each sequence to compensate for the growth in size that takes place. Dashed lines cross correlate the same stage in diagrams at different magnifications. (After diagrams by N. Prakash, in* Australian Journal of Botany, *17: 97, 1969.)*

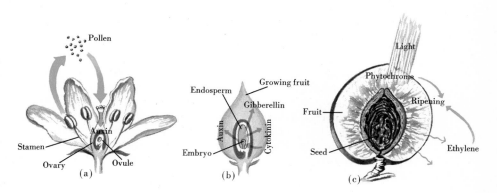

Fig. 10-2 *Diagram of the development of a simple fruit (peach) from the ovary of the flower, illustrating roles of growth regulators. For simplicity the ovary of the flower is shown as containing one ovule although it actually contains two, only one of which normally develops into a seed. Note that other fruits may contain several to many seeds derived from similar numbers of ovules. Fully grown fruit is much larger, relative to flower, than is shown in diagram.*

tractive to animals. This results from a conversion of organic acids and starch to sugar, a softening of the fruit structure due to partial breakdown of cell walls by hydrolytic enzymes such as cellulase and pectinase, and a formation of conspicuous pigments that signal the state of ripeness to interested animals. These changes are rather similar to those involved in the senescence and abscission of leaves (page 168).

Fruit ripening proves to be under primary control of the gaseous growth regulator *ethylene*, which is also implicated in the induction of leaf abscission (page 169). Fruits can be induced to ripen precociously by treating them with ethylene. In the normal course of events we can observe a sudden acceleration of ethylene production by the fruit itself just as natural ripening commences, and it has been proved in certain cases that this ethylene is sufficient of itself to set the ripening process in motion. By suitable ventilation arrangements to remove ethylene during storage it is possible to keep unripe fruits for extended periods and to induce them to ripen at will by treatment with ethylene; this has important commercial applications. Like many technological substitutes for the natural thing, however, this artificial ripening often leaves something to be desired in the quality of the produce. Among other reasons this may be because *phytochrome* is involved in the ripening process, for example, in inducing the pigmentation changes (page 173), and the requirement for light-induced phytochrome action may not be adequately satisfied during commercial ethylene-stimulated ripening.

These hormonal mechanisms for regulation of fruit development are summarized in Figure 10-2.

SEED GERMINATION   When the embryo plant within the seed resumes growth, now on its own in the world, its primary problem is to achieve enough growth and development of root system and photosynthetic organs to make it self-sufficient for water, minerals, and photosynthetic production. For its initial growth the seedling depends upon nutrient reserves that were furnished it within the seed, and the utilization of these reserves depends in turn upon mechanisms that bring about a regulated transformation of reserve products into a form that can be transported to the growing regions of the seedling. This mobilization is due first of all to action in the storage tissue (endosperm or cotyledons) of hydrolytic enzymes (hydrolases) such as amylases that convert starch to sugars, proteases that break down proteins to amino acids, nucleases that hydrolyze nucleic acids to nucleotides, and lipases that split fats into glycerol and fatty acids. The activity of such hydrolases in the seed rises during the earliest stages of germination, leading to a rapid breakdown of reserve materials. This is illustrated by data given in Figure 10-3.

Fat-storing seeds such as castor bean, watermelon, and flax convert their stored fats, which are insoluble, into soluble sugar in order to mobilize and translocate these reserves to the centers of growth. This conversion is accomplished by the *glyoxylate cycle* of biochemical reactions mentioned on page 21 which depends upon special enzymes *isocitrate lyase* and *malate synthetase*. During germination a striking rise in the activity of these enzymes, due to enzyme syn-

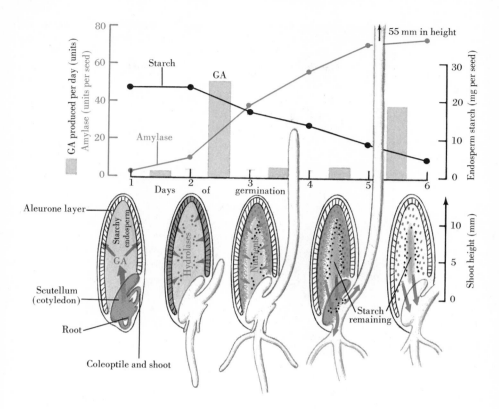

Fig. 10-3 *Germination of a seed of barley, illustrating the gibberellin-controlled formation of hydrolases that leads to release and translocation of nutrients (sugars, amino acids, and nucleotides, derived from the action of amylase on starch, protease on reserve protein, and ribonuclease on RNA, respectively). Data are given for synthesis of gibberellin by the embryo, for gibberellin-dependent synthesis of amylase by the aleurone cells, and for breakdown of starch by amylase. (Data of Russell L. Jones and Janet Armstrong, University of California.)*

thesis, occurs in the fat-storing tissue as illustrated by the data in Figure 10-4. These enzymes appear within the special organelles called *glyoxysomes* (page 21) which makes possible an efficient conversion of fat to sugar. After the reserve fats are used up, the glyoxylate cycle enzymes are no longer needed and are broken down (Figure 10-4).

Hormonal Control of Mobilization   In certain seeds the induction of enzyme formation during germination is known to be under hormonal control. The most extensively studied example is the induction by gibberellin of synthesis of amylase and other hydrolases (page 164) during germination of cereal seeds such as barley and rice.

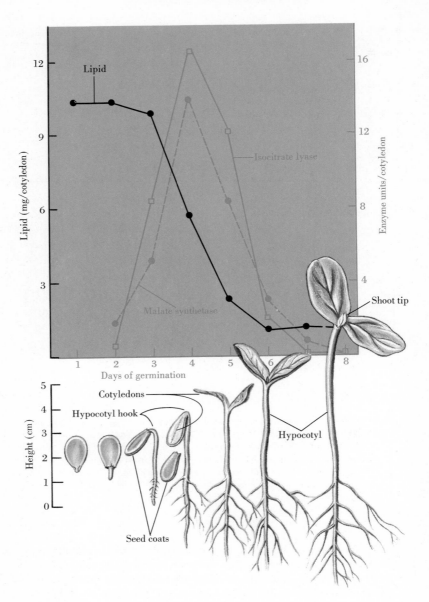

Fig. 10-4 *Germination of watermelon* (Citrullus vulgaris) *seed, showing changes in glyoxylate cycle enzymes (isocitrate lyase and malate synthetase) and in total lipid stored in the cotyledons. In the germination of this species the cotyledons are brought above ground and after fulfilling their storage role they expand and function in photosynthesis (compare with pea seedling, Figure 9-10, whose cotyledons remain below ground and serve only a storage function). (Unpublished data of Douglas I. McGregor and Harry Beevers, See B. Hock and H. Beevers,* Zeitschrift für Pflanzenphysiologie, **55:** *405, 1966.)*

These enzymes are synthesized by a special cell layer called the *aleurone* tissue which is found in the seeds of grasses (Figure 10-3). The aleurone cells secrete the hydrolases that they produce into the endosperm where the enzymes attack reserve materials releasing soluble nutrients. During normal germination, hydrolase synthesis by aleurone cells is induced by the embryo; if the embryo is removed, the aleurone cells fail to produce hydrolases, but they can be induced to do so by supplying gibberellin. Apparently gibberellin released by the embryo provides the natural signal for hydrolase synthesis. In this way the growth and associated hormone output of the embryo induce the release from the endosperm of nutrients required for the embryo's own growth. This regulatory phenomenon is summarized in Figure 10-3.

Gibberellin control of enzyme formation is not general for germinating seeds; for example, the synthesis of amylase that occurs during germination of pea seeds is not influenced by gibberellin. During germination of squash seeds, cytokinins act as inducers of hydrolases, seemingly playing here the same role that gibberellin serves in grass seeds. Gibberellin has been reported to induce the synthesis of glyoxylate cycle enzymes in the fat-storing seeds of hazel nut (*Corylus*) during germination, but such an effect has not been found with the better-studied examples of fat-storing seeds such as castor bean and watermelon; the means by which glyoxylate cycle enzyme synthesis is controlled in these latter cases is not yet understood.

CONTROL OF   As the seed matures the embryo enters a state of
SEED GERMINATION   dormancy that prevents the seed from germinating within the fruit that produced it. This condition disappears more or less rapidly after shedding of the seeds of many tropical and agricultural plants, presumably by processes of metabolic inactivation of growth inhibitors derived from the fruit; this phenomenon is called "after-ripening."

Once after-ripening is completed, germination may be initiated if moisture is supplied and certain critical temperature requirements are met. Given species or geographic races thereof show characteristic minimum and maximum temperatures between which seed germination will occur. These characteristics can be important in determining in what part of the seasonal temperature cycle particular wild or weedy species make their appearance and in which particular crop plants may be planted.

The seeds of wild plants adapted to cold-temperate climates often possess a persistent dormancy that can be terminated only by exposure to a period of cold temperature. This kind of dormancy resembles winter bud dormancy (page 167) and like the latter is presumably due to the accumulation of growth inhibitors such as abscisic acid which can be inactivated biochemically at near-freezing temperatures without replacement by continued biosynthesis.

Requirement for a cold period prevents germination of seeds shed in summer or fall, at which time the seedlings would have little chance to become established before the onset of unfavorable conditions. Instead, the seeds lie dormant through the winter and as a result of this cold treatment germinate early the following spring with the whole growing season ahead of them.

Various other kinds of seed dormancy are known, most of which cannot be discussed here. Annual plants adapted to desert climates may produce seeds whose dormancy can be broken only by exposure to a certain minimum amount of rainfall. This requirement prevents the seeds from germinating except when enough water has entered the ground to allow the plant to complete its developmental cycle. In years of insufficient rainfall such plants are not seen at all; their seeds can lie dormant in the soil for years at a time. In certain cases it has been found that this dormancy is caused by water-soluble chemical inhibitors in the seed, which must be washed out before the seed can germinate.

Germination may also be controlled chemically by the presence of other vegetation, because many plants produce inhibitory or toxic by-products such as tannins and other phenolic compounds, terpenes, or alkaloid drugs. These become released from the roots, leaves, or leaf litter into the soil where they can prevent germination of the seeds of the same or different species. Some ecologists consider that this kind of "chemical warfare" among plants plays an important role in the composition and density of natural plant communities.

Light Responses in Germination

Germination of many seeds is induced by light. The classic example is lettuce seed, which will germinate only if planted shallowly enough for some light to reach the seeds through the soil. This response is most sensitive to red light, whereas far-red light, given after a treatment with white or red light, reverses the effect and prevents germination. This evidence indicates that perception of light by seeds is due to phytochrome; indeed the far-red reversal phenomenon that is diagnostic for phytochrome was first discovered in studying the light-sensitivity of seeds.

The requirement for light in germination is generally encountered in *small* seeds. Its value is no doubt to ensure that the seed will not germinate when too deeply buried to grow into a successful seedling. By preventing the germination of buried seeds the requirement for light also allows a store of seeds to accumulate in the soil; these will then germinate when brought to the surface by disturbance or tillage of the soil. This helps weeds, for example, to persist despite the farmer's efforts to eradicate them by cultivation.

The inhibitory action of far-red light on seed germination may have adaptive usefulness to plants also. When light-requiring seeds are illuminated with sunlight that has been passed through green leaves, this light *inhibits* their germination because the red component of sunlight has been absorbed by chlorophyll while the far-red passes on through (see Figure 3-1). This inhibition tends to ensure that such seeds germinate only at a time and place when they are not heavily shaded by other vegetation and thus have a chance of carrying on effective photosynthesis.

The germination process involves some interesting kinds of light-controlled behavior that help with the problems of getting the young shoot out of the ground.

The phytochrome-controlled etiolation response (discussed on pages 169-172) serves to ensure that the shoots of seeds that germinate some distance below the soil surface elongate rapidly without leaf expansion until they emerge from the soil into the light.

Seedlings of grasses exhibit a particularly interesting system of phyto-chrome-controlled positioning responses which can be seen in action when a lawn or a cereal or maize crop is planted. The bullet-shaped coleoptile, whose phototropic behavior was discussed on pages 155–158, encloses the young leaves and shoot apical meristem. The coleoptile serves as a shield and drill for opening a path into the air for elongation of the leaves, which are too delicate to be forced directly through the soil. As illustrated in Figure 10-5, if the seed germinates well below the soil surface the stem beneath the coleoptile first elongates,

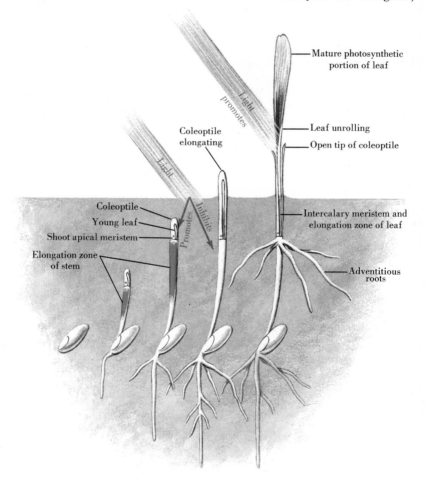

Fig. 10-5 *Germination of a grass seed, illustrating phytochrome-mediated responses to light that position the seedling relative to the soil surface. Actively growing regions of the shoot are indicated with color. For simplicity only one leaf is shown although several leaf primordia are actually developing around the apical meristem.*

pushing ahead of it the coleoptile with enclosed shoot. Growth of the stem is so sensitive (via phytochrome) to inhibition by light that the dim light which penetrates some distance into the soil stops stem elongation when the coleoptile has not quite reached the surface. This light, however, promotes elongation of the coleoptile, which drills the remaining distance to the surface and after emerging into full light ceases to grow and splits open at its tip, allowing the leaf inside to elongate freely into the air without friction against the soil. As it emerges the leaf unrolls, a light response that is also controlled by phytochrome. Adventitious roots form on the stem just below the level of the shoot apex. These light responses thus position the root and shoot systems of the grass seedling properly relative to the soil surface irrespective of the depth at which the seed germinates.

The shoots of most seedlings other than grasses have no mechanical protection; in order to get the growing point to the surface, the elongating zone of the stem typically emerges from the seed in the shape of a *hook* (illustrated by the seedlings in Figure 10-4). As elongation of the stem occurs in the vicinity of the elbow, it drags the unprotected young leaves and shoot apex up *backward* through the ground, thus exposing them to relatively mild mechanical action. When the shoot appears above the ground, the hook abruptly straightens out, turning the shoot apex upward. Straightening of the hook is another phytochrome response, sensitive to red light and antagonized by far-red light. This response can be seen in Figure 9-11, and was indeed selected for illustration of the action spectra for P_R and P_{FR} responses in Figure 9-4.

The hook-straightening response is interesting, further, as another example of a developmental phenomenon that is regulated by ethylene (see page 168. The hook produces ethylene, ethylene powerfully inhibits hook straightening, and light (via phytochrome) depresses ethylene production, thus allowing the hook to escape from this self-imposed inhibition.

PHOTOPERIODIC CONTROL OF FLOWERING   Experience tells us that plant reproduction is tied to the seasons, different wild and cultivated plants flowering at characteristically different times during the year. In 1918 W. W. Garner and H. A. Allard of the U. S. Department of Agriculture discovered the primary principle by which the timing of flowering is determined: plants are *sensitive to the length of the day*. It is a familiar fact that the length of the day varies with the seasons (Figure 10-6), increasing during spring to a maximum on June 21 and decreasing thereafter during summer and autumn to a minimum on December 21 (in the Northern Hemisphere; vice versa in the Southern Hemisphere). The length of the "day" or light period is called the "photoperiod," and the ability to respond to photoperiods of different lengths (actually to dark periods as we shall see below) is termed *photoperiodism*.

Two principal types of photoperiodic flowering responses, called "long-day" and "short-day" responses, are illustrated in Figure 10-7. A *long-day plant* flowers when the photoperiod *exceeds* a certain critical value, generally in the

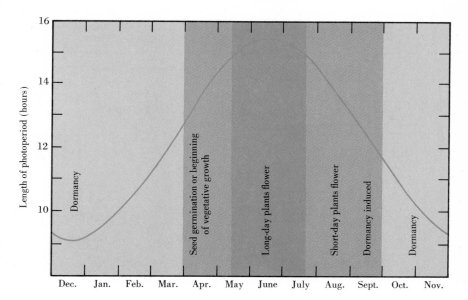

Fig. 10-6   *Yearly variation in length of the day, showing its relation to photoperiodic responses of plants in nature. Day-length data are given for 43 degrees north latitude. The growing season indicated is approximately what prevails in northeastern United States. The positions of boundaries separating different types of behavior are, of course, approximate. At different latitudes and under different climates the photoperiodic responses of plants are adapted to the prevailing growing season and day-length regime and will differ from what is shown here.*

neighborhood of 12 to 14 hours and characteristic of the particular species or strain of plant; under photoperiods less than the critical it either grows only vegetatively or else flowers much more tardily. A *short-day plant* flowers when the day length is *less than* a critical value, and grows vegetatively or flowers only tardily under days longer than the critical day length. Data showing these characteristics of long- and short-day responses are plotted in Figure 10-8.

Facultative short- or long-day plants are species whose flowering is merely accelerated by inductive photoperiods, while *obligate* short- and long-day plants absolutely require an inductive photoperiod for flowering and will grow indefinitely in the vegetative state under noninductive photoperiods, as is the case with *Xanthium* and *Hyoscyamus* illustrated in Figure 10-8. At the other extreme are plants whose flowering is indifferent to day length; these are called "day-neutral" plants. This class includes many agricultural plants, although a fair number of cultivated plants are photoperiodic, for example, soybean (short-day plant) and wheat and rye (facultative long-day plants).

In nature long-day plants pass from the vegetative to the reproductive phase when the days are lengthening, that is, in spring or early summer (see Figure 10-6). Short-day plants grow vegetatively during the long days of spring and early summer and flower when the days are shortening, from midsummer to

Photoperiod treatment

Response of short-day plant

Response of long-day plant

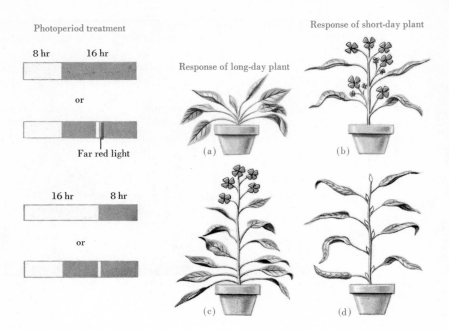

8 hr   16 hr

or

Far red light

(a)

(b)

16 hr   8 hr

or

(c)

(d)

Fig. 10-7   *Responses of typical long- and short-day plants to short days (above), to long days (below), to short days with interrupted night (below), and with night interruption followed by far red (above, far-red period shown by color).*

autumn. The shorter the critical day length, the later in the year a short-day plant flowers, because more of the season must elapse before the natural day gets shorter than the critical day length. It is worth noting that since critical day lengths for many short-day plants are considerably *greater* than 12 hours (see Figure 10-8), these plants flower *before* the day length has decreased to be equal to the night length, as shown in Figure 10-6. In other words, in nature many short-day plants become induced to flower under "long days" (day longer than night), contrary to what would appear to be implied by the term "short-day plant." However, these plants do flower rapidly under artificial short days; for example, a cycle of 8 hours of light followed by 16 hours of darkness is often employed in experiments to induce flowering of short-day plants.

The genetic instructions for development of flowers and execution of their reproductive function constitute an important part of the genetic heritage of a species. The photoperiodic response represents, therefore, a striking example of environmental induction of the expression of genetic information.

As noted previously (page 167) photoperiodism is involved in other responses of plants besides flowering. Induction of dormancy and leaf abscission in cold-temperate climates are short-day responses. In some species of trees termination of dormancy in the spring is a long-day response. Moreover in at least some cases *vegetative* (asexual) reproduction is regulated by photoperiod; for example, formation of tubers by potato and certain other tuber-producing plants is promoted by short days.

Mechanism of   An experiment illustrated in Figure 10-7 shows
Photoperiodism   that the length of the *night* is critical to the decision made by the plant. If a short-day plant is put
on a cycle of 8 hours light–16 hours dark, it will flower. However, if a short exposure to light is given in the middle of the dark period, flowering is completely
prevented, just as if the plant were being kept on a long-day cycle such as 16
hours light–8 hours dark. A night interruption of as little as 1 minute of light
from a 25-watt bulb is enough to prevent flowering of some short-day plant species. Evidently the requirement for induction of flowering in a short-day plant is
an *uninterrupted* dark period longer than a certain number of hours. A night interruption has the opposite effect on a long-day plant: it *promotes* flowering; thus
here too the plant appears to be measuring the length of the dark period.

The night-interruption experiment provides a very convenient way of determining the sensitivity of flowering to different wavelengths of light (action
spectrum) and hence of detecting what type of pigment is responsible for light

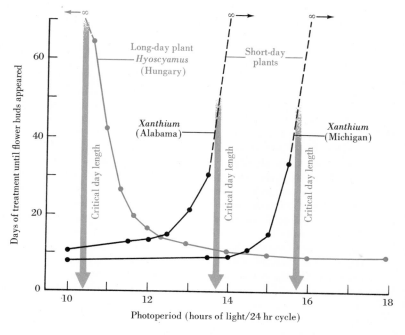

Fig. 10-8   *Photoperiodic response as seen in a long-day plant,* Hyoscyamus *(henbane),
and in two strains of a short-day plant,* Xanthium *(cocklebur), native to different latitudes. Groups of plants were maintained under each of the photoperiod treatments indicated by a data point, which records the number of days before visible flower buds appeared (*Xanthium*) or bolting began (*Hyoscyamus, *in which bolting corresponds with
time of flower bud initiation). The symbol ∞ means that no flower buds were ever formed
at the indicated photoperiod or those beyond it. (*Xanthium *data from P. M. Ray and W.
E. Alexander,* American Journal of Botany, **53:** 806, 1966; Hyoscyamus *data from A.
Lang and G. Melchers,* Planta, **33:** 653, 1943.)*

perception in photoperiodism. With a considerable variety of both short-day and long-day plants it has been found that the strongest effect is given by red light of wavelength 630 to 660 nm: a night interruption with red light inhibits flowering of a short-day plant and promotes flowering of a long-day plant. And if a night interruption with white or red light is followed within a few minutes by a short exposure to far-red light of wavelength about 730 nm, the effect of the night interruption is completely canceled: a short-day plant will flower and a long-day plant will be prevented from flowering (Figure 10-7). These facts show that perception of light in photoperiodism depends upon phytochrome.

The critical day length of certain plants such as cocklebur is relatively unaffected by variations in temperature. This implies that the plant possesses a temperature-independent (or temperature-compensated) "biological clock" for measuring the length of the night and the day. The value of this temperature independence is in enabling the plant to time correctly its reproductive activities, dormancy, leaf fall, and so forth, relative to the march of the seasons despite yearly peculiarities in the weather with its unpredictable variations in temperature. But how is a temperature-independent biological clock possible when metabolic processes depend so strongly upon temperature?

Our best clue was provided by the German plant physiologist Erwin Bünning, who suggested years ago that photoperiodic behavior is based upon the occurrence of spontaneous internal fluctuations in physiological state called "endogenous rhythms." In plants such rhythms show themselves in phenomena such as the daily up and down movements of leaves (Figure 10-9) called "sleep movements" or "nyctinasty" (*nyctos*, night; *nastos*, pressing together). A particularly conspicuous example is the nocturnal folding of the leaves of the widespread weed called sorrel (*Oxalis*). Nyctinastic movements continue, on a cycle of about 24 hours duration, even under constant temperature and light. They are therefore endogenous (internal) in origin, although the rhythm may be shifted or modified or the movements accentuated by light. Because the "free-running" (in constant environment) period of such rhythms is about equal to the natural day-night cycle, they are called *circadian rhythms* (*circa*, about; *dia*, day).

A remarkable feature of circadian rhythms is that their free-running cycle length or period is only slightly influenced by wide variations in temperature, as between 10 and 30°C, even though their occurrence depends upon metabolism. A circadian rhythm can therefore serve as a temperature-independent biological clock for time measurement. Several kinds of experimental evidence support the view that photoperiodic plants make use of a circadian rhythm for measuring the length of the dark period. The biochemical nature of this circadian rhythm and the means by which phytochrome interacts with it remain unknown, however.

Hormones in With certain short-day plants a *single leaf* is all
Flowering that need be exposed to short day in order to cause the rest of the plant, even though kept under long day, to flower. The simplest interpretation is that some hormone is produced in the leaf in response to short day and moves to the apical meristems of the shoot causing these to produce flowers rather than vegetative shoots.

It is possible to induce a plant to flower by *grafting* onto it a shoot from a

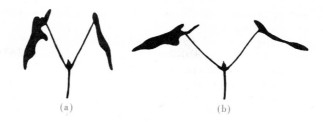

(a)   (b)

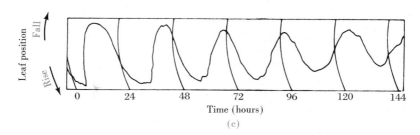

(c)

Fig. 10-9   *Day-night leaf movement (nyctinasty) in scarlet runner bean (*Phaseolus
multiflorus*). (a) Nocturnal position (blades lowered); (b) diurnal position (blades raised,
petioles spread); (c) a record of leaf rise and fall during 6 days under constant weak light
and constant temperature. The "free-running" period of the endogenous rhythm was 27
hr. (From E. Bünning,* The Physiological Clock, *2d ed. New York: Springer-Verlag, 1967,
with permission.)*

separate plant that has previously been induced to flower by the right photoperiod. For example, if we keep a short-day plant under long day, in which it
would not flower, but graft onto it a shoot taken from a short-day plant previously
exposed to short day, this shoot may cause the whole experimental plant to
flower. This experiment works just as well if the donor shoot is taken from a different strain or species of plant, provided the two can be successfully grafted
together. This suggests that different species use the same flowering hormone.
Moreover, the experiment works even if the receiver plant is a short-day plant
and the donor shoot is from a *long-day plant* exposed to *long* days. This indicates that a long-day plant produces the *same* kind of flowering stimulus when
exposed to long days as does a short-day plant when exposed to short days.

The hypothetical flowering hormone has been given various names, the
most popular being "florigen." It is believed to act on meristems to cause derepression of genes involved in flower morphogenesis. In support of this are observations that a burst of RNA synthesis occurs in the meristem at the time the
flowering stimulus arrives there from the leaves, and that the action of the flowering stimulus on the meristem can be blocked at this time by treating with an-
tagonists of transcription. However, efforts to isolate from plants a specific
flower-inducing chemical agent have not been convincingly successful so far,
implying that the "flowering hormone" is quite unstable, and impeding progress

toward a precise understanding of how the expression of genetic information for reproduction is regulated.

The most striking effects of known growth hormones on flowering have been obtained with gibberellins. Application of gibberellins to a number of long-day plants will cause them to flower under short days. In all such cases we are dealing with plants that grow vegetatively in the rosette form (page 163) and undergo a dramatic stem elongation or "bolting" prior to flowering. Gibberellin acts to induce stem elongation in such plants as previously mentioned, and its effect on flowering may be by this indirect route, as in some cases it induces elongation without flowering. Gibberellin has little effect on flowering of short-day plants under most conditions and thus cannot be the flowering hormone according to the evidence that the flowering hormone of long- and short-day plants is the same. However, gibberellin clearly seems to be involved in the flowering response of long-day rosette plants because the production of gibberellin is found to be promoted substantially by long-day treatment, and this leads to the stem elongation that is required for normal flowering.

CONTROL OF FLOWERING BY TEMPERATURE

Although, as already noted, the timing mechanism that underlies photoperiodic responses appears to be relatively temperature-independent, temperature does nevertheless influence profoundly the flowering behavior of many plants. The effects are quite various and include response to photoperiod at certain temperatures and not at others; acceleration of flowering under inductive or noninductive photoperiods by certain temperatures; and complete substitution of certain temperatures for inductive photoperiods. In the case of day-neutral plants flower initiation may be controlled largely or entirely by temperature considerations.

Experiments with controlled environments show that the day-time and night-time temperatures are usually separately important, the optimum night temperature usually being lower than the optimum day temperature. This situation has been called *thermoperiodism*, although there is no implication that the duration of the temperature periods is measured by the plant as in photoperiodism.

In a very rough way we can classify plants as "cool-night plants" or "warm-night plants" depending upon whether their flowering is favored by cool temperatures below some maximum or by warm temperatures above some minimum, night temperatures being generally of primary importance. "Cool-night plants" include plants adapted to early spring flowering, like the strawberry, and late summer-flowering short-day plants for which a positive response to cool temperature is of adaptive value in hastening reproduction if for any reason it becomes delayed until fall. This type of response is also observed in tuber formation by the potato plant, which is induced by either short days *or* cool night temperature. "Warm-night plants" on the other hand are adapted to mid-summer flowering.

In some cases flower development or seed and fruit set, rather than flower initiation, is the process that is especially sensitive to temperature and may control the occurrence of reproduction. For example, tomato plants, which are day neutral, set fruit well only if the night temperature is above about 50°F and are effectively "warm-night plants" even though they produce flowers under cooler temperatures. A somewhat similar situation is encountered with the much-studied short-day plant cocklebur (*Xanthium*).

Plants show comparable temperature preferences and tolerances for vegetative growth, preferences that may be complementary to temperature preferences for reproduction to the extent that vegetative growth occurs at the expense of flower initiation or vice versa. These temperature preferences and tolerances also vary in some cases with the stage of development or age of the plant. The constellation of such effects presumably constitutes an important part of what limits the climatic and geographical range over which different species are successful.

Vernalization   A period of exposure to temperatures near freezing induces or accelerates subsequent flowering of certain plants (see Figure 9-8). The induction of flowering competence by a cold treatment is called *vernalization*, in reference to the habit of such plants to flower in spring after the winter period of cold. The classic example is winter wheat, which is planted and germinates in the autumn, becomes vernalized during the winter, and as a result flowers promptly in spring to produce an early crop of grain. The vernalization phenomenon recalls the effect of cold in breaking bud and seed dormancy (pages 167, 183), but in vernalization development is switched from the vegetative to the reproductive mode and therefore, as in photoperiodic induction of flowering, vernalization presumably brings into action an array of genes that were not previously being expressed.

In nature plants that require vernalization commonly behave as *biennials*, that is, they complete their life cycle in two years. The first year the seed germinates and the plant grows vegetatively as a rosette, like the plant shown in Figure 9-8a. During the ensuing winter the cold requirement becomes satisfied; as a result the next spring the stem elongates and produces flowers, as in Figure 9-8c, and after fruiting the plant senesces and dies. If a biennial is maintained in the greenhouse without a cold treatment, it will grow vegetatively for years.

The value to the biennial plant of the cold requirement for flowering is to ensure that a whole season of vegetative growth elapses, during which the plant increases greatly in size and vigor, before reproduction commences. As a result much more seed can be produced per plant than would be the case if the plant flowered while it was young and weak; its reproductive potential is greatly increased.

With certain biennials treatment with gibberellin can substitute for the cold requirement and induce flowering (Figure 9-8b). It seems likely that the environmental signal (cold) is translated at least in part by activation of the gibberellin system but how this comes about is unknown.

Many vernalization-requiring biennial plants are also long-day plants; that is, vernalization makes them competent to flower but they do so only when subsequently induced by long days. An example is the carrot plant shown in Figure 9-8. This behavior ensures that the plants flower in late spring or early summer of their second year. These control relationships are summarized in Figure 10-10.

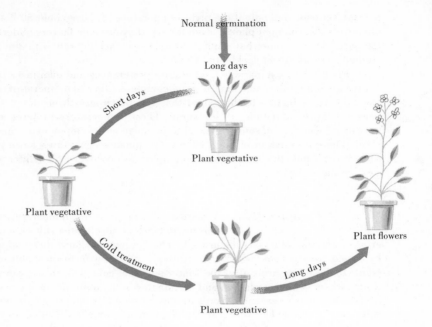

Fig. 10-10   *Interacting requirements for cold treatment (vernalization) and long days in flowering of biennial plants such as henbane (*Hyoscyamus*). Colored arrows indicate the normal sequence of environmental stimuli in nature.*

Many spring-flowering trees, shrubs, and perennial herbaceous plants initiate their flower primordia during the preceding growing season at or before the time of formation of dormant winter buds. These plants commonly exhibit a cold requirement for effective flowering that is not vernalization but simply an instance of the effect of cold in terminating winter dormancy (page 167). Apples, peaches, and various other fruit trees behave in this way, flowering erratically and bearing poorly or not at all except in climates that provide a sufficiently long period of near-freezing winter weather.

OTHER FACTORS INFLUENCING REPRODUCTION   Photoperiod and temperature are the principal determinants of flowering in plants of cold-temperate climates, but other controls both internal and environmental may be overriding in some plants and may take precedence entirely in plants adapted to tropical or arid climates.

Although various plants such as the cocklebur (*Xanthium*) can be photoperiodically induced to flower as soon as the seed has germinated, many plants do not become capable of initiating flowers until they reach a certain age, which may be weeks in the case of annual plants or up to several years in the case of perennials. This state of affairs is called attainment of "ripeness to flower"; it ensures that a definite amount of vegetative growth and level of vigor will precede the commencement of reproductive effort. More extreme examples are seen in many trees, seedlings of which typically go through a "juvenile phase" of many years' duration before beginning to flower. In some cases, as in *Eucalyptus, Acacia*, and many tropical trees, the size and shape of the leaves and form of vegetative shoot development exhibit a juvenile phase that alters abruptly to the adult form at the time of attainment of reproductive competence. This phenomenon can also be observed in common English ivy (*Hedera helix*). It clearly reflects an alteration of genetic expression in respect to morphogenetic controls in the shoot apical meristem.

The most spectacular delayed-reproduction behavior is seen in plants like "century plant" (*Agave*), many bamboos, and certain palms, which grow vegetatively for many years and then within a matter of weeks flower, fruit, and die. What determines the timing of their reproduction is a mystery.

Many plants and trees of tropical regions show seasonal flowering behavior in the absence of any substantial annual changes in mean temperature or photoperiod. Most tropical climates exhibit an annual cycle of wet and dry seasons, to which dormancy and leaf abscission are often coupled adaptively as noted on page 166. The dry season brings somewhat wider day–night temperature differences and one can imagine that either a very sensitive thermoperiodism or a response to water status could serve to time reproductive behavior; however, the actual mechanisms that control flowering of tropical plants are still largely unknown.

CONCLUSION   The phenomena of environmental control encountered in reproductive behavior of seed plants illustrate how regulatory mechanisms can bring about adaptive responses to environmental cues by modifying all aspects of development, from the immediate occurrence or nonoccurrence of growth processes to the expression of genetic information for alternative kinds of biochemistry and alternative patterns of development. As such these phenomena epitomize essentially all the levels of physiological function and its regulation that have been evolved by plants and constitute a suitable subject with which to conclude our study of functions of the living plant. In actuality we have as yet but a spotty understanding of these phenomena compared with vertebrate and human reproductive biology, and we may expect to learn much more of both fundamental and practical significance as the activities of plants are explored in greater depth and breadth in future research.

SUGGESTED READING

Borthwick, H. A., and S. B. Hendricks, "Photoperiodism in Plants," *Science*, **132**:1223–1228, 1960.

Bünning, E., *The Physiological Clock*, 2d ed. New York: Springer-Verlag, 1967.

Hillman, W. S., *The Physiology of Flowering*. New York: Holt, Rinehart and Winston, 1962. Chapters 1-6.

Hillman, W. S., "Photoperiodism and Vernalization," in *The Physiology of Plant Growth and Development*, M. B. Wilkins (ed.). New York: McGraw-Hill, 1969. Chapter 16.

Mayer, A. M., and A. Poljakoff-Mayber, *The Germination of Seeds*. New York: Pergamon Press, 1963.

O'Brien, T. P., and M. McCully, *Plant Structure and Development*. New York: Macmillan, 1969. Chapters 8 and 9.

Salisbury, F. B., "The Initiation of Flowering," *Endeavor*, **24:**74-80.

Salisbury, F. B., and C. Ross, *Plant Physiology*. Belmont, Cal.: Wadsworth, 1969. Chapters 24-27.

Sweeney, M., *Rhythmic Phenomena in Plants*. New York: Academic Press, 1969.

Wareing, P. F., and I. D. J. Phillips, *The Control of Growth and Differentiation in Plants*. New York: Pergamon, 1970. Chapters 9 and 10.

Went, F. W., *The Experimental Control of Plant Growth*. New York: Ronald, 1957. Chapters 17-19.

Index

A

Abscisic acid, 167, 173, 183
  effect on stomates, 54
Abscission, fruit, 168
  leaf, 166-169, 188
Accessory pigments, 32, 38
Acetabularia, 145
Action spectrum, of photo-
    morphogenesis, 169-171
  of photoperiodism, 189
  of photosynthesis, 30, 38
  of phototropism, 158
  of stomatal opening, 54
Active transport, 96, 117, 118
After-ripening, 183
Agave, 67, 90, 195
Ageing (*see* Senescence)

Air pollution, effects on plants, 69
Air spaces (*see* Intercellular gas system)
Aleurone cells, 165, 174, 183
Algae, 3, 21, 42, 173
  cell wall structure, 10
  chloroplasts, 32
  gas exchange, 49
  growth of, 133, 145
  ion relations, 97
  leaf structure of kelp, 120
  mineral requirements, 95
  nitrogen fixation by, 102
  pigments of, 32, 38
  translocation in, 119
Alkaloids, 184
Allard, H. A., 186
Amides, 105, 111
Amylase, 164, 168, 174, 181